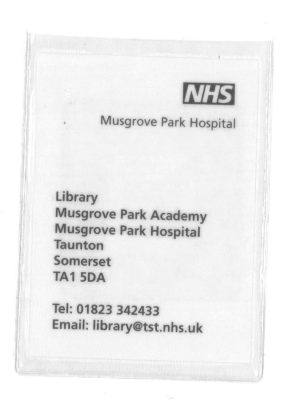

Emergency Ultrasound

Emergency Ultrasound

SECOND EDITION

O. John Ma, MD
Professor and Chair
Department of Emergency Medicine
Oregon Health & Science University
Portland, Oregon

James R. Mateer, MD, RDMS
Clinical Professor of Emergency Medicine
Department of Emergency Medicine
Medical College of Wisconsin
Milwaukee, Wisconsin
Staff Physician
Emergency Medicine
Waukesha Memorial Hospital
Waukesha, Wisconsin

Michael Blaivas, MD, RDMS
Professor of Emergency Medicine
Department of Emergency Medicine
Northside Hospital Forsyth
Cumming, Georgia

New York Chicago San Francisco Lisbon London Madrid
Mexico City Milan New Delhi San Juan Seoul Singapore
Sydney Toronto

Emergency Ultrasound, Second Edition

Copyright © 2008 by The McGraw-Hill Companies, Inc. All rights reserved. Printed in China. Except as permitted under the United States Copyright Act of 1976, no part of this publication may be reproduced or distributed in any form or by any means, or stored in a data base or retrieval system, without the prior written permission of the publisher.

1 2 3 4 5 6 7 8 9 0 CTP CTP 0 9 8 7

ISBN   978-0-07-147904-2
MHID   0-07-147904-X

This book was set in Times Roman by Aptara, Inc.
The editors were Anne M. Sydor and Peter J. Boyle.
The production supervisor was Catherine Saggese.
China Translation and Printing Services, Ltd., was printer and binder.

This book is printed on acid-free paper.

Cataloging-in-publication data is on file for this title at the Library of Congress.

As always, hunkering down to meet tight deadlines required tremendous assistance and sacrifice from my family. Elizabeth, Gabrielle, Tasha, and Davis showed their love by tolerating and humoring me throughout the project.
— O. John Ma —

"Patience" and Time. I appreciate the patience given to me by my family (Jody, Kristen, Shannon, and Sean) during the time I was focused on this project. I also thank the patients whose presenting conditions have shown us time and time again the clinical advantages of limited emergency ultrasonography.
—James R. Mateer —

Unwavering support and love from Laura, Roxy, and Scout continues to be my fuel and inspiration for this project and all others. None of this would have been possible without you.
— Michael Blaivas —

The editors would also like to dedicate this book to Bradley Frazee, MD, for his courage and strength.

CONTENTS

CONTRIBUTORS

Frédéric Adnet, MD
Universite Paris XIII
Hopital Avicenne
Bobigny, France
*Prehospital Ultrasound: Perspectives from Four
    Countries*

Chandra D. Aubin, MD, RDMS
Assistant Professor and Assistant Residency Director
Division of Emergency Medicine
Washington University School of Medicine
St. Louis, Missouri
Second- and Third-Trimester Pregnancy

Aaron E. Bair, MD, MS
Department of Emergency Medicine
University of California—Davis Medical Center
Sacramento, California
Vascular Access

Michael Blaivas, MD, RDMS
Professor of Emergency Medicine
Department of Emergency Medicine
Northside Hospital Forsyth
Cumming, Georgia
*Prehospital Ultrasound: Perspectives from
    Four Countries*
Testicular
Deep Venous Thrombosis
Ocular Ultrasound

Jörg Braun, MD
German Air Rescue, Filderstadt
*Prehospital Ultrasound: Perspectives from Four
    Countries*

Raoul Breitkreutz, MD
Department of Anesthesiology, Intensive Care
    and Pain Therapy
University Hospital, Johann Wolfgang Goethe-University
Frankfurt am Main, Germany
*Prehospital Ultrasound: Perspectives from
    Four Countries*

Franziska Brenner, MD
Frankfurter Institut für Notfallmedizin und
    Simulationstraining (FINEST)
Frankfurt, Germany
*Prehospital Ultrasound: Perspectives From Four
    Countries*

Thomas P. Cook, MD
Residency Program Director
Department of Emergency Medicine
University of South Carolina
Columbia, South Carolina
Abdominal Aortic Aneurysm

Andreas Dewitz, MD, RDMS
Director, Emcrgency Ultrasound
Department of Emergency Medicine
Boston Medical Center
Assistant Professor of Emergency
    Medicine
Boston University School of Medicine
Boston, Massachusetts
Soft Tissue
Additional Ultrasound-Guided Procedures

Giancarlo Fontana, MD
Niguarda Hospital Emergency Department
Milan, Italy
*Prehospital Ultrasound: Perspectives from Four
    Countries*

J. Christian Fox, MD, RDMS
Associate Professor of Emergency Medicine
Director of Emergency Ultrasound
Department of Emergency
    Medicine
University of California Irvine Medical
    Center
Director of Emergency and Trauma
    Ultrasound
University of California, Irvine
Gynecologic Concepts
Equipment

Bradley W. Frazee, MD
Associate Clinical Professor
Department of Medicine
UCSF Attending Physician
Alameda County Medical Center
Highland General Hospital
Oakland, California
Soft Tissue
Second- and Third-Trimester
   Pregnancy

Cristina Frigerio, MD
Niguarda Hospital Emergency Department
Milan, Italy
Prehospital Ultrasound: Perspectives from
   Four Countries

Jessica R. Goldstein, MD
Assistant Professor
Case Western Reserve University
Associate Director Emergency Ultrasound
MetroHealth Medical Center
Cleveland, Ohio
Additional Ultrasound-Guided Procedures

Carmela Graci, MD
Niguarda Hospital Emergency
   Department
Milan, Italy
Prehospital Ultrasound: Perspectives from
   Four Countries

Elena Guffanti, MD
Emergency Department
Niguarda Cà Granda Hospital
Milan, Italy
Prehospital Ultrasound: Perspectives from
   Four Countries

Lowell "Corky" Hecht, BA, RDMS, RDCS, RVT
Program Manager and Senior Clinical
   Instructor
Gulfcoast Ultrasound Institute, Inc.
St. Petersburg, Florida
Physics and Image Artifacts

William Heegaard, MD
Assistant Chief
Department of Emergency Medicine
Hennepin County Medical Center
Associate Professor
Department of Emergency Medicine
University of Minnesota Medical School
Minneapolis, Minnesota
Prehospital Ultrasound: Perspectives from
   Four Countries

Scott Joing, MD
Assistant Professor of Emergency Medicine
Department of Emergency Medicine
University of Minnesota Medical School
Faculty Physician
Department of Emergency Medicine
Hennepin County Medical Center
Minneapolis, Minnesota
Prehospital Ultrasound: Perspectives from Four Countries
Cardiac
First-Trimester Pregnancy

Robert A. Jones, DO, RDMS, FACEP
Assistant Professor
Department of Emergency Medicine
Case Western Reserve University
Director
Division of Emergency Ultrasound
Director
Emergency Ultrasound Fellowship MetroHealth
   Medical Center
Cleveland, Ohio
Additional Ultrasound-Guided Procedures

**Andrew W. Kirkpatrick, CD, MD, MHSc,
   FRCSC, FACS**
Associate Professor
Department of Surgery
Foothills Medical Centre
Associate Professor
Department of Critical Care Medicine
Foothills Medical Centre
Calgary, Alberta, Canada
Trauma

Thomas Kirschning, MD
Department of Anesthesiology
Johann Wolfgang Goethe-University
Frankfurt/Main, Germany
Prehospital Ultrasound: Perspectives from Four Countries

Frédéric Lapostolle, MD
Universite Paris XIII
Hopital Avicenne
Bobigny, France
Prehospital Ultrasound: Perspectives from Four Countries

Michael J. Lambert, MD, RDMS, FAAEM
Clinical Assistant Professor
Department of Emergency Medicine
University of Illinois College of Medicine
Fellowship Director, Emergency Ultrasound
Advocate Christ Medical Center
Oak Lawn, Illinois
Training and Program Development
Gynecologic Concepts

Matthew Lyon, MD, RDMS
Assistant Professor
Assistant Director, Section of Emergency
   Ultrasound
Department of Emergency Medicine
Medical College of Georgia
Augusta, Georgia
Ocular Ultrasound

O. John Ma, MD
Professor and Chair
Department of Emergency Medicine
Oregon Health & Science University
Portland, Oregon
Trauma

Diku Mandavia, MD, FACEP, FRCP
Attending Staff Physician
Department of Emergency Medicine
Cedars-Sinai Medical Center and Los Angeles
   County-USC Medical Center
Director of Emergency Ultrasound
Clinical Associate Professor of Emergency
   Medicine
Keck School of Medicine of the University of
   Southern California
Los Angeles, California
Renal

Ingo Marzi, MD
Department of Trauma Surgery
University of Saarland
Hamburg, Germany
*Prehospital Ultrasound: Perspectives from Four
   Countries*

James R. Mateer, MD, RDMS
Clinical Professor of Emergency
   Medicine
Department of Emergency Medicine
Medical College of Wisconsin
Milwaukee, Wisconsin
Staff Physician
Emergency Medicine
Waukesha Memorial Hospital
Waukesha, Wisconsin
Trauma

Luca Neri, MD
Prehospital Emergency
   Service
Niguarda Ca' Granda Hospital
Milan, Italy
*Prehospital Ultrasound: Perspectives from Four
   Countries*

Nadine Nieuwkamp, MD
Frankfurter Institut für Notfallmedizin und
   Simulationstraining (FINEST)
Frankfurt, Germany
*Prehospital Ultrasound: Perspectives from Four
   Countries*

Masaaki Ogata, MD
Director
Division of Emergency Medicine
Assistant Director
Department of Surgery
Kobe Nishi City Hospital
Kobe, Japan
General Surgery Applications

Aman K. Parikh, MD
Assistant Professor
Department of Emergency Medicine
University of California, Davis
Sacramento, California
Vascular Access

Michael A. Peterson, MD, FAAEM
Associate Professor of Medicine
David Geffen School of Medicine at UCLA
Director
Emergency Ultrasound Training Program and
   Fellowship
Department of Emergency Medicine
Harbor-UCLA Medical Center
Torrance, California
Training and Program Development
Pediatric Applications

Tomislav Petrovic, MD
Universite Paris XIII
Hopital Avicenne
Bobigny, France
*Prehospital Ultrasound: Perspectives from Four
   Countries*

Dave Plummer, MD
Department of Emergency Medicine
Hennepin County Medical Center
Minneapolis, Minnesota
Prehospital Ultrasound: Perspectives from Four Countries
Abdominal Aortic Aneurysm

Daniel D. Price, MD
Assistant Clinical Professor
University of California—San Francisco
Director, Emergency Ultrasound Fellowship
Alameda County Medical Center—Highland Campus
Oakland, California
Pediatric Applications

Robert F. Reardon, MD
Faculty
Department of Emergency Medicine
Hennepin County Medical Center
Assistant Professor
Department of Emergency Medicine
University of Minnesota
Minneapolis, Minnesota
Prehospital Ultrasound: Perspectives from Four Countries
Cardiac
Abdominal Aortic Aneurysm
First-Trimester Pregnancy

John S. Rose, MD
Division of Emergency Medicine
University of California—Davis Medical Center
Sacramento, California
Vascular Access

Will Scruggs, MD, RDMS
Director of Emergency Department Ultrasound
Hawaii Emergency Physicians Associated
Castle Medical Center
Kailua, Hawaii
Equipment

Dave Spear, MD, FACEP
Medical Director
Fire Department
Odessa Fire Department
Odessa, Texas
Emergency Ultrasound Director
Emergency Medicine
Parkland Hospital
Dallas, Texas
Prehospital Ultrasound: Perspectives from Four Countries

Enrico Storti, MD
Niguarda Hospital Emergency Department
Milan, Italy
Prehospital Ultrasound: Perspectives from Four Countries

Stuart Swadron, MD, FRCP(C), FACEP, FAAEM
Program Director
Residency in Emergency Medicine
Attending Staff Physician
Los Angeles County-USC Medical Center
Assistant Professor of Clinical Emergency Medicine
Keck School of Medicine of the University of Southern California
Los Angeles, California
Renal

Daniel Theodoro, MD, RDMS
Assistant Professor of Emergency Medicine
Washington University School of Medicine
St. Louis, Missouri
Hepatobiliary

Felix Walcher, MD, PhD
Department of Trauma Surgery
University Hospital Frankfurt
Hamburg, Germany
Prehospital Ultrasound: Perspectives from Four Countries

Jason Wilkins, MD
CEO
Mannequin and Network Teaching Associates
Springfield, Missouri
Physics and Image Artifacts

FOREWORD

Emergency practitioners are increasingly incorporating real-time ultrasound imaging into their practice, both for clinical decision-making and to guide procedural interventions. Drs. Ma, Mateer, and Blaivas are well known in emergency medicine for their educational and scientific contributions to the clinical application of emergency ultrasound. This second edition of their popular book on emergency ultrasound is welcomed by practitioners, educators, and clinical investigators. This work defines the state of current and future clinical practice using ultrasound in emergency medicine.

The editors and contributing authors provide valuable information related to the underlying principles of ultrasound physics, device application, and associated human anatomy. High-quality images bring home important teaching points, including the importance of developing familiarity with the operation of the device (i.e., the knobs, probes, and monitor), such that artifact and poor-quality images do not adversely impact the application of the technology to clinical decision making. An expanded role for this technology in clinical practice is highlighted, but will require considerable training and experience by the clinician. Hence, many of the expanded applications provided in this updated edition will be beyond the casual or novice user. Nonetheless, these applications emphasize the opportunities that exist for those emergency physicians still in training and the motivated current practitioner who will commit to obtaining the needed training and clinical experience with this modality.

Also in this edition, the authors have added content related to procedural guidance, one of the more common applications of ultrasound. Indeed this real-time application of ultrasound is recognized as an important means of reducing adverse events that can accompany clinical procedures. Performing procedures under ultrasound guidance will not eliminate all potential complications, even those for which image guidance is most valuable. Nonetheless, there is now ample evidence that when time permits, equipment is present, and ultrasound training sufficient, image-guided procedures are associated with fewer potentially avoidable procedural complications. That said, it is important that ultrasound fans and litigation attorneys appreciate that patient circumstances, equipment availability, operator experience, and other factors all contribute to whether there is a favorable risk/benefit for doing a clinical procedure under ultrasound guidance for a specific patient.

We expect that growing operator experience and equipment availability will move clinical practice toward more procedures being done with ultrasound guidance and being done more consistently under ultrasound guidance. Yet, practitioners must retain skills and use clinical judgment when weighing the likely benefit of reduced complications versus the urgency by which the procedure must be completed. It is likely that professional debate in this area will be with us through several more editions of this fine textbook.

The authors' inclusion of real-time image examples on the accompanying DVD will serve as a valuable teaching adjunct for current ultrasound users and the novice learner. The color images will also help these learners appreciate the static images and anatomic correlates. The chapter on ocular ultrasound provides exposure to an area of active inquiry, including the assessment of intraocular or intracranial pressure via this sonic window.

This is an exciting textbook that will get much use in clinical settings. Although designed for the emergency department, other critical care and ambulatory clinical settings will find the information of value. This book clearly highlights the opportunity for ultrasonography to guide the future clinical practice of ambulatory, emergency, and critical care medicine. The future is now!

Jerris R. Hedges, MD, MS, MMM
Professor of Emergency Medicine
Vice Dean, School of Medicine
Oregon Health & Science University
Portland, Oregon

PREFACE

Interest in emergency ultrasound continues to skyrocket. Clinicians who practice in the emergency department, the critical care setting, and other acute care settings have become increasingly familiar with how emergency ultrasound can improve and expedite patient care at the bedside. Moreover, its use in enhancing patient safety and reducing errors has been recognized. The application of emergency ultrasound has been incorporated into every emergency medicine residency program. The number of fellowship training programs has increased exponentially. Clinician investigators from nearly all medical specialties and from across the globe have published papers on bedside applications of emergency ultrasound.

This textbook was written by and for health care workers who are engaged in the practice of clinical medicine. We selected topics that represent those problems most commonly encountered in the emergency or acute care setting, thereby generating the greatest interest for the broadest readership. Our aim was to address the needs of clinicians with varied backgrounds and training. Emergency physicians certainly will find this book applicable to their daily practice. Physicians who practice in family medicine, internal medicine, critical care, and general surgery will also find this book to be of value for specific clinical scenarios.

We would like to thank the readers of the first edition of this textbook who offered us excellent feedback that helped us add several new features to this edition. For each chapter, as in the first edition, the clinical considerations and indications of the specific emergency ultrasound examination are discussed. Prior to presenting the technique for the focused emergency ultrasound examination, a new section on "Getting Started" is included to aid novice sonologists who may require additional information on the specific examination. Each chapter continues to emphasize the key aspects of the *focused* emergency ultrasound examination; this textbook does not attempt to cover every element of the normal comprehensive ultrasound examination. New chapters on prehospital care, ocular applications, and ultrasound-guided procedures are included. Another new feature in this edition is the inclusion of color figures throughout the book. Finally, we feel that if a picture is worth a thousand words, then a video clip may be worth a hundred thousand. A DVD that demonstrates several common emergency ultrasound examinations is included with each textbook.

Experts from six countries and a variety of medical specialties have contributed to this textbook. We would like to express our deep appreciation to the contributors for their commitment and hard work in helping to produce this textbook. We also would like to thank them for helping us collect the more than 900 figures that are included in this textbook. We would like to thank Lori Green and Gulfcoast Ultrasound for their support of this project and for providing us with numerous ultrasound images from their library. We are indebted to numerous individuals who assisted us with this project; in particular, we would like to thank Anne M. Sydor, Sarah Granlund, Martin Wonsiewicz, and Joe Rusko for their invaluable efforts.

O. John Ma, MD

James R. Mateer, MD

Michael Blaivas, MD

CHAPTER 1

Training and Program Development

Michael A. Peterson and Michael J. Lambert

Establishing a training program in focused point of care ultrasound is an exciting and rewarding experience. The impact of ultrasound on the clinical practice of medicine becomes so obvious that many clinicians, after acquiring basic ultrasound skills, wonder how they got along without this technology. This chapter outlines the process for developing a point of care ultrasound training program and addresses the common questions encountered when starting a new program. This chapter was written on the basis of our training experience in Emergency Medicine residency programs. The principles outlined could be applied to residencies in other specialties as well as to groups of practicing physicians who are interested in developing an ultrasound program for emergency and acute care settings.

Point of care ultrasound examinations are performed by the patient care provider to answer specific clinical questions in order to make patient care decisions in real time. "Comprehensive" examinations, generally done by imaging specialists, seek to completely evaluate a particular organ system or anatomical area. Point of care examinations, on the other hand, are focused in their scope and seek to answer only one or a few questions about an organ system or anatomical area (e.g., "are there gallstones or not?"). By virtue of their focused

interpretations, point of care examinations require less training for proficiency.

▶ STEPS TO ESTABLISHING A POINT OF CARE ULTRASOUND PROGRAM

The following are a set of steps for establishing a high-quality point of care ultrasound program. These steps should generally proceed in order. Early selection of the ultrasound director is preferable, as several of the steps are time consuming and would benefit by having a designated advocate to champion their completion.

1 Determine type of examinations to be performed.
2 Develop a program plan.
3 Select the point of care ultrasound director(s).
4 Obtain hospital approval of program plan.
5 Acquire an ultrasound machine.
6 Train the ultrasound director(s).
7 Train the group.
8 Perform problem solving and ongoing training.

▶ DETERMINE TYPE OF EXAMINATIONS TO BE PERFORMED

This step seems like an easy task. However, the number of focused ultrasound applications continues to expand along with technological advances in ultrasound and individual operator expertise. It makes sense to start with applications that will get the most use in a particular practice setting. Some acute care, emergency, and critical care settings provide excellent diagnostic ultrasound service so training might be best focused on services that are not offered or not offered in a time frame that is acceptable. Examples include most of the procedural applications, as well as the critically emergent diagnostic applications such as the focused assessment with sonography for trauma (FAST) examination, evaluation of cardiac arrest states, evaluation of undifferentiated hypotension, and the abdominal aortic aneurysm (AAA) examination. One advantage to starting with procedural applications is that they require less training than diagnostic examinations so they can be put into use quickly. Further more, there will likely be less political resistance to procedural ultrasound, which is now widely supported and utilized by a variety of clinicians. For a list of potential applications, see Table 1-1.

Emergency physicians and trauma surgeons can appreciate the benefits of point of care ultrasound when a trauma patient presents with an isolated penetrating injury to the chest. An echocardiogram is frequently required to exclude hemopericardium, which is the most potentially life-threatening condition. A trained echocardiography technician may be requested to perform an ultrasound examination that is then interpreted by a cardiologist. While during the day this process may be completed within a reasonable time frame, typically under 1 hour, after-hours echocardiograms can be significantly delayed. In the interim, if the patient's condition deteriorates because of cardiac tamponade, the treating physician may not be able to exclude pericardial effusion as a possible etiology. Delays in obtaining an echocardiogram can have serious consequences.

Focused ultrasound training in emergency medicine residency programs should cover all of the primary applications.[1] Although these primary applications are the foundation upon which emergency ultrasound was

▶ TABLE 1-1. SOME FOCUSED ULTRASOUND EXAMINATIONS

	Primary Applications	Additional Applications
Abdominal	Free abdominal fluid Abdominal aortic aneurysm Gallstones Hydronephrosis	Solid organ injuries Bladder volume/outlet obstruction
Obstetrics/gynecology	Early intrauterine pregnancy (to exclude ectopic pregnancy)	Adnexal masses Trauma in pregnancy IUD localization Fetal viability
Cardiothoracic	Pericardial effusion	Hypotension Cardiac activity during cardiac arrest Pleural effusion Valve failure
Soft tissue/orthopedic		Foreign body diagnosis Cutaneous abscess diagnosis Peritonsillar abscess diagnosis
Vascular		Deep venous thrombosis IVC—volume status
Ophthalmologic		Retinal detachment Vitreous hemorrhage

Procedural	Intravenous lines
	  Internal jugular
	  Femoral
	  Deep brachial
	Paracentesis
	Thoracentesis
		Bladder aspiration
		Fracture reduction
		Transvenous pacemaker placement
		Abscess drainage
		Foreign body removal
		Lumbar puncture
		Peritonsillar abscess drainage
		Arthrocentesis

Abbreviations: IUD – Intrauterine device; IVC – Inferior vena cava.

built, there are additional indications for point of care ultrasound that are applicable to many types of clinical practice (see Table 1-1). Procedural ultrasound and trauma ultrasound are excellent initial focused ultrasound applications that can make a significant impact on clinical decision-making.

A new point of care ultrasound program should strive to identify all of the ultrasound examinations that are of interest, both now and in the future. Making this decision early allows the program to seek hospital approval for all of these examinations from the beginning instead of having to apply for additional approval later. It also allows the program to define equipment needs prior to initial equipment purchase. Otherwise, additional purchases may have to be made as new applications are brought online. Such an approach may be logistically difficult in some settings where capital fund acquisition is difficult.

There are certain advantages to initially focusing training on just one or two ultrasound examinations, and honing these skills before adding more. This allows everyone time to concentrate their efforts on becoming proficient in the skills specific to that application. It also provides the trainees time to learn from the technical pitfalls inherent in those particular applications. Likewise, by keeping the entire training group on the same application(s), the ultrasound director can focus quality improvement efforts on those specific applications. Specific case study reviews of these applications can be beneficial to everyone involved. The entire group can learn from the success and mistakes of their peers. After competence is achieved, the next application can be introduced in a similar systematic fashion. There is no need to rush into all of the applications in a haphazard manner. Utilizing a systematic, one or two applications at a time, approach will ensure a safe, methodical, and effective implementation of focused ultrasound into daily clinical practice. Although diagnostic focused ultrasound examinations by definition are truncated examinations designed to answer a specific clinical question, the acquisition of these skills nevertheless requires significant education and experience.

▶ DEVELOP A PROGRAM PLAN

The program plan defines all aspects of the ultrasound training program. The plan guides the ultrasound director through all the administrative and teaching aspects of the program and serves as a reference for requirements in training. The easiest way to develop a plan is to model one after another group or institution's plan, adapting it for the local clinical and political environment. Many residency programs are willing to share their program plans. The program plan should, at a minimum, include the following elements:

- Definition of specific privileges
- Training and credentialing requirements
- Method of recording results
- Quality improvement plan
- Continuing medical education requirements

DEFINITION OF SPECIFIC PRIVILEGES

This section defines exactly how focused ultrasound examinations will be used. For example, a specific privilege may be: "Documentation of free abdominal fluid in trauma patients." This could also be shortened to "Documentation of free abdominal fluid" if there is an additional desire to diagnose ascites. Some institutions allow graduated privileges, meaning that physicians can do more with their ultrasound examinations as they gain experience (see Table 1-2). This approach is beneficial in that it allows implementation of point of care ultrasound for patient care with less training time. Earlier implementation helps maintain momentum in the training program as physicians see the benefits of their training sooner. The shortcoming is that graduated privileges create a more complex training program and physicians have a lesser overall understanding of ultrasound. Thus, confusion from atypical anatomy is more likely as well as missing atypically appearing pathology.

Privileges and training should be constructed toward the identification of *specific findings* (e.g., presence or absence of gallstones) and not toward the general evaluation of disease processes or anatomic structures (e.g., evaluation for "cardiac disease" or "right upper quadrant abdominal pain"). A useful resource for defining a particular examination is the Emergency Ultrasound Imaging Criteria Compendium.[2]

TRAINING AND CREDENTIALING REQUIREMENTS

Training

Scientific research into methods of training in focused ultrasound is still limited, so guidelines about how to train are typically based on expert consensus. We know that focused ultrasound accuracy rates that are comparable to imaging specialist accuracy rates have been achieved using current training methods. However, the minimal amount of training required to achieve these results has yet to be determined.

Some standards for training in ultrasound have been published. The American College of Radiology (ACR) and the American Institute of Ultrasound in Medicine (AIUM) have established guidelines[3,4] but their

▶ **TABLE 1-2. EXAMPLE OF THE GRADUATED PRIVILEGES APPROACH**

Level of User	Decision-Making Capabilities
Level 1	Able to accurately diagnose a live intrauterine pregnancy (LIUP) in the pregnant patient. Proficient in correctly locating live pregnancy in the uterus by verifying appropriate landmarks by transabdominal (TAS) technique (bladder, uterus, and vaginal stripe) or endovaginal (EV) technique (bladder and uterus). Accurately records images to support diagnosis. Credentialed to disposition the patient with documented LIUP and arranging either follow-up diagnostic study in the Department of Radiology or with the patient's personal physician. If LIUP not clearly identified must have gold standard diagnostic study obtained while the patient in the emergency department (ED).
Level 2	Able to accurately diagnose an intrauterine pregnancy (IUP) and an abnormal intrauterine pregnancy (ABNIUP) in a pregnant patient. Proficient in correctly locating IUP or ABNIUP in the uterus by verifying appropriate landmarks. Accurately records images to support diagnosis. May disposition the patient with documented IUP or ABNIUP with confirmatory study arranged in the Department of Radiology or with the patient's personal physician. If IUP or ABNIUP not clearly identified must have confirmatory diagnostic study obtained while the patient in the ED.
Level 3	Able to accurately diagnose no definitive intrauterine pregnancy (NDIUP) in a pregnant patient. Proficient in evaluating adnexa and abdomen for possible extrauterine gestation (EUG), adnexal mass or free fluid in the pelvis. Has obtained Doppler skills necessary to evaluate ovaries for cysts and ruling in ovarian torsion. Accurately records images to support diagnosis. May disposition the patient with documented NDIUP, and ovarian cysts for outpatient workup if stable. Obtains consultation in NDIUP, EUG, or Ovarian torsion cases with appropriate OB colleagues. Proficient in instructing patients with ectopic precautions, NDIUP protocols, and arranging for any necessary outpatient laboratorics and imaging.

guidelines are targeted at learning comprehensive examinations, a goal that is different from that of focused ultrasound. In 1994, a model curriculum for training in emergency ultrasound requiring fewer training examinations than either the ACR or the AIUM was published.[5] This model curriculum represented the best opinion at the time; however, now these criteria are felt to be excessive by some authors.[6,7] Most recently, the American College of Emergency Physicians (ACEP) published an expert consensus on ultrasound training that has become the current standard for emergency medicine, recommending specific didactic and experiential training.[1] Ultrasound directors still have some degree of latitude in designing their individual programs, but a well-constructed program should at least meet the ACEP Training Guidelines. A program should also include minimum requirements for each of the following areas:

- Minimum overall didactic hours
- Minimum overall didactic content
- Minimum number of overall ultrasound examinations performed
- Minimum didactic content pertaining to the specific examination
- Minimum number of examinations performed to look for the specific finding (either positive or negative)
- Minimum number of positive examinations

Credentialing

Credentialing applies mainly to hospital-based or clinic-based physicians who wish to perform focused ultrasound examinations on patients in the hospital. Standard methods of credentialing are crucial to safely and effectively implement a successful ultrasound program. The cornerstone of the credentialing processes revolves around a required number of technically proficient scans and interpretations, as outlined in the training requirements. Until the training requirements are achieved, the physician is in "training status" and cannot use any information from ultrasound examinations to manage patients. Physicians are also cautioned against discussing any of their results with either patients or consultants during the training period to avoid any misunderstandings about the accuracy of results. After the training requirements are met, physicians are credentialed by the hospital and may begin using examinations for patient care. If a graduated credentialing program is used, the physician may be able to use some findings for patient care, but is considered "in training" for other findings.

METHOD OF RECORDING RESULTS

Numerous methods are available to document the results of the ultrasound examinations. Two questions that need to be answered are as follows: (1) How will interpretations be documented and (2) How will images be documented? The answer to the latter question is especially important, as it will influence the type of ultrasound equipment purchased. Documentation of interpretations can be as limited as writing results on the chart, or as complete as entering them in the hospital information system so they are available to all interested health care providers. For billing purposes, a "separately identifiable written report" must be generated for each ultrasound performed, although this report can be part of the emergency department record.[8] One solution is to develop a form for the sole purpose of reporting emergency ultrasound results. These forms can then be included in the medical record. The advantage of the form is that it can be devised so as to restrict interpretations to those findings that physicians are privileged and help physicians avoid making interpretations beyond their level of skill. An example of such a report form is included as Figure 1-1.

Several options exist for the documentation of images. Options include videotape, radiograph film, digital archives, and thermal imaging. If results are to be included in the medical record, thermal imaging is a reasonable option. For some applications, images need to be posted to the medical record in order to bill.[8] If images are to be archived separately from the medical record, digital storage or videotaping can be used. Archiving images outside the medical record creates problems with compliance with medical record confidentiality and lack of access by other physicians. Some programs use videotaping or DVD recording for quality assurance and teaching purposes only. Point of care ultrasound programs do not typically use radiographic film to archive images.

QUALITY IMPROVEMENT PLAN

Any department implementing a new ultrasound program should place a strong emphasis on quality improvement (QI). No other area of emergency ultrasound training will provide as many teaching opportunities as a well-run QI program. If the resources or experience are lacking initially to overread all of the program's ultrasound images, then finding a trained colleague in other specialties to assist with this endeavor is an option. There are pitfalls common to every application of ultrasound that can serve as a springboard for providing feedback and teaching within the program. This is clearly one of the most advantageous methods of enhancing both the technical and interpretative skills of sonologists.

The cornerstone of the QI program is review of examinations by the program's director. For a very active group of physicians performing focused ultrasound examinations, it will be logistically difficult to review every ultrasound examination so a method for selecting examinations for review must be decided upon. Examinations can be reviewed on either an *indicated* basis or a *random* basis. Indicated reviews occur when a certain indicator is met, such as a reported discrepancy between the focused ultrasound examination and another definitive study or procedure, or when a case is referred by a colleague because of questions regarding the accuracy of the examination. Random reviews are conducted by randomly selecting a predetermined number, or percentage, of examinations to assess the overall performance of the group.

Problems that are encountered during the QI process should be categorized as to their importance. The following represents one method of categorization.

LEVEL I: minor

Level I deviations usually consist of some problem with the technical component of the examination (e.g., gain too high) or disagreement on diagnostic criteria (e.g., labeling a common bile duct as mildly dilated at 6.5 mm when for the patient's age, this was a normal measurement.). Level I problems have no direct bearing upon the medical management of the patient. Typically, when this level of disagreement is found, a documented written or electronic copy of the disagreement is sent to the recipient.

LEVEL II: moderate

Level II deviations consist of discrepancies in interpretation between the sonologist's recorded image(s) and the QI review. In these cases, the undiagnosed or misdiagnosed pathology is nonemergent. For example, the sonologist may record a gallbladder examination in which gallstones were diagnosed. Upon review, the QI review discovers a classic novice pitfall of a hyperechoic duodenal area that is mistaken for gallstones. Typically, when this level of disagreement is found, a chart review is undertaken to determine if subsequent care of the patient was appropriate. Depending upon the follow-up that was provided and the patient's clinical condition at the time of disposition, the action taken can range considerably.

LEVEL III: major

These problems consist of significant discrepancies between the sonologist's recorded image(s) and the QI review. For example, sonologist records a pelvic ultrasound examination on a pregnant patient as an intrauterine pregnancy. The QI review finds no evidence of an intrauterine pregnancy, but does note free fluid in the pelvis and a 3 × 4 cm adnexal mass. In this case, the

---

LIMITED EMERGENCY ULTRASOUND EXAM
Emergency Department, _____ Medical Center

Date: _____

Provider: _____
(PRINT NAME)

_____
(SIGN)

LEVEL I

Trauma
- ☐ Intra-abdominal fluid
- ☐ Indeterminate
- ☐ No fluid noted

Gallbladder
- ☐ Gallstones
- ☐ Indeterminate
- ☐ No gallstones noted

Cardiac
- ☐ Pericardial fluid
- ☐ Indeterminate
- ☐ No pericardial fluid noted

Pelvic
- ☐ Definite IUP
  (IU fetal pole or IU cardiac activity)
- ☐ Indeterminate

Aorta
- ☐ Aneurysm_____cm
- ☐ Indeterminate
- ☐ No AA noted

(ATTACH IMAGES TO REVERSE SIDE OF MEDICAL RECORD COPY ONLY)

LEVEL II

Trauma
- ☐ **Visualization adequate**
- ☐ **Visualization inadequate**
- ☐ Intra-abdominal fluid
- ☐ No free fluid

Gallbladder
- ☐ **Visualization adequate**
- ☐ **Visualization inadequate**
- ☐ Gallstones
- ☐ Pericholecystic fluid
- ☐ None of above
  CBD _____ mm
  Wall thickness _____ mm

Cardiac
- ☐ **Visualization adequate**
- ☐ **Visualization inadequate**
- ☐ Pericardial fluid
- ☐ No pericardial fluid

Pelvic
- ☐ **Transabdominal**
- ☐ **Transvaginal**
- ☐ **Visualization adequate**
- ☐ **Visualization inadequate**
- ☐ Definite IUP
  (IU fetal pole or IU cardiac activity)
- ☐ Definite ectopic
  (Ectopic fetal pole or cardiac activity)
- ☐ Adnexal mass
- ☐ Pelvic/abdominal fluid
- ☐ None of above findings

Aorta
- ☐ **Visualization adequate**
- ☐ **Visualization inadequate**
- ☐ Aneurysm_____cm
- ☐ No aneurysm detected

Hydronephrosis
- ☐ **Visualization adequate**
- ☐ **Visualization inadequate**
- ☐ Hydronephrosis present R/L
- ☐ No hydronephrosis

Additional Comments:
(Findings in this section are preliminary and require confirmation when clinically indicated)

_____

_____

_____

All Emergency Ultrasounds are considered "Limited Exams."
Exams do not exclude findings other than those recorded above.
Practitioners should procure comprehensive ultrasound
examinations when findings not listed here or findings listed under
"additional comments" are of concern.

Figure 1-1. Example Bedside Ultrasound Report Form

chart is immediately pulled and reviewed. Depending upon the follow-up provided or whether a confirmatory study was obtained, the patient may be immediately contacted. The patient is then given follow-up instructions appropriate to the changed diagnosis.

Feedback on reviews, both positive and negative, should be provided to the sonologist in confidence, along with constructive suggestions for improvement. On occasion, mandated remedial education or training may be appropriate at the discretion of the program's director. The ultrasound director is also responsible for recommending to the department chief limitation, suspension, or termination of ultrasound privileges. Records should be kept on providers so that concerning trends can be recognized and addressed. Actions taken to address such problems as well as the outcome of such actions should be recorded. These records are confidential peer-review in nature and should be labeled as such. Results of QI activities should be regularly reported to the appropriate QI organization in the department, hospital, or clinic.

CONTINUING MEDICAL EDUCATION

As with training requirements, there are no well-established guidelines to dictate the amount of continuing medical education (CME) one needs to maintain competency in focused ultrasound. A reasonable number of education hours, along with continued bedside ultrasound use, should easily maintain skill levels and, preferably, even advance them. "Reasonable" should be determined in light of all the other requirements for continuing education within a specialty. If physicians normally receive 50 hours a year of continuing education in all areas of their specialty, then it would seem excessive to insist that 20 or even 10 of those hours be specific to ultrasound. Likewise, in a residency program, it does not make sense to require 15–20 hours a year of ultrasound didactic education if the entire didactic curriculum is only 200 hours per year. In a poll of 42 academic emergency department ultrasound programs, the question was asked, "How much CME is needed to keep ultrasound skills up" Responses varied from 0 to 30 hours, with a median of 8 hours.[9] Ultrasound directors should consider all the above factors when making a decision about CME requirements.

► SELECTING THE ULTRASOUND DIRECTOR(S)

The ultrasound program's director is an individual with expertise in focused ultrasound that oversees the training program at an institution or a clinic. Generally, this is a person with ultrasound experience who is hired into the group, or more typically, is an existing member of the group who is selected for the position and then trained. Valuable resources for this position are residents or ultrasound fellows graduating from an established ultrasound program. In a busy program, the ultrasound director's duty may be shared.

In some instances, the ultrasound director is someone from outside the group who is hired on an hourly basis. Whenever possible, it is advantageous to establish this role within the group because the process of training other group members is continuous and easier to accomplish when the ultrasound director is readily available. The group should acknowledge that the ultrasound director will invest a considerable amount of time on initial training, often 100 hours or more, and this time should be fairly compensated.

► OBTAIN HOSPITAL APPROVAL OF THE PROGRAM

When performing focused ultrasound examinations in a hospital setting, the program must be hospital approved and credentialing has to be in place. Going through such an approval process increases the scrutiny of the program by individuals outside the department and may generate valuable additional input into the program structure. Closer scrutiny by others will also lead to a more careful internal review of the program before presentation to the hospital, invariably leading to a better constructed program and tighter control of point of care ultrasound use. Approval also ensures that in the event of a significant problem, it will be more difficult for others outside the department to unilaterally persuade hospital governance to restrict the ultrasound program's activities. As with the overall program design, a hospital proposal can be modeled after a successful one from another institution.

Obtaining hospital approval of an ultrasound program should be seen as a political process, especially since there has been some resistance to point of care ultrasound programs from imaging specialists.[10–13] Knowing which physician groups side with the proposal and which oppose it before open discussion occurs may guide the process. Physicians who tend to be most supportive are those who also want to establish ultrasound programs. This group includes emergency physicians, surgeons, nephrologists, and family physicians, among others. However, ultrasound allies and enemies vary from hospital to hospital and making assumptions without investigation is not prudent. Clinicians who already use ultrasound in their practice, such as obstetrician-gynecologists and cardiologists, may also be allies in this process.

The following are helpful to refer to in a proposal:

1. Specialty society policy statements regarding use of focused ultrasound. In emergency medicine, for example, the Society for Academic Emergency Medicine,[14] the American Academy of Emergency Medicine,[15] and the American College of Emergency Physicians[16] have supported focused ultrasound use in the emergency department.
2. The American Medical Association's Policy H-230.960[17] states that individual specialties have the right to determine how to appropriately use ultrasound in their practice.
3. The percentage of residency programs in the individual specialty, as well as clinicians in the region and nationally, who are training in and using ultrasound. Has ultrasound become or is it becoming the norm locally or regionally? Is it a resident training requirement? Performing and interpreting ultrasound is considered part of the core curriculum in emergency medicine.[18]
4. Some of the numerous articles attesting to the safety and efficacy of focused ultrasound, especially in comparison to ultrasound examinations performed by traditional imaging specialists.

▶ ACQUIRE AN ULTRASOUND MACHINE

This subject will be covered in detail in Chapter 2, "Ultrasound Equipment." When making the decision on a purchase of an ultrasound machine, the best advice is to compare different ultrasound machines "head to head." This can usually be accomplished at conferences that include ultrasound topics or specialty society meetings. Another approach is to simply have two or three companies leave an ultrasound machine with you at the same time for several days. Asking a trusted and experienced colleague is another option. Determine what they liked and disliked about their machines. What equipment did they get that they do not use and what do they wish they had gotten? What kind of service do they get from the manufacturer? The relationship with the manufacturer is almost as important as the machine itself. Company representatives may assist with scheduled maintenance, urgent repairs, equipment upgrades, and in many instances, actual training within the program. If you prefer not to purchase a machine, other options include renting or leasing a machine, or borrowing an older machine from a department that is upgrading its equipment.

▶ TRAINING THE ULTRASOUND DIRECTOR

Several training options are available for the ultrasound director. Most frequently, this person attends one of the many available ultrasound courses given by various specialty societies or commercial entities and then undergoes a period of training in his or her own clinical setting. The fastest way to become adept at focused ultrasound is to sit and practice with an experienced sonologist. A great teaching resource is the sonographer pool within a hospital. It may be possible for the director-in-training to sit with a sonographer and perform examinations during the sonographer's normal working hours. This approach has the advantage of minimal cost, but is less time efficient since the trainee will be required to sit through many examinations that may not be applicable to the interests of that trainee. In addition, there may be some examinations, like the FAST examination, that are not routinely performed by sonographers in the ultrasound suite. A better alternative is to hire a sonographer on an hourly basis to individually teach in the ultrasound director's own clinical setting.

The ultrasound director may require several months of training before they attain the expertise needed to train others within their group. It is imperative that the ultrasound director be well established before the rest of the group begins training. This is important to help facilitate the group through the "training doldrums," when the frustrations of training tend to peak. It should be emphasized that the learning curve is quite steep at the beginning of training but is actually relatively short in length so that examination competency can be achieved with a manageable number of ultrasound examinations.

▶ TRAINING THE GROUP

Initial training can be either brief or extensive, depending on the training approach that is taken. One training model is the "parallel" model, where individuals are training in several ultrasound examinations simultaneously. The other method is the "serial" model, where training occurs with one ultrasound examination at a time, without proceeding to another examination until a certain level of proficiency is achieved. The parallel model works best when individual trainees are able to dedicate a larger portion of their time away from patient care to learn a new set of skills, as is typical in residency training programs. The serial model has the advantage of requiring less time input to get a trainee to a minimum level of competency for one particular examination. Serial training is ideal for community-based practitioners who have less time for training and want to incorporate one set of ultrasound skills into their practice as rapidly as possible.

All training programs generally have the following components:

- An initial block of didactic instruction
- An initial "hands-on" exercise
- A required number of proctored examinations performed on actual patients

In addition, the ultrasound director should consider some type of competency assessment after the completion of training with a written test, observed examinations, or both.

INITIAL DIDACTIC INSTRUCTION

The initial didactic instruction is where members of the physician group get their "jump start" in training. Initial training may consist of anywhere from several hours of instruction, if training in only one examination type, to several days of instruction, if training in multiple examinations. At a minimum, an introduction to the basic physics of ultrasound is required to understand the capabilities and limitations of the technology. Understanding ultrasound physics, even at a basic level, is essential for acquiring and interpreting ultrasound images. In addition, there should be some specific didactic instruction on the examination(s) being taught. It is feasible for the ultrasound director to develop and perform the initial training block, especially if only one or two examinations are to be covered. If several examinations are being taught, then it may be more practical to have group members attend one of the commercially available introductory ultrasound courses. Planning and giving a large hands-on ultrasound instruction block is time consuming and is often better left to professional course organizers. It is important, however, that the ultrasound director ensure that any outside course meets the training requirements established for their program.

At an ultrasound course, 1 to 2 hours is generally spent on ultrasound physics and equipment instrumentation, and an additional hour or two on each specific examination type. Lectures should include discussions of the specific indications for the examination and review of the anatomy, including normal, normal variant, and abnormal ultrasound findings. Teaching should be "finding or problem based," concentrating on specific focused findings and problems rather than discussing all diseases related to a specific organ or anatomic area. The major finding for each examination type (e.g., gallstones) as well as other findings (e.g., common bile duct diameter, pericholecystic fluid, gallbladder wall thickness) should

be demonstrated, and the appropriate ways to use these findings for clinical decision making should be discussed. Indications for referral for more comprehensive imaging should be covered. A comprehensive listing of suggested content for didactic sessions is available in the Model Curriculum for Emergency Ultrasound and the Emergency Ultrasound Imaging Criteria Compendium.[2,5] Guidelines for an introductory course are outlined in the ACEP Training Guidelines.[1] Recently, the problem- and symptom-based approach to ultrasound education and patient evaluation has been recognized and is being used increasingly in a variety of clinical specialties, especially emergency and critical care ultrasound.

INITIAL HANDS-ON EXERCISE

The initial hands-on exercise is usually combined with the initial didactic instruction. During this exercise, image acquisition is practiced on normal models in a non-stressful, non-patient-care environment. There should be no more than four students and one instructor per ultrasound machine to maximize student scanning time. Topics covered should include basic operation of the ultrasound machine controls, techniques for maximizing image quality, normal ultrasound anatomy and systematic approaches to the examination types taught in the didactic sessions. Specific "pelvic" models are employed when transvaginal ultrasound is taught, and chronic ambulatory peritoneal dialysis (CAPD) patients may be employed to demonstrate free intraperitoneal fluid on ultrasound examination. CAPD patients can simulate a positive examination by infusing fluid into their peritoneal cavity at will, and can even vary the amount of fluid to give different appearances. In instances where budgetary or planning constraints exist, these sessions can be run with trainees examining each other. Although pathology will not (usually) be demonstrated using this approach, trainees can effectively learn techniques for good image acquisition and systematic examination.

A newer teaching method is the ultrasound simulator that uses a mannequin and a computer to simulate scanning. The advantage of a simulator is that it can be programmed to simulate pathology, thus giving the trainee a more varied and yet standardized training experience. Finding enough patients with actual pathology to examine is one of the biggest challenges during training. Simulator technology holds great promise for the future of ultrasound training. There are also various training "phantoms" and models, which are commercially available and can be used to practice skills such as vessel cannulation and foreign body localization. Models can also be home-made as well, using such materials as rubber tubing, gelatin, or even raw chicken or beef.

PROCTORED EXAMINATIONS

The goals of proctoring are to help establish basic ultrasound skills, solidify the approach to examination, verify the quality of images produced, and verify the accuracy of the examinations. Once a physician completes the initial training phase, the real learning begins. As the physician begins scanning a variety of patients in his or her own clinical environment, the relative complexity of the skill will become evident. The trainee needs to be mentally prepared for this predictably difficult period so that frustration will not inhibit training. "Real-time" proctoring is extremely helpful in assisting the physician through this period. Real-time proctoring involves having the proctor sit with and guide the trainee through examinations and is the best way to learn ultrasound. The ultrasound director can perform real-time proctoring, but this is quite time consuming. Real-time proctoring can be provided using a less expensive and sometimes more experienced sonographer.

Some programs choose to do "delayed" proctoring, meaning trainees perform examinations independently, and then an experienced individual judges the quality and accuracy of the examinations at a later time. A common delayed proctoring technique is to videotape examinations. This method results in slower training but is usually cheaper than hiring a sonographer for real-time proctoring and saves the ultrasound director from doing the real-time proctoring themselves. At least some proctoring, especially in the early training stages, will have to be "real-time" or the trainees will not be skilled enough to make their independent scanning time productive. A reasonable way to control costs, but provide high-quality training, is to employ a combination of both real-time and delayed proctoring.

Another delayed proctoring option is to keep track of how trainee ultrasound results compare with other clinical information, including ultrasound examinations performed by traditional imaging specialists, other imaging studies (such as computed tomography), or procedures. This method accomplishes verification of accuracy but does not fulfill the other goals of proctoring. If this method is used, trainees should occasionally undergo real-time proctoring as well. Reviewing static ultrasound images generated by trainees as the sole method to delayed proctoring is problematic, especially for negative examinations. Pathology may be visible in one imaging plane but not in another, and the inexperienced operator may simply fail to find and photograph the pathology. Static images that are clearly positive can be used for proctoring in a limited manner since it is more difficult to "create" a false positive image (though not at all impossible). If there is no one in the program with enough experience to confirm studies performed by the group, physicians may wish to "outsource" examination review to an expert reader. This kind of delayed proctoring is best done with videotapes of complete examinations. Details will depend on the requirements of the expert reader.

Proctoring is the longest phase of training, often taking several months to complete. The biggest challenge an ultrasound director faces is helping trainees to maintain enthusiasm for the training program as they begin to climb the steep, but short, learning curve.

▶ PERFORM PROBLEM SOLVING

Ultrasound directors often experience two major problems with their programs. The first is difficulty in convincing all members of the group to participate in training. The second is maintaining trainee enthusiasm during the long proctoring phase. Emergency physicians, faced with the difficulty of integrating ultrasound training examinations with patient care during busy emergency department shifts, will find it tempting to put off using ultrasound. The following are some strategies to help avoid these problems:

1. *Maintain easy access.* The easier the use of the ultrasound machine, the more it will be used. An ultrasound machine in a "safe" but inconvenient place will not be used. The ultrasound machine should be kept in close proximity to patient rooms and in full view. Not only will this remind physicians to use the machine, it will assist with security of the ultrasound machine since its absence will be noticeable. This is especially important in critical care settings, such as with hypotensive and cardiac arrest patients, where a machine that is not close at hand is infinitely far away.

2. *Examination efficiency.* Point of care ultrasound examinations can add 5–10 minutes to a patient encounter (although they tend to reduce overall length of stay in the emergency department), which can add up over the course of a shift. If physicians perceive the ultrasound examination as a major time drain, they will not perform them. Examination times can be reduced by bringing the machine to the patient's room at the time of first contact if an ultrasound examination is anticipated. The examinations should be focused. If it is clear early in the examination that the examination will be technically difficult, the examination should be terminated and referred to a traditional imaging specialist. The goal of focused ultrasound is not to do all examinations, but to do those that can be performed efficiently. With experience, the trainee will develop strategies for producing acceptable images on technically difficult patients.

3. *Make it easy to keep track of training examinations.* If trainees are required to bring or keep track of individual logbooks, then the program will likely flounder. Logbooks may be forgotten or lost, creating frustration on the part of trainees. Many programs keep centralized logbooks in the clinical area into which all trainees record their examinations. A centralized logbook has the advantage of keeping all records in one place and allowing proctors to keep records organized for videotape review sessions. Another approach is to have trainees submit individual $3'' \times 5''$ cards documenting each patient examined. This method avoids the tragedy of a lost logbook.

4. *Introduce competition.* Competition is an effective motivating factor if applied appropriately. Physicians tend to be competitive. Periodically publishing the progress of trainees so that they can see how they compare to their peers can encourage those who might otherwise be ambivalent. At a minimum, it serves to remind everyone to continue practicing their ultrasound skills. Introducing a stepped system of achievement is also beneficial, especially if the first level can be achieved in a reasonably short period of time. Being allowed to proctor less experienced trainees can also reward trainees who have achieved designated levels of training.

► REGISTRY OF DIAGNOSTIC MEDICAL SONOGRAPHERS

Most sonographers have been registered by the American Registry of Diagnostic Medical Sonographers and carry the title "RDMS" (Registry of Diagnostic Medical Sonographers). This is a certification that can be achieved after a prescribed period of training or experience, and satisfactory performance on a standardized examination. The RDMS certification is recognized nationally as the standard of training for sonographers. This certification is available to physicians as well and some propose it as a logical step in the acquisition of ultrasound skills. Tests are given in several specialty areas including the abdomen, adult echocardiography, and obstetrics and gynecology. This certification, however, is directed toward comprehensive examination rather than focused examinations. In order to be certified, an individual must pass both physics and instrumentation examinations and at least one specialty area examination. The advantage of RDMS certification is that it is a credential with which hospitals are familiar, and it may lend weight to the physician seeking credentialing in focused ultrasound.

► ELECTIVE TRAINING

An elective in ultrasound during residency is a superb way to accelerate ultrasound learning. Electives are typically 2–4 weeks long and offer a trainee dedicated time to learn ultrasound without the distraction of other patient care responsibilities. Setting objectives is the key to elective design. The elective director should be able to answer the question, "What should the trainee be able to do with ultrasound by the end of the elective?" Often, the objective is to perform a certain number of ultrasound examinations, or it may be to meet the requirements for a particular privilege level. The goals should be made clear to the trainee at the outset of the elective.

Example activities include the following:

1) Performance of a certain number of examinations under direct supervision or by post hoc review of video or static images.
2) Assigned reading, either from texts or from journals.
3) Involvement with administrative aspects of the ultrasound training program, including ultrasound machine maintenance, supplies, record keeping, and proctoring of other trainees. This is the contribution the trainee makes in return for the teaching time they receive. It is also an essential exercise for anyone considering directing an ultrasound program in the future.
4) Involvement with other special projects, including research, teaching, or creating teaching materials such as an ultrasound teaching file.
5) Testing, both written and practical.

Here are example requirements for a 2-week elective:

1) A pre-elective meeting outlining the objectives of the elective.
2) Four to 6 hours of directly supervised scanning distributed over the elective period.
3) An additional 56 hours of time spent independently scanning.
4) Assigned readings from an ultrasound textbook.
5) A written examination at the end of the elective.
6) Tape review sessions as needed for item (3) above.
7) Special projects amounting to an additional 4–8 hours (e.g., submit two cases to the ultrasound teaching file).

Ultrasound is a skill of great interest to residents in emergency medicine as well as medical students applying for emergency medicine residencies. Anecdotally, the enjoyment and satisfaction residents have received while doing emergency ultrasound electives has made it one of the most popular rotations in many departments.

▶ FELLOWSHIP TRAINING

To master the skills necessary to integrate this powerful imaging modality into clinical practice, and especially for those considering a position as an ultrasound program director, a fellowship in ultrasound should be considered. Fellowships provide a means for intensive ultrasound training beyond that which is currently possible within the curriculum of an existing residency program. There are currently a large number of ultrasound fellowships available to physicians who desire further training.

In order for a fellow to obtain a quality educational experience, programs will need a solid commitment from their departments to provide the necessary resources. Several vital elements are needed to foster this learning experience. First, there must be a physician who is qualified to mentor an ultrasound fellow. This person should invariably have an extensive experience in clinical ultrasound, along with a passion to teach. They should have research experience and academic involvement in one or more of their specialty's ultrasound committees. Second, the fellowship director's department must fully support their efforts to advance ultrasound education and provide protected academic time to mentor each fellow and train physicians within their own department. Departments should provide financial support for a quality ultrasound system and equipment, and administrative support for research. Third, the patient volume and demographics should be sufficient to provide the fellow with experience in all applications of focused ultrasound.

While the curriculum may vary somewhat, the foundation of each ultrasound fellowship program is fairly similar. They provide each ultrasound fellow with a core content of subject matter that is covered within the 1-year program along with several other educational experiences covered in the preceding sections. The Section of Emergency Ultrasound of the American College of Emergency Physicians produced a consensus document with recommended criteria for fellowship sites, director qualifications, and minimum criteria for graduation from the fellowship.[19] Some excerpts from the document follow:

Site Qualifications:

- Fellowship should be a minimum of 12 consecutive months.
- Ultrasound equipment should be owned or controlled by the emergency department.
- Fellow should be provided a minimum of five scanning shifts per month.
- All examinations should be videotaped for review.

Director Qualifications:

- Should have at least 4 years' ultrasound experience after residency

- Should have published at least three peer-reviewed emergency ultrasound articles in Medline indexed journals

Fellowship Criteria for Graduation:

- 800 completed examinations
- Initiation of at least one research project and involvement in a second
- Deliver three separate ultrasound lectures to the department of emergency medicine

CORE CONTENT OF THE FELLOWSHIP

The core content refers to the primary ultrasound applications, but can expand into additional applications, as the fellow's time and interest allow (see Table 1-1). Fellows may develop new applications and implement training for housestaff and faculty.

QUALITY IMPROVEMENT

Fellows should be involved in the department's ultrasound QI program. This activity offers a high educational return for time invested since the mistakes of others become lessons for the fellow. It also allows the fellow to see the structure and function of a QI program.

JOURNAL CLUB

Reviewing the literature is an important component of an ultrasound fellowship. Although the structure in which this is accomplished may vary, a working knowledge of the pertinent literature is an integral part of the educational process. Structured journal club meetings may also provide a means by which other members of the department can join in the educational development. Likewise, a review of the literature may also provide an avenue to formulate other research ideas.

TEACHING RESPONSIBILITIES

The ultrasound fellow should also be responsible for educating other physicians within the department. Depending upon the experience of the ultrasound fellow, this duty may vary considerably. Once the fellow has developed the skills necessary to supervise others safely and competently, he or she should be utilized to advance the ultrasound education of other physicians within the department. The fellow should have protected nonclinical time devoted to teaching. The fellow may have other elective teaching opportunities outside of the department, such as at local hospitals, society meetings, or

▶ TABLE 1-3. **COSTS OF A POINT OF CARE ULTRASOUND PROGRAM**

One-time costs	
Ultrasound machine[a]	Approximate range $16,000–$200,000
Program development	10–40 hours or more. May be much more if the ultrasound director prepares and delivers all initial training.
Initial training	1–3 days per physician. The cost per physician for commercial courses ranges from $500 to $1000. This cost will be reduced if the ultrasound director does the training.
Proctoring	Cost of online proctoring each physician in training (ultrasound technician cost estimated at $35–$45 per hour). The ultrasound director may perform this duty.
Recurring costs	
Supplies (paper, gel, etc.)	Approximate range $300–$1800/year.
Maintenance agreement[b]	Approximate range $700–$8000/year.
Administration of program	Highly variable, based on program structure
Continuing medical education	8 hours/year (median recommendation), per physician
Time spent examining[c]	10 minutes/examination (estimate)

[a]These figures are from the year 2000. Since that time several lower cost ultrasound machines targeted at the clinical ultrasound market have been introduced. An ultrasound machine should be seen as having about a 5- to 7-year useful life; a machine should work until the end of that period but technology and options will progress so that replacement of the machine should be planned. It is also possible that once the ultrasound program is established, a second ultrasound machine may be purchased as a backup to avoid long downtime periods when the primary machine is out of service.
[b]Highly recommended.
[c]This is included to determine how much income might be lost, especially in a busy emergency department, where time spent scanning is lost income due to fewer patients being seen. It is possible, though unproven, that ultrasound might actually increase the number of patients a physician can care for by narrowing the differential diagnosis sooner and moving patients through the clinical setting more swiftly.

national conferences, in which to hone their skills by lecturing and providing hands-on training.

FUTURE DIRECTORS

The goal of most ultrasound fellows is to start or direct an ultrasound program after graduating from the fellowship. This may involve implementing or enhancing an ultrasound program at an existing residency program or private hospital. The fellowship experience should include a road map for this important step. Part of this training should involve the fellow in the political arena in which they must interact. This includes the likes of departmental policies on credentialing, ultrasound system maintenance, billing, QI discrepancies, and intradepartmental policies. They will also need assistance in developing lectures, training courses, and various training aides for their program. The fellowship should also include networking with other leaders in their field who will provide them with an opportunity to share ideas, research projects, and shape the future of ultrasound.

▶ COST OF A POINT OF CARE ULTRASOUND PROGRAM

One of the most common questions posed by physician groups about ultrasound is "How much will it cost us?"

Little has been published about the costs of an ultrasound program, but after discussing costs with representatives of ultrasound programs at over 40 academic emergency medicine centers, several generalizations can be made.[9] Some of the costs are easy to define (e.g., equipment and supply costs, price of training courses) and some are not as easy to define (e.g., time spent developing a program plan or performing practice ultrasound examinations). Table 1-3 provides general estimates.

▶ BILLING

The second most common question asked by those who must make the balance sheet work for an office or department is "Can we bill for this service?" The short answer is "yes." A detailed discussion of the financial side of ultrasound is beyond the scope of this chapter, but there are certain issues worth mentioning. Performing a focused examination does not (at the time of chapter writing) exclude a traditional imaging specialist from performing and charging for a comprehensive ("complete") examination of the same area, even on the same visit. Serial focused ultrasound examinations, if medically indicated, can be billed individually (e.g., serial FAST examinations in a deteriorating patient) at this time. Emergency physicians do not have to meet the same reporting standard as radiologists in order to charge for ultrasound examinations, but they may, in some instances, be required to record images to receive full reimbursement. Hospital-based physicians generally cannot own an ultrasound machine to charge a "technical" fee in addition to their usual "professional" fee for an ultrasound examination. The American College of Emergency Physicians publishes detailed information on coding and billing for emergency ultrasound.[8]

▶ CONCLUSION

Over the last decade smaller and smaller ultrasound machines have been introduced and machine prices have dropped dramatically. This along with increasing evidence that clinicians can perform accurate focused ultrasound assessments in order to make important clinical decisions in real time has driven the growth in the number of emergency physicians who perform ultrasound. The American Board of Emergency Medicine estimated in 2004 that 34% of all emergency physicians were using ultrasound, a jump from 23% in 2003.[20] Learning ultrasound requires a significant commitment, but it is rapidly becoming a required skill for the practice of emergency medicine.

REFERENCES

1. American College of Emergency Physicians: ACEP emergency ultrasound guidelines-2001. *Ann Emerg Med* 38:470–481, 2001.
2. Kendall JL, Bahner DP, Blaivas M, et al.: *Emergency Ultrasound Imaging Criteria Compendium*. American College of Emergency Physicians, 2006.
3. American College of Radiology: *Resolution 22, Standard for Performing and Interpreting Diagnostic Ultrasound Examinations. American College of Radiology,* Reston, VA: 1996.
4. American Institute of Ultrasound in Medicine: *Training Guidelines for Physicians Who Evaluate and Interpret Diagnostic Ultrasound Examinations.* Official Statement. September 2003. *www.aium.org/publications/statements/_statementSelected.asp?statement=14* (6/2/06).
5. Mateer J, Plummer D, Heller M, et al.: Model curriculum for physician training in emergency ultrasonography. *Ann Emerg Med* 23:95–102, 1994.
6. Witting MD, Euerle BD, Butler KH.: A comparison of emergency medicine ultrasound training with guidelines of the Society for Academic Emergency Medicine. *Ann Emerg Med* 34:604–609, 1999.
7. Lanoix R, Leak LV, Gaeta T, et al.: A preliminary evaluation of emergency ultrasound in the setting of an emergency medicine training program. *Am J Emerg Med* 18:41–45, 2000.
8. Hoffenberg: Emergency ultrasound coding and reimbursement. *www.acep.org/NR/rdonlyres/9ECB1EA2–0EFB-496F-ABE4–0D7C41144065/0/emergUltrasoundCoding Reimb.pdf* (5/16/06).
9. Peterson M, Fischer T, Blaivas M: Survey: Cost of an ultrasound program. Preliminary results presented at the Ultrasound Section Meeting, Society for Academic Emergency Medicine Annual Meeting, May 2000.
10. Merritt CR: ER ultrasound services—some points to consider. *Soc Radiol Ultrasound Newslett* July 1999.
11. Hamper UM: Commentary on "Hertzberg BS, Kliewer MA, Bowie JD, Carroll BA, DeLong DH, Gray L, Nelson RC. Physician training requirements in sonography: How many cases are needed for competence. *AJR Am J Roentgenol* 174(5):1221–1227, 2000." *Soc Radiol Ultrasound Newslett.* June 2000.
12. Unknown author: Who can perform ultrasound imaging? *Soc Radiol in Ultrasound Newslett* March 2000.
13. Hertzberg BS, Kliewer MA, Bowie JD, et al.: Physician training requirements in sonography: How many cases are needed for competence? *AJR Am J Roentgenol* 174:1221–1227, 2000.
14. Society for Academic Emergency Medicine: *Ultrasound position statement.* October 2004. *www.saem.org/publicat/ultrasou.htm* (6/2/06).
15. American Academy of Emergency Medicine: *Performance of emergency screening ultrasound examinations. Position Statement.* February 1999. *www.aaem.org/positionstatements/ultra.shtml* (6/2/06).
16. American College of Emergency Physicians: *Use of ultrasound imaging by emergency physicians. Policy Statement.* June 2001. *www.acep.org/webportal/PracticeResources/PolicyStatements/pracmgt/UseofUltrasoundImagingby EmergencyPhysicians.htm* (6/2/06).
17. American Medical Association: *Privileging for ultrasound imaging.* House of Delegates Policy H-230.960, 2000. *www.ama-assn.org/apps/pf_new/pf_online?f_n=browse& doc=policyfiles/HnE/H-230.960.HTM* (6/2/06).
18. Allison EJ, Jr., Aghababian RV, Barsan WG, et al.: Core content for emergency medicine. Task Force on the Core Content for Emergency Medicine Revision. *Ann Emerg Med* 29:792–811, 1997.
19. American College of Emergency Physicians Section of Emergency Ultrasound: *Emergency ultrasound fellowship guidelines: An information paper.* January 2005. *www.acep.org/webportal/PracticeResources/issues/ultra/ultrasoundfellowshipguide.htm* (6/2/06).
20. American Board of Emergency Medicine: *Longitudinal Survey of Emergency Physicians.* 2004.

CHAPTER 2

Equipment

Will Scruggs and J. Christian Fox

Point-of-care ultrasound has grown rapidly over the last 10–15 years. What was once a very small and underserved section of medical imaging has now grown to more than $95 million in sales of compact ultrasound units annually and is predicted to grow to $330 million by 2010.[1] Companies are introducing more machines with greater options (Appendices A and B). In addition to the traditional large corporate entities, there are a host of upstart companies marketing to nontraditional markets such as emergency medicine, anesthesiology, critical care, and the multitude of office practices in medicine today.

▶ GENERAL CONSIDERATIONS

PORTABILITY

The decreased size and portability of ultrasound machines have made it possible to use the modality outside of the radiology department. Portability has increased to the point that providers are taking point-of-care ultrasound into the prehospital setting and even on the frontlines of military operations.[2,3] Size requirements for ultrasound equipment will change on the basis of the setting and the type of examination that will be performed.

Both cart-based and compact systems are available. In addition, many compact systems offer a small cart to which the handheld component can be connected and easily removed. This cart will contain peripherals such as a printer, video recorder, and additional transducers. In general, cart-based systems tend to be higher-end machines and offer more options and increased resolution and performance. However, the performance gap between cart-based machines and compact machines is narrowing.[4]

The emergency department (ED) generally requires some form of cart-based system, as several probes are necessary for the growing number of applications that are used. Also, finding a place to set down a handheld machine while scanning can be difficult. Cart-based machines have varying amounts of storage space for adjunct equipment commonly used with scanning such as ultrasound gel, probe sheaths, printers, recording devices, and cleaners.

A removable component of the machine can be beneficial when other areas of the hospital need to be covered for "code" situations or when a cart will not fit into the nooks and crannies of an ED overflowing with patients. Office-based clinicians who limit their ultrasound use to a single probe and health care professionals using their devices outside of the hospital may benefit by having the compact machine without a cart. These machines are very portable and require only limited storage space.

POWER

A discussion about power may seem superfluous in a discussion about a medical imaging device. How an ultrasound machine is powered and how quickly it boots up may be the difference between a diagnostic tool that is used regularly in practice and one that sits in the corner collecting dust.

Many companies offer products that are powered via both wall outlets and rechargeable battery packs. Furthermore, most products with batteries allow for the seamless use of the device as it is unplugged. This can be a huge advantage in situations where more than one patient must be scanned in rapid succession, such as a multiple trauma situation.

If powering via battery is not an option, close attention should be paid to the amount of time necessary to boot up a system. Ultrasound machines that take more than 30 seconds from depression of the power switch to general use are impractical in the ED and critical care units. Beyond the obvious drawbacks in critical situations, machines with long boot-up times will lead to physician aggravation and diminished use of the machine.

Another important consideration is the power cord itself. Machines in the ED are often moved rapidly and by many different people with varying levels of concern for the machine. The power cord and its connection to the machine take a lot of abuse when it is run over or pulled from the wall when the machine is used. It is important for devices to have the ability to retract the power cord or a specific area of the machine for its storage. Cords should be detachable and replaceable if they do become damaged.

POWER FOR ANCILLARY DEVICES

Another consideration regarding electrical power for ultrasound machines is outlets on the machine for supplementary devices. Most machines provide outlets that are used to power ancillary devices such as thermal printers, video recorders, or gel warmers. Some machines have outlets that require specialized adapters. This may not be a problem if only the storage devices provided by that company are used, but it may limit options if the outlets are too few or too specialized.

TRANSDUCER CHANGERS

Different ultrasound applications require different probes. While office practices may require only a single probe for one or two types of ultrasound examinations, clinical settings such as the ED or critical care unit require several probes for multiple applications. Many cart-based systems allow toggling between probes at the push of a button. These systems have several active ports. Machines that only allow one probe to fit into the machine at any given time have one active port and storage ports where other probes are held while not in use.

Multiple active ports are essential for the full use of an ultrasound machine in an ED or a critical care setting. Physicians in these settings typically perform many types of scans and often in rapid succession. Untangling cords and changing probes between patients and scans can be frustrating and time consuming.

▶ BASIC KNOBOLOGY

Ultrasound machines are like rental cars. While there are hundreds of different machines out there, they all have the same basic controls. Ignition, steering wheel, gas, brakes, transmission, windshield wipers, headlights... and you're off! Clinicians with ultrasound experience should be able to use any machine, no matter where they find it in the hospital or how many knobs are found on the control panel. This next section identifies the basic controls that are found on every machine from the most portable, inexpensive device to the most expensive, washing machine-sized behemoth.

CONTROL PANEL

Control panels on ultrasound machines vary widely. Machines with more bells and whistles tend to have more buttons and knobs on the control panel than very portable machines that are equipped with only the essentials. No matter how complicated the machine, any sonologist can work any machine. However, more complex control panels may scare off clinicians newer to ultrasound.

Along with the complexity of the layout, there are two other considerations when thinking about different control panels. Durability is an important issue. Machines with more buttons and knobs may also have more cracks and crevices through which fluids may enter and disrupt function. The durability testing that companies perform on their systems should always be checked. Another minor question relates to the difference between trackballs and trackpads. Trackballs may work more precisely and quickly than a trackpad, especially with gel-laden gloves. Trackballs, however, may become clogged with gel and lose function, requiring removal and cleaning.

ACOUSTIC POWER

The acoustic power (also called output power) relates to the amplitude of sound waves produced by the transducer and helps determine the brightness and quality of the image. Increasing the acoustic power results in higher transmitted amplitudes and stronger returning echoes. This may improve image quality by increasing the contrast between light and dark areas on the display. However, if the power setting is too high, lateral and longitudinal resolution will diminish. The Food and Drug Administration (FDA) tightly regulates power output by all diagnostic ultrasound machines, and only limited control over power levels is truly available.

Acoustic power is directly related to intensity. The intensity of the ultrasound beam, meaning the amount of energy in a given area, determines the bioeffects of ultrasound. As the intensity increases, the amount of heat produced in the tissue increases. Much of the concern regarding potential harmful effects of ultrasound is related to the production of heat. While no studies have provided solid evidence that diagnostic ultrasound has a deleterious effect on human tissue, including fetal tissue, practitioners using ultrasound work by the ALARA (**A**s **L**ow **A**s **R**easonably **A**chievable) principle. This means that the lowest possible power setting necessary should be used for obtaining the appropriate image.[5] This is particularly important when scanning pregnant women. Generally, the obstetric preset on a given machine adjusts the power output to FDA-approved levels. Most machines do allow the sonologist to adjust the acoustic power. With some more basic machines, the power is adjusted only by toggling through presets.

GAIN

The other control that affects brightness is gain. Gain refers to the control sonologists use to adjust the brightness with which returning sound waves are displayed by the ultrasound machine. When an echo returns from body tissue, it does so within an amplitude range. The

ultrasound device translates that amplitude range to a brightness, which it displays on the monitor. The overall gain allows the sonologist to adjust the brightness of all returning echoes. Decreasing the gain makes the overall image less bright, while increasing the gain makes the image more bright (Figure 2-1).

The concepts of acoustic power and gain may be confusing to some. One can use television as an example. Stations choose the output power with which they transmit the auditory component of their television shows. The volume on our television set allows us to change the volume ("gain") that is transmitted out of the television set to our ears. The stations actually increase the auditory power output of the transmission during commercials. This explains why commercials may be louder than the television shows even if the volume is not adjusted.

Both acoustic power and gain change the brightness of the image produced by the ultrasound device. Power changes the brightness by changing the strength of sound entering the body, thereby increasing the strength

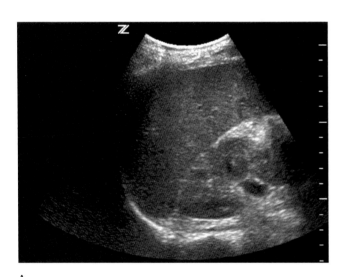

A

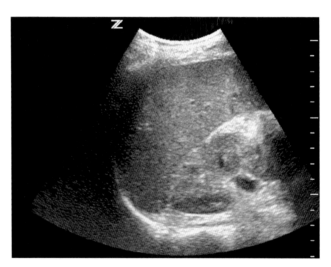

B

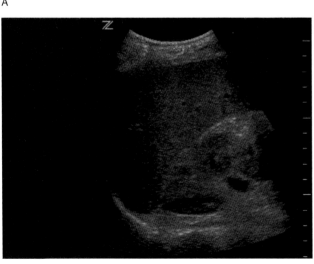

C

Figure 2-1. Gain–correct, over, under. (A) (Correct) This image is correctly gained. (B) (Over) The image has too much gain applied to the image. Compared with image A, echoes are found where there should be none. (C) (Under) The image is undergained. The image is too dark, potentially making it difficult for accurate diagnosis.

of returning echoes. Gain changes the brightness by adjusting the amplification of the electronic signals after the echoes have returned to the transducer. Working with the ALARA principle, the lowest possible power setting should be used. Therefore, when an image is not bright enough, the gain should first be adjusted to improve the image rather than the acoustic power. Care should be taken not to overgain images. Despite the perception of novice sonologists that brighter is better, increased gain can lead to loss of subtle information on the ultrasound screen.

TIME GAIN COMPENSATION

Time gain compensation (TGC) allows the sonologist to adjust the brightness of the image (gain) at different depths. To understand TGC, one must understand attenuation. Attenuation is the progressive weakening of the ultrasound beam as it passes through tissue. This occurs because of the energy absorption by tissues and reflection and scattering of sound waves after striking particles in the body. If the ultrasound device were to display the actual amplitude range of returning echoes, the image would become progressively darker from superficial to deep. Accordingly, machines are built to compensate for attenuation by increasing the brightness that is displayed for structures that are deeper in the body in order to create an ideal image—one that is of uniform echogenicity throughout.

Ultrasound devices often make this adjustment with slight inaccuracies because different tissues attenuate

sound at different rates. An example of this is the very bright image that is typically displayed posterior to a bladder in a transabdominal pelvic window. Sound does not attenuate much as it passes through fluid such as urine, so it returns to the probe with higher amplitude than sound waves that pass through soft tissue. The ultrasound machine misinterprets that to mean that there are stronger reflectors posterior to the bladder and therefore displays them much more brightly on the monitor.

Sonologists can adjust the time gain compensation on most ultrasound devices to correct for inaccurate assumptions by the device. The simplest method of adjustment is two knobs, one dedicated to the near field and the other dedicated to the far field. By using these levels, the sonologist is able to adjust the gain more quickly and smoothly throughout the image (Figure 2-2). Newer technology being introduced on many ultrasound machines allows the machine itself to evaluate tissue density under the ultrasound transducer and automatically make adjustments.

DEPTH

Next to the power switch, the most frequently used control feature on any ultrasound machine is depth. The control panel typically will contain either a single rotary knob or two buttons used to change how far into the body the machine images. There are two important reasons to optimize the depth. First, the display is a finite size and imaging at a greater depth means structures are made smaller because more area is being presented. If

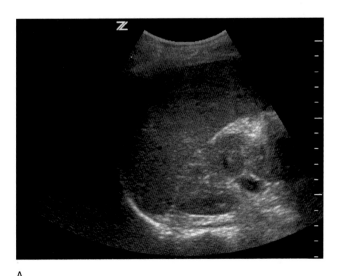

A

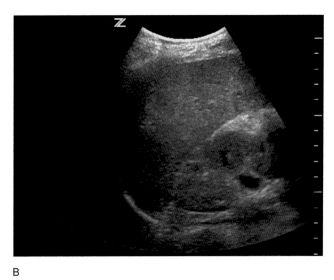

B

Figure 2-2. TGC—near field, far field. (A) The TGC through the near field segments of the image are decreased, resulting in poor visualization of the superficial liver tissues. (B) The TGC through the far-field segments of the image are decreased, resulting in poor visualization of the deep liver tissues. Compare these to Figure 2-1A, where the image has a correct application of TGC, with a uniform echogenicity throughout the liver.

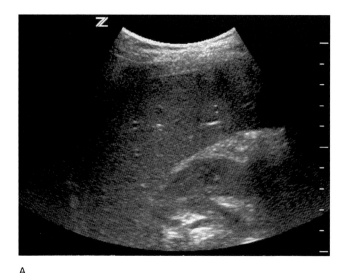

A

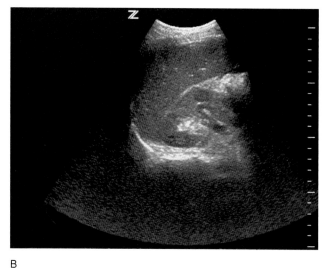

B

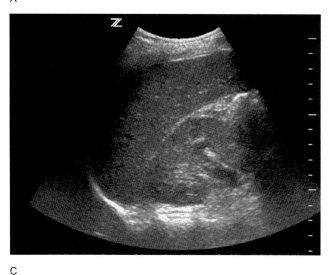

C

Figure 2-3. Depth—shallow, deep, correct. (A) Note that the depth is focused too shallow, leaving out important structures in the deeper field. (B) The depth is set too deep wasting valuable space in the far fields. (C) The depth is set correctly providing the balance of including all important structures, while utilizing the entire display.

the deeper structures are not important to the sonologist, that area of the display is simply "wasted real-estate." By reducing the depth, the machine will display only the necessary information and magnify the more superficial structures, thereby improving resolution and diagnostic ability (Figure 2-3). Second, adjusting the depth changes the amount of time the machine listens for returning echoes. If the depth is increased, the machine must listen for a longer period of time to collect data before it can display that frame. This may decrease the overall frame rate and temporal resolution, making the stream of images displayed less smooth to the eye. This may have a negative effect on diagnostic accuracy and the precision of procedure guidance.

The depth refresh rate refers to how long it takes a machine to create a new image after the sonologist adjusts the depth knob. High-end machines will refresh the image almost seamlessly, whereas lower-end machines

may have a noticeable delay. Among more portable machines, there is a wide spectrum of depth refresh times. While it is debatable whether this makes any clinical difference, a slow refresh rate certainly can be an irritation to the sonologist.

ZOOM

Most ultrasound machines offer a zoom function. The zoom function takes one section of the display and magnifies it. The resolution in the "zoomed" area remains the same, meaning that the number of pixels does not change. Rather, they are magnified to create the larger image resulting in a "pixilated" image that may appear somewhat blurry. The zoom function is most useful when the sonologist wants to focus on a deeper structure such as the common bile duct.

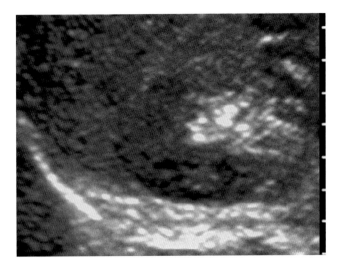

Figure 2-4. Zoom/depth. The image of the kidney has been created from the image shown in (Figure 2-3b) by using the Zoom function. It is magnified, but the overall resolution is not as sharp as the image created by decreasing the depth (Figure 2-3c) because there are fewer pixels creating the image.

Zoom and depth controls work by entirely different mechanisms. Whereas the zoom function magnifies the original data the device acquired (postprocessing), the depth function actually changes the way the image is acquired (preprocessing). Decreasing the depth allows the machine to dedicate more pixels to a smaller area. The temporal resolution improves because the machine spends less time listening for returning echoes. Whenever possible, sonologists should first change the depth to optimize the image. Zoom should be used only when deeper structures need to be magnified (Figure 2-4).

FREEZE

The freeze button allows the sonologist to hold a current image on the monitor. This is generally required to print images, save images, perform measurements and calculations, and add text. Most devices keep the last several seconds of images in memory (referred to as "cine loop") so when sonologists freeze the display, they are allowed to move through those saved images via left/right buttons or a roller-ball. The exact number of images saved in current memory varies with the machine.

MEASUREMENTS AND CALCULATIONS

The ability to measure structures is very important for any machine in a clinical setting. Almost all ultrasound devices produce electronic calipers that the sonologist may use to make measurements. Many machines also offer calculation packages that will use measurements

to make clinically important calculations such as area, volume, crown-rump-length, biparietal diameter, cardiac output, and others.

DATA ENTRY

The vast majority of ultrasound machines allow for patient data entry. The amount of data that may be entered varies widely, especially in portable machines. Some will allow for large amounts of text with specific locations for patient name, identification number, date of birth, indication for the study, sonologist, etc. Others allow for only a few lines of patient data or no data at all. Text and other identification devices such as arrows or body markers that can be added to an image are features most machines offer. A library of frequently used terms or schematic diagrams may also be available for the sonologist to toggle.

► ADVANCED KNOBOLOGY

M-MODE

M-mode (motion-mode) ultrasound is used to evaluate the movement of structures within the body. The sonologist focuses a narrow line through the structure in question. The machine maps echoes from that line through the tissue onto the vertical axis of a graph while time is depicted on the horizontal axis. The resulting image made up of lines of varying echogenicity moving across the display from right to left. Practically speaking, each line represents a tiny structure and its movement over time. Many machines will display this image adjacent to a smaller version of the original grayscale image. Cardiologists will often use M-mode ultrasound to precisely evaluate the movement of heart valves (Figure 2-5), while a common use in the emergency and acute care settings is to display and quantitate fetal cardiac activity (Figure 2-6).

DOPPLER

Doppler ultrasound uses the frequency shift created by the reflection of sound off a moving body to observe and describe that movement. Doppler shift is the change from the original frequency that occurs when the sound reflects off a moving structure. The amount of shift that occurs relates to the velocity of that structure. Doppler shift occurs in the range of audible sound. The simplest form of Doppler ultrasound audibalizes the Doppler shift. Palm-sized machines that "whoosh" in time with the pulsating flow of blood through peripheral vessels or the fetal heart are used in many parts of the

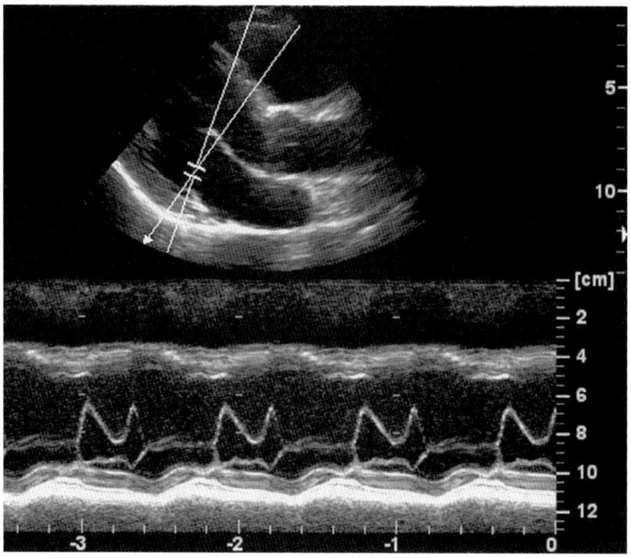

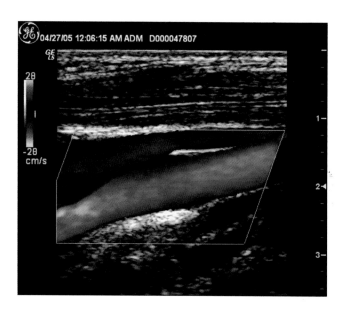

Figure 2-5. M-mode Cardiac. The cursor has been placed over the mitral valve. The graph below demonstrates the motion of the valve at the cursor over time. (Courtesy of GE Medical)

hospital. Diagnostic ultrasound devices offer more advanced Doppler that visually displays Doppler shift.

COLOR FLOW AND POWER DOPPLER

Bidirectional Doppler is probably the most recognizable form of Doppler ultrasound. The Doppler shift is de-

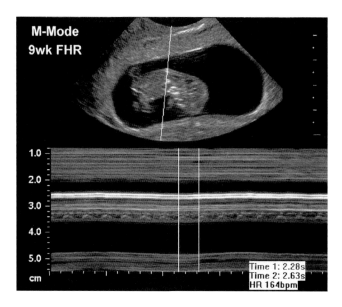

Figure 2-6. M-mode Fetal Heart. The M-mode line is placed through the fetal heart in this image. The movement of the heart is charted against time and can be seen at approximately 3.5 cm on the resulting graph. The movement calculates to 164 bpm. (Courtesy of Zonare)

Figure 2-7. Color Doppler. Color Doppler measures the frequency shift and displays it as color over the grayscale image. Note the color scale to the left of the ultrasound image. The blue at the top of the scale indicates that flow toward the probe is labeled blue. (Courtesy of GE Medical)

tected and movement toward and away from the probe is displayed in different color—generally in red and blue (but not limited to those colors). The color image is placed on the backdrop of the grayscale image so flow can be assessed related to the surrounding anatomy (Figure 2-7).

For inexperienced users of color Doppler ultrasound, it is important to note that red and blue have nothing to do with artery and vein. The ultrasound device generally will display a graph in one corner of the display when color Doppler is activated. The color displayed at the top of the graph refers to flow toward the probe, while the color at the bottom of the graph corresponds to flow away from the probe.

Viewing the speed of movement of substances toward and away from the probe is termed velocity mode. With this mode, the lighter shades of each color on the graph represent higher average flow rates. Variance mode may also be available on some machines. Variance mode demonstrates the presence of turbulence. Devices display turbulence by color and the representation is demonstrated on the same chart as the velocity. A mosaic pattern will generally be displayed by the ultrasound machine. The color to the right indicates turbulent flow. Variance mode is most often used by cardiologists evaluating blood flow around valves and within the proximal aorta or by radiologists and vascular surgeons for evaluation of flow through blood vessels (Figure 2-8).

Power Doppler displays flow without regard to direction. Rather than two colors distinguishing the direction of flow, the same color (frequently orange) with

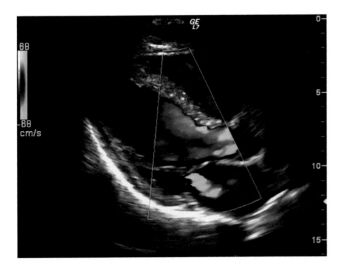

Figure 2-8. Variance mode. In the upper left corner of the display there is a legend referencing the colors to the echocardiogram. The left side of the legend shows that red indicates flow toward the probe and blue flow away from the probe. The right side of the legend demonstrates that green indicates turbulent flow throughout the image. (Courtesy of GE Medical)

▶ **TABLE 2-1. COMPARISON OF COLOR FLOW AND POWER DOPPLER**

Color Doppler	Power Doppler
Indicates relative speed and direction of flow	More sensitive
Less motion artifact	Less dependant on imaging angle

Doppler is less affected by the angle of the ultrasound beam relative to the direction of flow than is bidirectional color Doppler (Table 2-1).

Just as the brightness can be adjusted in B-mode ultrasound using the gain function, the amount of Doppler signal displayed by the device can be adjusted. On many machines, turning up the gain knob while in Doppler mode will display lower amplitude Doppler shifts. Other machines will have a second knob or button specifically for Doppler sensitivity. Increasing the sensitivity of Doppler will also make the image more prone to artifact created by subtle movements of the patient. Other factors that can change Doppler sensitivity include increasing or decreasing the power output, altering the Doppler scale, decreasing the Doppler angle, and adjusting the frequency.

Most machines that have a Doppler function allow the sonologist to adjust the size of the area they are monitoring for Doppler shift. The area is usually indicated by a parallelogram or sector on the ultrasound display. The area is limited because the larger the area the worse

a range of hues is applied to a grayscale image wherever a frequency shift (from movement or flow) is found (Figure 2-9). Power Doppler is more sensitive to subtle movement, thereby showing slower flow; however, this comes at the expense of more motion artifacts with subtle movements (such as respiration). Additionally, power

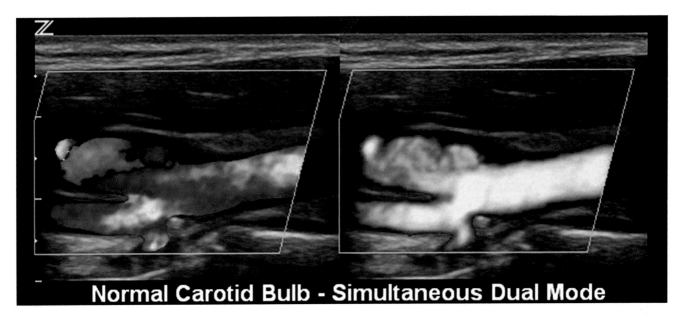

Normal Carotid Bulb - Simultaneous Dual Mode

Figure 2-9. Color flow Doppler vs. Power Doppler. The image on the left demonstrates normal flow in the carotid sinus with bidirectional color flow Doppler. The image on the right uses power Doppler. Note the single color for all directional flow in the power Doppler image versus the color Doppler image that uses two colors to indicate flow toward and away from the probe. (Courtesy of Zonare)

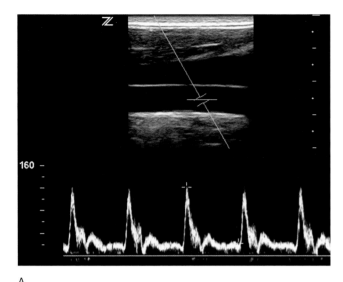
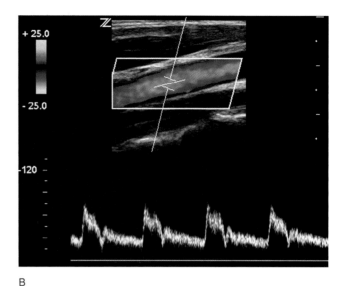

A   B

Figure 2-10. (a) Duplex spectral ultrasound. Duplex ultrasound consists of either the grayscale image with color Doppler, or the grayscale image with the spectral Doppler graph (A) (Courtesy of Zonare). (b) Triplex ultrasound. Triplex ultrasound displays (B) consist of a grayscale image, color Doppler, and spectral Doppler graph all on the same display. (Courtesy of Zonare)

the temporal resolution as the machine takes longer to listen for returning echoes. Larger areas will give more Doppler information, but will tend to be choppy and difficult to read.

Wall filtering is found on most machines that have Doppler as a function. Doppler typically is used to visualize the movement of red blood cells through the vasculature. However, when vasculature pulsates, the walls will move as well. Wall filters reject low-level Doppler shifts around the baseline flow within the vessel, such as the Doppler shifts that occur because of movement of the blood vessel wall. The purpose is to show less movement of flow that appears to extend into the tissue surrounding the vasculature created by these subtle movements.

PULSE WAVE OR SPECTRAL DOPPLER

Pulse wave is a type of spectral (or quantitative) Doppler that displays the velocity of moving structures (such as blood cells) on the vertical axis of a graph with time as the horizontal axis. The resulting graph accurately quantifies flow. It is useful when evaluating the flow of blood within a vessel or through a valve. This is most frequently used in detailed examinations of vasculature (such as carotid artery stenosis) and flow through the heart.

Duplex ultrasound combines the anatomic image of two-dimensional (2-D) ultrasound with either color Doppler or the graph representing the spectral Doppler analysis on the same display. Triplex scanning demonstrates the spectral Doppler waveform, the color Doppler

image, and the grayscale ultrasound image on the same display. The screen is split into two sections with the grayscale and overlying color Doppler image above and the spectral Doppler graph found underneath. Duplex and triplex ultrasound are useful tools in determining the location and flow patterns of vasculature (Figure 2-10). Common applications of duplex ultrasound include adjunctive use in the diagnosis of deep venous thrombosis (DVT) and determining flow in ovarian and testicular torsion. Common indications for triplex ultrasound are those in which spectral Doppler is used.

FOCUS

Through constructive and destructive interference, ultrasound probes effectively transmit an hourglass-shaped cone of sound. The greatest resolution is found at the narrowest portion of that hourglass shape—the focal zone. Many devices offer the ability to adjust that focal zone through electronic focusing. This can be a very helpful feature with subtle findings. The focus is usually represented by a small arrow or line to the left or right of the image. The greatest lateral resolution will be found at the level identified by the arrow.

Many machines offer the ability to create multiple focal zones within the image. Multiple arrows will be displayed and the overall lateral resolution of the image will improve. However, increasing the number of focal zones will also decrease temporal resolution as the device spends more time listening for returning echoes and processing each image.

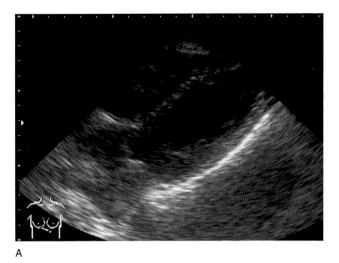

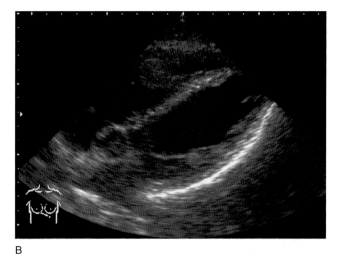

A

B

Figure 2-11. Harmonic imaging (subcostal cardiac view). Figure A demonstrates an image without harmonic imaging. Figure B shows the same image with harmonics. Note the improved detail of the left ventricular walls, endocardium, mitral subvalvular and aortic valve areas. (Courtesy of James Mateer, MD)

HARMONICS

All ultrasound devices send pulses of sound into the body at a primary frequency and then listen for echoes at that same frequency. The crystals "hear" echoes that are directly "aimed" at, but they also receive echoes that are scattered from other points in the image. These scattered echoes decrease the overall quality of the image.

When echoes are reflected, they are reflected at the primary frequency and at harmonic frequencies, which are at multiples (2×, 4×, 8×, etc.) of the original frequency. Harmonic frequencies produce less scatter and side-lobe artifact creating a cleaner image. They are attenuated less by tissue than the primary harmonic frequency. Thus, higher frequency waves can reach further through tissue and potentially yield a higher resolution image. The THI (Tissue Harmonic Imaging) function tells the machine to filter the echoes returning at the primary frequency and use the harmonic frequency to create the image (Figure 2-11). This can be a very useful option for viewing certain structures or when patient specific image quality is difficult. The tissue harmonic function is usually activated with a single button on the control panel labeled "THI." In some patients the quality of the image may actually decrease. Sonologists should be just as willing to turn it off as they are to turn it on.

OPTIMIZATION BUTTON

Many newer machines offer an "Optimization" button. This function may be noted by several other terms, but they all refer to the same basic idea. This feature allows the processor within the machine to use all of the above functions as well as a few more advanced techniques to create the "ideal image" (Figure 2-12). This can be a very simple and effective way to improve image quality. It should not, however, be the sole means to improve image quality.

PRESETTINGS

Presets use adjustments of acoustic power, gain, focal zones, lines per sector, sector size, and other settings to create an image generally most useful for that particular type of imaging. Obstetrical settings are notable in that they decrease the power output to FDA-accepted levels for ultrasound of the fetus. Cardiac settings work to increase the frame rate at the expense of image quality. Aside from imaging differences, some machines allow for different calculations while using certain presets. An example of this is biparietal diameter and crown-rump length in obstetrics mode. Many machines also allow the operator to create their own presets.

VOLUMETRIC ULTRASOUND/ THREE-DIMENSIONAL ULTRASOUND

Technological advances in ultrasound are being made as the speed of computer processors improves. Volumetric scanning is now being made available for widespread commercial use. In a volume scanning protocol, the probe is held in place while an ultrasound beam is steered through a wide scanning plane by the ultrasound device and data are collected through the entire

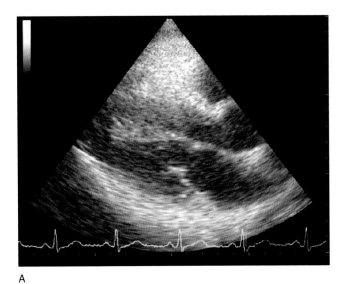

A

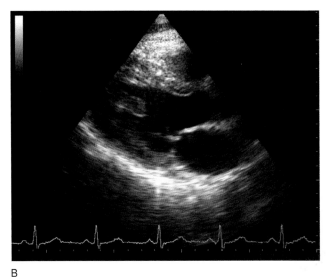

B

Figure 2-12. Image "optimization" (parasternal long-axis view). Figure A is an image without "optimization." Figure B shows the same image with "optimization." (Courtesy of Biosound Esaote)

volume through which the beam passed. Operators can then make cuts through any portion of the resulting data set (Figure 2-13). The technology has the potential to revolutionize ultrasound in the same way multidetector computed tomography (CT) has revolutionized conventional radiography.

Three-dimensional ultrasound imaging for diagnostic purposes and procedure guidance is currently in its infancy (Figure 2-14). It is also based on volume data collection. Obstetrics and cardiology are at the forefront in the use of 3-D ultrasound for diagnostic purposes.[6,7] However, current diagnostic use of 3-D ultrasound is very limited even in these fields. The American Institute of Ultrasound in Medicine (AIUM) considers 3-D ultrasound to be an adjunct to 2-D ultrasound.[8]

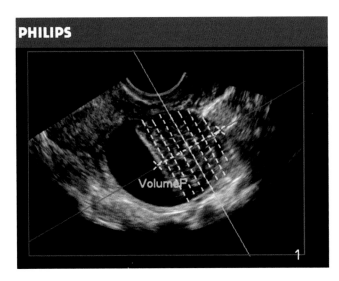

Figure 2-13. Volumetric scanning. Volume scan collects data over an entire volume rather than a slice. The resulting data set can be manipulated to display an image through any plane in the volume. (Courtesy of GE Medical)

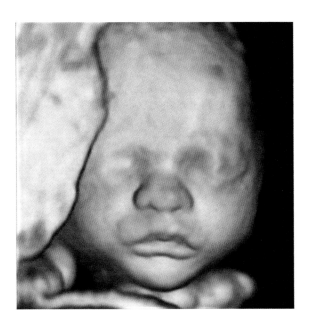

Figure 2-14. Three-dimensional Ultrasound. Three-dimensional technology provides incredible ultrasound images, but has limited emergency diagnostic value at this time. (Courtesy of Philips)

▶ PROBES

BASICS

Ultrasound utilizes piezoelectric crystals that convert electrical energy to mechanical energy in the form of sound waves, which are projected into the body. When the sound waves return to the probe, it is converted back into electrical energy.

There are several layers to an ultrasound probe. The piezoelectric crystals form the active element of the probe. A matching layer directly covers the piezoelectric crystals and provides impedance (resistance to movement of sound through a substance) in between the crystals and the body. The matching layer is important because large differences in impedances cause reflection. Piezoelectric crystals have impedance 20 times that of tissue. Such a difference would cause 80% of sound to be reflected away from the body, leaving almost no sound waves to use diagnostically.[9] The matching layer drastically reduces this effect.

The backing material suppresses crystal vibration. By damping the vibration caused by the application of electricity to the crystal, the backing material improves the ability of the crystal to listen. Finally, the covering to the probe protects the internal mechanisms within the probe from trauma and insulates the patient and the sonologist from electrical shock.

Probe maintenance is very important. A probe should never be used when cracked. A compromised cover may expose the sonologist and the patient to electrical current. Any damaged probe should be replaced or returned to the manufacturer for repair.

Durability is a very important factor in probe selection, especially in rougher environments such as an ED. Depending on the setting, the probe itself may be dropped or run over frequently and the cord may take abuse as well. Probes are expensive and it is important to consider whether or not they fit well into a specific practice setting.

PROBE CLEANING

Piezoelectric substances are polarized and stabilized at high heats and pressures, meaning that they will no longer change shape with pressure or voltage rendering them useless. They should never be autoclaved.

General ultrasound probes (those not used on mucous membranes) should be cleaned with water and a nonabrasive soap after each use. After cleaning, a low- or intermediate-level disinfectant should be used such as quaternary ammonium sprays or wipes as directed by the manufacturer.[10] Further cleaning may be necessary in the case of contact with blood or with drug-resistant micro-organisms or highly virulent viruses.[11]

Ultrasound probes designed for contact with mucus-membranes (endocavitary probes) require more stringent measures. Probes should be cleaned with nonabrasive soap and water, followed by a high-level disinfectant such as gluteraldehyde products or Cidex OPA.[11,12] Proper disinfection may require soaking the probe in an approved substance. More information regarding FDA-approved high-level disinfectants can be found at the FDA Web site: http://www.fda.gov/cdrh/ode/germlab.html (Table 2-2).[13] Probes in contact with

▶ TABLE 2-2. **FOOD AND DRUG ADMINISTRATION-CLEARED HIGH-LEVEL DISINFECTANTS**

Manufacturer	Active Ingredient(s)	Conditions
Acecide™ High Level Disinfectant		
Healthpoint LTD	8.3% hydrogen peroxide	10 min at 25°C
	7.0% peracetic acid	5 days Max. Reuse
Aldahol III High-Level Disinfectant		
Healthpoint LTD	3.4% gluteraldehyde	10 min at 20°C
	26% isopropanol	14 days Max. Reuse
Banicide® Advanced for Sterilization and High-Level Disinfection		
Pascal Company, Inc.	3.5% gluteraldehyde	45 min at 25°C
		30 days Max. Reuse
Cidex® OPA Solution		
Advanced Sterilization Products	0.55% *ortho*-phthaldehyde	12 min at 20°C
		14 days Max. Reuse
Sporicidin Sterilizing and Disinfecting Solutions		
Sporicidin International	1.12% gluteraldehyde	20 min at 25°C
	1.93% phenol/phenate	14 days Max. Reuse
Cetylcide-G® Concentrate and Diluent Concentrate		
Celylite Industries, Inc.	3.2% gluteraldehyde	40 min at 20°C
		28 days Max. Reuse

▶ **TABLE 2-2. (CONTINUED) FOOD AND DRUG ADMINISTRATION-CLEARED HIGH-LEVEL DISINFECTANTS**

Manufacturer	Active Ingredient(s)	Conditions
MedSci 3% Gluteraldehyde MedSci, Inc.	3% gluteraldehyde	25 min at 25°C 28 days Max. Reuse
Endospor™ Plus Sterilizing and Disinfecting Solution Cottrell Limited	7.35% hydrogen peroxide 0.23% peracetic acid	15 min at 20°C 14 days Max. Reuse
Sporox Sterilizing & Disinfection Solution Reckitt & Colman Inc.	7.5% hydrogen peroxide	30 min at 20°C 21 days Mx. Reuse
Peract™ 20 Liquid Sterilant/Disinfectant Minntech Corporation	1.0% hydrogen peroxide 0.08% peracetic acid	25 min at 20°C 14 days Max. Reuse
Procide® 14 N.S. Cottrell Limited	2.4% gluteraldehyde	45 min at 20°C 14 days Max. Reuse
Omnicide™ Long Life Activated Dialdehyde Solution Cottrell Limited	2.4% gluteraldehyde	45 min nat 20°C 28 days Max. Reuse
Omnicide™ Plus Cottrell Limited	3.4% gluteraldehyde	45 min at 20°C 28 days Max. Reuse
Metricide Plus 30® Long-Life Activated Dialdehyde Solution Metrex Research, Inc.	3.4% gluteraldehyde	90 min at 25°C 28 days Max. Reuse
Metricide® 28 Long-Life Activated Dialdehyde Solution Metrex Research, Inc.	2.5% gluteraldehyde	90 min at 25°C 28 days Max. Reuse
Metricide® Activated Dialdehyde Solutions Metrex Research, Inc.	2.6% gluteraldehyde	45 min at 25°C 14 days Max. Reuse
Cidex™ Activated Dialdehyde Solution Johnson & Johnson Medical Products	2.4% gluteraldehyde	45 min at 25°C 14 days Max. Reuse
Cidex Formula 7™ Long-Life Activated Dialdehyd Solution Johnson & Johnson Medical Products	2.5% gluteraldehyde	90 min at 25°C 28 days Max. Reuse
Cidex Plus™ 28 Day Solution Johnson & Johnson Medical Products	3.4% gluteraldehyde	20 min at 25°C 28 days Max. Reuse
Wavicide® - 01 Wave Energy Systems	2.5% gluteraldehyde	45 min at 22°C 28 days Max. Reuse

ODE Device Evaluation Information - FDA Cleared Sterilants and High Level Disinfectants with General Claims for Processing Reusable Medical and Dental Devices - September 28, 2006.

mucus-membranes should be covered with an imperme-able barrier prior to the use and the sonologist should use universal precautions as well.

FREQUENCY

Most diagnostic ultrasound probes are broadband de-vices made to work over many frequencies (see Chapter 3, Physics and Image Artifacts, for further discussion). General-purpose probes allow users to toggle between 2 and 3 preset frequencies. An example would be a 2- to 4-MHz abdominal probe that can be switched to 2 MHz, 3 MHz, or 4 MHz. Lower frequencies improve penetra-tion, but sacrifice resolution. What is gained in depth will be lost in image quality.

FOOTPRINT

The footprint is the area through which sound leaves and returns to the probe. It is the window the ultra-sound device uses to view the world. Larger footprints allow for better deep imaging, but present greater diffi-culty in working around sound-resistant barriers at the skin surface, such as ribs. Intracostal imaging can be very difficult with large footprint probes that can dis-play 2-3 rib shadows on a given image. Smaller foot-print probes pass the ultrasound beam through a smaller aperture, making it easier to direct the beam between structures such as the ribs, but sacrifice resolution in the far fields as the beam diverges from the focus (Figure 2-15).

MECHANICAL TRANSDUCERS

Mechanical sector probes are used on some older ma-chines. A single piezoelectric element is moved across the scanning plane while pulses of electrical energy are applied, producing and receiving echoes. The probe ac-tually vibrates because of the movement of the crystal. Mechanical sector probes are not extensively used in

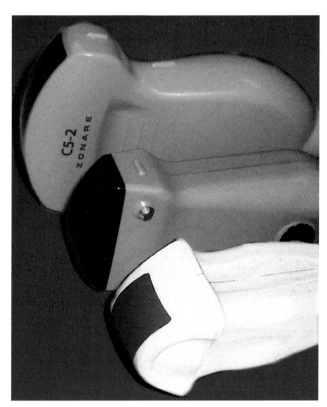

A

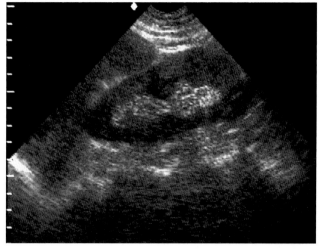

B

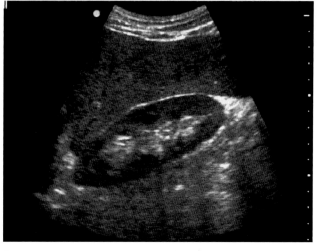

C

Figure 2-15. Curved Probes, C15, C30, C60. These three curved array probes each have different footprint sizes (A). Note that the smaller footprint probes have a tighter curvature. The image created by each is pie shaped. The smaller footprint probe (B) has a much smaller near-field image allowing greater intercostal ac-cess than the large footprint probe (C).

▶ TABLE 2-3. COMPARISON OF STANDARD PROBE STRUCTURES

Probe	Advantages	Disadvantages
Linear array	Very detailed superficial images Wide superficial field-of-view	Poor penetration with high-frequency probes Sector size limited to footprint
Large-curved array	Wide superficial and deep fields-of-view Excellent deep structure imaging	Difficult intercostal imaging Poor superficial resolution
Small-curved array	Wide deep field-of-view Excellent intercostal imaging	Narrow superficial field-of-view Deep structure imaging not as clear as large, curved probe
Phased array	Excellent intercostal imaging Wide deep field-of-view Excellent penetration for large patients	Narrow superficial field-of-view Deep structure imaging not as clear as large, curved probe Poor focus at periphery of image
Endocavitary	Very detailed images of superficial/ internal structures	Poor deep field imaging
Vector array	Very detailed superficial images Wide superficial and deep fields-of-view	Poor penetration

newer machines as the focus of the probe is fixed and Doppler ultrasound is not possible.

ARRAY TRANSDUCERS

Modern ultrasound probes use electronic array technology. Array transducers sequentially arrange crystals or groups of crystals along the footprint of the probe.[14] By varying the timing of activation of the groups of crystals, the ultrasound device can electronically steer and focus the ultrasound beam. This is possible because sound waves from different groups of crystals predictably interact through constructive and destructive interference. Precise timing is required and malfunction of a single

group of crystals can alter the direction and focus of the entire beam. Array transducers are produced in multiple forms, each with their own advantages and disadvantages (Table 2-3).

LINEAR ARRAY PROBES

Linear array probes have a flat face along which a sequence of crystals is arranged. The sector size of the linear probe is identical to the footprint of the probe itself and the resulting image is rectangular or square (Figure 2-16). Linear probes are generally used to view superficial structures and are therefore constructed to produce higher frequencies. Linear probes are used for

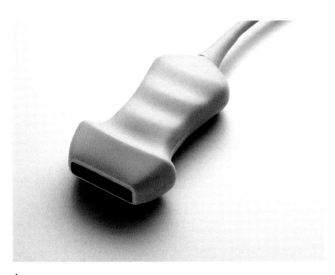

A

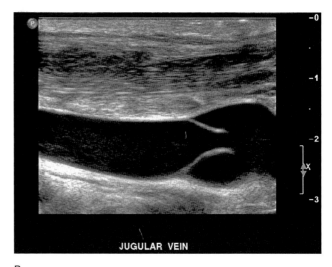

B

Figure 2-16. Linear probe, linear image. The linear probe with high frequency provides excellent superficial resolution (A) (Courtesy of Sonosite). Note that the sector size is equal to the footprint of the probe (B) (Courtesy of Philips).

venous and arterial cannulation, testicular and thyroid ultrasonography, subcutaneous foreign body identification and retrieval, diagnosis and procedure guidance of subcutaneous abscesses, peripheral nerve blocks, evaluation of appendicitis and pneumothorax, and various musculoskeletal applications.

Linear probes come in many sizes. Larger linear probes (made with lower frequencies) are sometimes used for 2nd- and 3rd-trimester pregnancy examinations as well as deeper abdominal examinations. Probes solely used for procedure guidance are generally smaller, on the order of 25 mm, with frequencies greater than 8 MHz.[15,16] General use linear probes used for the full spectrum of emergency ultrasound applications are closer to 40 mm with frequencies ranging from 5 to 10 MHz.

CONVEX ARRAY PROBES

The crystals in convex arrays are arranged along a curved face. The resulting image has a sector size larger than the footprint of the probe. There are many variations of curved probes. Lower frequency curved probes are used for deep imaging in the thorax, abdomen, and bladder. Higher frequency curved probes are used for endocavitary scanning, such as transvaginal and transrectal applications.

The range of frequencies and overall construction of curved array probes are important determinants regarding where they are most beneficial. Larger footprint probes with less curvature typically provide greater lateral resolution at a given frequency in the far fields. However, smaller footprint probes with a tighter curvature allow for easier access through the intercostal spaces.

Endocavitary probes are basically curved array probes on a stick. They can be inserted through an orifice to get closer to the organ(s) of interest. They have a very wide field of view, up to 180 degrees, and are higher frequency probes (8-13 MHz) because they require little penetration to access the desired organs (Figure 2-17). The resolution is generally outstanding. While endovaginal scanning is the most common use for endocavitary probes, urologists use similar probes for endorectal prostate imaging. In the ED, intraoral ultrasound for the evaluation of peritonsillar abscess and procedure guided drainage is another promising use for endocavitary probes (Figure 2-18).[17]

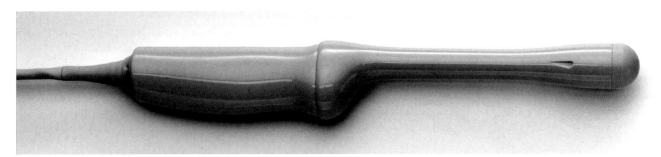

A

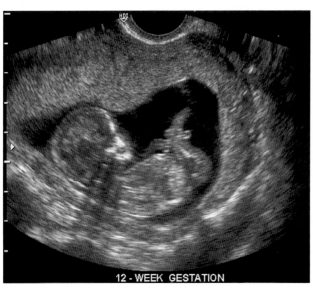

12 - WEEK GESTATION

B

Figure 2-17. Endocavitary probe, endovaginal image. The endocavitary probe has a very wide field-of-view (A) (courtesy of Sonosite). Note the near 180 degree view in this ultrasound of a 12-week IUP (B).

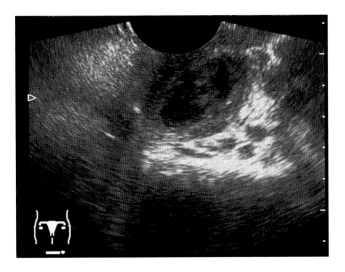

Figure 2-18. PTA image. Endocavitary probes are used beyond the pelvis. Peritonsillar abscess identification and procedure-guided drainage are another use.

PHASED ARRAY PROBES

Phased array probes have a flat footprint much like linear array probes. However, the crystals are grouped into a very small cluster. Phased array probes use every element with each ultrasound pulse. This is the major difference between this type of probe and curved and linear array probes. The device varies the timing and sequencing of the application of electrical pulses to the crystals to create a sector shaped image (Figure 2-19). Phased array probes are often used in echocardiography as the small footprint allows for easy intercostal imaging and the small, flat probe makes excellent skin contact with minimal pressure. Furthermore, phased array probes provide excellent deep Doppler capabilities.[14]

Abdominal imaging is also possible with phased array probes in lower frequencies. Emergency physicians find them useful for the same reasons as cardiologists—they provide good image quality with a very small footprint for intercostal imaging. Phased array probes have a small superficial field of view and poor peripheral focusing capabilities, which can limit intra-abdominal use. They offer good penetration, which is helpful in patients with a challenging body habitus.

VECTOR ARRAY PROBES

Vector array probes are linear probes that use array technology to steer and focus ultrasound to an area larger than the probe itself. The sector that is created is trapezoidal in shape and wider than the footprint of the probe (Figure 2-20). Vector array probes are useful for superficial structures that are larger than the footprint of the linear probe. These probes can be useful in the ED to image the testicles, large abscesses, or other soft tissue structures.

▶ ACCESSORIES

GEL

Gel is used between ultrasound devices and the skin or mucus membranes to decrease the amount of air

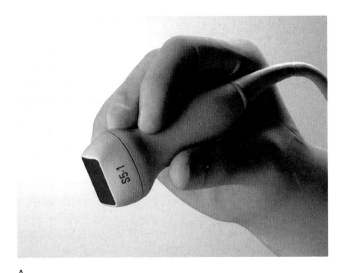

A

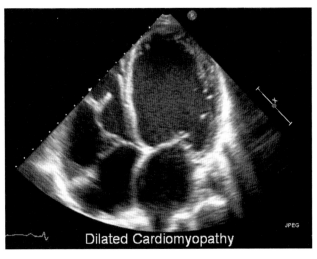

Dilated Cardiomyopathy

B

Figure 2-19. Phased array probe, phased array image. Phased array probes have a small, flat footprint and create a pie-shaped sector (A) (Courtesy of Sonosite). The resulting image has a very narrow superficial field-of-view with a large far field (B) (courtesy of Philips).

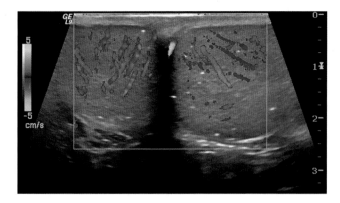

Figure 2-20. Vector array. Vector array technology creates a trapezoidal image from a linear probe. This image views both testicles with color Doppler (courtesy of GE Medical).

between the probe and the patient. Air has a very different impedance than both the probe and the skin, which causes tremendous reflections at the probe–air interface. By providing a coupling medium with an impedance between the matching layer and the skin, gel allows more sound waves to pass from the probe into the body similar to the way the matching layer improves transmission of sound from the crystal.

There are two situations when standard ultrasound gel should not be used. First, commercially available gels may be irritating to mucous membranes.[18] Generally, they are for external use only. Sterile, nonirritating gels should be used for endocavitary examinations. Gels that are made for contact with mucous membranes, such as sterile packets used for rectal and pelvic examinations, are more appropriate. Second, gels for standard ultrasound use are not sterile and any procedure that involves breaking the skin should utilize only sterile gels unless the site is marked and the probe is removed from the site prior to sterilization of the field.[19] Several companies offer sterile gels for ultrasound-guided procedures. Gel found in the small packets provided for rectal and pelvic examinations are sterile and bacteriostatic.

SHEATHS

Probe sheaths are an essential part of ultrasound when performing sterile procedures and endocavitary scanning. Low rates of perforation and contamination have been found with standard latex condoms, making them an inexpensive and useful adjunct.[20] Commercial sheaths are available, but have been associated with higher rates of perforation and contamination.[21] Whatever cover is to be used, care should be taken to identify patients with latex allergies since severe reactions can occur if latex comes in contact with the mucous membranes of these patients.[22]

STERILITY

Standard sterile precautions such as gowns, masks, and gloves should be used for ultrasound-guided procedures. Packets containing sterile covers and gels are available for purchase. Ultrasound-guided procedures are most easily performed with covers and gels specific to that purpose and are particularly helpful as they most often extend to cover the cord connecting the probe to the machine (Figure 2-21).

Many physicians use sterile gloves as probe covers along with sterile gels found in their own departments. If gloves are to be used, extra care must be used to protect the sterile field from the nonsterile cord that the glove

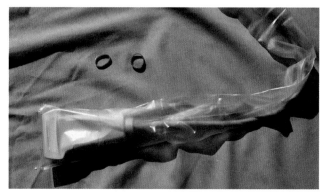

A

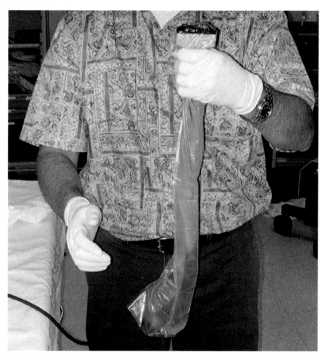

B

Figure 2-21. Sterile sheaths. Sterile sheaths specifically made for ultrasound probes will extend over the probe and cord.

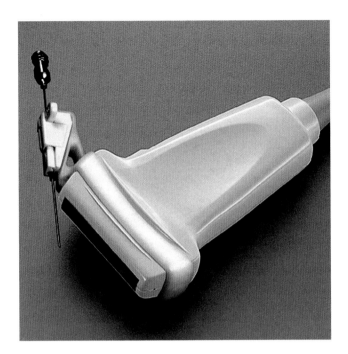

Figure 2-22. Needle guide attachment. Many companies offer attachments that provide needle guidance to their small parts probes.

does not cover. It may be advantageous to use a second operator to assist with this process.

NEEDLE GUIDANCE

Many companies offer disposable accessories that attach specifically to their probes to provide directional and depth assistance with needles during procedures (Figure 2-22). The attachments direct the needle to the middle of the probe in the long axis, enabling the operator to more easily see the entire length of the needle. In the short axis, different attachments are used for structures at different depths so the tip of the needle will not pass beyond the plane of the ultrasound beam. Attachments are not necessary for ultrasound-guided procedures, but they may be beneficial to some.

HEAD-MOUNTED DISPLAYS

Procedure guidance can be very cumbersome and technically challenging. In the single-operator method, clinicians hold the probe in one hand, the needle in the other, and must continually turn their head between the skin and the ultrasound machine. Head-mounted displays are becoming available that minimize head turning and the potential for complications due to excessive movement. The image is displayed onto a small monitor positioned just above the eyes. The eyes can move more easily between the skin and display rather than moving the head and shoulders to visualize the screen.

ULTRASOUND CONTRAST AGENTS

Ultrasound contrast agents are microbubbles that are administered intravenously. The microbubbles vibrate strongly at the high frequencies used in diagnostic ultrasonography, which makes them several thousand times more reflective than normal body tissues. This characteristic allows microbubbles to enhance both grey scale images and flow-mediated Doppler signals. Intravenous contrast for cardiac imaging is readily available and frequently used in echocardiography laboratories. For body imaging, initial investigations of ultrasound contrast utility have focused on evaluation of tumors in the liver and other solid organs. There is also great potential for contrast use in trauma patients since contrast makes detection of solid organ injury in the absence of hemoperitoneum possible.

▶ IMAGE VIEWING AND DATA STORAGE

The ability to view and store images is essential to any ultrasound program. Monitor attributes are important to consider as they affect the quality of imaging and the number of people who may view the image at a given time. Storing images or video is important for quality assurance, archiving for patient records, and teaching. Digital storage is becoming more prevalent and convenient for archiving and quality assurance.

MONITORS

High-quality monitors are available on most machines. Considerations include flat panel versus cathode-ray tube (CRT) monitors, viewing angle, and overall monitor size. Flat panel displays can offer high-quality images and weigh much less than CRT monitors. However, they tend to cost more than CRT monitors of similar quality.

Particularly with flat-panel monitors, the angle at which a sonologist can review the display is important. Lower quality machines may make it difficult for those at the periphery of the screen to view the image. Higher quality machines can offer almost 180 degrees of viewing.

The size of the display varies greatly among machines. Compact machines have small, liquid crystal displays 5-8 inches in size. Larger machines offer 12- to

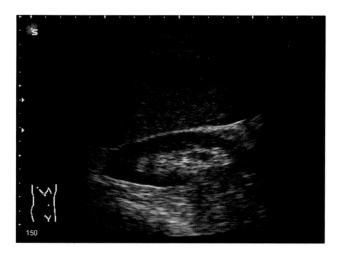

Figure 2-23. B-color ultrasound. A feature that allows various shades of color (magenta in this example) assigned to the grayscale image, which can provide better recognition of more subtle pathology. This may be particularly helpful when full-room lighting is required for patient care, as grayscale images are more difficult to interpret under these conditions.

15-inch displays that are much easier to view. Some handheld compact machines are able to connect to larger monitors when on the cart.

Regardless of the type of monitor used, it is important to remember to adjust the room lighting to a low setting when performing a bedside ultrasound. It is difficult to adjust the brightness of the image correctly and appreciate more subtle findings when you are looking at the monitor in a fully illuminated room. When treating a critically ill or injured patient, however, turning the lights down may not be an option. For these cases, it can be helpful to utilize B-color ultrasound (Figure 2-23). This is a feature that is often available on compact ultrasound machines, but infrequently utilized. Various shades of color are assigned to the grayscale image that can provide better recognition of more subtle pathology in full-room lighting situations. This is an option to consider if you find that you are frequently required to scan under these conditions.

PRINTERS

Printing devices associated with portable ultrasound machines are limited to thermal printers. Thermal printers offer low-cost and high-quality copies of ultrasound images that can be maintained for review, teaching, or archiving in medical records. Color printers are also available. Anecdotally, typical films used in thermal printing will save a high-quality image for 10+ years if stored correctly. Film used in radiology departments are much more costly, but have a much longer shelf life.

VIDEO STORAGE

Ultrasound examinations can be archived in video form. Many machines now allow users to record video clips ranging from several seconds to minutes. The majority of machines will allow a connection to an external device such as a video, CD, or DVD recorder. Video allows those reading the scans later to experience the ultrasound examination in the same way the sonologist saw the images. This can be valuable in education as well as overall quality assurance.

Most ultrasound machines work with a combination of analog and digital data processing. Conversion to a digital format is most useful for transferring images for the purposes of teaching and for efficient storage. Digital VCRs and DVD recorders can accomplish such a conversion. Users can store video in analog form on a standard VCR. However, image quality suffers and the transfer of data between users is made more difficult. Digital data are easily stored on and transferred between computers.

ELECTRONIC STORAGE AND TRANSMISSION

The most recent additions to the point-of-care ultrasound market have made tremendous strides in advancing the ability to digitally transfer images and video. Whereas older machines were limited to analog data transfer through S-video or VGA ports, newer models support digital data transfer via USB, IEEE, HD ports, and even wireless systems. Such a variety of communication ports allows users a seemingly limitless number of electronic storage options including CD, DVD, digital video, CF/SD cards, and the hospital's picture archiving and communication system (PACS) system.

The PACS system is a collection of digital technologies used to store and transmit medical imaging.[23] Radiology departments are the primary users of PACS systems, but clinicians are integrating their ultrasound images into the PACS systems at some hospitals. This technology may allow clinicians to share the images and interpretations of their ultrasound examinations with other health care professionals. Digital imaging and communication in medicine (DICOM) is a standard format to which images and data can be coded for transmission and electronic storage.[24] It is the standard data format used within PACS. Many of the new generation of portable ultrasound machines are manufactured with the ability to encode in the DICOM format along with many others.

REFERENCES

1. U.S. Ultrasound Markets. 12:34–37, 2004.
2. Walcher F, et al.: Prehospital ultrasound imaging improves management of abdominal trauma. *Br J Surg* 93(2):238–242, 2006.
3. Rozanski TA, Edmondson JM, Jones SB: Ultrasonography in a forward-deployed military hospital. *Mil Med* 170(2):99–102, 2005.
4. Blaivas M, Brannam L, Theodoro D: Ultrasound image quality comparison between an inexpensive handheld emergency department (ED) ultrasound machine and a large mobile ED ultrasound system. *Acad Emerg Med* 11(7):778–781, 2004.
5. Barnett SB, et al.: International recommendations and guidelines for the safe use of diagnostic ultrasound in medicine. *Ultrasound Med Biol* 26(3):355–366, 2000.
6. Benacerraf BR, et al.: Three- and 4-dimensional ultrasound in obstetrics and gynecology: proceedings of the american institute of ultrasound in medicine consensus conference. *J Ultrasound Med* 24(12):1587–1597, 2005.
7. van den Bosch AE, Krenning BJ, Roelandt JR: Three-dimensional echocardiography. *Minerva Cardioangiol* 53(3):177–184, 2005.
8. AIUM Official Statement: *3D Technology.* November 12 2005 Available from: http://www.aium.org/publications/statements/_statementSelected.asp?statement=23.
9. Kremkau F, ed.: *Diagnostic Ultrasound: Principles and Instruments.* 7th ed. St. Louis, MO: Saunders, 2006.
10. AIUM Official Statement: *Recommendations for Cleaning Transabdominal Transducers.* June 22, 2005.
11. Sterilization and Disinfection of Medical Devices: *General Principles. Centers for Disease Control, Division of Healthcare Quality Promotion.*
12. AUIM Official Statement: *Guidelines for Cleaning and Preparing Endocavitary Ultrasound Transducers Between Patients.* June 4, 2003.
13. ODE Device Evaluation Information—*FDA Cleared Sterilants and High Level Disinfectants with General Claims for Processing Reusable Medical and Dental Devices.* September 28, 2006.
14. Middleton WD, KA, Hertzberg BS, ed.: *Ultrasound: The Requisites.* 2nd ed. *The Requisites,* ed. T. JH. St. Louis, MO: Mosby, 2004.
15. Purohit RS, et al.: Imaging clinically localized prostate cancer. *Urol Clin North Am* 30(2):279–293, 2003.
16. Nicholls SJ, et al.: Intravascular ultrasound in cardiovascular medicine. *Circulation* 114(4):e55–E59, 2006.
17. Lyon M: Intraoral ultrasound in the diagnosis and treatment of suspected peritonsillar abscess in the emergency department. *Acad Emerg Med* 12(1):85–88, 2005.
18. Villa A, Venegoni M, Tiso B: Cases of contact dermatitis caused by ultrasonographic gel. *J Ultrasound Med* 17(8):530, 1998.
19. Wooltorton E: Medical gels and the risk of serious infection. *Cmaj* 171(11):1348, 2004.
20. Amis S., et al.: Assessment of condoms as probe covers for transvaginal sonography. *J Clin Ultrasound* 28(6):295–298, 2000.
21. Milki AA, Fisch JD: Vaginal ultrasound probe cover leakage: Implications for patient care. *Fertil Steril* 69(3):409–411, 1998.
22. Fry A, Meagher S, Vollenhoven B: A case of anaphylactic reaction caused by exposure to a latex probe cover in transvaginal ultrasound scanning. *Ultrasound Obstet Gynecol* 13(5):373, 1999.
23. Doi K: Diagnostic imaging over the last 50 years: Research and development in medical imaging science and technology. *Phys Med Biol* 51(13):R5–R27, 2006.
24. Graham RN, Perriss RW, Scarsbrook AF: DICOM demystified: A review of digital file formats and their use in radiological practice. *Clin Radiol* 60(11):1133–40, 2005.

APPENDIX A

Ultrasound Manufacturers with Offices in the United States

Aloka
10 Fairfield Boulevard
Wallington, CT 06492
Telephone: 800-872-5652
Fax: 203-269-6075
www.aloka.com

B-K Medical Systems, Inc.
250 Andover St.
Wilmington, MA 01887
Telephone: 800-876-7226
Fax: 978-988-1478
www.bkmed.com

Biosound Esaote, Inc.
8000 Castleway Drive
Indianapolis, IN 46250
Telephone: 800-428-4374
Fax: 317-841-8616
www.biosound.com

GE Medical Systems
P.O. Box 414
Milwaukee, WI 53201
Telephone: 888-202-5528
Fax: 414-544-3384
www.gehealthcare.com/usen/ultrasound/

Medison America, Inc.
11075 Knott Avenue, Suite C
Cypress, CA 90630
Telephone: 714-889-3000
Fax: 714-889-3030
www.medisonusa.com

Philips Medical Systems, N.A.
22100 Bothell Everett Highway
P.O. Box 3003
Bothell, WA 98041–3003
Telephone: (800) 722-7900 Ext. 0
Fax:(425) 485-6080
www.medical.philips.com/main/products/ultrasound/

Siemens Medical Solutions USA, Inc.
51 Valley Stream Parkway
Malvern, PA 19355
Telephone: 888-826-9702
Fax: 800-932-5667
www.medical.siemens.com

Sonosite, Inc.
21919 30 th Drive SE
Bothell, WA 98021-3904
Telephone: 888-482-9449
Fax: 425-951-1201
www.sonosite.com

Toshiba America Medical Systems, Inc.
2441 Michelle Drive
Tustin, CA 92781
Telephone: 800-421-1968
Fax: 714-734-0362
www.medical.toshiba.com

Ultrasonix
8312 254 th Ave NE
Redmond, WA 98052
Telephone: 425-284-1821
Fax: 425-284-1825
www.ultrasonix.com

Zonare Medical Systems, Inc.
20 North Bernardo Ave.
Mountain View, CA 94043
Telephone: 1-877-zonare-1
Email: info@zonare.com
www.zonare.com

APPENDIX B

There are many non-traditional ultrasound systems available to radiology and nonradiology clinicians alike. Where traditional machines tend to be large machines with tremendous imaging capabilities, nontraditional systems tend to be smaller, more portable, and relatively inexpensive. The systems listed in Appendix B are many of the ultrasound devices marketed to ED physicians today. The number of nontraditional options is growing rapidly, leading to increased competition and improved value. The machines are listed alphabetically by company. We do not endorse any one machine.

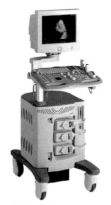
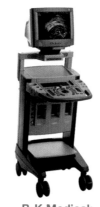
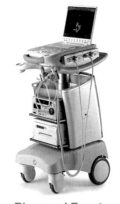
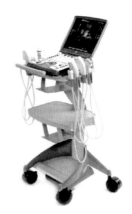

	Aloka: Prosound SSD-3500	B-K Medical: Pro Focus	Biosound Esaote: MyLab 30CV	GE: Logic e
Cart dimensions (inches)	W19 × D31 × H58	W21 × D31 × H59	W20 × D20 × H39	Info not provided
Cart weight (lb)	225	170	99	Info not provided
Handheld dimensions (inches)	N/A	N/A	H6 × W14 × D20 in	W13 × D11 × H2
Handheld weight (lb)	N/A	N/A	20	10
Battery?	N/A	No	Yes	Yes
Length of charge	N/A	N/A	30 min	1 hr continuous
Boot-up time	45	Info not provided	60	20
Ancillary outlets	3	Info not provided	3	3
Display dimensions (inches)	15	15	15	15
Analog/Digital display	Digital	Info not provided	Digital	Digital
Degrees of visualization		Info not provided	130	160
Max shades of gray	256	256	256	256
Max resolution		512 × 480	1024 × 768	1024 × 768
Flat panel available?	No	No	Standard	Standard
Depth refresh rate	<1 sec	Info not ptovided	0.1	<0.5
Trackball/trackpad	Trackball	Trackball	Trackball	Trackball
Adjustable acoustic output	Yes	Info not provided	Yes	Yes
Levels of TGC control	8	Info not provided	7	6
Adjustable focus	Yes	Yes	Yes	Yes
Max focal points	4	25	8	8
Zoom	Standard	Standard	Standard	Standard
Split screen function	Standard	Standard	Standard	Standard
Automated image enhancement	Standard	Standard	None	Standard
Tissue harmonic imaging	Standard	Standard	Standard	Standard
3D rendering	Optional	Optional	None	Optional
M-mode	Standard	Standard	Standard	Standard
Bidirectional Doppler	Standard	Standard	Standard	Standard
Power Doppler	Standard	Standard	Standard	Standard
Quantitative Doppler	Standard	Standard	Standard	Standard
Triplex	Standard	Standard	Standard	Standard
Max # Calipers	10	Info not provided	1	9
#Active Transducer ports	2	4	2	1
				3 with cart
#Storage ports	1	Info not provided	1	Cart dependent

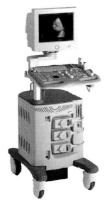 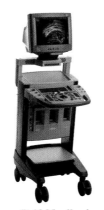 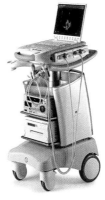 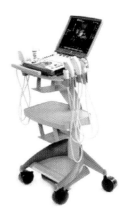

	Aloka: Prosound SSD-3500	B-K Medical: Pro Focus	Biosound Esaote: MyLab 30CV	GE: Logic *e*
Available transducers	Curved array Linear array Phased array Endocavitary	Curved array Linear array Endocavitary	Curved array Phased array Linear array Endocavitary	Curved array Phased array Linear array Endocavitary
Transesophageal capability	Yes	None	Yes	None
Storage memory	999 images	30 GB	60 GB	25 GB
Cine loop length	2048 frames	3000 frames	400 frames/Unlimited	1000 frames
B/W printer	Optional	Optional	Optional	Standard
Color printer	Optional	Optional	Optional	Optional
CD/DVD burner	CD R/RW Standard	DVD: none CD: Optional	Standard	Standard
CF/SD card/USB	No	USB (3)	USB	USB
Format of stored images	JPEG TIF BMP DICOM	BMP html AVI BK3d	Native DICOM AVI BMP JPEG	JPG, AVI, Raw
DICOM compatibility	Optional	Optional	Standard	Standard
Communication ports		Firewire (2) Ethernet RS232 serial channel	SVHS VHS XVGA	SVHS Composite SVGA
Warranty	1 year	Contact company	1 year	1 year
Price Range	Contact company	Contact company	Contact company	$40–60,000

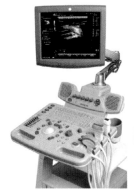 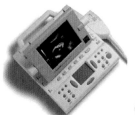 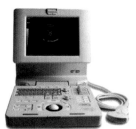 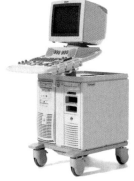

	GE: LOGIQ P5	Medison: Mysono201	Medison: SonoAce PICO	Philips: EnVisor
Cart dimensions (inches)	W17 × D25 × H53	N/A	Optional	Info not provided
Cart weight (lb)	161	N/A	Optional	220
Handheld dimensions (inches)	N/A	W11 × D12 × H4	W13 × D14 × H8	N/A
Handheld weight (lb)	N/A	8	20	N/A
Battery?	Yes	Yes	No	None
Length of charge	20 min	2 hrs	N/A	N/A
Boot-up time	80	45	45	<60
Ancillary outlets	4	0	0	Info not provided
Display dimensions (inches)	15	6.4	10.4	15
Analog/digital display	Digital	Digital	Digital	Digital
Degrees of visualization	170	45	45	Info not provided
Max shades of gray	256	64	256	256
Max resolution	800×600	640×480	640×480	Info not provided
Flat panel available?	Standard	N/A	N/A	Standard
Depth refresh rate	<0.2	Info not provided	Info not provided	Info not provided
Trackball/trackpad	Trackball	Trackpad	Trackball	Trackball
Adjustable acoustic output	Yes	No	Yes	Yes
Levels of TGC control	8	3	6	6
Adjustable focus	Yes	Yes	Yes	Yes
Max focal points	8	Info not provided	3	4
Zoom	Standard	Info not provided	Standard	Standard
Split screen function	Standard	Info not provided	Standard	Standard
Automated image enhancement	Standard	Standard	Standard	Standard
Tissue harmonic imaging	Standard	No	Standard	Standard
3D rendering	Standard	No	Standard	Optional
M-mode	Standard	Standard	Standard	Standard
Bidirectional Doppler	Standard	No	Standard	Standard
Power Doppler	Standard	No	Standard	Standard
Quantitative Doppler	Standard	No	Standard	Standard
Triplex	Standard	No	Standard	Standard
Max # Calipers	8	Info not provided	2	8
#Active Transducer ports	3	1	1	4
#Storage ports	0	0	0	Info not provided

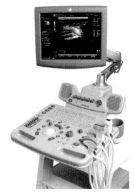 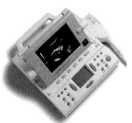 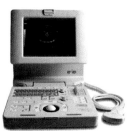 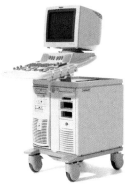

	GE: LOGIQ P5	Medison: Mysono201	Medison: SonoAce PICO	Philips: EnVisor
Available transducers	Curved array Linear array Phased array Endocavitary	Curved Array Linear array Endocavitary	Curved array Linear Array Endocavitary	Curved array Phased array Linear Array Endocavitary
Transesophageal capability	No	No	No	Yes
Storage memory	25 GB	64 frames	30 GB	80 GB
Cine loop length	1000 frames	32 frames	256 frames	1000 frames
B/W printer	Standard	Optional	Optional	Optinoal
Color printer	Optional	No	No	Optinoal
CD/DVD burner	Standard	No	No	CD R/RW Standard MOD Standard 3.5in floppy
CF/SD card/USB	USB	CF	CF	USB
Format of stored images	JPG, AVI, Raw	JPEG	JPEG	JPEG AVI DICOM
DICOM compatibility	Standard	No	Standard	Standard
Communication ports	SVHS Composite SVGA	VHS	VHS S-VHS	Info not provided
Warranty	1 year	1 year	1 year	1 year
Price range	$40–60,000	Contact company	Contact company	Contact company

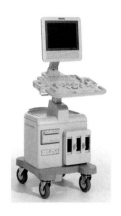 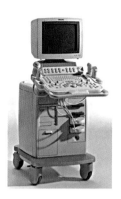 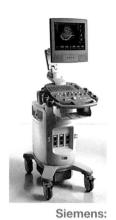 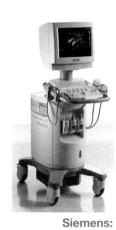

	Philips: HD3	Philips: HD11	Siemens: Acuson X300	Siemens: Sonoline G40
Cart dimensions (inches)	W20 × D31 × H40	W22 × D41 × H51	W20 × D35 × H54	W20 × D34 × H53
Cart weight (lb)	150	220	225	205
Handheld dimensions (inches)	N/A	N/A	N/A	N/A
Handheld weight (lb)	N/A	N/A	N/A	N/A
Battery?	None	None	No	N/A
Length of charge	N/A	N/A	N/A	N/A
Boot-up time	<60	<60	60	130
Ancillary outlets	1	Info not provided	2	2
Display dimensions (inches)	11	17	15	15
Analog/digital display	Digital	Digital	Digital	Digital
Degrees of visualization	Info not provided	Info not provided	Info not provided	Info not provided
Max shades of gray	256	256	256	Info not provided
Max resolution	Info not provided	Info not provided	1024×768	800×600
Flat panel available?	Standard	Standard	Standard	No
Depth refresh rate	Info not provided	Info not provided	Info not provided	Info not provided
Trackball/trackpad	Trackball	Trackball	Trackball	Trackball
Adjustable acoustic output	Yes	Yes	Yes	Yes
Levels of TGC control	6	6	8	8
Adjustable focus	Yes	Yes	Yes	Yes
Max focal points	Info not provided	4	Info not provided	Transducer dependent
Zoom	Standard	Standard	Standard	Standard
Split screen function	Standard	Standard	Standard	Standard
Automated image enhancement	Standard	Standard	Optional	Optional
Tissue harmonic imaging	Standard	Standard	Optional	Optional
3D rendering	Optional	Optional	Optional	Optional
M-mode	Standard	Standard	Standard	Standard
Bidirectional Doppler	Standard	Standard	Standard	Standard
Power Doppler	Standard	Standard	Standard	Standard
Quantitative Doppler	Standard	Standard	Standard	Standard
Triplex	Standard	Standard	Standard	Standard
Max # Calipers	Multiple	Multiple	8	8
#Active Transducer ports	3	4	2 Standard/ 3rd Optional	2/3rd optional
#Storage ports	Info not provided	Info not provided	6	6

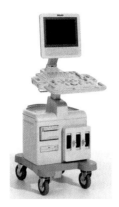 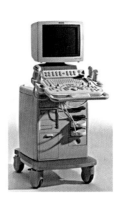 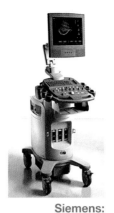 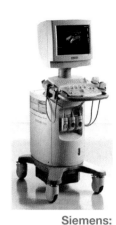

	Philips: HD3	Philips: HD11	Siemens: Acuson X300	Siemens: Sonoline G40
Available transducers	Curved array	Curved array	Curved array	Curved array
	Phased array	Phased array	Linear array	Linear array
	Linear Array	Linear Array	Phased Array	Phased array
	Endocavitary	Endocavitary	Endocavitary	Endocavitary
Transesophageal capability	No	Yes	No	No
Storage memory	75 GB	80 GB	80 GB	40 GB
Cine loop length	Info not provided	1000 frames	120 sec/545 frames	545 frames
B/W printer	Optional	Optional	Optional	Optional
Color printer	Optional	Optional	Optional	Optional
CD/DVD burner	CD R/RW Standard	CD R/RW Standard	Standard	CDR/RW Standard
	MOD Standard	MOD Standard		
CF/SD card/USB	No	No	USB (2)	USB (2)
Format of stored images	PC Format	JPEG	TIFF	TIFF
	DICOM	AVI	DICOM	DICOM
		DICOM		
DICOM compatibility	Optional	Standard	Optional	Optional
Communication ports	Info not provided	Info not provided	Ethernet	Ethernet
			RS232	RS232C
Warranty	1 year	1 year	1 year	1 year
Price range	Contact company	Contact company	Contact company	Contact company

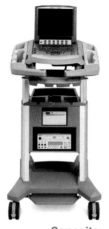 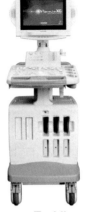 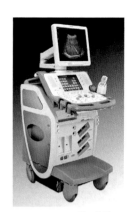

	Sonosite: MicroMaxx	Toshiba: Nemio XG	Toshiba: Xario
Cart dimensions (inches)	W32 × D23 × H33	W19 × D31 × H54	W21×32D × H57
Cart weight (lb)	79	220	331
Handheld dimensions (inches)	W12 × D11 × H3	N/A	N/A
Handheld weight (lb)	7.5	N/A	N/A
Battery?	Yes	No	No
Length of charge	2 hrs	N/A	N/A
Boot-up time	14	45	230
Ancillary outlets	5	4	4
Display dimensions (inches)	10.4	15	17
Analog/Digital display	Digital	Digital	Digital
Degrees of visualization	85	150	150
Max shades of gray	256	256	256
Max resolution	640×480	640×480	Info not provided
Flat panel available?	N/A	Standard	Standard
Depth refresh rate	<0.5	Info not provided	Info not provided
Trackball/trackpad	Trackpad	Trackball	Trackball
Adjustable acoustic output	With presets	Yes	Yes
Levels of TGC control	2	8	8
Adjustable focus	With presets	Yes	Yes
Max focal points	8	8	8
Zoom	Standard	Standard	Standard
Split screen function	Standard	Standard	Standard
Automated image enhancement	No	Standard	Standard
Tissue harmonic imaging	Standard	Standard	Standard
3D rendering	No	No	Standard
M-mode	Standard	Standard	Standard
Bidirectional Doppler	Standard	Standard	Standard
Power Doppler	Standard	Standard	Standard
Quantitative Doppler	Standard	Standard	Standard
Triplex	No	Standard	Standard
Max # Calipers	8	8	8
#Active transducer ports	1/3 optional with cart	3	3
#Storage ports	1/ 4 optional with cart	3	2

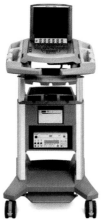
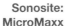
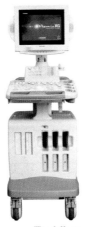
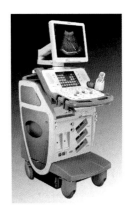

	Sonosite: **MicroMaxx**	Toshiba: **Nemio XG**	Toshiba: **Xario**
Available transducers	Curved array Linear array Phased array Endocavitary	Curved array Linear array Phased array Endocavitary	Curved array Linear array Phased array Endocavitary
Transesophageal capability	Yes	Yes	Yes
Storage memory	4 GB	160 GB	80 GB
Cine loop length	120 frames/6 seconds	120 sec/512 frames	37 sec/ 4095 frames
B/W printer	Optional	Optional	Standard
Color printer	Optional	Optional	Optional
CD/DVD burner	Optional	Optional	No
CF/SD card/USB	CF, USB	USB	No
Format of stored images	BMP MJPEG	DICOM, JPEG, BMP, AVI	DICOM, JPEG, TIFF, AVI
DICOM compatibility	Standard	Standard	Optional
Communication ports	Ethernet S-Video DVI	RGB VGA S-Video Audio Composite RS232 USB Ethernet	S-Video Audio Composite SVGA RS232 Ethernet
Warranty	5 years	1 year	1 year
Price range	Base $45,000	$42–70,000	Contact company

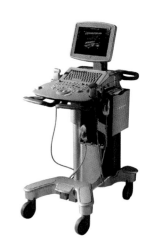

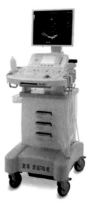

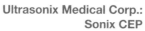

	Ultrasonix Medical Corp.: Sonix CEP	Zonare: z.one
Cart dimensions (inches)	W21 × D24 × H57	miniCart W22 × D22 × H47
		Supercart W24 × D33 × H50
Cart weight (lb)	185	miniCart 119
		Supercart 187
Handheld dimensions (inches)	N/A	W10 × D10 × H8
Handheld weight (lb)	N/A	5.5
Battery?	Yes	Handheld yes
		Carts no
Length of charge	20 min scanning	1 hr
	30 min standby	
	60 min sleep	
Boot-up time	20	20
Ancillary outlets	2	miniCart 1
		Supercart 4
Display dimensions (inches)	17	Handheld 5.8
		Carts 13
Analog/Digital display	Digital	Handheld/miniCart digital
		Supercart analog
Degrees of visualization	160	170
Max shades of gray	256	Handheld 64
		Carts 256
Max resolution	1024×768	Handheld 800×480
		Carts 600×480
Flat panel available?	Standard	Standard
Depth refresh rate	<1	0.5
Trackball/Trackpad	Trackball	Trackball
Adjustable acoustic output	Yes	Yes
Levels of TGC control	5	8
Adjustable focus	Yes	Yes
Max focal points	5	102
Zoom	Standard	Standard
Split screen function	Standard	Standard
Automated image enhancement	Standard	Standard
Tissue harmonic imaging	Standard	Standard
3D rendering	Optional	No
M-mode	Standard	Standard
Bidirectional Doppler	Standard	Standard
Power Doppler	Standard	Standard
Quantitative Doppler	Standard	Standard

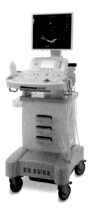

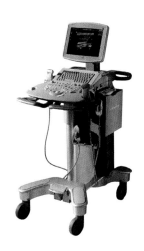

	Ultrasonix Medical Corp.: Sonix CEP	Zonare: z.one
Triplex	Standard	Standard
Max # Calipers	>30	4
#Active Transducer ports	3	1
#Storage ports	1	6
Available transducers	Curved array	Curved array
	Phased array	Phased array
	Linear array	Linear array
	Endocavitary	Endocavitary
Transesophageal capability	None	None
Storage memory	80 GB	8 GB
Cine loop length	1024 frames/ 2 min	180 frames
B/W printer	Optional	Optional
Color printer	Optional	Optional
CD/DVD burner	Standard	Optional
CF/SD card/USB	CF	USB (4)
	SD	
	USB (2)	
Format of stored images	PNG	DICOM
	JPEG	
	BMP	
	AVI	
DICOM compatibility	Optional	Optional
Communication ports	S-video	Ethernet
	Composite	HDMI
	RGB	
	SVGA	
	DVI	
	RJ45 NIC	
Warranty	1 year, 5 year optional	1 year
Price range	$60,000	$55–110,000

CHAPTER 3

Physics and Image Artifacts

Corky Hecht and Jason Wilkins

Diagnostic ultrasound has experienced tremendous technological advances. Over the past 50 years, ultrasound has evolved from a single specialty tool with large bulky machines to a technology that is highly compact and portable. The development of smaller, less expensive ultrasound systems has increased the number of medical specialties utilizing ultrasound. Many are discovering the benefits of "point of care" diagnostic ultrasound. Medical students, nurses, and physicians have embraced ultrasound as a tool to facilitate patient evaluation and improve outcomes of invasive procedures. However, these increased applications introduce a level of potential risk if the operator is not appropriately trained. The operator must have a basic understanding of the physical principles of ultrasound. It is these principles upon which ultrasound rests its ability to be an effective tool in medical imaging.

▶ UNDERSTANDING SOUND AND ULTRASOUND

HISTORY

The simplest way to describe ultrasound is in the pulse-echo principle. SONAR can be used as an example of the forerunner of diagnostic ultrasound. A submarine that possesses sonar capability can precisely control when an acoustic pulse is generated. It assumes a relative propagation speed as it travels through a specific medium (water). The amount of elapsed time required for the "echo" to return subsequent to striking an object allows the relative distance to be calculated to the target of interest.

Diagnostic ultrasound uses the same concept of the pulse-echo principle. Electric current is passed though crystals in the transducer creating a sound wave. This piezoelectric effect generates a constant pulse of high-frequency, longitudinal, mechanical sound waves that can be measured and used in calculations. This pulse travels at a relatively constant speed until it encounters a reflective surface, at which time a fraction of the sound is reflected back toward the transducer crystal. When the returning echo strikes the crystal, it generates an electrical impulse that is eventually converted into information that is processed into diagnostic images. Sound is calculated to travel through human tissue at body temperature at approximately 1,540 m/s. The ultrasound system measures the round-trip time and intensity of the returning "echo." The amount of time required for the returning echo determines its relative distance from the transducer while the returning intensity is proportional to the grayscale assignment of the pixel. This information may then be represented as a pixel (dot) of information on the display device.

Sound waves are actually a series of repeating mechanical pressure waves that propagate through a medium. These pressure waves are measured in hertz (cycles/second). Typically, audible sound ranges between 16,000 and 20,000 Hz. Ultrasound is technically defined as a "sound" having a frequency in excess of 20,000 Hz. In medicine, ultrasound used for diagnostic purposes incorporates frequencies that generally range between 2 and 20 MHz (megahertz), or 2 and 20 million cycles/second, well above the range of human hearing. While diagnostic ultrasound frequencies extending beyond 15 MHz are available for medical imaging, they are often used in catheter-based technology.

► BASIC DEFINITIONS

A variety of methods are often used to convey an understanding of specific terms. Definitions are often expressed via graphs, charts, and formulas. The text that follows is designed to introduce the reader to the components of an acoustic wave and its terminology (Figure 3-1).

AMPLITUDE

Amplitude is the peak pressure of the wave (height). This may be simply interpreted as the loudness of the wave. Amplitude correlates with the intensity of the returning echo. A loud sound has large amplitude while a soft sound has small amplitude.

PERIOD

Period is the time required to complete a single cycle.

FREQUENCY

Frequency is the number of times per second the wave is repeated. The range of frequencies typically discussed here is between 2 and 15 MHz.

SPATIAL PULSE LENGTH

Spatial pulse length is the distance or length of each pulse that is determined by the frequency and pulse duration.

Transducer technology is based upon the piezo-electric effect. *Piezoelectric* is defined as "pressure-electricity" and refers to materials that have a dual function of converting electric energy into mechanical energy (pressure) and conversely mechanical energy (returning echo) into electrical energy. While quartz is a naturally occurring crystal, the crystal elements in modern transducers are synthetic. The arrangement and the number of crystals within a transducer vary depending upon the manufacturer, transducer design, and its intended application.

Transducer frequency has a direct effect on image quality and resolution. Generally speaking, high frequencies result in higher resolution and image quality improves. While resolution may increase, penetration will decrease. Lower frequencies result in lower resolution, but have better penetration.

Consider this analogy to help explain this concept. A person has enough energy to walk 10 paces. In one case their stride is a yard (so they can walk 10 yards). In the other instance their stride is a foot so with the same energy applied they can only walk 10 feet. The higher frequency will travel a shorter distance in soft tissue than a lower frequency beam because each wave covers a shorter distance.

Resolution is the result of the stride distance or spatial pulse length as well. In the case of the yard stride, there are two reference points far apart both of which indicate that the surface under their foot is concrete. The assumption is that the entire area in between must be concrete and therefore the conclusion is that it must be a sidewalk, for instance. However, with a foot stride there are more points of reference over the same distance traveled and although there is concrete at the end points there is grass in between so it becomes apparent that it is a patio stone walkway and not a sidewalk. Higher frequency gives you more reference points or pixels over a similar spatial distance and thus produces higher resolution by displaying smaller tissue segments. However, the trade-off is that the higher frequency will not travel as far or penetrate deep tissue.

The ultrasound beam is affected in part by the frequency being emitted by the transducer, with each transducer emitting a "center" frequency during the transmit portion of the cycle. A range of frequencies exists on either side of the center frequency and is known as the bandwidth (Figure 3-2).

Many ultrasound systems make use of these bandwidth frequencies during the receive portion of the cycle and thus incorporate broadband transducers. Technology may allow the operator to select one of multiple "center" frequencies available from a single transducer. This selection allows the operator to easily maximize the transmit frequency of the transducer that offers the best resolution or best penetration for the area of interest. Regardless of which type of transducer technology is utilized, the highest frequency should be used that will penetrate the area of interest and that offers the best resolution. Image resolution is based upon many transducer factors including the spatial pulse length of the wave.

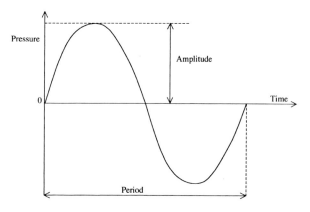

Figure 3-1. Time vs. pressure graph of a sound wave. Amplitude: peak pressure of a wave. Period: time required to complete a single cycle. (Courtesy of SonoSite)

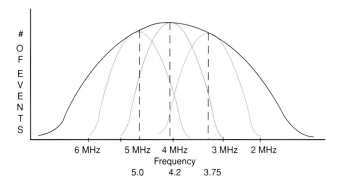

Figure 3-2. Broad bandwidth or multi-frequency selectable transducers.

The spatial pulse length is dependent on specific transducer characteristics set by the manufacturer. This may explain why simply increasing the transmit frequency of a transducer may not consistently result in improved resolution or improved image quality.

VELOCITY

Velocity of sound is defined as the speed of the wave. The velocity of sound is dependent on the material through which the wave is traveling. Velocity is independent of frequency. Since the speed of ultrasound through a given medium is constant, the closer the molecules are in position to one another, the better the propagation. Therefore, sound travels faster in bone than in human soft tissue. When molecules become less dense (gases), the velocity of the sound slows even further or may not propagate at all as is the case with a vacuum.

WAVELENGTH

Wavelength (propagation speed/frequency) is the distance the wave travels in a single cycle.

ATTENUATION

The attenuation of sound begins the instant the pulse is generated inside the transducer and continues until it returns to the transducer to be registered. There are several factors that contribute to attenuation. These factors include the wavelength of the emitted sound, the medium through which the sound is traveling, and the number of interfaces it encounters.

The type and density of tissue combined with its degree of homogeneity or heterogeneity contribute to the rate of attenuation. Tissue of the same type and density will facilitate the ability to assist in the transmission of the sound rather than inhibit its progression. A combination of varying tissues would weaken energy at an

accelerated rate. This is one of the reasons why transabdominal ultrasound scanning of the uterus and ovaries is facilitated by a distended urinary bladder. The fluid inside the bladder provides an acoustic window for the sound wave and allows an efficient use of the transmitted sound to visualize the posterior anatomy.

Reflection is a form of attenuation. It is the redirection of part of the sound wave back to its source. Reflection is the foundation upon which ultrasound scanning is based. The ultrasound beam should evaluate the anatomy of interest at 90 degrees to maximize the reflection and visualization of the anatomical structures. Manipulating the transducer so the area of interest is positioned directly under the transducer in the center of the display offers improved visualization and the ability to better appreciate the surrounding anatomical structures.

Refraction is the redirection of part of the sound wave as it crosses a boundary of mediums possessing different propagation speeds. This condition worsens with nonperpendicular incidence (Figure 3-3).

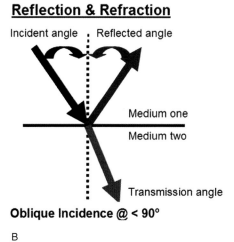

Figure 3-3. Reflection and refraction.

Scattering occurs when the ultrasound beam encounters an interface that is smaller than the sound beam or irregular in shape.

Absorption occurs when the energy of the sound wave is contained within the tissue. When the acoustic energy is converted to thermal energy, it dissipates as heat within the tissue. This forms the foundation for therapeutic ultrasound. Therapeutic ultrasound employs a different range of frequencies compared with diagnostic ultrasound.

INTERFACES

When sound crosses a boundary of tissues in contact with one another having different acoustic impedance, an interface is said to occur.

ACOUSTIC IMPEDANCE

Acoustic impedance refers to the resistance of the tissue to molecular movement. Acoustic impedance is directly related to tissue density. Blood, urine, fat, and muscle all have sufficient differing acoustic impedances to generate a reflection. The greater the density difference between tissues the greater or stronger the reflection. The intensity of the reflection (how loud the echo is) is determined by how much of a difference exists between the tissues in contact. A small density difference (acoustic impedance) results in a small echo being generated. A large difference in density results in a large echo generated with much of the energy lost to reflection. Therefore, little energy remains available to continue for visualization of deeper structures. This explains why diagnostic ultrasound cannot "see" through bowel gas or bone, as there is too large a difference in acoustic impedance that exists between these types of interfaces and soft tissue. This phenomenon is referred to as "acoustic mismatch" and will be covered further in the section on artifacts.

IMAGE RESOLUTION

Resolution refers to the quality of the image produced by the machine. It is the ability to differentiate the anatomical and pathological areas of interest with greater detail. While there are several factors that contribute to the overall image quality, we will limit our discussion to axial, lateral, temporal, and contrast resolution.

AXIAL RESOLUTION

Axial resolution is the ability to differentiate two closely spaced echoes that lie in a plane parallel to the direction of sound wave propagation. The ability to distinguish these echoes in greater number improves the resolution. If we consider the dpi (dots per inch) setting commonly available on a computer printer, the greater the dpi setting provides us with greater image resolution and a higher quality image.

There are several factors that contribute to the quality of the axial resolution; however, the rate-limiting step under control by the operator is the ultrasound beam and transducer frequency. In general, the higher the transducer frequency the better the resultant image quality (Figure 3-4).

LATERAL RESOLUTION

Lateral resolution is the ability to differentiate two closely spaced echoes that are positioned perpendicular to the direction of propagation of the ultrasound beam. Generally, lateral resolution will be inferior to axial resolution. The primary equipment control that improves lateral resolution is adjusting the "focal zone" to the area of interest. Some equipment manufacturers slave the transducer frequency with the "focal zone" and changing the frequency may aid in improving lateral resolution because it adjusts the focal zone to a new segment of the image closer to the area of interest. Ultrasound beam width contributes to this side-to-side resolution. The width of an average beam emitting from a transducer is approximately 1–1.5 mm at a focal depth. For transducers incorporating an internal focusing capability, a user selectable adjustment is often available. This adjustment allows the operator to vary the width of the ultrasound beam relative to depth within the image. If this "focal zone" is positioned on the screen adjacent to the area of interest on the ultrasound image, then the ultrasound beam will in theory be the narrowest at this point allowing for improved lateral resolution. Multiple focal zones may be selected on a single ultrasound image in an attempt to maximize the resolution at specific depths. Since this action requires additional processing time, a slower frame rate will occur and the image will appear to have less of a real-time appearance. Single focal zone capabilities are generally sufficient for most abdominal and cardiac examinations. Multiple focal zones are often of greater value when examining superficial structures when transducer movement is at a minimum and additional signal processing time is of less concern.

Adjusting the focal zone also narrows the "in and out of plane dimension" of the beam or the "slice thickness" at the point of interest. This can prevent "slice thickness artifacts" that result from the beam being thicker than the structure being imaged and averaging larger volumes of tissue than intended and thus reducing or decreasing the azimuthal type of lateral resolution.

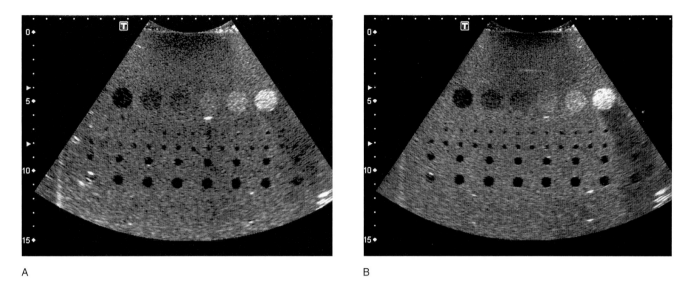

A   B

Figure 3-4. Axial and lateral resolution Note how grainy and pixilated the lower frequency (1.9 MHz) image is (A) compared to the smoother characteristics of the higher resolution (5.0 MHz) image (B). Both images were obtained using a multipurpose phantom (Model 539 Multipurpose, ATS Laboratories, Inc.).

For instance, when trying to visualize a blood vessel (like the inferior vena cava), if the beam thickness is wider than the blood vessel, it may get reflected signal from the tissue on either side of the blood vessel and the averaged signal display may make the lumen appear to have some tissue component producing a slice thickness artifact.

In more sophisticated equipment an additional control that greatly impacts the "in plane" lateral resolution is "line density or vector density." This feature adjusts the number of scan lines used to create a composite frame.

The greater the number of scan lines used to build the image the smaller the space between the pulse lines, which results in a better lateral resolution. This also requires more processing time to scan the increased number of lines and will slow the frame rate proportionally (Figure 3-5).

The operator can also affect frame rate by adjusting the width of the sector from wide to narrow or vice versa. As the sector width narrows, the frame rate increases (Figure 3-6). This adjustment can be especially important when scanning to detect motion such as

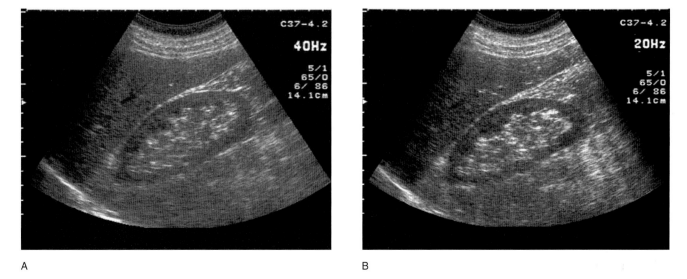

A   B

Figure 3-5. Line density vs. frame rate. Image resolution does not vary greatly between the low line density (A) and the high line density settings (B), but frame rate is significantly affected: 40 Hz (A) vs. 20 Hz (B).

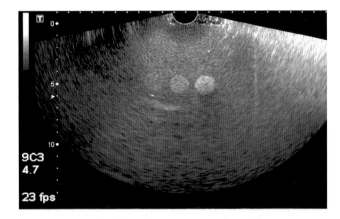

A

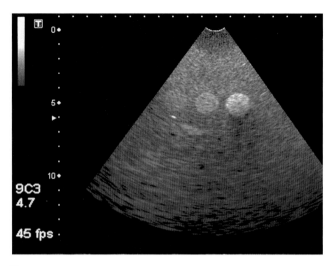

B

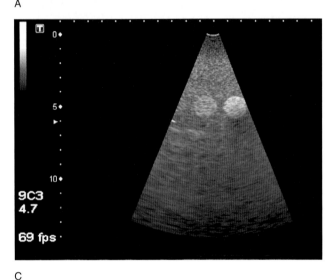

C

Figure 3-6. Sector width vs. frame rate. The more narrow the sector, the faster the frame rate as noted for: wide sector (A) frame rate = 23fps, medium sector (B) frame rate = 45fps, narrow sector (C) frame rate = 69fps.

in early pregnancy using a wide-angled Endovaginal transducer.

TEMPORAL RESOLUTION

Temporal resolution refers to the acquisition rate of a composite frame expressed as frame rate (frames per second) or sometimes expressed as Hz (cycles per second). A frame rate of 15 Hz is required to see structures move in "real time" such as a fetal heart beat or other adult cardiac structures. Adjusting sector width or decreasing line density will have the greatest impact on increasing temporal resolution or frame rate because in both situations the system is scanning fewer lines that require less time.

CONTRAST RESOLUTION

Contrast resolution refers to the ultrasound system's ability to assign a grayscale value to returning echoes of varying amplitudes. Many diagnostic ultrasound systems

today allow an assignment of 256 shades of gray, which facilitates the ability to discriminate between the subtle differences that exist between tissues. A higher contrast (less shades of gray) may be more pleasing to the human eye but may, in fact, contain less diagnostic information. This dynamic range of information (measured in decibels or db) is often a programmable feature on ultrasound systems and may be examination specific. The optimum setting allows a clear differentiation between the area of interest and the surrounding anatomy and typically the more shades of gray the better the contrast resolution.

To better understand the principle of contrast resolution, picture someone throwing a tennis ball at a plywood partition. Contrast resolution is equivalent to measuring the change in strength of the returning "bounce" based upon changes in the thickness of the plywood; for instance, being able to differentiate if it was 1″ plywood or ³/₄″ or ¹/₂″ plywood. That is how contrast resolution enables the sonologist to detect subtle changes in tissue compliance and detect disease at an early stage (Figure 3-7).

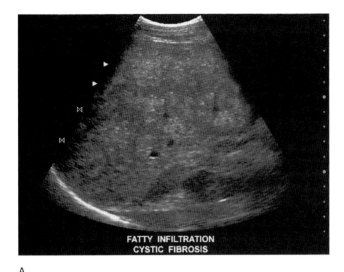

A

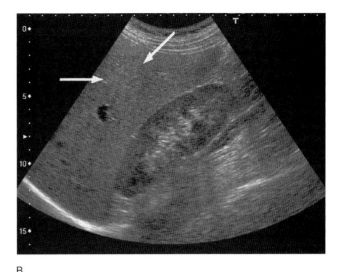

B

Figure 3-7. Contrast resolution. In (A) the pathology is quite dramatic but in (B) the "fatty infiltrate" is much more subtle and is apparent only because the system has good contrast resolution and a wide dynamic range.

▶ MODES

A Mode, or "Amplitude," provided one of the original evaluations of the human body using sound. A Mode ultrasound included an oscilloscope display for returning amplitude information and a traditional picture did not exist. The peak amplitude information on the horizontal axis provided information regarding the strength or "loudness" of the wave, while the vertical axis provided reflector distance information from the transducer (Figure 3-8a).

B Mode, or "Brightness," converts amplitude waveforms into an image allowing better correlation with anatomical structures. Returning signals are assigned a gray-scale pixel based on amplitude. Grayscale scanners display up to 256 shades of grayscale information. These shades of gray allow subtle differences within tissues to be visualized The ultrasound system's ability to divide and display the returning echoes into different shades of gray (64 vs. 256 shades, for instance) corresponds to the ultrasound system's contrast resolution or dynamic range (Figure 3-8a).

M Mode, or "Motion," permits a simultaneous display of the two-dimensional (2-D) B Mode image and a characteristic waveform (Figure 3-8b). This waveform depicts the motion or deflection of the tissue relative to the transducer on the vertical axis and represents time or changes in the cardiac cycle on the horizontal axis. M Mode technology can be of value in the emergency and acute care setting during pregnancy examinations and permits measurement and documentation of fetal cardiac activity. It can also be useful to demonstrate timing of events during changes in the cardiac cycle such as identifying right ventricular diastolic collapse secondary

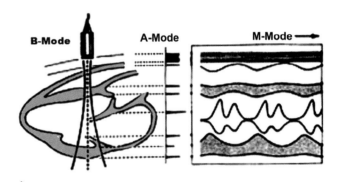

A

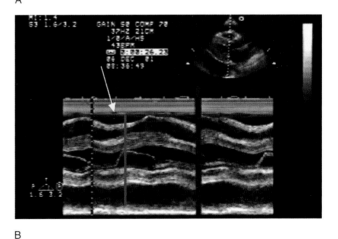

B

Figure 3-8. Comparison of modes. The diagram (A) depicts the image display for each of three modes: B-mode, A-mode, and M-mode. The mitral valve is open during ventricular diastole and closed during systole. M-mode ultrasound of pericardial effusion (B). The arrow shows that the RV collapses during early diastole (MV open on right as indicated by red time-line).

to pericardial effusion. Similarly, documentation of lung sliding or similar applications can also be achieved using M-mode.

D Mode, or "Doppler," is presented in a few different forms. Doppler technology relies on the interpretation the "frequency shift" that exists between the transmitted and received Doppler signal, while the anatomy (blood within the vessel) is moving as it is imaged.

For example, as a train whistle is engaged, the pedestrian at the crossing will experience an increase in the pitch (Doppler shift) of the whistle as the train approaches and a decrease in the pitch as the train continues to move away. The train engineer does not experience this shift in sound since he is traveling with the sound, and an audible shift in frequency does not occur.

Doppler ultrasound technology makes use of this "frequency shift" and the angle of interrogation of a vessel is a prominent factor in the quality and accuracy of the Doppler signal. Sources moving toward the receiver produce higher reflected frequencies, while sources moving away produce lower frequency shifts.

Spectral Doppler provides a characteristic waveform and allows a quantitative assessment for blood flow analysis consisting of Continuous or Pulsed Wave technologies. Pulsed Wave Doppler produces short bursts of sound. It uses the same crystal to generate and receive the signal. By the transducer listening at specific intervals, it can control precisely where the reflected sound is coming from and thus has "range gate resolution." The limitation of Pulsed Wave techniques is that it can only display certain maximum or peak velocities before the signal will alias and become nonquantifiable. The maximum velocity it can display is limited by the transducer's Doppler frequency and the depth of the moving target. Continuous Wave Doppler uses different crystals to send and receive signals. One crystal constantly sends signals while another receives the reflected signal. It has no depth or range gate resolution but it does not alias and can quantify much higher velocities. Aliasing or wraparound occurs if the velocity is too high to display. The peaks are cut off and displayed below baseline.

Color Doppler utilizes the pulse-echo principle to generate color images. The color image is superimposed on the 2-D image. The red and blue displays provide information regarding direction and *mean* velocity of flow. It cannot display instantaneous peak velocities and is not truly quantifiable. The color at the top of the display represents flow toward the transducer, and color at the bottom of the display represents flow away from the transducer. It is sensitive to probe position (Figure 3-9).

Whether using Pulsed Wave Doppler or Color Doppler Imaging, if the sound pulse strikes the blood vessel or blood flow at an angle over 60 degrees, it can

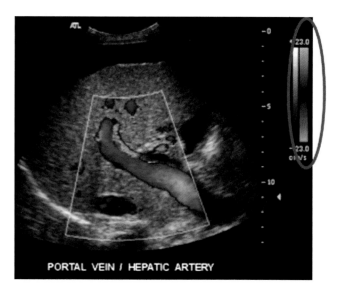

Figure 3-9. Color Doppler of portal vein. Red circle emphasizes color key for direction and/or mean velocity of flow.

result in inaccurate velocity readings and may even suggest that there is no flow when in fact it is due to poor Doppler angle.

Power Doppler images are based on amplitude or strength of the motion. Color maps in Power Doppler are represented by one continuous color. It provides better sensitivity for slow flow or low blood volume states like ovarian or testicular torsion. It accomplishes this because it compares or averages several frames storing the accumulated flow over a number of cardiac cycles. This does take additional processing time and slows the acquisition frame rate. It is less angle dependent, but more sensitive to motion artifacts.

Each form of Doppler consists of benefits and limitations; however, its operation appears deceptively simple. A complete understanding of Doppler physics and velocity components is beyond the scope of this chapter, and it is strongly recommended that the reader pursue additional educational pathways for learning this valuable addition to ultrasound imaging.

▶ TWO-DIMENSIONAL IMAGING

ECHOGENICITY

Echogenicity refers to the amplitude or brightness display of the returning echoes. If a structure presents as hyperechoic, it is said to be more echogenic (of increased amplitude) than the surrounding anatomy. Conversely, hypoechoic structures appear less echogenic (of decreased amplitude). Isoechoic information has the same echogenicity as the surrounding structures. Finally, anechoic refers to the absence of echoes. Typically,

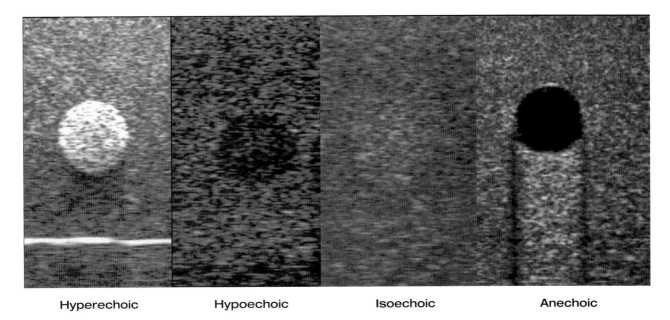

| Hyperechoic | Hypoechoic | Isoechoic | Anechoic |

Figure 3-10. (Courtesy of SonoSite)

fluid-filled structures appear anechoic (Figures 3-10 and 3-11).

▶ IMAGE ARTIFACTS

Unrecognized artifacts are frequently the source of misleading information and misdiagnosis. The ability to recognize and interpret echo information not only includes the anatomical reflections we expect to visualize, but also includes the formation of echoes that appear as a result of image artifacts. Artifacts will be defined as any echo information that does not correspond to the anatomical information as it is positioned and reflected from within the patient. The origin of these artifactual echoes may occur from within the patient, as a result of attenuation or refraction, from an external source, or operator error.

SHADOWING

Acoustic shadowing is one of the most common and frequently encountered imaging artifacts in diagnostic ultrasound. Shadowing may occur for several different reasons, including anatomical, pathological, or changes undergone by the ultrasound beam.

Acoustic shadowing frequently occurs when the sound encounters a highly reflective (high-attenuation) surface. The reflected energy is returned to the transducer with little acoustic energy available to continue traveling to deeper structures. Gallstones, renal stones, ribs, or tissue calcifications are some of the reasons a "clean shadow" from attenuation may exist. "Dirty shadowing" is caused by an "acoustic mismatch" such as when sound interacts with air (Figures 3-12 and 3-13).

REFRACTION — "EDGE SHADOWS"

Shadows may also occur because of changes in the ultrasound beam. A change in the sound beam direction results when there is an oblique incidence of the sound beam as it crosses a boundary of tissue with different propagation speeds or strikes a curved structure. As the sound crosses this boundary, a change in the beam direction occurs and an acoustic shadow results. When an

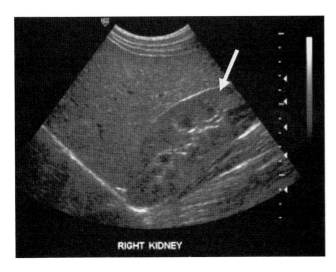

Figure 3-11. Renal parenchyma texture (arrow) is *hypoechoic* as compared with the adjacent liver texture.

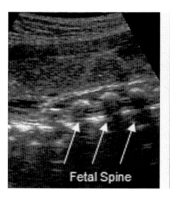
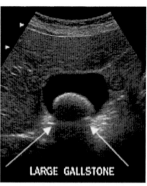

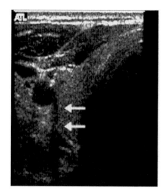
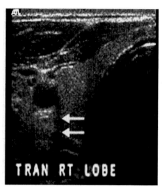

Figure 3-12. Clean shadowing from attenuation. Bone density objects such as this fetal spine and a large gallstone, generally result in a darker more homogenous ("clean") shadow (arrows).

acoustic shadow presents, it is wise to map out the path so we may appreciate its origin (Figure 3-14).

ACOUSTIC ENHANCEMENT

As sound crosses a boundary where less signal attenuation occurs, acoustic enhancement of the beam is often the result. The effects of acoustic enhancement are quite simply the opposite of high-attenuating objects.

As sound encounters ultrasound friendly objects (e.g., simple cysts, distended normal gallbladder, urinary bladder, some types of solid tissue, etc.), less attenuation of the signal occurs, which results in a greater amount of acoustic energy available to continue its journey along

Figure 3-14. Transverse view of the thyroid. The arrows indicate the "edge artifact" that is seen in both images despite moving away from the density seen on the first image of the carotid artery. The sound is refracted off the side of the vessel, thus creating the acoustic shadow.

the same path. This increase in acoustic energy results in a similar increase in echogenicity (hyperechoic) immediately posterior to the area where less attenuation of the signal occurred. This type of imaging artifact is commonly used to confirm the presence of areas suspected to be fluid-filled in etiology and is also referred to as increased through transmission (Figure 3-15).

GAS

The presence of gas is the enemy of ultrasound. The large differences in density that exists between gas and soft tissue disperse the sound waves. Diagnostic

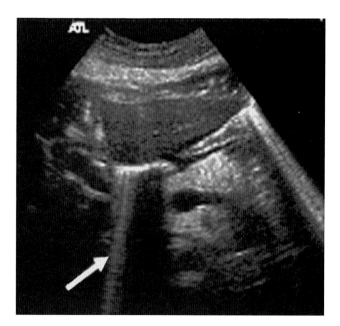

Figure 3-13. Dirty shadowing from air (arrow). Gas density objects such as bowel gas produce a shadow containing lighter, irregular gray level ("dirty") echoes.

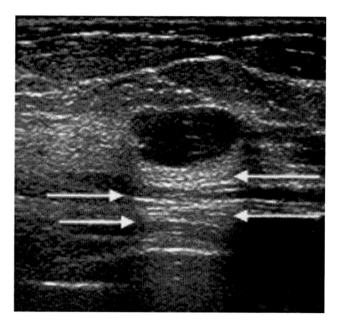

Figure 3-15. Acoustic enhancement. This artifact (arrows) is also referred to as "increased through transmission."

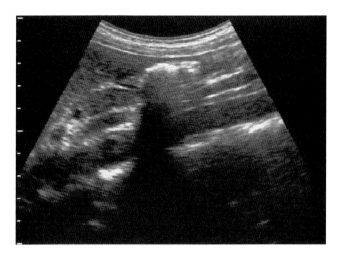

Figure 3-16. Longitudinal aorta is partially obscured by bowel gas. (Courtesy of SonoSite)

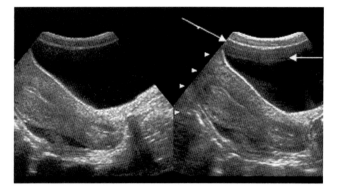

Figure 3-17. Longitudinal suprapubic view of the bladder and uterus. The arrows on the right image indicate a reverberation artifact. The TGC was adjusted on the left image to reduce this artifact.

ultrasound is not equipped to handle these large differences and much of the acoustic energy is scattered with little or no appreciable diagnostic information visualized. Slight transducer pressure or a change in patient and/or transducer positioning may minimize the obstacle. Experience will typically dictate when additional views may not prove of benefit (Figure 3-16).

REVERBERATION

When sound "bounces" between two highly reflective objects, reverberation artifacts appear as recurrent bright arcs displayed at equidistant intervals from the transducer. This artifact will frequently appear at the anterior aspect of the distended urinary bladder or near the layers of the abdominal wall and become more of a nuisance when interrogating structures that are positioned in close proximity. Adjusting the Time Gain (TGC) or Depth Gain (DGC) controls corresponding to this area or changes in transducer positioning, patient positioning, or transducer transmit frequency may reduce their appearance; however, their presence is not likely to be confused with a pathologic condition (Figure 3-17).

MIRRORING

Mirror artifacts are displayed as objects that appear on both sides of a strong reflector. These artifacts can be confusing in appearance and occur because of changes in the reflected beam. Ultrasound assumes that sound is traveling in a straight line and the distance (or depth) of the reflector is proportional to the travel time necessary to make the return trip. When the ultrasound beam undergoes multiple reflections as it returns, an incorrect interpretation of the signal timing ensues and results in a

duplication of structures. The more posterior echo information is the "false" echo. Mirror artifacts are common around the diaphragm and may depict hepatic structures appearing on both sides of the diaphragm. Changes in transducer or patient positioning should alleviate any real threat to misdiagnosis (Figure 3-18).

MOTION ARTIFACTS

Motion artifacts can be generated from a variety of sources. Patient movement, transducer movement, patient respirations, and transmitted pulses from cardiac activity may all contribute to blurring of the image as the "freeze" button has been depressed. Frequently, this fuzzy image may be improved through a function called "cine memory" that allows the operator to view a number of frames that preceded the frozen image. The exact number of available image frames will vary by

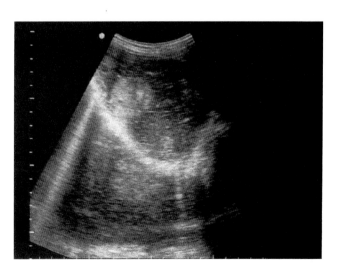

Figure 3-18. Mirror image artifact. Liver tissue and hyperechoic liver lesion are duplicated above the diaphragm. (Courtesy of SonoSite)

ultrasound product and other parameters set forth by the manufacturer. In fact, often it is less than 1 second of information remaining in memory. This may not sound like an abundance of time; however, at 20–30 frames/second, a frame of information free of motion artifact is generally available. Cine memory is particularly helpful when Doppler is performed since the area demonstrating the specific frame of interest may be identified.

SIDE LOBES

It is easy to envision one ultrasound beam being emitted from the probe along a plane parallel to the central axis of the transducer. In reality, ultrasound beams of lower intensity, called "side lobes," may originate at angles to the primary beam and are generally of little consequence. Highly reflective interfaces return echoes via this pathway of side lobes and present as false information. This false information may be introduced as an oblique line of acoustic reflection. Changes in the scanning angle often confirm these returning echoes as side lobes (Figure 3-19).

NOISE

Electronic noise may obscure the primary echo information as it is displayed. Electronic noise occurs when these signals disturb the primary signal of information. Sources of electronic noise vary and include electronic devices, other devices that are supplied by the same electrical

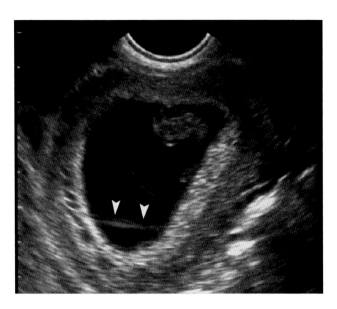

Figure 3-19. Side lobes. Endovaginal image reveals intrauterine gestation with embryonic pole and thin amniotic membrane. Side lobe artifact is demonstrated within the gestational sac (arrowheads). (Courtesy of SonoSite)

service, and radio frequency signals traveling through the air. Shielding these devices is often difficult and understanding noise as an occasional artifact in imaging is necessary.

TECHNIQUE

Incorrect TGC and gain settings can create confusing image patterns. Incorrect settings can diminish quality of the image displayed, hide pathologic variants, and limit the use of the machine (Figure 3-20). Noise caused by the excess gain can easily be corrected by adjusting the controls on the machine. Incorrect depth selection can limit the field of view on the patient and cause the focus of the examination to be lost. Depth markers are found on the display and can be changed on the control panel. Incorrect probe marker position will misrepresent the image being displayed. The operator must be aware of the position of the probe and use it properly for the ultrasound examination being performed.

▶ QUALITY ASSURANCE

Quality assurance is a topic often interpreted as the "quality" of the ultrasound examination that is solely dependent on the skill level of the operator. While the operator is in direct control over the views obtained and system settings to perform a quality examination, the consistency with which the ultrasound system produces quality examinations over time cannot be overlooked.

Diagnostic ultrasound phantoms exist in part to allow a reproducible standard to be documented that ensures the ultrasound system and its components are operating at the performance level defined by the product manufacturer. Ultrasound system and transducer performance may change over time. General purpose ultrasound phantoms allow evaluation of transducer parameters, measurement calibration, focal zone, axial and lateral resolution, sensitivity, functional resolution, and grayscale displays. Specialty phantoms are available to examine transducer beam profile and slice thickness in addition to Doppler phantoms. Scheduled performance evaluations should be incorporated at regular intervals to ensure the ultrasound system and documentation devices are operating at peak performance.

▶ BIOLOGICAL EFFECTS

Risk factors do exist in diagnostic ultrasound and their effects over time have yet to be determined. The American Institute of Ultrasound in Medicine (AIUM) has adopted an acronym termed ALARA: As Low As Reasonably Achievable. The term reminds the sonologist that the amount of time for an examination, along with

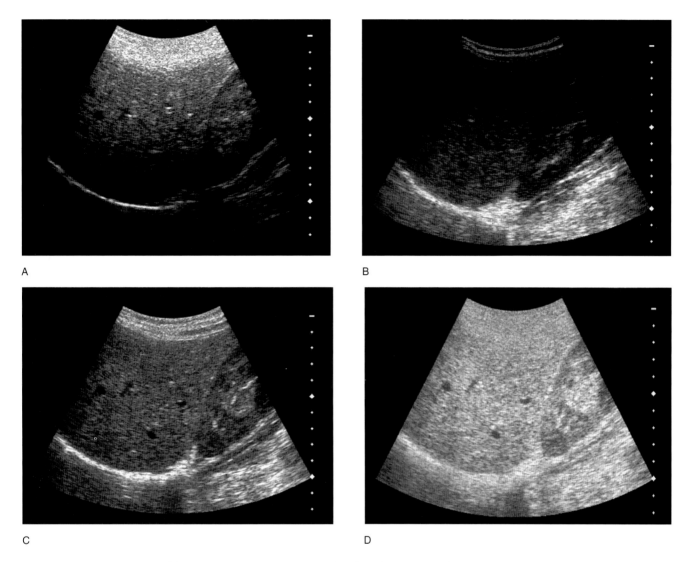

Figure 3-20. Incorrect TGC settings (A). Maladjusted far field/posterior TGC setting does not permit visualization of posterior structures. Incorrect TGC settings (B). Maladjusted near field/anterior TGC setting does not permit visualization of structures positioned closer to the transducer. Correct TGC and gain settings (C). By balancing the display of echogenic information, one can appreciate the subtleties which occur among tissues. Excessive gain settings (D) reduce the ability to differentiate subtleties among various tissues. (Courtesy of SonoSite)

equipment settings, contributes to prudent use of diagnostic ultrasound. The receiver controls (i.e., TGC, Gain, etc.) need to be optimized before increasing Acoustic Power capabilities in an attempt to secure or improve the desired image (see Appendix A).

▶ SUMMARY

A basic understanding of ultrasound physics must be attained before the operator may enjoy the benefit of bedside sonography and reduce any of its potential risks. By implementing emergency ultrasound, there remains a responsibility to the patient community that diagnostic ultrasound examinations include our understanding and

implementation of physics and image artifacts. This is the first step in ensuring that a quality ultrasound examination is performed while minimizing any potential risk to the patient or the operator.

REFERENCES

1. Gill K: *Abdominal Ultrasound: A Practitioner's Guide.* Philadelphia, PA: WB Saunders, 2000.
2. Goodsit MM, Carson JY, Witt TG, et al.: Real Time B-mode ultrasound quality control test procedures. Report of AAPM Ultrasound task Group No. 1. *Am Assoc Phys Med* 27:23–25, 1998.
3. Kurtz AB, Middleton AB: *Ultrasound: The Requisites.* Philadelphia, PA: WB Saunders, 1996.

4. Kremkau FW: *Diagnostic Ultrasound: Principles and Instruments.* 6th ed. Philadelphia, PA: WB Saunders, 2002.

5. Lin GS, Milburn DT, Briggs S: Power Doppler: How it works, its clinical benefits and recent technological advances. *JDMS* 14:45–48, 1998.

6. Nielsen TJ, Lambert MJ: Physics and Instrumentation. *Emergency Ultrasound.* Ma OJ, Mateer JR, ed. McGraw Hill, 2003:Chapter 3.

7. Nilsson A, Ingemar Loren I, Nirhov N, et al.: Power Doppler sonography: Alternative to computed tomograph in abdominal trauma patients. *JUM* 18:129–132, 1999.

8. Rumack CM, Charboneau JW, Wilson SR: *Diagnostic Ultrasound,* 2nd ed. Philadelphia, PA: WB Saunders 1998.

9. Stephen E, Felkel S: Ultrasound Safety Mechanical and Thermal Indices: A Primer. *JDMS* 15:98–100, 1999.

10. Tempkin BB: *Ultrasound Scanning: Principles and Protocols,* 2nd ed. Philadelphia, PA: WB Saunders, 1998.

APPENDIX

Further reading materials includes the American Institute of Ultrasound In Medicine (AIUM) publications listed below on ultrasound safety and are available by contacting AIUM:

American Institute of Ultrasound in Medicine
www.aium.org
800-638-5352
14750 Sweitzer Lane
Suite 100
Laurel, MD 20707

Ultrasound Safety Publications

Bioeffects and Safety of Diagnostic Ultrasound

Evaluation of Research Reports: Bioeffects Literature Reviews (1962–1982)

Evaluation of Research Reports: Bioeffects Literature Reviews (1985–1991)

Evaluation of Research Reports: Bioeffects Literature Reviews (1992–1998)

How to Interpret the Ultrasound Output Display Standard for Higher Acoustic Output Diagnostic Ultrasound Devices (technical bulletin)

Mechanical Bioeffects from Diagnostic Ultrasound: Consensus Statements

Medical Ultrasound Safety

What You Should Know about the Safety of Your Ultrasound Examination (patient pamphlet).

CHAPTER 4

Prehospital Ultrasound: Perspectives from Four Countries

Clinical accuracy and timeliness are essential for successful decision-making and problem-solving in out-of-hospital medical care. The prehospital use of ultrasonography can improve initial data gathering, which enhances the delivery of acute care in a timely and effective fashion.

Emergency ultrasound has greatly improved patient care since the first published reports by emergency physicians. Emergency ultrasound has been shown to reduce morbidity and mortality in critically ill patients, and multiple studies have shown that it can be efficiently and effectively performed by clinicians, provided that adequate training and quality assurance programs are in place.

Over the last decade, investigators have begun evaluating the use of ultrasound in a wide variety of prehospital, civilian, and military settings. Several case studies and case series have suggested that its use is cost-effective and enhances care. Ongoing prospective studies are providing additional evidence of its impact on patient management (clinical effectiveness) and on the overall service and health care system performance (organizational and social effectiveness). Efforts are being made to identify its most appropriate applications in the prehospital setting, the technical feasibility and reliability of its use, prehospital provider training and competency requirements, and the impact of prehospital ultrasound on patient outcomes and community health.

To highlight the growing evidence in support of prehospital ultrasound, this chapter will review the overall applications undergoing studies throughout the world, focusing on the experience of the German, French, Italian, and American helicopter and ground-based emergency medical services (EMS).

▶ OUT-OF-HOSPITAL ULTRASOUND

The term "out-of-hospital ultrasound" refers to sonographic examinations performed in a wide variety of settings outside of traditional hospital departments, laboratories, and freestanding imaging centers. "Prehospital ultrasound" is synonymous, even though this term is mostly used in reference to EMS and tactical medicine applications. Prehospital ultrasound examinations are generally not performed by radiologists or sonographers; caregivers incorporate the use of ultrasound into the initial patient assessment at the point of care in the prehospital setting. The images obtained provide real-time morphologic and functional clinical information.

In the current emergency and critical care literature, "point-of-care ultrasound" most commonly refers to "bedside emergency ultrasound" since the scientific debate has been originally focused on patients being cared for in the emergency department; the resuscitation, operative, or recovery room; the intensive care unit; the medical imaging department; or other medical and surgical wards. Diagnostic and therapeutic advances have allowed "critical care" to be taken outside of the hospital setting to the scene of illness and injury in a wide variety of settings (Table 4-1)

In all of these settings, ultrasonography provides a visual extension of the clinical examination, permitting more accurate assessment of anatomic and

▶ TABLE 4-1. OUT-OF-HOSPITAL ULTRASOUND SETTINGS AND PROVIDERS

US SETTINGS	US PROVIDERS

Prehospital EMS care
  Accident scenes
  Aboard helicopters, planes, ambulances
  Others
Mass casualties and disaster medicine
  Nature-born catastrophes
  Building collapses
  Car, train, air accidents
  Explosions, terrorist attacks
  Others
Remote, austere and wilderness medicine
  Mountain, rural, forest, desert areas
  Ship-travels, air flights, space flights
  Scarce-resource health services
  Humanitarian operations
  Others
Tactical medicine
  Combat fields
  Field hospitals
  Peace-keeping operations
  Others
Sports medicine
  Sport stadiums, Winter Olympic Games
Primary care
  General practice
  Primary health care
	• Emergency physicians
	• Critical care physicians/intensivists
	• Anesthesiologists
	• Emergency/trauma surgeons
	• Orthopedists
	• Sport physicians
	• Other "system-based" specialists
	• General practitioners
	• Nurses
	• Midwives
	• Paramedics
	• Technicians
	• Lay personnel

physiologic integrity in complex states of illness and injury (Figures 4-1 and 4-2). Prehospital applications are generally incorporated into defined problem-based clinical pathways rather than organ-based categorizations (i.e., "shock assessment" rather than "liver assessment").

Germany

Felix Walcher, Franziska Brenner, Nadine Nieuwkamp, Jörg Braun, Thomas Kirschning, Ingo Marzi, and Raoul Breitkreutz

The German emergency system takes advantage of a close alliance between emergency physicians and the rescuing service staff prior to transportation to the hospital. The overriding principle of on-scene care is "stay and play" in contrast to the "scoop and run" principle prevalent in most prehospital systems. The implementation of ultrasonography into such a system is supported by the development of two major concepts and training programs—Prehospital Focused Abdominal Sonography for Trauma and Focused Echocardiographic Evaluation in Resuscitation—for emergency physicians, critical care physicians, and paramedics.

▶ PREHOSPITAL FOCUSED ABDOMINAL SONOGRAPHY FOR TRAUMA

Prehospital Focused Assessment with Sonography for Trauma (P-FAST) is related to prehospital trauma care. Clinical estimates of intraperitoneal bleeding at the trauma scene are difficult to accurately assess. A blunt trauma patient with normal vital signs and an unremarkable physical examination may have massive intraperitoneal bleeding that requires urgent operative management for hemorrhage control. Data from several studies support the role of prehospital ultrasound in enhancing detection of intraperitoneal hemorrhage.

The 2001 Frankfurt/Main pilot study and a subsequent prospective multicenter study of P-FAST investigated the feasibility of prehospital ultrasound in trauma care. Five air rescue centers in southwestern Germany and one ground ambulance rescue team in Frankfurt/Main took part in these studies. The entire P-FAST examination took about 2 minutes when results were negative, whereas positive intraperitoneal sonographic findings could be detected within seconds. Prehospital diagnosis of intraperitoneal injury by ultrasound was made approximately half an hour prior to arrival at the emergency department. In more than 90% of the cases, there was enough time to complete the P-FAST examination on the scene or during

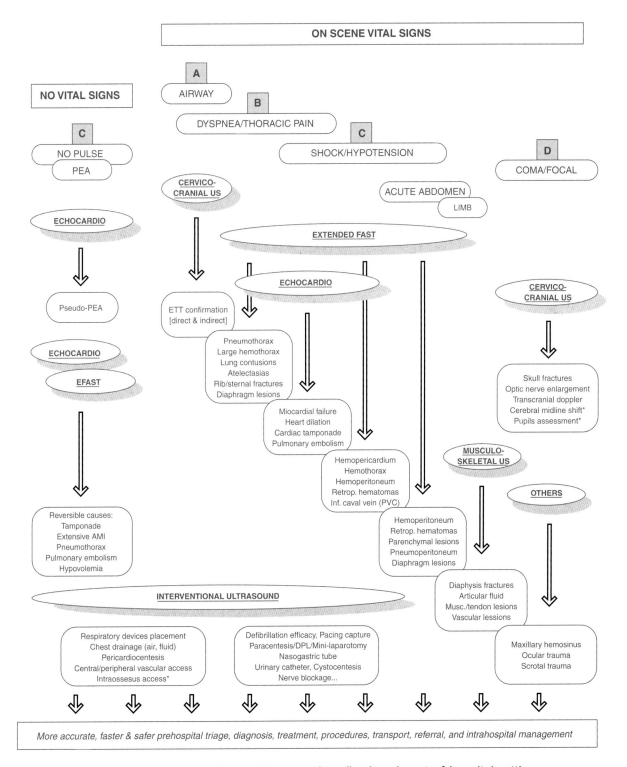

Figure 4-1. ABCD-conformed ultrasound applications in out-of-hospital setting.

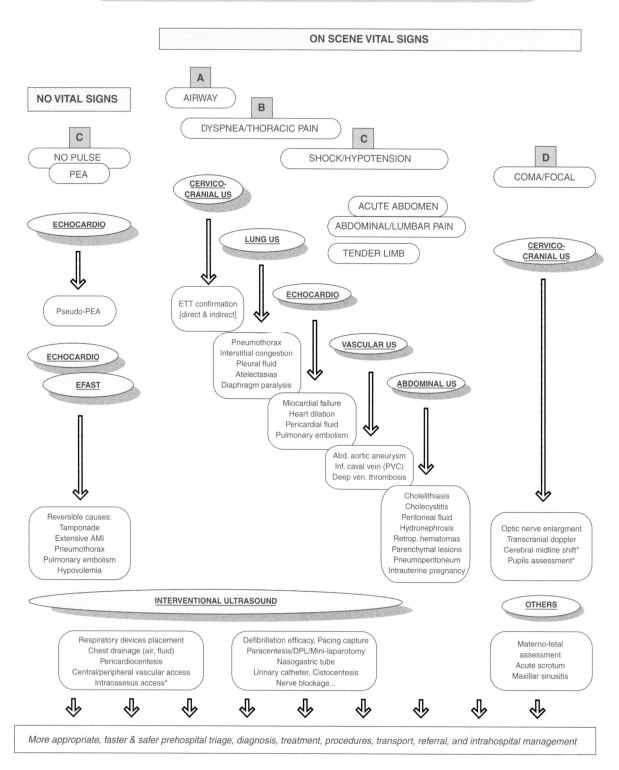

Figure 4-2. Current Level 1 ultrasound applications in out-of-hospital setting: ABDCE-conformed pathways for the acute medical and surgical patient.

transportation. In a few cases ultrasound could not be completed because of suboptimal conditions (e.g., subcutaneous emphysema, patient obesity, or lack of time). The P-FAST examination had a sensitivity of 93% for the detection of intraperitoneal hemorrhage. The investigators concluded that P-FAST had potential as a useful, reliable diagnostic tool in surgical triage at the trauma scene.

All rescue teams involved in the multicenter study stated that P-FAST had an important impact on decision making. In approximately one third of the cases, the findings of P-FAST had an influence on trauma management at the scene. Whenever intraperitoneal bleeding was detected, the prehospital phase of care was minimized to enable immediate transportation, either by ground or by helicopter. In contrast, if the findings of P-FAST were negative, the routine algorithm for trauma care at the scene was followed by completion of the primary and secondary surveys in accordance with the principles of advanced trauma life support (ATLS). The ultrasound findings led to a change in the choice of admitting hospital in approximately 20% of the cases. In addition, the results of P-FAST gave surgeons additional information that allowed appropriate planning of the hospital phase of care.

► FOCUSED ECHOCARDIOGRAPHIC EVALUATION IN RESUSCITATION

Focused Echocardiographic Evaluation in Resuscitation (FEER) addresses the development of skills for emergency physicians in the assessment of nontraumatic patients. Time-dependent scenarios occur in preresuscitation care, cardiopulmonary resuscitation, and postresuscitation care. Suspected myocardial insufficiency due to acute global left-sided or right-sided heart failure, pericardial tamponade, and hypovolemia should be identified during the initial resuscitation. Another major challenge is recognizing return of spontaneous circulation when no central pulse is palpable. New evidence suggests that echocardiography can identify a "subclinical" return of spontaneous circulation (i.e., mechanical cardiac output).

The FEER algorithm is a structured process of transthoracic echocardiography that can be applied at the point of care. The 2005 American Heart Association resuscitation guidelines recommend high-quality cardiopulmonary resuscitation with minimal interruptions to reduce no-flow intervals. The identification and treatment of reversible causes or complicating factors are recommended as well.

Studies have evaluated the FEER examination for its ease of implementation into the cardiopulmonary resuscitation process and its ability to identify characteristic pathologies. The FEER examination is a 10-step procedure (Table 4-2) designed to be performed during cardiopulmonary resuscitation cycles in order to reduce unwanted interruptions. Prehospital indications for performing FEER are listed in Table 4-3.

In a prospective, observational trial in the prehospital setting, we tested (a) the capability of FEER to differentiate pulseless electrical activity (PEA) states and (b) the feasibility of FEER using a mobile, battery-powered ultrasound system. Trained emergency physicians

► TABLE 4-2. THE 10-STEP FOCUSED ECHOCARDIOGRAPHIC EVALUATION IN RESUSCITATION (FEER) ALGORITHM

Phase	FEER Step
High-quality CPR, preparation, team information	1. Perform immediate and accurate BLS and ACLS according to AHA guidelines, at least five cycles of chest compression/ventilation 2. Tell the CPR Team: "I am preparing an echocardiogram." 3. Prepare portable ultrasound (allow prepare) and test it. 4. Accommodate situation (e.g., best position of patient and doctor, removal of clothes, etc.), be ready to start
Execution, obtaining the echocardiogram	5. Tell CPR Team to count down 10 seconds and to perform a pulse check simultaneously 6. Command: "Interrupt at the end of this cycle for echocardiography." 7. Put the probe gently onto the patient's subxiphoid region during chest compressions 8. Perform a subcostal (long axis) echocardiogram as quickly as possible. If you cannot identify the heart after 3 seconds, stop the interruption and repeat again after five cycles and/or with the parasternal approach.
Resuming CPR Interpretation and consequences	9. Command after 9 seconds at the latest: "Continue CPR" and control it. 10. Communicate (after continuation of chest compressions only): the findings to the CPR team (e.g., "wall motion, heart is squeezing," "cardiac stand still," "(massive) pericardial effusion," "no conclusive finding," "suspected pulmonary artery embolism," "hypovolemia" and explain consequences as well as follow-up procedures.

▶ **TABLE 4-3. PREHOSPITAL INDICATIONS TO PERFORM FOCUSED ECHOCARDIOGRAPHIC EVALUATION IN RESUSCITATION (FEER)**

"Preresuscitation" Care
    Penetrating trauma, blunt trauma
    Postcardiotomy due to cardiac surgery
    Hypotension, shock of unknown origin
    Unconsciousness, unresponsiveness
    Acute severe dyspnea
    Syncope in young adults
    Vein thrombosis
    Acute myocardial infarction (AMI), mechanical
       complications of AMI
    "Atypical" chest pain: suspected aortic-dissection,
       suspected aortic abdominal or thoracic aneurysm,
       nontraumatic cardiac rupture
    Iatrogenic complications following invasive
       procedures (e.g., insertion of an artificial pace maker,
       pulmonary artery catheter, electrophysiologic
       investigative procedures)
    Great-vessel disease
Cardiopulmonary resuscitation (CPR)
    Pulseless electrical activity
    Bradycardia-asystole, pacemaker-ECG
    Performance of CPR
    Suspected cardiac tamponade
    Early detection of return of spontaneous circulation
    Effectiveness of chest compressions
Postresuscitation Care
    Hypotension, adaptation of vasopressors

applied the FEER examination as described in prehospital cardiac arrest patients who were being resuscitated. In 77 out-of-hospital arrests, PEA was diagnosed in 30 patients. In 19 of these PEA cases, cardiac wall movement was detected and correctable causes, such as pericardial tamponade (3), poor ventricular function (14), and hypovolemia (2), were diagnosed and treated. Thirteen patients survived to hospital admission. In terms of feasibility, the quality of ultrasound image was considered as being "good" in 11 examinations, "sufficient" in 21, and "poor" in 5, and most were adequate using the subxiphoid window (23/39).

▶ **EDUCATION AND TRAINING**

Before 2002, a uniform course to teach P-FAST was unavailable in Germany or other parts of Europe. Prior to the P-FAST studies, it was necessary to set up a structured educational program for emergency physicians and paramedics. We developed a P-FAST course concept on the basis of several studies that had been performed in the 1990s with respect to the use of ultrasound in

the clinical setting. Some groups had investigated which type of education programs were required to gain competency in performing the FAST examination and had assessed the learning curve. The recommended duration of didactic training, including hands-on experience, ranged from 2 to 30 hours.

The main goal of the P-FAST training is to prepare participants for uncommon situations in trauma scenarios under field conditions. The 1 day course in P-FAST includes both didactic and hands-on training. The didactic session includes a general introduction to ultrasound, physics of ultrasound, and the causes and relevance of artifacts and shadows that may be encountered during an ultrasound examination. Participants are introduced to the rationale for performing ultrasound as part of trauma management and are taught how to integrate P-FAST into the prehospital algorithm for trauma care. Numerous photographs and videos provide an overview of the physiologic and pathologic situations. During the hands-on training, participants perform the P-FAST examination under the supervision of experienced sonologists. The ratio of instructors to students is 1:2. During the course, a trainee performs 30–40 ultrasound examinations under the supervision of the instructors.

In the first part of hands-on training, participants perform the standardized procedure of P-FAST on healthy and patient volunteers. Patient volunteers have positive findings for free intraperitoneal fluid secondary to peritoneal dialysis or ascites. In the second part of the hands-on training, students learn how to perform the ultrasound examination under difficult circumstances, such as on patients found in challenging prehospital conditions. In the third part, real-time scenarios are presented with healthy or patient volunteers found in critical situations following a traumatic event. These scenarios include surgical triage of three or more victims or volunteers trapped in the wreckage of a vehicle. Our evaluation of the course program is consistent with data from other training evaluations in the literature, which have shown that these programs produce competent examiners and are associated with a steep learning curve. We found no significant differences between emergency physicians and paramedics in terms of sensitivity, specificity, and accuracy of P-FAST examinations.

We also evaluated a 1-day course on focused echocardiography for emergency physicians and critical care physicians who had no previous experience in performing echocardiography. Our course emphasizes basic echocardiography, rapid evaluation, and documentation skills. In addition, training in lung sonography and the detection of central vessels are included. An emergency physician's ability to obtain a correct subxiphoid 4-chamber view was evaluated. We also evaluated an emergency physician's ability to interpret a

5-second echocardiogram MPEG movie at a glance and provided clips on normal and pathologic findings such as pericardial effusion, reduced ventricular function, cardiac arrest, PEA, hypovolemia, and normal examinations. We found that emergency physicians could learn to identify some simple pathologic findings on very short video clips.

▶ MOBILE ULTRASOUND DEVICES

Prior to the German P-FAST multicenter study, the fire department and the Department of Trauma Surgery at the University of Frankfurt used PRIMEDIC HandyScanTM (Metrax Company, Rottweil, Germany). This device is based on Esaote TringaTM (Esaote Company, Genora/Florence, Italy) and especially developed for EMS needs. It weighs 2.2 kg, has a 5″ monitor, and can be operated with a 3.5 MHz or 5 MHz ultrasound sector probe. The screen resolution is 320 × 240 pixels with 256 different shadows of gray; it has a memory capacity of 160 pictures and a battery capacity of up to 6 hours. This mobile device can be held with one hand; the adjustments necessary during an examination can be made with the thumb.

The compact ultrasound machine SonoSite 180 Plus (SonoSite Corporation, Bothell, Wshington, USA) is used by the German army and in the MediVac system operating worldwide. This device has a color Power Doppler, a spectral- and pulse-waved Doppler, and an ECG module. The SonoSite MicroMaxx includes a wide variety of probes, including a high-frequency linear probe and a multiplanar transesophageal probe for use during intensive care transport.

▶ PROPAGATION OF PREHOSPITAL ULTRASOUND IN AIR AND GROUND RESCUE SERVICE

Since 2003, the German Air Rescue Organization (Deutsche Rettungsflugwacht) has incorporated P-FAST into the algorithm for trauma management. By 2007, 29 helicopters and 3 fixed wing air crafts will be equipped with portable ultrasound devices and most of the emergency physicians and paramedic crews will be trained. The other main provider of air rescue services, the German Automobile Club, also has adopted P-FAST.

Some air rescue centers of the German federal police have implemented P-FAST; in addition, the German air force also have equipped their international mobile medical crews and supplied their aircraft for multinational flights with mobile ultrasound devices. Their crews have been trained in our courses.

P-FAST and FEER have been integrated into ground-based services as well. The region of Darmstadt adopted the prehospital FEER examination in 2002. In Frankfurt/Main, the five ground-based ambulances staffed by emergency physicians have been equipped with portable ultrasound devices with financial support from the city's public health department.

France

Tomislav Petrovic, Frédéric Lapostolle, and Frédéric Adnet

The feasibility and usefulness of prehospital ultrasound have been explored since the beginning of the 1980s in France. These early investigations utilized bulky equipment requiring very skilled operators; as a result, they had limited applicability to most prehospital systems. In the early 1990s, technological advances produced lighter ultrasound machines that were much more practical to use in the prehospital setting.

French prehospital clinicians have been interested in broad applications of prehospital ultrasound. French investigators have studied the detection of free intraperitoneal fluid, assessment of cardiac function in shock and arrest states, evaluation of thoracic injuries, and the detection of deep venous thrombosis. Other ongoing investigations include the assessment of long diaphysis fractures and optic nerve enlargement.

The methods of training and the level of performance of emergency physicians using ultrasound in prehospital settings in France were evaluated. The ultrasound training was scheduled for one half-day session that included didactic and practical instruction. Like our German colleagues, didactic sessions reviewed the guiding principles of ultrasonography and normal and pathological images. The practical training consisted of performing examinations on healthy subjects or on patients with pertinent findings on ultrasound examinations (e.g., patients with ascites). The training focused on examinations pertinent to the French prehospital setting, which included the assessment for pneumothoraces, pleural effusions, abdominal or pericardial effusions, or deep venous thrombosis of the lower limbs.

Eight physicians of the SAMU 93 (EMS department) were trained on the emergency use of a portable ultrasound device (SonoSite 180). The number of training sessions varied from 1 to 6, according to the experience level of the operators. Each operator determined a clinical diagnostic probability (before ultrasonography) noted on an analog visual scale from 0 (*absence of lesion*) to 10 (*presence of lesion*). According to the same principle, the operator determined a second probability after ultrasonography. The hospital follow-up of the patients made it possible to obtain the final diagnosis (0 for absent and 10 for present lesion) that was compared with the pre- and posttest probabilities.

The initial analysis of 83 ultrasound examinations carried out on 40 patients revealed a median time of examination of 5 minutes, 100% sensitivity, 98% specificity, a positive predictive value of 92%, and a negative predictive value of 100%. In our analysis of the learning curve for ultrasound proficiency by prehospital providers, we found that the number of ultrasound examinations required to achieve desired proficiency was approximately 25 examinations.

The absolute difference between the probabilities before and after ultrasound was calculated and compared with the final diagnosis (0 or 10). When ultrasound had brought the operator closer to it, a positive value was allotted to the obtained number; conversely, a negative value was allotted when ultrasound had moved the operator away from the final diagnosis. For example, if a diagnostic probability was 3 before and 8 after ultrasonography, the absolute difference was 5 (8 − 3). If the final diagnosis was positive (presence of a lesion), ultrasound would have brought the operator closer to the final diagnosis. The value allotted to ultrasound would then be +5. Conversely, if the final diagnosis was negative (absence of lesion), ultrasound would have moved away the operator from the final diagnosis. The value allotted to ultrasound would then be −5.

The results of 302 ultrasound examinations were analyzed. The median impact of ultrasound on the final diagnosis was +2. The diagnostic performance was improved by ultrasound in 67% of the cases; it was not modified in 25% of the cases and it was degraded in 8% of the cases. Our results were consistent with the use of ultrasound as a "complement" to the clinical examination.

In France, prehospital ultrasound has established itself as a legitimate clinical adjunct. Just as the stethoscope serves as an extension of the physician's ears, the ultrasound probe serves as an extension of her hands and eyes. If the indications are focused, the procedure is codified, and the operators are properly trained, then the level of performance approaches that of a medical imaging expert. The rapidity of the examinations provides additional diagnostic information without delaying transport or definitive care. As experience with this modality increases and technological advances produce improved portability and resolution, we believe that the use of ultrasound will gain broad acceptance in prehospital venues around the world.

Italy

Luca Neri, Cristina Frigerio, Carmela Graci, Elena Guffanti, Enrico Storti, and Giancarlo Fontana

The use of ultrasound in the Italian EMS system was initiated in 2005 following the demonstration of feasibility by German, French, and North American investigators. Multiple Italian medical centers are studying the optimal use for prehospital ultrasound applications in the assessment (triage, diagnosis) and management (treatment and transporation) of critically ill or injured patients. In Milan, a helicopter and two ground units ("S.S.U.Em. 118 - Milano") are staffed with advanced medical teams using a SonoSite 180 Plus portable ultrasound machine. Like our European colleagues, the Italian system is focusing on three clinical scenarios: cardiac arrest (level 1 echocardiography to differentiate between PEA and pseudo-PEA and to detect rapidly reversible causes of PEA), thoracoabdominal trauma (extended FAST examination to assess for free pericardial, pleural, and intraperitoneal free fluid and pneumothorax), and the acutely dyspneic patient (level 1 lung ultrasound to differentiate between pulmonary edema and emphysema).

Another area of interest is disaster medicine, particularly mass casualty events in urban and rural settings. Although theoretically ultrasound may be of tremendous benefit in this scenario, no definitive data have demonstrated its optimal use. In the Milan prehospital system, portable ultrasound units have been used on the helicopter and ground units to evaluate patients in a simulated terrorist attack on Milan's railway and subway systems. Use of ultrasound during the initial triage phase would allow more appropriate triage and distribution of patients to facilities best able to provide definitive care.

Because of the operator-dependent nature of ultrasound, any EMS system that plans to implement prehospital ultrasound should first design an educational program for the system that reflects a competency needs assessment. A second fundamental step is collaboration with the "intra-hospital" critical and intensive care communities in order to design an "Ultrasound Curriculum for Critical Care Medicine." A model for different levels of ultrasound practice, proficiency, and training in prehospital and critical care medicine should be designed, with some specifications about the main settings of implementation (field triage, ICU, and tactical medicine). Minimal requirements for acquiring and retaining competency should be outlined, and key competencies categorized according to an outcome and problem-based approach, with priorities aimed at the primary stabilization of the ABCs.

The ultimate goal is to implement an international multicenter study aimed at developing and validating a prehospital ultrasound curriculum and testing and studying training outcomes. The overall aim is to facilitate and bolster international training programs. In the future, the international prehospital ultrasound community should identify and highlight the core competencies and specifications that should be part of all EMS-oriented ultrasound applications.

United States of America

William Heegaard, Robert Reardon, Dave Spear, Dave Plummer, Scott A. Joing, and Michael Blaivas

Prehospital ultrasound in the United States is presently in its infancy because the goal of American EMS systems traditionally has been to expeditiously transport ill or injured patients to the receiving medical center for definitive care. The published data available on prehospital ultrasound are either case reports or prospective observational studies. No large prospective, randomized study analyzing outcomes derived from prehospital ultrasound use has been published in the American medical literature even though ultrasound has been utilized in two broad prehospital areas, helicopter EMS and ground ambulances.

▶ AIR AND GROUND MEDICAL TRANSPORT

Air medical transport is a logical area to investigate prehospital ultrasound, given the critical and time-sensitive nature of patients using this transport modality. The rapid growth of helicopter EMS transport in the United States has mandated that we evaluate improved methods for the care of critically ill or injured patients. Conservative estimates suggest that there are 300,000 helicopter transports and 150,000 fixed wing transports per year in the United States. At least three United States helicopter EMS programs are utilizing or have utilized ultrasound (Oregon Health and Science University, Portland, Oregon; MetroHealth Medical Center, Cleveland, Ohio; and LifeLinkIII, Minneapolis, Minnesota).

In 2000, Price and colleagues demonstrated that the FAST examination could be performed rapidly and with relative ease in the helicopter. Using a SonoSite 180 ultrasound machine with a 3.5 MHz probe, 10 flight sonologists performed 21 FAST examinations on 14 patients. Nine patients were simulated. They reported no effect on avionics and were able to complete the standard FAST examination in a mean time of 3 minutes. In 2004, Heegaard and coinvestigators applied a focused template for didactic ultrasound training with additional hands-on training in an emergency department. They found that flight clinicians could perform a wide variety of ultrasound examinations with good long-term retention (>90%) over 1 year. Ultrasound examinations were performed proficiently in the helicopter, although time and space constraints limited the clinicians' ability to perform the complete FAST examination. Finally, a case series examined the use of ultrasound to perform a screening examination on obstetric patients transported by helicopter. Monitoring the fetus in the helicopter using traditional methods of Doppler auscultation has always been difficult and unreliable. The Fetal Evaluation for Transport with Ultrasound is a screening examination that evaluates fetal heart rate, position, and movement and general condition of the placenta. The examination can be performed serially in flight with no acoustic distortion from rotor noise. The additional information can be advantageous when transport decisions need to be made or when conditions do not allow Doppler stethoscope use.

Potential applications of helicopter EMS and ground ambulance ultrasound in the United States include, but are not limited to,

- FAST examination on trauma patients to expedite definitive care and early operating room activation, especially in rural areas;
- focused cardiac ultrasound examination in hypotensive patients to place them in one of four shock states (severe hypovolemia, cardiogenic, pericardial tamponade, or right ventricular obstruction), which helps guide therapy;
- fetal monitoring and evaluation in obstetrical patients. In addition, evaluation of pregnant trauma patients for fetal viability and gestational age can be performed;
- early detection of mainstem intubations;
- early detection of pneumothorax with the extended FAST examination;
- early evaluation of cardiac arrest and PEA; and
- confirmation of death by documentation of patients in asystole.

Most studies on prehospital ultrasound in the United States have utilized the SonoSite 180, a 2.4-kg compact ultrasound machine with 3.5 MHz probe. One helicopter EMS program (LifeLink III. Minneapolis, MN) utilized the SonoSite iLook ultrasound machine (1.4 kg) with a 3.5 MHz probe, which was mounted in the helicopter for ease of use.

In the United States, there is a paucity of data on the use of ultrasound in ground ambulances. It remains to be seen whether the European experience will impact the implementation of ultrasound in ground ambulances in the United States. The first American ground EMS system to utilize prehospital ultrasound was in Odessa, Texas. However, obstacles to implementing prehospital ultrasound programs include lack of reimbursement for ultrasound imaging, difficulty in maintaining ultrasound competency among numerous EMS personnel, and the cost of ultrasound machines.

▶ TACTICAL MEDICINE

In addition to its use on helicopter and ground EMS units, prehospital ultrasound has been applied in tactical medicine scenarios. Unlike a hospital, tactical medicine presents unique environmental challenges. Medical providers may be under fire and have to operate in an unsecured environment. Military and police medics typically practice scoop and run of injured suspects, bystanders, and team members. In some instances, however, diagnosis and intervention cannot wait for a victim to be removed from the scene and transported to a hospital for evaluation. Many critical disease entities such as pericardial effusion and pneumothorax may require expeditious diagnosis and treatment. The actual ultrasound applications utilized in tactical medicine scenarios are identical to those found in emergency department and critical care settings.

The working environment of a tactical physician who will be utilizing compact ultrasound for patient care is foreign to many clinicians. Tactical physicians are frequently armed to protect themselves and their patients. This also means the use of heavy and cumbersome protective gear such as a ballistic vest and helmet. Carrying a gas mask, pepper spray, radio, restraints, flashlights, knives, and assorted other gear makes the job more difficult. Most tactical physicians prefer to have all the critical equipment to handle one or two serious trauma patients on their back. This will include equipment required for endotracheal intubation, ventilation, vascular access, thoracostomy, thoracotomy, hemostasis, and medical resuscitation. Thus, any ultrasound unit carried has to be lightweight.

The durability and versatility of tactical ultrasound machines is a critical issue. Potential damage to the machine is high. Because of the space and weight limitations, the tactical physician is best served utilizing a microconvex transducer. This transducer will provide adequate images of the abdominal organs as well as the heart. While a linear transducer is preferable in evaluating for a pneumothorax, a microconvex transducer has been utilized with good success in a previous study of trauma patients. This micro-convex transducer also offers some assistance in vascular access and optic nerve sheath evaluation. A phased array transducer may be substituted, but it is not as proficient for evaluating for a pneumothorax, measuring optic nerve sheath, and assisting with vascular access as the micro-convex transducer. The use of a curved linear transducer or linear array is not recommended.

Ease of use and rapid boot-up time are also critical features of an ultrasound machine in tactical medicine conditions. Although some compact units now boot up in less than 15 seconds that may still seem like an eternity in a tactical situation. The majority of currently available compact equipment may take 45 seconds or more to boot up, which is unacceptable to the tactical sonologist. The ideal ultrasound machine would be light and, compact, provide excellent images in a variety of applications with just one transducer, and boot up within several seconds. The ability to function on battery power is a prerequisite as well.

The utility of having a tactical physician present during high-risk military and police operations is becoming clear to a variety of local, state, federal, and military agencies around the globe. Few other "patient care areas" are in as much need of rapid and accurate diagnostic imaging as the tactical medicine environment.

BIBLIOGRAPHY

1. Breitkreutz R, Walcher F, Seeger F: Focused echocardiographic evaluation in resuscitation management (FEER): Concept of an advanced life-support-conformed algorithm. *Crit Care Med* 2006 (in press).
2. Heegaard W, Plummer D, Dries D, et al.: Ultrasound for the air medical clinician. *Air Med J* 23(2):20–23, 2004.
3. Lapostolle F, Petrovic T, Catineau J, et al.: Out-of-hospital ultrasonographic diagnosis of a left ventricular wound after penetrating thoracic trauma. *Ann Emerg Med* 43:422–423, 2004.
4. Lenoir G, Petrovic T, Galinski M, et al.: Influence de l'échographie préhospitalière sur le diagnostic porté par le médecin urgentiste. Congres Urgences 2003 (Paris), *JEUR* 16:1S49, 111, 2003.
5. Melanson SW, McCarthy J, Stromski CJ, et al.: Aeromedical trauma sonography by flight crews with a miniature ultrasound unit. *Prehospital Emerg Care* 5:399–402, 2001.
6. Plummer D, Brunette D, Asinger R, et al.: Emergency department echocardiography improves outcome in penetrating cardiac injury. *Ann Emerg Med* 21:709–712, 1992.
7. Polk JD: Fetal evaluation for transport by ultrasound performed by air medical teams: A case series. *Air Med J* 23(4):32–34, 2004.
8. Price DD, Wilson SR, Murphy TG: Trauma ultrasound feasibility during helicopter transport. *Air Med J* 19:144–146, 2000.

9. Rodgerson J, Heegaard W, Plummer D, et al.: Emergency department right upper quadrant ultrasound is associated with a reduced time to diagnosis and treatment of ruptured ectopic pregnancies. *Acad Emerg Med* 8:331–336, 2001.

10. Walcher F, Kortüm S, Kirschning T, et al.: Optimierung des Traumamanagements durch präklinische Sonographic [Optimized management of polytraumatized patients by prehospital ultrasound]. *Der Unfallchirurg* 105(11):986–994, 2002.

11. Walcher F, Weinlich M, Conrad G, et al.: Prehospital ultrasound imaging improves management of abdominal trauma. *Br J Surg* 93:238–242, 2006.

CHAPTER 5

Trauma

O. John Ma, James R. Mateer, and Andrew W. Kirkpatrick

Over the past 30 years, trauma surgeons in Europe and Japan have demonstrated the proficient use of ultrasonography in evaluating blunt trauma patients.[1-9] During the 1990s, emergency physicians and trauma surgeons in North America have prospectively evaluated the applications of ultrasonography in trauma and have presented results comparable with those of other investigators worldwide.[10-18]

The focused assessment with sonography for trauma (FAST) examination is a bedside screening tool to aid clinicians in identifying free intrathoracic or intraperitoneal fluid. The underlying premise behind the use of the FAST examination is that clinically significant injuries will be associated with the presence of free fluid accumulating in dependent areas. The FAST examination was originally developed as a limited ultrasound examination, focusing primarily on the detection of free fluid, and was not designed to universally identify all sonographically detectable pathology. While a number of groups have subsequently recommended additions or modifications to the standard FAST examination, such as evaluating for pneumothoraces, quantifying the degree of free intraperitoneal fluid present, or following the accumulation of the free fluid, the essence of the examination remains identifying findings that can be interpreted by clinicians in a clinical context.

▶ CLINICAL CONSIDERATIONS

The rapid and accurate diagnosis of injuries sustained by trauma patients can be difficult, especially when they are associated with other distracting injuries or altered mental status from head injury or drug or alcohol use. In the United States, the three generally accepted diagnostic techniques for evaluating abdominal trauma patients are diagnostic peritoneal lavage, computed tomography (CT) of the abdomen, and ultrasonography. Each of these diagnostic modalities has its own advantages and disadvantages.

Diagnostic peritoneal lavage remains an excellent screening test for evaluating abdominal trauma. The advantages of diagnostic peritoneal lavage include its sensitivity, availability, relative speed with which it can be performed, and low complication rate. A unique advantage of diagnostic peritoneal lavage is its ability to detect early evidence of bowel perforation. Disadvantages, however, include the potential for iatrogenic injury, its misapplication for evaluation of retroperitoneal injuries, and its lack of specificity.

Computed tomography of the abdomen has a greater specificity than diagnostic peritoneal lavage, thus making it the initial diagnostic test of choice at many trauma centers. Oral and intravenous (IV) contrast material should be given to provide optimal resolution. Advantages of CT include its ability to precisely locate intra-abdominal lesions preoperatively, to evaluate the retroperitoneum, to identify injuries that may be managed nonoperatively, and its noninvasiveness. The disadvantages of CT are its expense, time required to perform the study, need to transport the trauma patient to the radiology suite, the need for contrast materials, and a radiation exposure that may be quite significant in the typically young trauma population if this modality is used liberally.

Ultrasonography offers several advantages over diagnostic peritoneal lavage and abdominal CT. Numerous studies have demonstrated that the FAST examination, like diagnostic peritoneal lavage, is an accurate screening tool for abdominal trauma.[1–19] Advantages of the FAST examination are that it is accurate, rapid, noninvasive, repeatable, and portable, and involves no nephrotoxic contrast material or radiation exposure to the patient. There is limited risk for patients who are pregnant, coagulopathic, or have had previous abdominal surgery. The average time to perform a complete FAST examination of the thoracic and abdominal cavities is 2.1 minutes[20] to 4.0 minutes.[12] In addition, investigators have demonstrated that a massive hemoperitoneum may be quickly detected with a single view of Morison's pouch in 82%–90% of hypotensive patients with an abdominal source of bleeding,[18,21] and this required an average of 19 seconds to determine in one study.[18] One major advantage of the FAST examination is the ability to also evaluate for free pericardial and pleural fluid and for pneumothorax. Disadvantages include the inability to determine the exact etiology of the free intraperitoneal fluid and the operator-dependent nature of the examination. Other potential disadvantages of the FAST examination are the difficulty in interpreting the images in patients who are obese or have subcutaneous air or excessive bowel gas, and the inability to distinguish intraperitoneal hemorrhage from ascites.[22] The FAST examination also cannot evaluate the retroperitoneum as well as CT.

In light of the evolving nonoperative approach to certain types of solid-organ injuries, a positive diagnostic peritoneal lavage by itself is becoming less of an indication for immediate exploratory laparotomy than the amount of hemorrhage and the clinical condition of the patient. Since the FAST examination can reliably detect small amounts of free intraperitoneal fluid and can be used to estimate the rate of hemorrhage through serial examinations, ultrasonography has essentially replaced diagnostic peritoneal lavage for most indications in blunt abdominal trauma in the majority of North American trauma centers.[23]

► CLINICAL INDICATIONS

The clinical indications for performing the FAST examination are

- acute blunt or penetrating torso trauma,
- trauma in pregnancy,
- pediatric trauma,
- subacute torso trauma, and
- undifferentiated hypotension.

► ACUTE BLUNT OR PENETRATING TORSO TRAUMA

At Level 1 trauma centers, the primary utilization of the FAST examination has been for the rapid detection of free intraperitoneal fluid in patients who have sustained significant blunt torso trauma. More recently, trauma programs have begun to incorporate the FAST examination into the primary patient assessment for detecting the presence, amount, and location of intracavitary hemorrhage in general.

With blunt trauma, the FAST examination is particularly useful for patients who (1) are too hemodynamically unstable to leave the emergency department for CT scanning; (2) have a physical examination that is unreliable secondary to drug intoxication, distracting injury, or central nervous system injury; and (3) have unexplained hypotension and an equivocal physical examination.

With penetrating trauma patients, the FAST examination should be performed when it is not certain that immediate surgery is indicated. In patients with multiple wounds, the FAST examination can be used to quantify and locate the source of internal hemorrhage. When the trajectory of a penetrating wound is uncertain, the FAST examination may quickly identify the course by the presence of free fluid within the compartments involved.[24] This is particularly helpful when the entry location is the precordium, lower chest, or epigastrium. Inappropriate surgical sequencing has been reported to occur in 44% of patients with wounds in multiple body cavities.[25] In a review of patients with injuries to both the thoracic and abdominal cavities, the investigators regretted their limited use of early FAST examinations in directing surgical sequencing and strongly recommended its increased use in the initial patient evaluation.[25] The FAST examination can therefore be used to prioritize such life-saving interventions as pericardiocentesis, pericardiotomy, thoracostomy, thoracotomy, laparotomy, or sternotomy. The FAST examination is useful in evaluating patients who have sustained stab wounds to the abdomen where local wound exploration indicates that the superficial muscle fascia has been violated. Also, the FAST examination may be useful in confirming a negative physical examination when tangential or lower chest wounds are involved.

In non-Level 1 trauma centers, emergency physicians and surgeons often lack the immediate availability of CT scans and formal two-dimensional (2D) echocardiograms. The availability of bedside ultrasonography and physicians trained to perform the FAST examination in these settings will significantly improve patient evaluation, initial treatment, consultation, and the timely transportation of patients to trauma centers when indicated. When the FAST examination demonstrates intracavitary fluid in these settings, surgeons and operating room personnel can be consulted immediately and/or transportation to a Level 1 trauma center can be initiated. When the diagnostic imaging personnel and surgeons are out of the hospital, and the severity of the patient's injuries is not clinically evident, a positive FAST examination could save up to an hour or more of time to definitive surgical treatment.[26-28]

Although the FAST examination is used most commonly to detect free intraperitoneal fluid, it may also aid in the rapid identification of pneumothorax and free pericardial or pleural fluid, and the evaluation of the fetus in the pregnant trauma patient. In addition, the FAST examination has been evaluated in the management of pediatric trauma patients and can be utilized in patients who present with subacute trauma but with a significant mechanism of injury or concerning physical examination.

▶ DETECTION OF FREE INTRAPERITONEAL FLUID

By the latter half of the 1990s, for patients who had sustained blunt or penetrating abdominal trauma, the FAST examination's utility for detecting free intraperitoneal fluid had been universally recognized. While CT remained the gold standard for detecting specific intra-abdominal pathology, the FAST examination had gained acceptance as a rapid screening tool for identifying free intraperitoneal fluid.

During the 1980s, surgeons in Germany developed bedside utilization of ultrasonography for evaluation of trauma patients. Although excellent results were reported in early studies, with the sensitivity ranging from 84 to 100% and the specificity from 88 to 100%, these findings went largely unnoticed in the United States in part since the articles were not initially translated into English.[2-7]

In the 1990s, a number of prospective studies (with study sizes greater than 100 patients) had been reported on this issue in the English literature.[1,8-19] The majority of these studies focused on the FAST examination

for the evaluation of free intraperitoneal fluid in blunt abdominal trauma patients only. These studies reported the sensitivity and the specificity to range from 69% to 90% and 95% to 100%, respectively.

Tiling *et al.* were the first investigators to suggest that the FAST examination could provide comprehensive evaluation for significant areas of hemorrhage, including pericardial, pleural, intraperitoneal, and retroperitoneal. Their prospective study of 808 blunt trauma patients found a sensitivity of 89% and a specificity of 99% for free intraperitoneal fluid. Their clinical algorithm incorporates the FAST examination during the initial patient evaluation (Figure 5-1).[1]

In one of the first North American trauma ultrasound studies, Rozycki *et al.* demonstrated the FAST examination to have an overall sensitivity of 79% and specificity of 95.6%. They concluded that appropriately trained surgeons could rapidly and accurately perform and interpret FAST examinations and that ultrasound was a rapid, sensitive, and specific diagnostic modality for detecting intraperitoneal fluid and pericardial effusion.[10] In another study, they successfully used ultrasound as the primary adjuvant modality to detect hemoperitoneum and pericardial effusion in injured patients. In the FAST examinations of 371 patients, they had 81.5% sensitivity and 99.7% specificity. The authors stated that ultrasound should be the primary adjuvant instrument for the evaluation of injured patients because it was rapid, accurate, and potentially cost-effective.[11]

In 1995, Ma and Mateer prospectively demonstrated that the FAST examination could serve as a sensitive, specific, and accurate diagnostic tool in the detection of free intraperitoneal and thoracic fluid in patients who

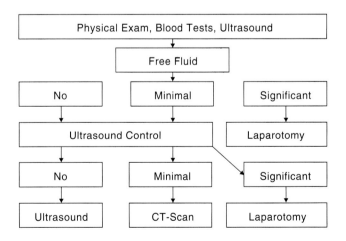

Figure 5-1. Tiling's algorithm for managing blunt abdominal trauma. (From Tiling T, Bouillon B, Schmid A, et al. Ultrasound in blunt abdomino-thoracic trauma, in Border JR, Allgoewer M, Hansen ST, et al. (eds.): *Blunt Multiple Trauma: Comprehensive Pathophysiology and Care.* New York, Marcel Dekker, 415–433, 1990; with permission.)

had sustained major blunt or penetrating trauma. Overall, the FAST examination had a sensitivity of 90%, specificity of 99%, and accuracy of 99%. In evaluating the subgroup of blunt trauma patients, which consisted of 165 of the 245 patients, the FAST examination was 90% sensitive, 99% specific, and 99% accurate. In evaluating the subgroup of penetrating trauma victims, which consisted of 80 of the 245 patients, the FAST examination was 91% sensitive, 100% specific, and 99% accurate.[12] Since emergency physicians performed all the FAST examinations, it became the first prospective study to support that appropriately trained emergency physicians could accurately perform and interpret FAST examinations. The results reiterated that a FAST examination of the entire torso could successfully provide early and valuable information for the presence of free fluid in both the peritoneal and thoracic cavities. In addition, the FAST examination was found to be equally sensitive, specific, and accurate for both blunt and penetrating torso trauma. Penetrating trauma patients could benefit from the rapid and accurate information yielded by ultrasonography.[18,19,24] The identification and localization of significant hemorrhage in penetrating trauma patients would allow physicians "to prioritize resources for resuscitation and evaluation."[10] Most studies have utilized a multiple view FAST examination for evaluation of trauma patients. Some investigators have employed a single view technique, examining only Morison's pouch for free intraperitoneal fluid.[29-31] In one study, all patients were placed in the Trendelenburg position and the perihepatic (Morison's pouch) was the single area examined. The results of this technique were reported to be 81.8% sensitive, 93.9% specific, and 90.9% accurate.[29]

The single-view (perihepatic) imaging technique was compared with the multiple-view technique of the FAST examination for the identification of free intraperitoneal fluid in patients who had sustained major blunt or penetrating torso trauma. For detecting free intraperitoneal fluid, when comparing the multiple-view FAST examination of the abdomen to the gold standard, the multiple-view FAST examination technique had a sensitivity of 87%, a specificity of 99%, and an accuracy of 98%. When comparing the perihepatic single view of the abdomen to the gold standard, the single view FAST examination technique had a sensitivity of 51%, a specificity of 100%, and an accuracy of 93%.[13] Based on this and other studies, the more sensitive and accurate FAST examination method for detecting free intraperitoneal fluid was determined to be the multiple-view technique.[13]

DETECTION OF SOLID ORGAN INJURY

The concept of contrast-enhanced ultrasound may assist clinicians to identify specific organ injuries on the FAST examination.[32-35] Contrast enhanced ultrasound is the application of ultrasound contrast agents to complement or augment traditional sonography. Ultrasound contrast agents are microbubbles that are administered intravenously. The microbubbles vibrate strongly at the high frequencies used in diagnostic ultrasonography, which makes them several thousand times more reflective than normal body tissues. This characteristic allows microbubbles to enhance both grey scale images and flow-mediated Doppler signals. Microbubbles, which are filled with an inert gas, have been found to be as safe as conventional agents in radiography and magnetic resonance imaging.[36] Preliminary reports have demonstrated contrast-enhanced ultrasound as a promising tool for detecting solid organ (liver and spleen) injuries after blunt abdominal trauma. When an ultrasound contract agent was administered immediately before performing the traditional FAST examination, studies have demonstrated that the examination correlated appreciably better than unenhanced sonography for detecting hepatic and splenic injuries and estimating the extent of their injuries.[32-34] Contrast enhanced ultrasound may potentially guide clinicians with the nonoperative management of patients with solid organ injuries after blunt trauma.

CLINICAL ALGORITHMS

Clinical pathways and protocols have been derived from the use of the FAST examination and incorporated with other diagnostic methods commonly used for trauma evaluation in North America (Figure 5-2). An ultrasound-based key clinical pathway has been shown to reduce the number of diagnostic peritoneal lavage procedures and CT scans required to evaluate blunt abdominal trauma without increased risk to the patient. Using the key clinical pathway, diagnostic peritoneal lavage procedures were reduced from 17 to 4%, and CT scans reduced from 56 to 26%. The injury severity score increased from 11.6 to 21.5 for diagnostic peritoneal lavage patients and from 4.6 to 8.3 for CT scan patients. FAST examinations were used exclusively in 65% of the patients. This ultrasound-based key clinical pathway was found to result in significant reductions in the utilization of diagnostic peritoneal lavage and CT scanning in the evaluation of blunt abdominal trauma without increased risk to the patient (Figure 5-3). The investigators estimated cost savings of $450,000 per year, using this key clinical pathway.[37] The issue of cost savings of the FAST examination has also been addressed in another study. For blunt trauma patients, the FAST examination was found to be more efficient and cost-effective than CT scanning or diagnostic peritoneal lavage. There was a significantly shorter time to disposition at approximately one third the cost in the ultrasonography group.[38]

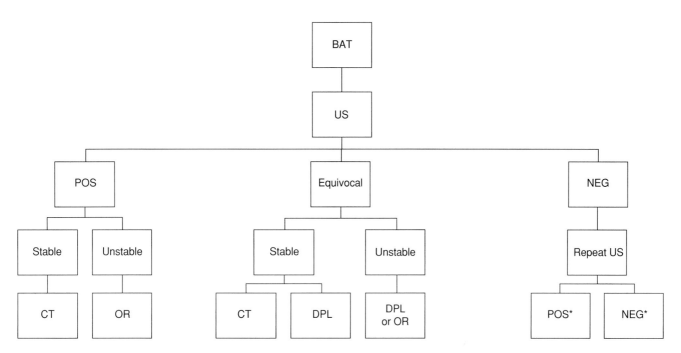

Figure 5-2. Suggested algorithm for the use of ultrasonography in the evaluation of the patient with blunt abdominal trauma. (From Rozycki GS, Shackford SR: Ultrasound: What every trauma surgeon should know. *J Trauma* 40:2, 1996, with permission.)

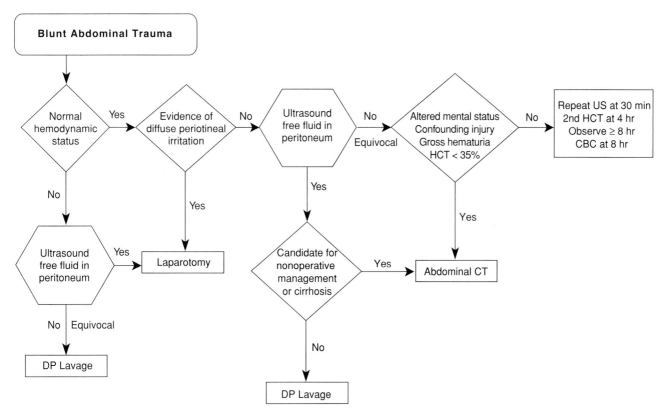

Figure 5-3. Key clinical pathway for the evaluation of blunt abdominal trauma. (From Branney SW, Moore EE, Cantrill S, et al.: Ultrasound-based key clinical pathway reduces the use of hospital resources for the evaluation of blunt abdominal trauma. *J Trauma* 42:1086–1090, 1997, with permission.)

An ultrasound-based scoring system has been developed to quantify the amount of intraperitoneal blood in blunt abdominal trauma patients and to assess the need for therapeutic exploratory laparotomy. Scores ranged from 0 to 8. The system assigned two points for significant fluid collections ≥2 cm and one point for fluid collections ≤2 cm. A score of 3 correlated with 1000 mL of fluid. In the study, of those patients who had a score of 3 or more, 24 of 25 patients (96%) required therapeutic laparotomy. Of those who had a score of less than 3, therapeutic laparotomy was required in only 9 of 24 patients (38%). The FAST examination was found to be a useful adjunct in helping to make clinical decisions during the resuscitation period.[39] In another study evaluating the role of the FAST examination in determining the need for therapeutic laparotomy, none of the patients with negative FAST examination results died or sustained identifiable mortality as a consequence of their negative scans.[40]

DETECTION OF PERICARDIAL FLUID

In the hypotensive patient who has sustained penetrating trauma to the torso, the echocardiographic portion of the FAST examination may prove to be the most beneficial aspect. Echocardiography remains the gold standard diagnostic procedure for detecting pericardial effusions. The classic physical examination findings of acute cardiac tamponade—distended neck veins, hypotension, and muffled heart tones—are present in less than 40% of patients with surgically proven cardiac tamponade.[41] Timely emergency department procedures and expeditious transportation of the patient to the operating room may be accomplished by ultrasound diagnosis of hemopericardium.

In 1992, Plummer and coinvestigators evaluated the effect of bedside echocardiography performed by emergency physicians on the outcome of 49 patients with penetrating cardiac injuries over a 10-year period. Compared to a retrospective control group, the use of bedside echocardiography significantly reduced the time of diagnosis and disposition to the operating room from 42.4 ± 21.7 minutes to 15.5 ± 11.4 minutes while the actual survival improved from 57.1 to 100%.[42]

The accuracy of emergency ultrasound has been evaluated after it was introduced into five Level I trauma centers for the diagnosis of acute hemopericardium. Surgeons or cardiologists (four centers) and technicians (one center) performed pericardial ultrasound examinations on patients with penetrating truncal wounds. By protocol, patients with positive examinations underwent immediate operation. In 261 patients, pericardial ultrasound examinations were found to have a sensitivity of 100%, specificity of 96.9%, and accuracy of 97.3%. The mean time from ultrasound to operation was 12.1 ±

5 minutes. This further demonstrated that ultrasound should be the initial modality for the evaluation of patients with penetrating precordial wounds because it is accurate and rapid.[43]

Over the years, numerous studies have examined the role of echocardiography in blunt cardiac trauma. The utility and role of ultrasound, particularly with the diagnosis of cardiac contusion, remain unclear (see chapter 5, "Cardiac," for a comprehensive review of this topic).

DETECTION OF PLEURAL FLUID

Since patients who have sustained major trauma routinely present to the emergency department immobilized on a long spine board, clinicians may have difficulty identifying bilateral hemothoraces or a small unilateral hemothorax on the initial supine chest radiograph. The FAST examination can detect hemothorax before the completion of a chest radiograph or can be used as additional information when the chest radiograph is equivocal.

Of the six anatomic areas scanned by the FAST examination, only two are required to identify the presence of free pleural fluid in the two pleural cavities. Thus, tube thoracostomy for trauma patients may be expedited with the use of ultrasonography.

Ma and Mateer demonstrated that the FAST examination could serve as a sensitive, specific, and accurate diagnostic tool in detecting hemothorax in major trauma patients. When comparing the FAST examination and the chest radiograph to the criterion standard definitions, both diagnostic tests had an equal sensitivity (96.2%), specificity (100%), and accuracy (99.6%) for detecting pleural fluid. They concluded that ultrasonography was comparable to the chest radiograph for identifying hemothorax.[44]

Ultrasonography can detect smaller quantities of pleural fluid than the chest radiograph. It is estimated that an upright chest radiograph can accurately detect a minimum of 50–100 mL of pleural fluid[45] and that a supine chest radiograph can detect a minimum of 175 mL of pleural fluid.[46] By contrast, it is estimated that ultrasonography can detect a minimum of 20 mL of pleural fluid.[9] Also, ultrasonography can help differentiate between pleural fluid and pleural thickening or pulmonary contusion when the supine chest radiograph is equivocal.

Although the FAST examination cannot completely replace the chest radiograph, it can complement chest radiograph findings by rapidly identifying hemothorax in the supine patient. By utilizing the FAST examination to initially identify hemothorax, the standard chest radiograph of the trauma patient can be performed after tube thoracostomy, thereby sparing the patient an additional chest radiograph.

DETECTION OF PNEUMOTHORAX

Not only can the FAST examination detect a hemothorax, it can also identify a pneumothorax before the completion of a chest radiograph. This is especially relevant since the reported proportion of pneumothoraces that are occult compared to those actually seen on the chest radiograph ranges from 29 to 72%.[47–52] The concept of using ultrasound to exclude the presence of a pneumothorax relies on the simple premise that if the two pleural surfaces are normally in apposition, then an intrapleural collection of air (pneumothorax) cannot be separating them. The focused goal is to identify the contiguity of the visceral and parietal pleura using simple sonographic signs to exclude the presence of a pneumothorax. This diagnostic test is considered to be an extended FAST (EFAST) examination.[51] With experience, a pneumothorax can be expeditiously excluded in the vast majority of cases.[53]

Detecting a pneumothorax with ultrasound may initially appear to be paradoxical since air has the highest acoustic impedance of normal body substances, with almost complete reflectance of sounds waves at commonly used frequencies.[54] Thus, only artifacts are normally seen deep to the pleural interface in the normal lung.[55] Both hemothoraces and pneumothoraces, however, are superficial pleural-based diseases and, therefore, lend themselves to sonographic examination.

Unless there are pleural adhesions from previous disease or injury (a condition that reduces the risk of pneumothorax), normal respiration is associated with a physiologic sliding of the two pleural surfaces upon one another. The most common normal sign on sonography, which in essence excludes the presence of a pneumothorax, is lung sliding.[48,51,53] For this physiologic "lung sliding" along the visceral–parietal pleural interface to be seen, both surfaces must be accessible for imaging and must be either contiguous or separated by a layer of fluid.[50,51,56] This movement is better visualized at the lung bases and less so at the apices.[53] A notable exception is when subcutaneous emphysema superimposes itself between the skin and parietal pleura, a clinical situation that is associated with a specificity of 98% for underlying occult pneumothorax.[57] Examining the pleural interfaces with the color power Doppler mode can enhance the depiction of this sliding movement due to power Doppler's ability to detect motion, a finding that has been designated the "Power Slide."[49] Power Doppler is superior to conventional color Doppler in determining the presence or absence of flow at the expense of direction and speed information and thus has the ability to identify low-velocity and low-volume flow (or motion).[49,58,59] It also documents a real-time physiologic process as occurring in a single image, allowing for simpler archiving and tele-transmission. In a similar way, the use of M mode imaging documents either the presence of lung sliding ("seashore sign") or its absence when a pneumothorax is present ("stratosphere sign") since the pleural movement will normally generate a homogenous granular pattern in this mode.[53,60] An intermediate sign that is best documented in M mode is the "lung point" sign, which is visualized when the lung intermittently contacts the parietal pleura with inspiration, thus alternating between the seashore and stratospheric signs.

Another normal sign is the comet tail artifact, which is a reverberation artifact that arises from distended water-filled interlobular septae under the visceral pleura. Comet tail artifacts are presumed to be the ultrasound equivalents of Kerley B lines seen on a chest radiograph.[53,61] Being related to the visceral pleura, comet tail artifacts can be seen only when the visceral pleura is in apposition to the parietal pleura. When a pneumothorax is present, the intrapleural air will separate the two pleural surfaces, and the "normal" signs will not be seen. Instead, the only images that will appear to be deep to this level are horizontal reverberation artifacts, which are often seen as a "mirror image" of the chest wall.

Lichtenstein and coworkers have described a standardized, but hierarchal thoracic examination whose scope depends on the clinical status and mobility of the patient. They designate the A-line as a brightly echogenic line between the rib shadows recurring at an interval that exactly replicates the interval between the skin and pleural line, and represents the horizontal reverberation artifact generated by the parietal pleura.[53]

If both lung sliding and comet tail artifacts are present, then the clinician can confidently exclude the presence of a pneumothorax. If lung sliding and comet tail artifacts are not visible, then the examiner should suspect the presence of a pneumothorax, a suspicion further heightened by the presence of the horizontal reverberation artifact (A-line).[62,63] In 200 consecutive undifferentiated ICU patients who went on to CT scanning, Lichtenstein and coworkers were able to note absent lung sliding in all patients with occult pneumothoraces; 41 of 43 patients had an A-line sign. The absence of lung sliding alone had 100% sensitivity, but only 78% specificity for diagnosing an occult pneumothorax. When an A-line was seen with absent lung sliding, there was 95% sensitivity and 94% specificity for diagnosing an occult pneumothorax.[60] The presence of a lung point had 100% specificity for an occult pneumothorax. Kirkpatrick and coinvestigators prospectively evaluated a handheld ultrasound device in the real-time resuscitation of critically ill patients.[51] This study focused on the most difficult-to-diagnose subset of pneumothoraces, as any patient with a clinically evident pneumothorax was treated without any imaging and those patients with clear-cut pneumothoraces on chest radiograph were excluded as well. In the remaining clinically stable patients, when comparing EFAST directly to chest radiography, the EFAST examination was more sensitive for the detection of occult pneumothoraces after trauma (49% versus 21%). Using CT corroboration, there were 22 false negative studies with EFAST compared to 34 with chest radiography.[51] Blaivas and coworkers studied 176 patients by systematically examining four thoracic locations, ranging from the 2nd intercostal space in the midclavicular line to the 6th intercostal space at the posterior axillary line. They searched for lung sliding, supplemented by color power Doppler when lung sliding was not easily detected, and assessed the relative size of the pneumothorax by correlating the relative topography of lung sliding. Overall, they noted the sensitivity and specificity of ultrasound to be 98% and 99%, respectively, compared with 76% and 100%, respectively, for chest radiography in this setting.[64]

Reflecting on basic principles, the EFAST technique has an inherent advantage over chest radiography due to the physiologic behavior of pneumothoraces in the supine patient. Because of the effect of gravity, the supine lung tends to hinge dorsally, with free air collecting anteromedially.[65–69] Supine pneumothoraces are reported to be most commonly located at the anterior (84%), apical (57%), basal (41%), medial (27%), lateral (24%), and never posterior (0%) lung locations.[70] The standard imaging anatomic sites for the EFAST were chosen to correspond to the recommended auscultatory locations from the Advanced Trauma Life Support course.[71]

Despite the fact that pneumothoraces are often dynamic processes, clinical management is often based on the perceived size of a pneumothorax. Allowing for other factors such as the need for transport and positive pressure ventilation, many small pneumothoraces are managed expectantly, whereas large ones are drained. Thus, it is pertinent to ask whether ultrasound may be of help in determining the size of pneumothoraces. While it was once believed that sonography was of no use in determining the volume of a pneumothorax,[55] it is now suggested that sonography may actually have utility in determining not only the presence, but actual extent of a pneumothorax.[68]

The presence of a "lung point" sign is not only 100% specific for pneumothorax, but the location of this sign roughly correlates with the radiographic size of the pneumothorax.[63] A "partial sliding" sign has been described to represent the same phenomenon whereby smaller or occult pneumothoraces might be detected.[72] Also, a good correlation between the estimates of pneumothorax size and CT findings using the relative thoracic topography of lung sliding has been noted.[64]

▶ TRAUMA IN PREGNANCY

Trauma continues to be one of the leading causes of nonobstetrical mortality in pregnant patients.[73] Moreover, it contributes to fetal death more frequently than maternal death.[74–78] Ultrasonography may be a valuable

adjunct for rapid diagnosis of traumatic injuries for both the mother and the fetus.[79–81]

The pregnant trauma patient presents unique diagnostic and management issues for the emergency physician and trauma surgeon. Maternal shock carries a high fetal mortality rate.[77] Although there are two lives at stake, proper assessment and stabilization of the mother will provide the best opportunity for fetal stability. Therefore, rapid assessment of the pregnant trauma patient is essential for early identification of life-threatening injuries. The FAST examination clearly may play a role in the timely assessment of pregnant trauma patients.

In this setting, ultrasonography offers several advantages over abdominal CT scan and diagnostic peritoneal lavage. The FAST examination may aid in the timely identification of pregnant trauma patients who need exploratory laparotomy immediately, and may help avoid delays in management while other diagnostic tests are obtained. The FAST examination can be performed at the bedside and involves no contrast material or radiation exposure to the mother or the fetus. Sonography can rapidly assess the pregnant trauma patient for hemoperitoneum and intrathoracic hemorrhage, and can assess the fetus for fetal heart tones, activity, and approximate gestational age. While ultrasonography is useful for identifying fetal heart tones and fetal movement, it is not as accurate in diagnosing uterine rupture or placental abruption, and it may be more technically difficult for advanced third-trimester pregnancy.[82]

The identification of free intraperitoneal fluid may be related to hemorrhage from solid organ injuries or amniotic fluid from uterine rupture or both. Ultrasonography should not be considered a reliable method for the specific identification of uterine rupture. The presence of an intrauterine organized hematoma and/or oligohydramnios, however, may suggest this diagnosis. Finally, although ultrasonography can be utilized to confirm immediate fetal viability, it cannot be used to rule out fetal–placental injury. While ultrasonography is used as an adjunct for the diagnosis of placental abruption, it is not sufficiently sensitive to exclude this diagnosis.[82] Continuous cardiotocographic monitoring, which has been demonstrated to accurately detect significant placental abruption, should be utilized as early as possible for all pregnant patients with significant blunt trauma.[83] (Please see chapter 13, Second and Third-Trimester Pregnancy, for further reading.)

▶ PEDIATRIC TRAUMA

The precise role of the FAST examination in evaluating pediatric trauma patients has not been as well defined as in adults. The utilization of bedside ultrasonography in a pediatric trauma center setting was pioneered in Montreal, Quebec, Canada, in the late 1970s. Their accuracy for detecting splenic and hepatic injuries approached 90% with experience. Bedside ultrasonography has become their initial diagnostic procedure of choice unless multiple organs are involved (particularly head trauma) in which case CT is initially utilized.[84] Later reports from their medical center (1993) confirmed the continued utilization of the FAST examination. In children, the bedside FAST examination holds several advantages. It obviates the need for sedation prior to CT. The thin abdominal wall of children enhances the resolution of the ultrasound image. Also, CT can be more difficult to interpret in children because of the relative lack of intraperitoneal fat stripes.[85]

Subsequent studies, primarily performed by radiologists, have not been as optimistic with their results for pediatric trauma. Two studies demonstrated that 31–37% of children with solid organ injuries do not have associated hemoperitoneum.[86,87] This finding potentially would limit the utility of the FAST examination in this setting since the underlying premise of the technique is to detect free fluid. Other studies have shown the sensitivity of the FAST examination in children to range from 30 to 80% and the specificity to range from 95% to 100%.[88–90] A surgeon-performed FAST examination demonstrated a sensitivity of 81%, specificity of 100%, and accuracy of 97% in 85 children who sustained blunt abdominal trauma.[91] The FAST examination's sensitivity in children appears to fall short of the results found in adult trauma patients, and this may be due to the unique pathophysiology of pediatric trauma patients. As further clinical studies are performed, investigators should consider the opinion by Luks *et al.*, "The use of ultrasound in the primary evaluation of blunt abdominal trauma does not require it to surpass other modalities in diagnostic accuracy, as long as it identifies all potentially life-threatening conditions." Although ultrasound alone was not always diagnostic, there were no false positive or false negative results when used in conjunction with a clinical protocol.[85] Since the vast majority of solid organ injuries are managed nonoperatively in the pediatric population, the important applicability of serial examinations with ultrasonography may be further demonstrated in the future.

▶ SUBACUTE TRAUMA

Patients occasionally present one or more days after the traumatic event with complaints of chest or abdominal pain. The issues of evolving hemothorax, hemoperitoneum, or subcapsular organ hemorrhage should be considered. When solid organ injuries are strongly considered, CT scanning is the preferred diagnostic method. When the index of suspicion is lower, bedside ultrasonography can be utilized to confirm the absence of unexpected abnormalities. A common scenario is a patient with suspected left-sided rib injuries who has left upper quadrant abdominal tenderness on examination. With subacute trauma, a splenic injury is likely to have evolved to the point where it could be detected by ultrasonography. The confirmation of a normal perisplenic ultrasound examination (without hemoperitoneum or subcapsular hemorrhage) would validate the clinician's suspicion of an isolated ribcage injury. In this case, an unexpected abnormal ultrasound examination would significantly alter the patient's treatment and disposition.

▶ UNDIFFERENTIATED HYPOTENSION

Patients who present with a history of trauma and hypotension should be managed as hemorrhagic shock until proven otherwise. In some cases, however, the initial assessment and FAST examination may not be consistent with hemorrhage as the etiology of shock. A classic example is the "trauma" patient with a minor mechanism for injury but further history determines the event was preceded by syncope. In patients with a negative FAST examination and no significant external hemorrhage, bedside ultrasound may be of further use for determining the cause of hypotension. A patient presenting to the emergency department with unexplained or undifferentiated hypotension often represents a highly stressful situation for the clinician. In nontrauma patients, emergency physicians determine the diagnosis in only 24% of cases of undifferentiated hypotension.[92] Patient survival often depends upon making a rapid diagnosis to direct specific therapy since sustained hypotension is the greatest predictor of adverse outcome[93] and instituting the wrong therapy can be catastrophic.

Recognizing that bedside ultrasound, especially utilizing FAST examination principles, can address the detection of multiple life-threatening conditions, a number of groups have recently formalized resuscitative protocols for the patient with undifferentiated hypotension. In 2001, Rose and colleagues described the combination of an abdominal evaluation, a qualitative cardiac assessment, and an evaluation of the abdominal aorta to assess for hemoperitoneum, pericardial effusion, and ruptured abdominal aortic aneurysm, respectively.[94] The protocol was based on the underlying premise that acute sonographic findings would not be subtle in the hypotensive patient. The examination was meant to be a focused, goal-directed, and systematic approach, with an emphasis on ruling in obvious pathology rather than definitively excluding conditions not seen.[94]

Another study examined the incorporation of a goal-directed ultrasound protocol in evaluating undifferentiated hypotension. Patients who underwent immediate ultrasound examinations had a significantly smaller number of viable diagnoses, and more often the correct one, after 15 minutes of care than those patients who had a delayed ultrasound examination.[95] The majority of patients were found to have diagnoses that warranted specific treatments beyond fluid resuscitation. In addition to the views utilized by Rose, this protocol included an assessment of the degree of inferior vena cava collapse with inspiration as an indicator of intravascular volume status as well as parasternal long cardiac and apical four-chamber views for a qualitative estimation of left ventricular function. Each view used was intended to answer a binary question regarding the obvious presence of pericardial tamponade, left ventricular dysfunction, right ventricular dilatation, intravascular volume depletion, intraperitoneal free fluid, and the presence of an aortic aneurysm. Despite the more detailed examination, the time taken per examination averaged 5.8 minutes. A hyperdynamic left ventricular function was found to be a strong independent predictor of sepsis among these patients, performing better than traditional markers such as the white blood cell count or fever.[96] Studies support that physicians with basic ultrasound skills who undertake limited but focused training in echocardiography can estimate left ventricular function with accuracy when assessed as poor (ejection fraction < 30%), moderate (30% < ejection fraction < 55%), or hyperdynamic/normal (ejection fraction > 55%).[92,97]

▶ ANATOMIC CONSIDERATIONS

The shape of the peritoneal cavity provides three dependent areas when a patient is in the supine position. These areas are divided by the spine longitudinally and the pelvic brim transversely. The site of accumulation of intraperitoneal fluid is dependent on the position of the patient and the source of bleeding.[13] Free intraperitoneal fluid has the propensity to collect in dependent intraperitoneal compartments formed by peritoneal reflections and mesenteric attachments (Figure 5-4).

The main compartment of the peritoneal cavity is the greater sac, which is divided into the supramesocolic and inframesocolic compartments. These two compartments are connected by the paracolic gutters. The right paracolic gutter connects Morison's pouch with the pelvis. Morison's pouch is the potential space between the liver and the right kidney. The left paracolic gutter is more shallow than the right and its course to the splenorenal recess is blocked by the phrenicocolic ligament. Thus, free fluid will tend to flow via the right paracolic gutter since there is less resistance. In the supine patient, the most dependent area of the supramesocolic compartment is Morison's pouch. Overall, however, the rectovesical pouch is the most dependent area of the supine male and the pouch of Douglas is the most dependent area of the supine female.[98]

In the supine patient, free intraperitoneal fluid in the right upper quadrant will tend to accumulate in Morison's pouch first before overflowing down the right paracolic gutter to the pelvis. In contrast, free intraperitoneal fluid in the left upper quadrant will tend to accumulate in the left subphrenic space first, and not the splenorenal recess, which is the potential space between the spleen and the left kidney. Free fluid overflowing from the left subphrenic space will travel into the splenorenal recess and then down the left paracolic gutter into the pelvis. Free fluid from the lesser peritoneal sac will travel across the epiploic foramen to Morison's pouch. Free intraperitoneal fluid in the pelvis will tend to accumulate in the rectovesical pouch in the supine male and the pouch of Douglas in the supine female (Figure 5-5).[98]

Positioning of the patient during the FAST examination may allow redistribution of free fluid in some cases but it may require patient angles of 30° to 45° (decubitus or Trendelenburg) for fluid to flow completely over the spine or pelvic brim. In addition, intraperitoneal hemorrhage often results in a combination of liquid and clotted blood. The organized hemorrhage may not redistribute to another compartment with patient repositioning.

If an initial abbreviated FAST examination is required, the data from one study suggest that for supine patients, an isolated pelvic view may provide a slightly greater yield (68% sensitivity) than does an isolated view of Morison's pouch (59% sensitivity) in the identification of free intraperitoneal fluid.[13]

The quantity of free intraperitoneal fluid that can accurately be detected on ultrasound has been reported to be as little as 100 mL.[8] Tiling considered a small anechoic stripe in Morison's pouch to represent about 250 mL of fluid and a 0.5-cm anechoic stripe to correspond to more than 500 mL of fluid within the peritoneum.[1]

▶ GETTING STARTED

The FAST examination consists of multiple ultrasound views of the abdomen and lower thorax. The standard examination is performed with the patient in the supine position. In general, the sonologist should stand on the right side of the patient's bed next to the ultrasound machine. Left-handed dominance, room configuration, or other ongoing procedures may alter this arrangement. The patient's torso should be exposed from the clavicles to the symphysis pubis.

A standard 3.5 MHz microconvex probe is commonly used because the footprint of the transducer can scan between the ribs during the evaluation of the thorax and upper quadrant views. Although they may have some limitations for this examination, a phased array, mechanical sector, or standard curved array probe

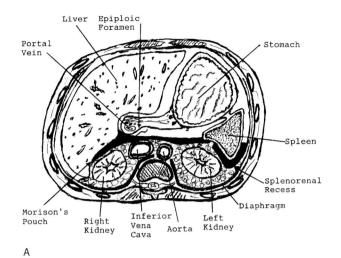

A

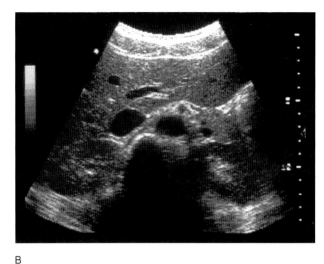

B

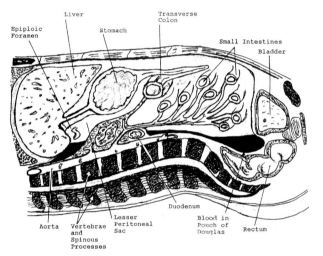

C

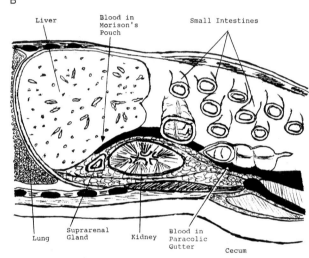

D

E

Figure 5-4. Transverse illustration of the upper abdomen that demonstrates the dependent compartments where free intraperitoneal fluid may collect (A). A transverse ultrasound view of the normal upper abdomen is depicted for comparison (B). Longitudinal illustration of the midline (C) and right paramedian abdomen (D) which demonstrate the dependent compartments where free intraperitoneal fluid may collect. A longitudinal ultrasound view of the normal right upper abdomen is depicted for comparison (E). (Courtesy of Lori Sens and Lori Green, *Gulfcoast Ultrasound*; (B),(E); Mark Hoffmann, MD, (A),(C),(D))

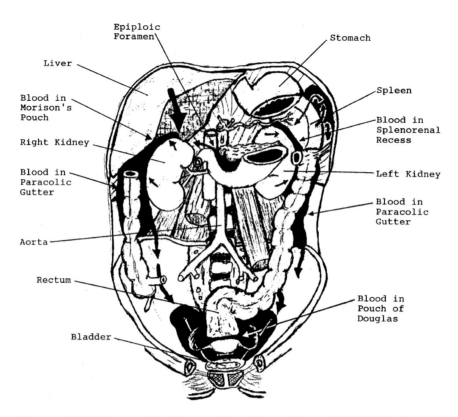

Figure 5-5. Movement patterns of free intraperitoneal fluid within the abdominal cavity. (Courtesy of Mark Hoffmann, MD)

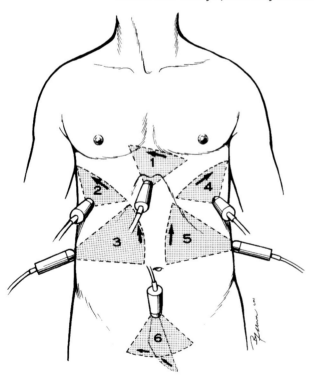

Figure 5-6. Ultrasound probe positions for the focused assessment with sonography for trauma (FAST) examination. (Reprinted with permission from Ma OJ, Mateer JR, Ogata M, et al.: Prospective analysis of a rapid trauma ultrasound examination performed by emergency physicians. *J Trauma* 1995;38:879–885.)

also may be used. A sweeping motion of the transducer should be used for each view to maximize the information obtained. The scan planes are longitudinal (sagittal), transverse, and coronal. Figure 5-6 demonstrates the six areas of the basic FAST examination protocol. The sonologist should perform each FAST examination in a systematic manner. We recommend that the FAST examination be performed using a standard sequence whenever possible: begin by examining the subxiphoid four-chamber view of the heart, move next to the right intercostal oblique and right coronal views, then examine the left intercostal oblique and left coronal views, and conclude by examining the pelvic (longitudinal and transverse) views. For the EFAST examination, the transthoracic views should be assessed after these standard views.

The sensitivity of the FAST examination may be influenced by a number of factors, which include the experience of the sonographer, type of equipment, timing of the FAST examination during the resuscitation, performance of serial examinations, the number of anatomical areas examined, and the position of the patient.

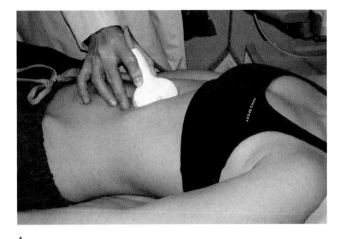

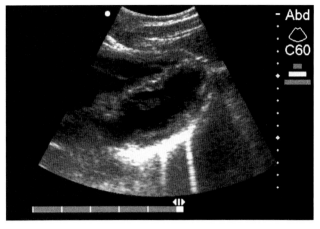

A

B

Figure 5-7. Subxiphoid four-chamber view of the heart. Probe position (A) and corresponding ultrasound image (B). The normal pericardium is seen as a hyperechoic (white) line surrounding the heart.

▶ TECHNIQUE AND NORMAL ULTRASOUND FINDINGS

The subxiphoid four-chamber view of the heart (Figure 5-6, area 1) should be used to examine for free pericardial fluid. For this pericardial view, the ultrasound probe is placed in the subxiphoid area and angled toward the patient's left shoulder. A coronal section of the heart should provide an adequate four-chamber view of the heart. From this view, global cardiac function and chamber size can be inspected briefly. The normal pericardium is seen as a hyperechoic (white) line surrounding the heart and, by using an anterior to posterior sweeping motion, the pericardium can be fully evaluated (Figure 5-7).

Next, the right intercostal oblique and right coronal views (Figure 5-6, areas 2 and 3, respectively) should be used to examine right pleural effusion, free fluid in Morison's pouch, and free fluid in the right paracolic gutter. From these views, the right diaphragm, the right lobe of the liver, and the right kidney also should be inspected briefly. For these perihepatic views, the ultrasound probe is placed in the mid-axillary line between the 8th and 11th ribs with an oblique scanning plane. The probe indicator should be pointing toward the right posterior axilla at the proper angle to keep the image plane between the ribs. The liver, right kidney, and Morison's pouch should be readily identified (Figure 5-8). The angle of the probe can be directed more cephalad to examine for pleural fluid superior to the right diaphragm. The right diaphragm appears as a hyperechoic structure; pleural fluid can be identified as an anechoic stripe superior to the diaphragm. The right pararenal retroperitoneum and paracolic gutter are viewed by rotating the transducer to the coronal imaging plane (probe indicator toward the axilla) and positioning the probe caudally below the 11th rib in the mid- to posterior axillary line (Figure 5-9).

The left intercostal oblique and left coronal views (Figure 5-6, areas 4 and 5, respectively) should be used to examine left pleural effusion, free fluid in the subphrenic space and splenorenal recess, and free fluid in the left paracolic gutter. From these views, the left diaphragm, the spleen, and the left kidney also should be inspected briefly. For these perisplenic views, the ultrasound probe is placed at the left posterior axillary line between the 8th and 11th ribs with an oblique scanning plane. The probe indicator should be pointing toward the left posterior axilla. If the left kidney is identified first, then the probe should be directed slightly more cephalad to locate the spleen (Figure 5-10). The angle of the probe can then be directed more cephalad to examine for pleural fluid superior to the left diaphragm. The left diaphragm appears as a hyperechoic structure; pleural fluid can be identified as an anechoic stripe superior to the diaphragm. The left pararenal retroperitoneum and paracolic gutter are viewed by rotating the transducer to the coronal imaging plane (probe indicator toward the axilla) and positioning the probe caudally below the 11th rib in the mid- to posterior axillary line. The left kidney is often more difficult to visualize than the right kidney because it is positioned higher in the abdomen and can be obscured by overlying gas in the stomach and colon (Figure 5-11). Another reason why the left kidney may be more difficult to visualize is that the spleen is a smaller organ than the liver, thus providing a much smaller acoustic window. Renal imaging may be facilitated in some patients by initiating a deep inspiration during this portion of the examination.

The pelvic (longitudinal and transverse) views (Figure 5-6, area 6) should be used to examine for free

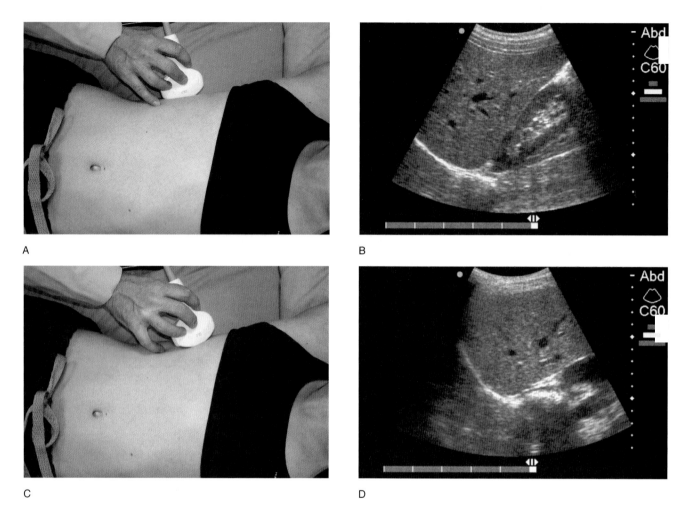

Figure 5-8. Right intercostal oblique view. Probe position (A) and corresponding ultrasound image (B). The liver, right kidney, and Morison's pouch are readily identified. Right intercostal oblique view. Probe position (C) and corresponding ultrasound image (D). The right diaphragm appears as a hyperechoic structure.

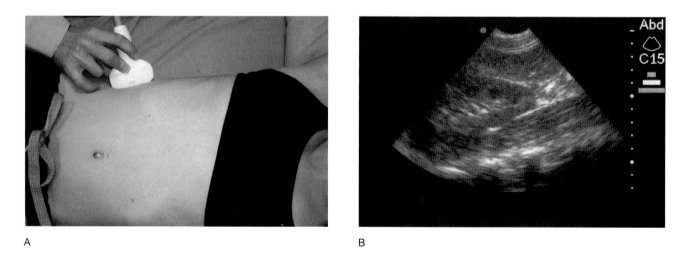

Figure 5-9. Right coronal view. Probe position (A) and corresponding ultrasound image (B). The right pararenal retroperitoneum and paracolic gutter areas are identified above the psoas muscle in this view.

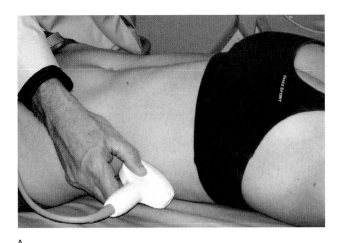

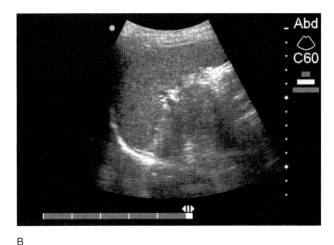

A

B

Figure 5-10. Left intercostal oblique view. Probe position (A) and corresponding ultrasound image (B). A longitudinal view of the spleen, a portion of the diaphragm and surrounding areas are visualized.

fluid in the anterior pelvis or cul-de-sac (pouch of Douglas). Ideally, these views should be obtained before the placement of a Foley catheter. From these views, the bladder, the prostate or uterus, and the lateral walls of the pelvis also should be inspected briefly (Figure 5-12). For these pelvic views, the ultrasound probe should be placed 2 cm superior to the symphysis pubis along the midline of the abdomen with the scanning plane oriented longitudinally and the probe aimed caudally into the pelvis. The probe indicator should be pointing toward the patient's head. The probe is then rotated 90° counterclockwise to obtain transverse images of the pelvis. Fluid in a filled bladder appears as a well-circumscribed and contained fluid collection that appears anechoic. In women, the uterus will be seen posterior to the bladder. A partially filled bladder can be differentiated from free peritoneal fluid by emptying the bladder (Foley catheter) or by retrograde bladder filling and repeating the examination.

Finally, to evaluate for a pneumothorax in the EFAST examination, the use of a high-frequency linear array transducer whose footprint fits well between the rib spaces is advisable since it provides the best resolution of the pleural interface. However, the performance of the EFAST examination for pneumothorax is most practically initiated using the same probe as was used for the FAST examination. In fact, some diagnostic artifacts are more obvious with a lower frequency transducer (3.5 MHz) as opposed to the high-frequency linear array (7.5+ MHz).

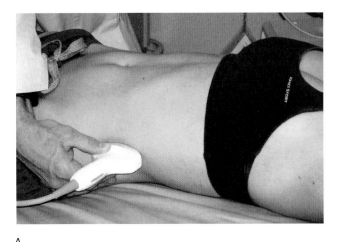

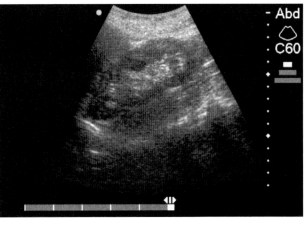

A

B

Figure 5-11. Left coronal view. Probe position (A) and corresponding ultrasound image (B). The left pararenal, paracolic gutter areas and kidney are examined in this view.

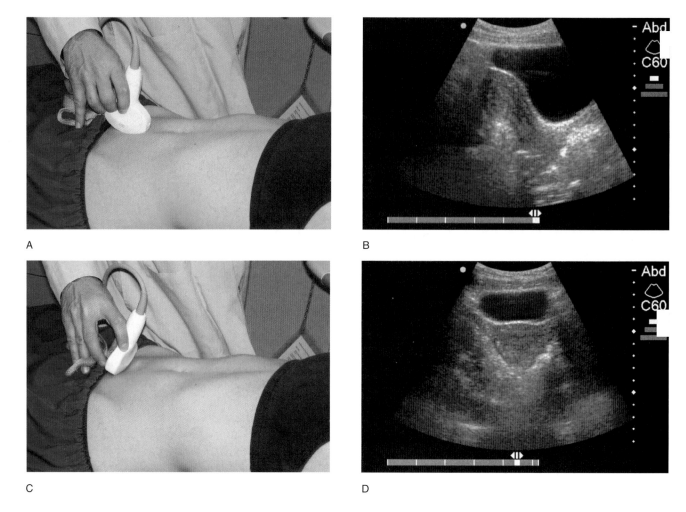

A

B

C

D

Figure 5-12. Pelvic longitudinal views. Probe position (A) and corresponding ultrasound image (B). Ideally, these pelvic views should be obtained before the placement of a Foley catheter. Pelvic transverse views. Probe position (C) and corresponding ultrasound image (D). In addition to potential fluid spaces, the bladder, the prostate or uterus, and the lateral walls of the pelvis can also be inspected briefly.

Regardless of which transducer is selected, the probe should first be oriented longitudinally on the anterior chest wall at the mid-clavicular line. This produces an image perpendicular to the ribs to identify the echogenic pleural interface in reference to the overlying (and acoustically impervious) ribs (Figure 5-13). The image of the two ribs separated by the pleural line is known as the "bat-sign" and is a basic landmark of lung sonography. Once this view is obtained, the sonologist should look for respiratory motion at the interface (lung sliding) and for the presence of normal comet tail artifacts and the A-line (Figure 5-14). Power Doppler (Figure 5-15) and M-mode analysis (Figure 5-16) may further document normal lung sliding. Estimating the size of a pneumothorax can be facilitated by rotating the probe orientation parallel to the ribs and sliding the probe laterally within successive rib interspaces (Figure 5-17). Detection of an image where partial sliding or a lung point is present marks the lateral aspect of a pneumothorax. For some patients, use of a high-frequency linear array probe (when available) may enhance visualization of the pleura and detection of normal lung sliding.

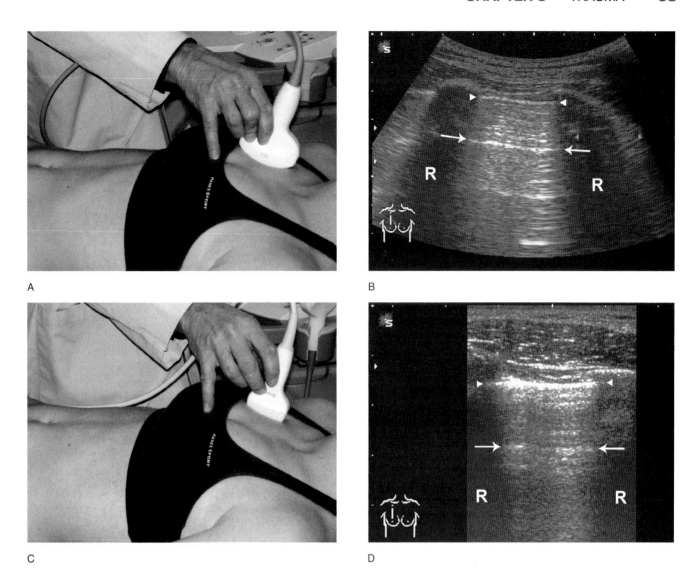

A

B

C

D

Figure 5-13. Longitudinal view: "Bat sign." Normal lung with 3.5 MHz curved array probe. Probe position (A) and corresponding ultrasound image (B). This probe may allow a view of more than one rib interspace and can show normal artifacts more consistently. The A-line (arrows) is obvious and repeats at regular intervals. Normal lung with 7.5–10 MHz linear array probe. Probe position (C) and corresponding ultrasound image (D). This probe provides more detail of the pleural interface (arrowheads) and better visualization of sliding in real time. R = rib shadow.

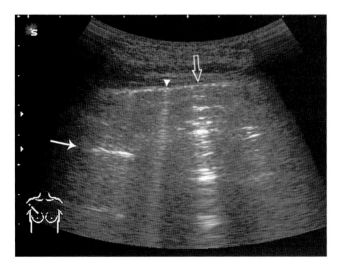

Figure 5-14. Normal lung artifacts (3.5 MHz). The A-line represents the horizontal reverberation artifact generated by the parietal pleura (arrow). Comet tail artifacts arise from the pleura and project to the depth of the image. They move back and forth along with the pleura in real time and may vary between a narrow (arrowhead) or wider (open arrow) appearance.

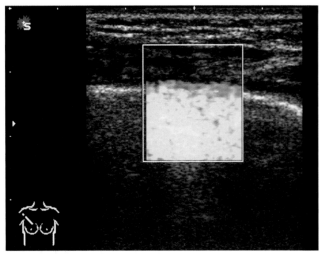

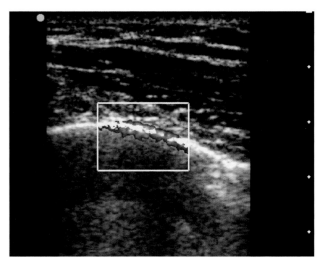

A   B

Figure 5-15. Power Doppler of normal lung (7.5–10 MHz). Power Doppler is very sensitive to movement. In (A) the color gain is set higher and both pleural and lung movement artifact are detected (entire color box is filled in below pleural line). In (B), the color gain is low so that only movement along the pleural interface is demonstrated. Avoid setting the gain too high, as general patient respiratory motion will be detected.

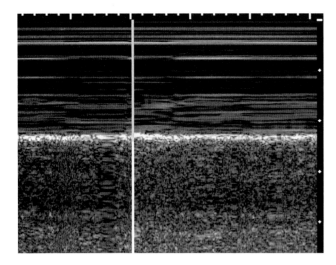

Figure 5-16. M-mode ultrasound of normal lung at 7.5–10 MHz ("seashore sign"). Granular artifacts below the bright pleural line represent normal pleural sliding and lung motion on M-mode.

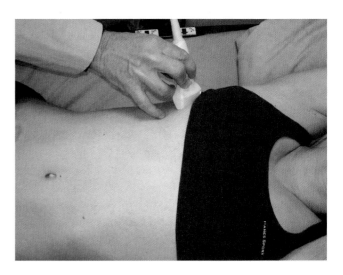

Figure 5-17. Extended lung examination. In a supine patient, the extent of a pneumothorax can be outlined by orienting the probe parallel to the ribs and sliding it laterally along successive rib interspaces.

► COMMON AND EMERGENT ABNORMALITIES

On ultrasound images, free fluid appears anechoic (black) or hypoechoic (if the blood is clotted) and, since it is not contained within a viscus, will have sharp edges as opposed to rounded edges.

Hemopericardium. Free pericardial fluid is identified as an anechoic stripe surrounding the heart within the parietal and visceral layers of the bright hyperechoic pericardial sac (Figure 5-18).

Free pleural fluid. The right or left diaphragm appears as a bright hyperechoic structure; free pleural fluid can be identified as an anechoic stripe superior to the diaphragm (Figure 5-19).

Hemoperitoneum. Morison's pouch is a common site for blood to accumulate when any solid intra-abdominal organ has been injured. Free fluid appears as an anechoic stripe in Morison's pouch (Figure 5-20) or within the right paracolic gutter (adjacent to the lower pole of the right kidney) (Figure 5-21a). For comparison, fluid contained within the retroperitoneal pararenal

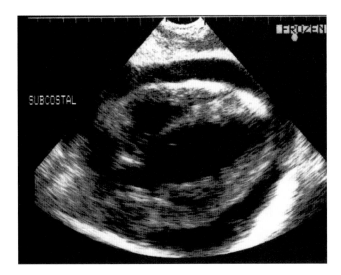

Figure 5-18. Hemopericardium. Free pericardial fluid is identified as an anechoic stripe surrounding the heart between the parietal and visceral layers of the bright hyperechoic pericardial sac.

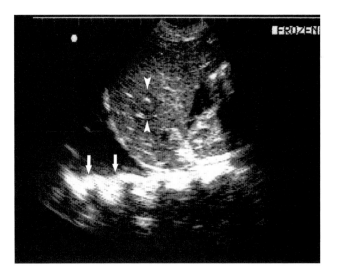

Figure 5-19. Free pleural fluid. The right diaphragm appears as a bright hyperechoic structure along the border of the liver. Free pleural fluid can be identified as an anechoic stripe superior to the diaphragm. The pleural fluid allows visualization of the lateral chest wall (arrows) that cannot be visualized when the air-filled lung is normally present. The patient also has a circular defect in the liver (arrowheads) from a bullet wound, and fluid in Morison's pouch.

space appears as a hypoechoic stripe adjacent to the psoas muscle (Figure 5-21b).

In the perisplenic region, free fluid appearance and location are similar to the description for the perihepatic area (Figure 5-22). Free intraperitoneal fluid appears as an anechoic stripe in the subdiaphragmatic space, splenorenal recess, or the left paracolic gutter. Since the splenorenal recess is not the most common site for free intraperitoneal fluid to accumulate in the left upper quadrant, it is essential to visualize the left diaphragm and left subphrenic space.

Free intraperitoneal fluid often accumulates in the pelvis because it is the most dependent area of the peritoneal cavity (Figure 5-23). Liquid blood or ascites floats above the bowels and will be located adjacent to the bladder and anterior peritoneum. Blood clots in the pelvis are located in the cul-de-sac and may distort the contour of the bladder (Figure 5-24).

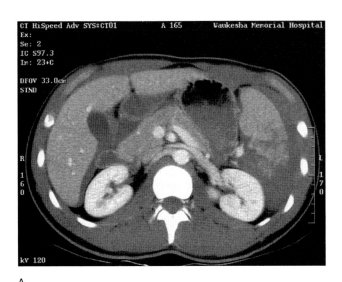

A

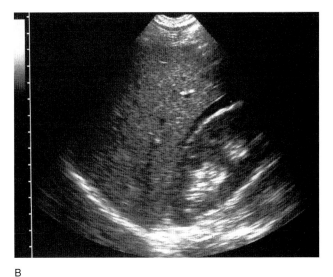

B

Figure 5-20. Hemoperitoneum. The abdominal contrast CT (A) demonstrates a fractured spleen with surrounding hematoma but a small stripe of fluid is also present above the right kidney in Morison's pouch. A right intercostal oblique ultrasound view from the same patient reveals a thin stripe of free fluid in Morison's pouch (B).

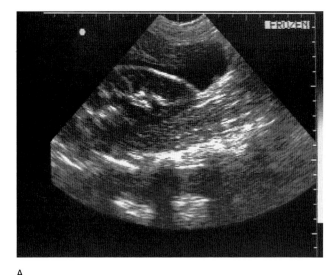

A

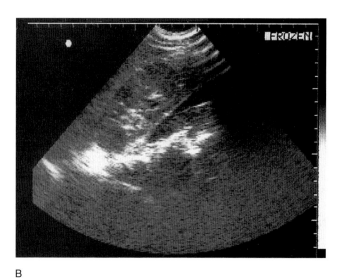

B

Figure 5-21. Free fluid vs. retroperitoneal fluid. Right coronal views. Image (A) demonstrates free peritoneal fluid in the paracolic gutter (adjacent to the lower pole of the right kidney). For comparison, image (B) shows contained retroperitoneal fluid (pararenal space) overlying the psoas muscle stripe and medial to the kidney.

Pneumothorax. Ultrasound diagnosis of a pneumothorax is based on the **absence** of the normal findings—sliding sign and comet tail artifacts—along the pleural interface (see Figures 5–13 to 5–15). When these are absent, the specificity for the diagnosis may be further enhanced by documenting the presence of an A-line (a reverberation artifact from the pleural interface that is found at twice the distance from the skin to pleura) (Figure 5-25). In one study, lung sliding alone had 100% sensitivity, but only 78% specificity for diagnosing an occult pneumothorax. When an A-line was seen with absent lung sliding, there was 95% sensitivity and 94% specificity for diagnosing an occult pneumothorax.[60] The size of the pneumothorax may be estimated if the ultrasound examination reveals the lung point. This represents the lateral aspect of the pneumothorax in a supine patient and may be seen in real time as intermittent normal findings with respiration and documented with M-mode (Figure 5-26). The presence of a lung point had 100% specificity for an occult pneumothorax.[60]

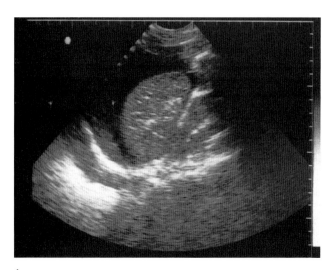

A

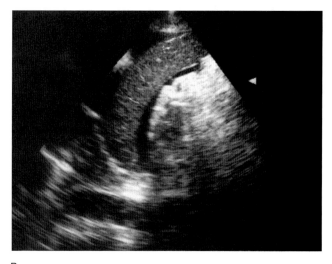

B

Figure 5-22. Left intercostal oblique views reveal the spleen surrounded by hypoechoic fluid in the subdiaphragmatic space (A). A small amount of clotted blood is also noted adjacent to the bright curvilinear diaphragm. Image (B) shows free intraperitoneal fluid as an anechoic stripe in the splenorenal recess. The tubular fluid-filled object at the bottom of the image is the aorta. (Courtesy of Lori Sens, Gulfcoast Ultrasound, (B))

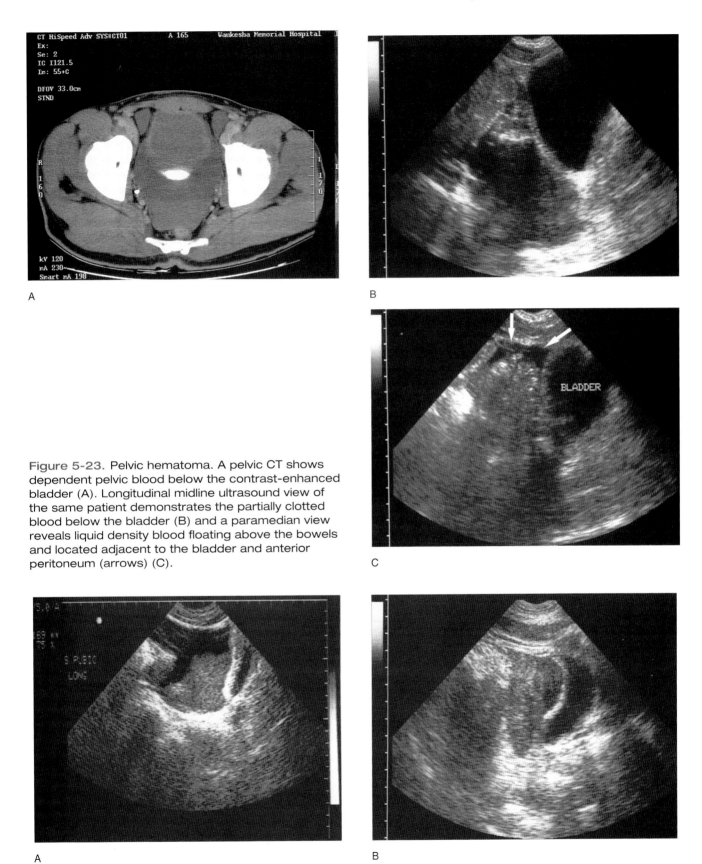

Figure 5-23. Pelvic hematoma. A pelvic CT shows dependent pelvic blood below the contrast-enhanced bladder (A). Longitudinal midline ultrasound view of the same patient demonstrates the partially clotted blood below the bladder (B) and a paramedian view reveals liquid density blood floating above the bowels and located adjacent to the bladder and anterior peritoneum (arrows) (C).

Figure 5-24. Longitudinal pelvic views demonstrate a collapsed bladder and dependent clotted blood in the cul-de-sac with liquid blood above (A). Blood clots in the pelvis may distort the contour of the bladder. The uterus-like object in the center of the image in this male patient, is actually a hematoma (B).

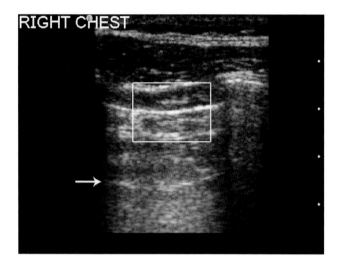

Figure 5-25. Pneumothorax (7.5–10 MHz). Power Doppler is activated and the gain adjusted correctly by comparison to the normal left hemithorax. The patients right hemithorax showed a negative pleural sliding sign, no comet tail artifacts and no power Doppler signal at the pleural interface. The specificity for pheumothorax is improved when an A-line is also visible (arrow).

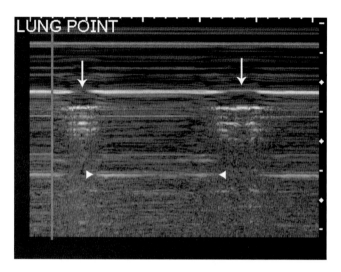

Figure 5-26. Lung point. The probe is located on the chest at the edge of a pneumothorax. During the M-mode sweep the patient has taken 2 breaths allowing normal pleural movement to be documented briefly (arrows) as the "seashore sign." The remainder of the M-mode sweep shows the "stratosphere sign" of pneumothorax. Note: A-line (arrowheads).

▶ COMMON VARIANTS AND SELECTED ABNORMALITIES

When performing the FAST examination, it is essential to recognize common normal variants that may mimic positive findings. When examining the perihepatic views, fluid in the gallbladder, duodenum, hepatic flexure of the colon and other regions of the bowel, or inferior vena cava (IVC) may be erroneously identified as free intraperitoneal fluid. When examining the perisplenic views, fluid in the stomach or splenic flexure of the colon or blood within the vena cava or portal veins may be erroneously identified as free intraperitoneal fluid (Figure 5-27). When examining the pelvic views, fluid within a collapsed bladder or an ovarian cyst may be incorrectly identified as free intraperitoneal fluid. In the male patient, the seminal vesicles may be incorrectly identified as free intraperitoneal fluid. Also, premenopausal women occasionally may have a small baseline amount of free fluid in the pouch of Douglas.[99]

Occasionally, when performing the FAST examination, the clinician may directly detect injury in a solid organ, which is usually the spleen or liver. While this is not the specific goal of the FAST examination, it is helpful to understand some of the sonographic features of solid organ injury. When the patient is stable and serial follow-up examinations (control examinations) are being performed, the clinician has more time to evaluate for possible obvious solid organ injuries. Acute solid organ lacerations may appear as fragmented areas of increased or decreased echogenicity. Contained intraparenchymal or subcapsular hemorrhages may appear initially as isoechoic or slightly hyperechoic; this can make them difficult to reliably detect (Figure 5-28). The examiner must pay close attention to contour and organ tissue irregularities to observe these injuries (Figure 5-29). CT is more sensitive for acute organ injuries and should be ordered when these are suspected (Figure 5-20a). Over time, contained hemorrhage will become hypoechoic, with the area lacking sharp margins. A subcapsular hemorrhage may appear as a crescent-shaped hypoechoic stripe surrounding the organ (Figure 5-30).

Intraperitoneal fat is usually hyperechoic but in some cases is relatively hypoechoic. When the fat is present in the perinephric areas, it can be mistaken for intraperitoneal fluid or hematoma. Intraperitoneal fat (as opposed to hematoma) will be a consistent density throughout and will not move independently with respirations compared to the adjacent organ. Intraperitoneal hematoma contains grey level echoes but often will be accompanied by hypoechoic fluid areas as well. Clotted blood tends to move with respirations independent of surrounding structures.

A pericardial fat pad can be hypoechoic or contain grey level echoes. The pericardial fat pad is almost always located anterior to the right ventricle and is not present posterior to the left ventricle (Figure 5-31). Pericardial fluid or hemorrhage will be located in both the anterior and posterior pericardial spaces. A small amount of fluid (<5 mm) may be present within the dependent

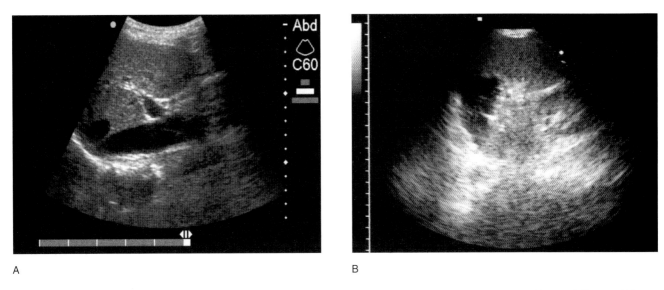

A   B

Figure 5-27. Fluid pitfalls. Oblique view of the liver shows fluid below that is contained within the IVC (A). When examining the perisplenic views, fluid in the stomach (or other bowels) may be erroneously identified as free intraperitoneal fluid (B).

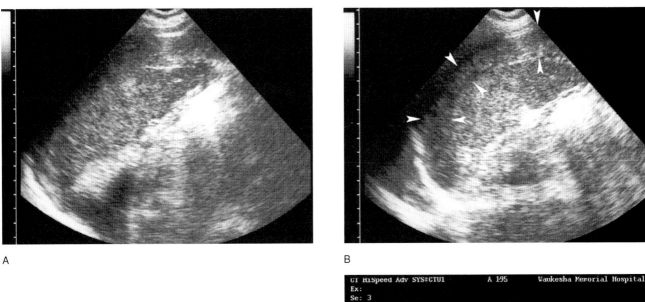

A   B

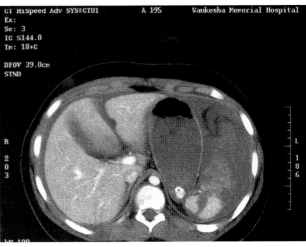

Figure 5-28. Intercostal oblique views of the spleen. The initial view (A) showed only a questionable area of isoechoic tissue between the spleen tip and the ultrasound probe. The spleen does not have obvious injuries. A slightly different view of the spleen (B) reveals a 1.5- to 2-cm echogenic stripe (arrowheads) around the spleen (contained hematoma) and an irregular echo pattern from the splenic tissue (the hemispleen closest to the diaphragm is hyperechoic). CT of the same patient (C) shows a large intraparenchymal and perisplenic hematoma with contrast enhanced spleen fragments posteriorly.

C

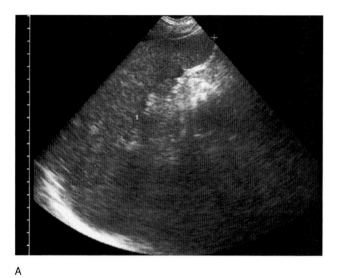

A

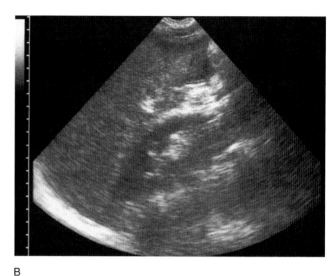

B

Figure 5-29. Initial oblique view of the spleen (A) showed enlargement (long axis is 17 cm) and a contour irregularity (narrow inferior tip). A slightly different view of the same patient revealed clots and liquid blood near the spleen tip (B). Compare these ultrasound findings with the CT findings from the same patient in Figure 5-20a. The splenic fractures were not apparent on the ultrasound views.

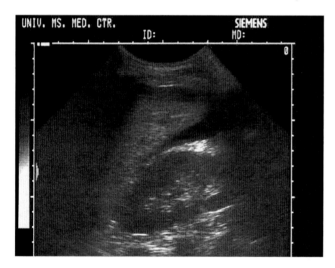

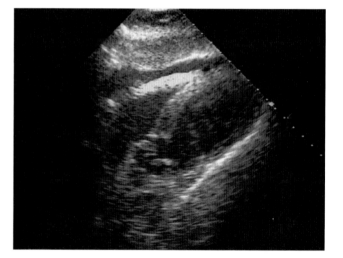

Figure 5-30. Subcapsular hemorrhage. This intercostal oblique view of the liver appears to have free fluid in Morison's pouch and a hypoechoic stripe between the probe and the liver tissue. There was no other evidence for free fluid on ultrasound. The patient's CT revealed a contained subcapsular hematoma of the liver and no free fluid. (Courtesy of Verena Valley, MD)

Figure 5-31. Subcostal long axis view of the heart and pericardium. A pericardial fat pad can be hypoechoic or contain grey level echoes. The pericardial fat pad is almost always located anterior to the right ventricle and is not present posterior to the left ventricle.

pericardium, but is usually considered to be physiologic when it is visualized during systole only.

▶ PITFALLS

1. **Contraindication**. The only absolute contraindication to performing the FAST examina-

tion is when immediate surgical management is clearly indicated, in which case the FAST examination could delay patient transportation to the operating room.

2. **Overreliance on the FAST examination**. A clinical pitfall is the overreliance of an initial negative FAST examination in caring for the trauma patient. There is still no substitute for sound clinical judgment. Each FAST examination is a single

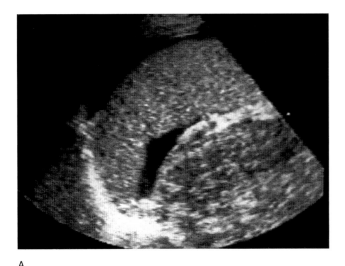

A

B

C

Figure 5-32. Cirrhosis of the liver. This oblique view of the right lobe demonstrates the findings of contracted size, increased echogenicity, and irregular texture of the liver (A). There is surrounding echo-free ascites (Contributed by Simon Roy, MD). An oblique right upper quadrant view of the abdomen (B) shows a contracted liver, massive ascites, and generalized thickening of the gallbladder wall. This gallbladder finding is common with chronic liver disease and ascites. Long axis view of the spleen (C) measures more than 17 cm. (Courtesy of Simon Roy, MD, (A); Lori Sens, Gulfcoast Ultrasound, (C))

data point in the overall clinical picture of the trauma patient. When mandated by the mechanism of injury or an evolving physical examination, serial FAST examinations or an abdominal CT scan should be performed on the patient. Serial FAST examinations are a common practice in Germany and are gaining acceptance in the United States.[100] They are used to determine if new intraperitoneal fluid has developed or if existing intraperitoneal fluid is expanding.

3. **Limitations of the FAST examination.** Limitations include difficulty in imaging patients who are morbidly obese or have massive subcutaneous emphysema. Also, in a patient at risk for ascites, it may be difficult to determine whether the free intraperitoneal fluid is ascites or blood. To help distinguish between the two, general ultrasound findings that point to ascites secondary to chronic liver disease include nodular cirrhosis of the liver, a contracted and hyperechoic liver, generalized thickening of the gallbladder wall,

enlargement of the caudate lobe, enlargement of the spleen, or engorgement of the portal venous system (Figure 5-32). The clinician could also clarify the issue by performing an ultrasound-directed needle paracentesis of the fluid to distinguish ascites from hemoperitoneum. Another limitation is that ultrasound is not as reliable as CT in distinguishing and grading precise solid organ injury. In the future, contrast-enhanced ultrasound may improve identification of specific organ injuries on the FAST examination.

4. **Limitations associated with pregnancy.** There are limitations of the FAST examination in pregnant trauma patients that should be noted. Evaluating the pouch of Douglas for hemoperitoneum in the presence of a gravid uterus requires careful consideration. The distortion of usual landmarks and the difficulty with differentiating between intra-uterine versus extra-uterine fluid can make this a challenging examination for the inexperienced sonologist.

Also, the dependent portions of the peritoneal cavity may become further distorted with advanced third-trimester pregnancy, making the diagnosis of free intra-peritoneal fluid versus intra-uterine fluid more difficult.[81] As previously discussed, the FAST examination alone cannot exclude uterine rupture or placental abruption.

5. **Technical difficulties with the FAST examination**. (A) Most clinicians have little difficulty locating Morison's pouch but have greater difficulty locating the splenorenal recess and left pleural space. One common technical error is not placing the ultrasound probe posterior or superior enough. The probe often must be placed in the posterior axillary line at the 8–9th intercostal space to visualize these structures. (B) With some patients, visualizing the pericardium can be difficult. Placing the probe as close to the xiphoid as possible and depressing the probe toward the spine can facilitate the subcostal cardiac view. Even so, the patient may have to take a deep breath or the depth of the image adjusted to visualize the entire pericardium. If subcostal views are ineffective, then parasternal or apical views should be attempted (see Chapter 6, Cardiac). (C) Breathing or ventilation can interfere with the examination (from lung or rib artifact) or enhance the examination when it brings organs closer to the ultrasound probe (diaphragm, heart, liver, spleen, or kidneys). (D) Fluid in a partially emptied bladder can be mistaken for free intraperitoneal fluid. This scenario can be clarified with complete catheter emptying of the bladder or by retrograde bladder filling and repeat examination.

6. **Injuries undetected by ultrasound**: Certain injuries may not be detected initially by the FAST examination. These include perforation of a viscus, bowel wall contusion, pancreatic trauma, or renal pedicle injury. Newer ultrasound imaging techniques such as power color Doppler may be used to evaluate renal tissue perfusion in patients with suspected renal pedicle injury. The entire diaphragm also cannot be visualized using ultrasonography.

▶ CASE STUDIES

CASE 1

Patient Presentation

A 48-year-old man presented to the emergency department after he slid into a telephone pole when his motorcycle skidded on a patch of ice. He was wearing a helmet but lost consciousness at the scene of the crash. The patient complained of abdominal pain but denied any chest pain, shortness of breath, headache, or nausea and vomiting. He admitted to drinking "at least a dozen" beers earlier in the evening.

On physical examination, his blood pressure was 88/48 mmHg; pulse rate, 122 beats per minute; respirations, 18 per minute; and temperature, 37.0°C. He was arousable but drowsy and slurring his words. He had a strong odor of alcohol on his breath. His head, neck, pulmonary, and cardiovascular examinations were unremarkable. The abdominal examination was soft, diffusely tender, and without peritoneal signs. His extremities revealed diffuse deep abrasions but without bony injury. His neurologic examination was unremarkable except for his depressed mental status.

Management Course

After being infused 2 L of intravenous crystalloid fluid, the patient's blood pressure was 92/60 mmHg and his pulse was 116 beats per minute. A supine chest radiograph was normal. Urinalysis revealed gross hematuria. His serum ethanol level was 342 mg/dL. A FAST examination of the abdomen performed by the emergency physician revealed a large quantity of free intraperitoneal fluid in Morison's pouch (Figure 5-33), the right paracolic gutter, and in the pelvic cul-de-sac. The decision to perform an abdominal CT scan or diagnostic peritoneal lavage was deferred by the attending trauma surgeon. Instead, a head CT scan was performed in 10 minutes, which was negative for intracranial pathology. The patient was then taken directly to the operating room for an

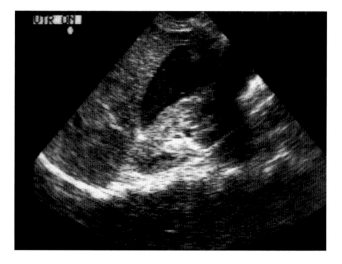

Figure 5-33. Case 1. A large quantity of free intraperitoneal fluid is present in Morison's pouch. The fluid is mildly echogenic because of the clotting of the blood.

exploratory laparotomy, which revealed large liver and right kidney lacerations and 1.5 L of hemoperitoneum.

Commentary

Case 1 was an example of a patient presenting to the emergency department hypotensive after sustaining blunt abdominal trauma. His profound alcohol intoxication and possible closed head injury complicated his examination and evaluation. Since the patient was too hemodynamically unstable to leave the trauma room, the FAST examination was an ideal diagnostic study to evaluate the patient. The FAST examination revealed gross free intraperitoneal fluid. The information provided by the FAST examination in this case negated the need for an abdominal CT scan or diagnostic peritoneal lavage. Instead, time was saved by the expeditious use of a head CT scan to evaluate for intracranial pathology followed by the direct transportation of the patient to the operating suite.

CASE 2

Patient Presentation

A 21-year-old man was critically injured after his small motor vehicle was hit by a tractor-trailer at highway speeds. The patient was noted to be in profound shock, with a GCS of 5, a systolic blood pressure of 60 mmHg, and a pulse of 130 beats per minute when first assessed by the responding air ambulance. He was intubated at the scene and underwent a needle decompression of his chest. He was transported to a small rural hospital where he continued to be hypotensive and was administered 5 L of crystalloid fluid, 3 units of packed red blood cells, and had bilateral chest tubes inserted. There was evidence of marked bruising and swelling to the right hip and thigh. A Foley catheter was inserted and produced 400 mL of bloody urine. He was then transported to a tertiary care trauma center. En route, he was reported to have no detectable blood pressure and dilated, minimally reactive pupils bilaterally despite in-flight fluid and blood resuscitation.

Management Course

On arrival at the trauma center, he had a blood pressure of 80/50 mm Hg, and GCS of 5, and temperature was 34.5°C. Portable radiographs of the chest and pelvis were obtained. The FAST examination revealed no obvious free intraperitoneal fluid. The AP pelvis radiograph revealed a widened sacroiliac joint consistent with a vertically unstable, type C pelvic fracture and bilateral inferior and superior pubic rami fractures (Figure 5-34A,B). On the basis of the patient's hemodynamic instability and the functional layout of the treating hospital in which the angiography suite was geographically sep-

arate from the CT scanner and the operating room, the patient was prioritized to undergo emergent angiography because it was felt that the likely source of bleeding was retroperitoneal and related to his multiple pelvic fractures. The patient had an angioembolization of his right internal iliac artery, which established control of his massive bleeding (Figure 5-34c). On arrival in the intensive care unit, he was cold and coagulopathic, despite being administered fresh frozen plasma, cryoprecipitate, platelets, and activated Factor VIIa. He went on to develop an abdominal compartment syndrome, which necessitated urgent laparotomy for decompression. The laparotomy revealed a massive, but contained retroperitoneal hematoma and a minor liver laceration. The patient eventually recovered after a complicated intensive care unit course notable for multiple reoperations, lung injury, ventilator-associated pneumonia, and the delayed closure of his abdominal wound.

Commentary

Case 2 demonstrated the critical importance of interpreting the FAST examination in the clinical context. In the context of a near-moribund trauma patient who required expeditious control of the primary source of hemorrhage (internal iliac bleeding source), the "negative" FAST examination directed therapy away from exploratory laparotomy and toward angiography. In the future, as resuscitative operating rooms evolve to provide both operative and interventional capabilities, the decision to go to the operating room or angiography suite may not be a life-or-death decision; presently, however, fatal results may occur if the wrong decision is made. In this case, the FAST examination may have been considered technically "wrong," or a false negative since a minor liver laceration was present, if the test was being performed to detect all intraperitoneal injuries. The FAST examination is clearly not as sensitive as CT for this purpose, and clinically insignificant injuries are frequently detected on CT that are not suspected by ultrasound.[27,101,102] But for this patient, the clinical question being asked was: is the major source of hemorrhage in the peritoneal cavity? This is a question which the FAST examination is very accurate at answering as long as indeterminate images are not accepted as negative.[21,27,103]

CASE 3

Patient Presentation

A 45-year-old man was thrown from his motorcycle after being struck by a car. He was unconscious and intubated at the scene by the responding paramedics. On arrival at the trauma center, he had a blood pressure of 110/70 mmHg and a heart rate of 110 beats per minute. He was being ventilated at 12 breaths per minute, but

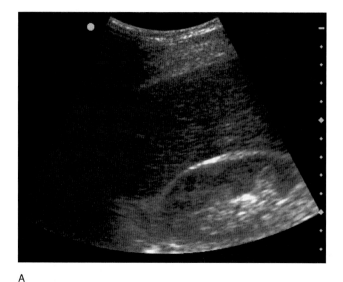

A

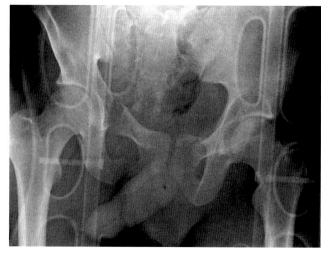

B

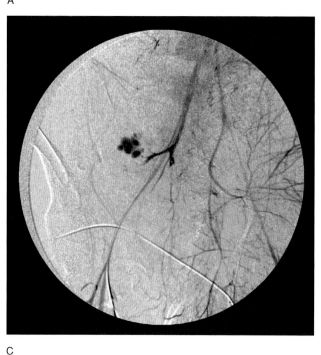

C

Figure 5-34. Case 2. Morison's pouch view (A). The FAST examination revealed no obvious free intraperitoneal fluid. The AP pelvis radiograph (B) revealed a widened sacroiliac joint consistent with a vertically unstable, type C pelvic fracture and bilateral inferior and superior pubic rami fractures. Angiography of the right internal iliac artery (C).

marked resistance to ventilation was noted. On physical examination, no obvious chest deformity or subcutaneous emphysema was noted, but the patient had diminished breath sounds in the left chest.

Management Course

An EFAST examination of the chest revealed lung sliding, moving comet tail artifacts, and a power Doppler signal localized to the pleural interface (Power Slide) on examination of the right chest. Examination of the left chest revealed the presence of comet-tail artifacts localized to the pleural interface, but without evidence of lung sliding or a Power Slide from the pleural interface

(Figure 5-35A). While the examination was considered negative for the determination of a pneumothorax, it was definitely abnormal. Upon interpretation of the portable chest radiograph (Figure 5-35B), it became apparent that there was in fact a right mainstem intubation and the left lung was not being adequately ventilated. Upon endotracheal tube repositioning, appropriate lung sliding, comet tail artifacts, and a Power Slide returned to the left chest (Figure 5-35C).

Commentary

Case 3 demonstrated that the EFAST examination for pneumothoraces must be interpreted in the clinical

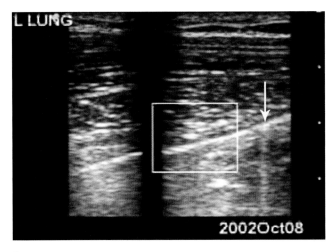

A

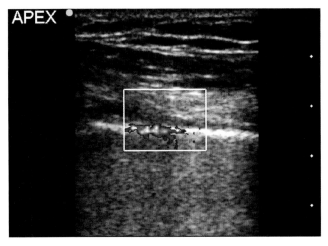

C

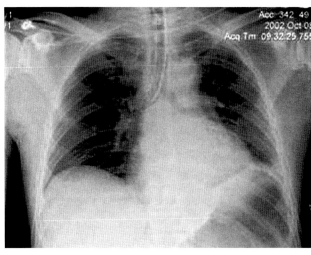

B

Figure 5-35. Case 3. Examination of the left lung (A) revealed a comet-tail artifact (arrow), but no motion documented on power Doppler (negative "power slide"). Portable chest radiograph (B) revealed a right mainstem intubation. Power slide returned to the left chest after endotracheal tube repositioning (C).

context like all other focused sonographic examinations. While the absence of lung sliding is most often associated with the presence of pneumothorax, the presence of comet tail artifacts also excludes pneumothorax with a greater predictive ability.[61] The thoracic role of the EFAST in practically guiding resuscitation is still in evolution and must be carefully assessed to prevent iatrogenic injuries. Whereas only a surgeon can perform a laparotomy on an unstable patient with a positive FAST examination, any clinician with appropriate training can insert a chest tube to treat a pneumothorax. The sonographic findings of absent sliding and comet tail artifacts after traumatic injury should be promptly addressed. When found on the left chest, the positioning of the endotracheal tube should be quickly verified. If the patient is stable, chest radiography or preferably CT scanning of the chest should be obtained. If the patient is unstable, chest tube insertion should be performed. The complications of chest drainage are not negligible,[104] but are far

outweighed by the consequences of an untreated tension pneumothorax.

REFERENCES

1. Tiling T, Bouillon B, Schmid A, et al.: Ultrasound in blunt abdomino-thoracic trauma, In: Border JR, Allgoewer M, Hansen ST, et al. eds.: *Blunt Multiple Trauma: Comprehensive Pathophysiology and Care.* New York, Marcel Dekker, 1990:415–433.
2. Halbfass HJ, Wimmer B, Hauenstein K, et al.: Ultrasonic diagnosis of blunt abdominal injuries. *Fortschr Med* 99:1681, 1981.
3. Aufschnaiter M, Kofler H: Sonographic acute diagnosis in polytrauma. *Aktuel Traumatol* 13:55, 1983.
4. Hoffman R, Pohlemann T, Wippermann B, et al.: Management of blunt abdominal trauma using sonography. *Unfallchirurg* 92:471, 1989.
5. Seifert M, Petereit U, Ortmann G: Sonographs of the

diagnostic multi-system trauma patients. *Zentrlbl Chir* 114:1012, 1989.

6. Kohlberger VEJ, Strittmatter B, Waninger J: Ultrasound diagnostic technique after abdominal trauma. *Fortschr Med* 107:244, 1989.
7. Wening JV: Evaluation of ultrasound, lavage and computed tomography in blunt abdominal trauma. *Surg Endosc* 3:152, 1989.
8. Kimura A, Otsuka T: Emergency center ultrasonography in the evaluation of hemoperitoneum: A prospective study. *J Trauma* 31:20–23, 1991.
9. Rothlin MA, Naf R, Amgwerd M, et al.: Ultrasound in blunt abdominal and thoracic trauma. *J Trauma* 34:488–495, 1993.
10. Rozycki GS, Ochsner MG, Jaffin JH, et al.: Prospective evaluation of surgeons' use of ultrasound in the evaluation of the trauma patient. *J Trauma* 34:516–527, 1993.
11. Rozycki GS, Ochsner MG, Schmidt JA, et al.: A prospective study of surgeon-performed ultrasound as the primary adjunct modality for injured patient assessment. *J Trauma* 39:492–500, 1995.
12. Ma OJ, Mateer JR, Ogata M, Kefer MP, et al.: Prospective analysis of a rapid trauma ultrasound examination performed by emergency physicians. *J Trauma* 38:879–885, 1995.
13. Ma OJ, Kefer MP, Mateer JR, et al.: Evaluation of hemoperitoneum using a single- vs multiple-view ultrasonographic examination. *Acad Emerg Med* 2:581–586, 1995.
14. Hoffman R, Nerlich M, Muggia-Sullam M, et al.: Blunt abdominal trauma in cases of multiple trauma evaluated by ultrasonography: A prospective analysis of 291 patients. *J Trauma* 32:452–458, 1992.
15. Tso P, Rodriquez A, Cooper C, et al.: Sonography in blunt abdominal trauma: a preliminary progress report. *J Trauma* 33:39–44, 1992.
16. Lentz KA, McKenney MG, Nunez DB, et al.: Evaluating blunt abdominal trauma: Role for ultrasonography. *J Ultrasound Med* 15:447–451, 1996.
17. McElveen TS, Collin GR: The role of ultrasonography in blunt abdominal trauma: A prospective study. *Am Surg* 63:184–188, 1997.
18. Rozycki GS, Ochsner MG, Feliciano DV, et al.: Early detection of hemoperitoneum by ultrasound examination of the right upper quadrant: A multicenter study. *J Trauma* 45:878–883, 1998.
19. Bode PJ, Edwards MJ, Kruit MC, et al.: Sonography in a clinical algorithm for early evaluation of 1671 patients with blunt abdominal trauma. *AJR Am J Roentgenol* 172:905–911, 1999.
20. Thomas B, Falcone RE, Vasquez D, et al.: Ultrasound evaluation of blunt abdominal trauma: Program implementation, initial experience, and learning curve. *J Trauma* 42:384–388, 1997.
21. Wherrett LJ, Boulanger BR, McLellan BA, et al.: Hypotension after blunt abdominal trauma: The role of emergent abdominal sonography in surgical triage. *J Trauma* 41:815–820, 1996.
22. Boulanger BR, Brenneman FD, Kirkpatrick AW, et al.: The indeterminate abdominal sonogram in multisystem blunt trauma. *J Trauma* 48:52–56, 1998.
23. Boulanger BR, Kearney PA, Brenneman FD, et al.: FAST utilization in 1999: Results of a survey of North American trauma centers. *Am Surg* 66:1049–1055, 2000.
24. Boulanger BR, Kearney PA, Tsuei B, et al.: The routine use of sonography in penetrating torso injury is beneficial. *J Trauma* 51:320–325, 2001.
25. Asensio JA, Arroyo H, Veloz W, et al.: Penetrating thoracoabdominal injuries: Ongoing dilemma—which cavity and when? *World J Surg* 26:539–543, 2002.
26. Kirkpatrick AW, Simons RK, Brown DR, et al.: Digital hand-held sonography utilised for the focussed assessment with sonography for trauma: A pilot study. *Ann Acad Med Singapore* 30:577–581, 2001.
27. Kirkpatrick AW, Sirois M, Laupland KB, et al.: The hand-held FAST exam for blunt trauma. *Can J Surg* 48:453–460, 2005.
28. Brooks A, Davies B, Connolly J: Prospective evaluation of handheld ultrasound in the diagnosis of blunt abdominal trauma. *J R Army Med Corps* 148:19–21, 2002.
29. Jehle D, Guarina J, Karamanoukian H: Emergency department ultrasound in the evaluation of blunt abdominal trauma. *Am J Emerg Med* 11:342–346, 1993.
30. Hilty WE, Wolfe RE, Moore EE, et al.: Sensitivity and specificity of ultrasound in the detection of intraperitoneal fluid. *Ann Emerg Med* 22:921, 1993.
31. Branney SW, Wolfe RE, Moore EE, et al.: Quantitative sensitivity of ultrasound in detecting free intraperitoneal fluid. *J Trauma* 39:375–380, 1995.
32. Valentino M, Serra C, Zironi G, et al.: Blunt abdominal trauma: Emergency contrast-enhanced sonography for detection of solid organ injuries. *AJR* 186:1361–1367, 2006.
33. Catalano O, Lobianco R, Raso MM, et al.: Blunt hepatic trauma: Evaluation with contrast-enhanced sonography: Sonographic findings and clinical application. *J Ultrasound Med* 24:299–310, 2005.
34. Catalano O, Lobianco R, Sandomenico F, et al.: Splenic trauma: Evaluation with contrast-specific sonography and a second-generation contrast medium. *J Ultrasound Med* 22:467–477, 2003.
35. Blaivas M, Lyon M, Brannam L, et al.: Feasibility of FAST examination performance with ultrasound contrast. *J Emerg Med* 29:307–311, 2005.
36. Nanda NC, Carstensen C: Echo-enhancing agents: Safety. In: Nanda NC, Schlief R, Goldberg BB eds. *Advances in Echo Imaging Using Contrast Enhancers*. Dordrecht: Kluwer, 1997:115–131.
37. Branney SW, Moore EE, Cantrill S, et al.: Ultrasound-based key clinical pathway reduces the use of hospital resources for the evaluation of blunt abdominal trauma. *J Trauma* 42:1086–1090, 1997.
38. Arrillaga A, Graham R, York JW, et al.: Increased efficiency and cost-effectiveness in the evaluation of the blunt abdominal trauma patient with the use of ultrasound. *Am Surg* 65:31–35, 1999.
39. Huang MS, Liu M, Wu JK, et al.: Ultrasonography for the evaluation of hemoperitoneum during resuscitation: A simple scoring system. *J Trauma* 36:173–177, 1994.
40. Porter RS, Nester BA, Dalsey WC, et al.: Use of ultrasound to determine the need for laparotomy in trauma patients. *Ann Emerg Med* 29:323–330, 1997.

41. Carrel R, Shaffer M, Franaszek J: Emergency diagnosis, resuscitation and treatment of acute penetrating cardiac trauma. *Ann Emerg Med* 11:504–517, 1982.

42. Plummer D, Brunette D, Asinger R, et al.: Emergency department echocardiography improves outcome in penetrating cardiac injury. *Ann Emerg Med* 21:709–712, 1992.

43. Rozycki GS, Feliciano DV, Ochsner MG, et al.: The role of ultrasound in patients with possible penetrating cardiac wounds: A prospective multicenter study. *J Trauma* 46(4):543–551, 1999.

44. Ma OJ, Mateer JR: Trauma ultrasound examination versus chest radiography in the detection of hemothorax. *Ann Emerg Med* 29:312–316, 1997.

45. Rubens MB: The pleura: Collapse and consolidation. In: Sutton D ed. *A Textbook of Radiology Imaging*, 4th ed. Edinburgh, Churchill Livingstone, 393, 1987.

46. Juhl JH: Diseases of the pleura, mediastinum, and diaphragm. In: Juhl JH, Crummy AB eds. *Essentials of Radiologic Imaging*, 6th ed. Philadelphia, PA: JB Lippincott Company, 1993:1026.

47. Dulchavsky SA, Schwarz KL, Kirkpatrick AW, et al.: Prospective evaluation of thoracic ultrasound in the detection of pneumothorax. *J Trauma* 50:201–205, 2001.

48. Kirkpatrick AW, Nicolaou S: The sonographic detection of pneumothoraces. In: Kharmy-Jones R, Nathens A, Stern E, eds. *Thoracic Trauma and Critical Care*. Boston, MA: Kluwer Academic Publishers, 2002:227–234.

49. Cunningham J, Kirkpatrick AW, Nicolaou S, et al.: Enhanced recognition of "lung sliding" with power color Doppler imaging in the diagnosis of pneumothorax. *J Trauma* 52:769–771, 2002.

50. Kirkpatrick AW, Nicolaou S, Rowan K, et al.: Thoracic sonography for pneumothorax: The clinical evaluation of an operational space medicine spin-off. *Acta Astronautica* 56:831–838, 2005.

51. Kirkpatrick AW, Sirois M, Laupland KB, et al.: Handheld thoracic sonography for detecting post-traumatic pneumothoraces: The extended focused assessment with sonography for trauma (EFAST). *J Trauma* 57:288–295, 2004.

52. Rowan KR, Kirkpatrick AW, Liu D, et al.: Traumatic pneumothorax detection with thoracic US: Correlation with chest radiography and CT—Initial experience. *Radiology* 225:210–214, 2002.

53. Lichtenstein DA: Pneumothorax and introduction to ultrsound signs in the lung. In: *General Ultrasound in the Critically Ill*. 1st ed. Berlin: Springer, 2002:105–115.

54. Merritt CRB. Physics of ultrasound. In Rumak CM, Wilson SR, Charboneau JW, (eds.), *Diagnostic Ultrasound*. 2nd ed. St. Louis, MO: Mosby, 1998:3–33.

55. Sistrom CL, Reiheld CT, Gay SB, et al.: Detection and estimation of the volume of pneumothorax using real-time sonography: Efficacy determined by receiver operating characteristic analysis. *AJR* 166:317–321, 1996.

56. Kirkpatrick AW, Ng AK, Dulchavsky SA, et al.: Sonographic diagnosis of a pneumothorax inapparent on plain chest radiography: Confirmation by computed tomography. *J Trauma* 50:750–752, 2001.

57. Ball CG, Kirkpatrick AW, Laupland KB, et al.: Incidence, risk factors, and outcomes for occult pneumothoraces in victims of major trauma. *J Trauma* 59:917–925, 2005.

58. Lencioni R, Pinto F, Armillotta N, et al.: Assessment of tumour vascularity in hepatocellular carcinoma: Comparison of power Doppler US and color Doppler US. *Radiology* 201:3583–358, 1996.

59. Rubin JM, Bude RO, Carson PL, et al.: Power Doppler US: A potentially useful alternative to mean-frequency based color Doppler US. *Radiology* 190:853–856, 1994.

60. Lichtenstein DA, Meziere G, Lascols N, et al.: Ultrasound diagnosis of occult pneumothorax. *Crit Care Med* 33:1231–1238, 2005.

61. Lichtenstein D, Meziere G, Biderman P, et al.: The comet-tail artifact: An ultrasound sign of alveolar-interstitial syndrome. *Am J Respir Crit Care Med* 156:1640–1646, 1997.

62. Lichtenstein D, Meziere G, Biderman P, et al.: The comet-tail artifact: An ultrasound sign ruling out pneumothorax. *Intensive Care Med* 25:383–388, 1999.

63. Lichtenstein D, Meziere G, Biderman P, et al.: The "lung point": An ultrasound sign specific to pneumothorax. *Intensive Care Med* 26:1434–1440, 2000.

64. Blaivas M, Lyon M, Duggal S: A prospective comparison of supine chest radiography and bedside ultrasound for the diagnosis of traumatic pneumothorax. *Acad Emerg Med* 12:844–849, 2005.

65. Rhea JT, vanSonnenberg E, McLoud TC: Basilar pneumothorax in the supine adult. *Radiology* 133:593–595, 1979.

66. Moskowitz PS, Griscom NT: The medial pneumothorax. *Radiology* 120:143–147, 1976.

67. Lams PM, Jolles H: The effect of lobar collapse on the distribution of free intrapleural air. *Radiology* 142:309–312, 1982.

68. Cooke DA, Cooke JC: The supine pneumothorax. *Ann R Coll Surg Engl* 6(9):130–134, 1987.

69. Tocino IM, Miller MH, Fairfax WR: Distribution of pneumothorax in the supine and semirecumbent critically ill adult. *AJR* 144:901–905, 1985.

70. Ball CG, Kirkpatrick AW, Laupland KB, et al.: Factors related to the failure of radiographic recognition of occult posttraumatic pneumothoraces. *Am J Surg* 189:541–546, 2005.

71. American College of Surgeons: *Advanced Trauma Life Support Course for Doctors*. Committee on Trauma. Instructors Course Manual. Chicago, IL, 1997.

72. Sargsyan AE, Hamilton DR, Nicolaou S, Kirkpatrick AW, et al.: Ultrasound evaluation of the magnitude of pneumothorax: A new concept. *Am Surg* 67:232–236, 2001.

73. Varner MW: Maternal Mortality in Iowa from 1952 to 1986. *Surg Gynecol Obstet* 168:555–562, 1989.

74. Lane PL: Traumatic Fetal Deaths. *J Emerg Med* 7:433–435, 1989.

75. Agran PF, Dunkle DE, Winn DG, et al.: Fetal Death in Motor Vehicle Accidents. *Ann Emerg Med* 16:1355–1358, 1987.

76. Pepperell RJ, Rubinstein E, MacIsaac LA: Motor-car accidents during pregnancy. *Med J Aust* 1:203–205, 1977.

77. Stafford PA, Biddinger PW, Zumwalt RE: Lethal intrauterine fetal trauma. *Am J Obstet Genecol* 159:459–459, 1988.

78. Crosby WM, Costiloe JP: Safety of lap-belt restraint for pregnant victims of automobile collisions. *N Engl J Med* 284:632–636, 1971.

79. Pearlman MD, Tintinalli JE, Lorenz RP: Blunt trauma during pregnancy. *N Engl J Med* 323:1609–1613, 1990.

80. Sherer DM, Schenker JG: Accidental injury during pregnancy. *Obstet Gynecol Surg* 44:330–338, 1989.

81. Drost TF, Rosemury AS, Sherman HF, et al.: Major trauma in pregnant women: Maternal/fetal outcome. *J Trauma* 30:574–578, 1990.

82. Ma OJ, Mateer JR, DeBehnke DJ: Use of ultrasonography for the evaluation of pregnant trauma patients. *J Trauma* 40:665–668, 1996.

83. Pearlman MD, Tintinalli JE, Lorenz RP: A prospective controlled study of outcome after trauma during pregnancy. *Am J Obstet Gynecol* 162:1502–1510, 1990.

84. Filiatrault D, Longpre D, Patriquin H, et al.: Investigation of childhood blunt abdominal trauma: A practical approach using ultrasound as the initial diagnostic modality. *Pediatr Radiol* 17:373–379, 1987.

85. Luks FI, Lemire A, St-Vil D, et al.: Blunt abdominal trauma in children: The practical value of ultrasonography. *J Trauma* 34:607–610, 1993.

86. Taylor GA, Sivit CJ: Posttraumatic peritoneal fluid: Is it a reliable indicator of intraabdominal injury in children? *J Pediatr Surg* 30:1644–1648, 1995.

87. Coley BD, Mutabagani KH, Martin LC, et al.: Focused abdominal sonography for trauma (FAST) in children with blunt abdominal trauma. *J Trauma* 48:902–906, 2000.

88. Thourani VH, Pettitt BJ, Schmidt JA, et al.: Validation of surgeon-performed emergency abdominal ultrasonography in pediatric trauma patients. *J Pediatr Surg* 33:322–328, 1998.

89. Patel JC, Tepas JJ: The efficacy of focused abdominal sonography for trauma as a screening tool in the assessment of injured children. *J Pediatr Surg* 34:44–47, 1999.

90. Mutabagani KH, Coley BD, Zumberge N, et al.: Preliminary experience with focused abdominal sonography for trauma (FAST) in children: Is it useful? *J Pediatr Surg* 34:48–54, 1999.

91. Soundappan SV, Holland AJ, Cass DT, et al.: Diagnostic accuracy of surgeon-performed focuaed abdomial sonography (FAST) in blunt paediatric trauma. *Injury* 36:970–975, 2005.

92. Moore CL, Rose GA, Tayal VS, et al.: Determination of left ventricular function by emergency physician echocardiography of hypotensive patients. *Acad Emerg Med* 9:186–193, 2002.

93. Jones AE, Aborn LS, Kline JA: Severity of emergency department hypotension predicts adverse hospital outcome. *Ann Emerg Med* 22:410–414, 2004.

94. Rose JS, Bair AE, Mandavia D, et al.: The UHP ultrasound protocol: A novel ultrasound approach to the empiric evaluation of the undifferentiated hypotensive patient. *Am J Emerg Med* 19:299–302, 2001.

95. Jones AE, Tayal VS, Sullivan M, et al.: Randomized, controlled trial of immediate versus delayed goal-directed ultrasound to identify the cause on nontraumatic hypotension in emergency department patients. *Crit Care Med* 32:1703–1708, 2004.

96. Jones AE, Craddock PA, Tayal VS, et al.: Diagnostic accuracy of left ventricular function for identifying sepsis among emergency department patients with nontraumatic symptomatic undifferentiated hypotension. *Ann Emerg Med* 24:513–517, 2005.

97. Randazzo MR, Snoey ER, Levitt MA, et al.: Accuracy of emergency physician assessment of left ventricular ejection fraction and central venous pressure using echocardiography. *Acad Emerg Med* 10:973–977, 2003.

98. Meyers MA: The spread and localization of acute intraperitoneal effusion. *Radiology* 94:547–554, 1970.

99. McKenney KL, Nunez DB, McKenney MG, et al.: Ultrasound for blunt abdominal trauma: Is it free fluid? *Emerg Radiol* 5:203–209, 1998.

100. Henderson SO, Sung J, Mandavia D: Serial abdominal ultrasound in the setting of trauma. *J Emerg Med* 18:79–81, 2000.

101. Miller MT, Pasquale MD, Bromberg WJ, et al.: Not so Fast. *J Trauma* 54:52–60, 2003.

102. Chiu WC, Cushing BM, Rodriguez A, et al.: Abdominal injuries without hemoperitoneum: A potential limitation of focused abdominal sonography for trauma (FAST). *J Trauma* 43:617–625, 1997.

103. Kirkpatrick AW, Simons RK, Brown DR, et al.: The hand-held FAST: Experience with hand-held trauma sonography in a level-I urban trauma center. *Injury* 33:303–308, 2002.

104. Etoch SW, Bar-Natan MF, Miller FB, et al.: Tube thoracostomy: Factors related to complications. *Arch Surg* 130:521–526, 1995.

CHAPTER 6

Cardiac

Robert F. Reardon and Scott A. Joing

Echocardiography is the gold standard for the diagnosis of many cardiac and pericardial abnormalities.[1] Echocardiography provides critical information about cardiac structure and function in real time. Since it is impossible for expert echocardiographers to be present in a timely manner for most critical resuscitations, emergency physicians have begun to incorporate focused bedside echocardiography into their daily clinical practice.[2-7] During the past 20 years, there is a growing body of evidence that noncardiologists can use focused echocardiography safely and accurately in a variety of clinical settings.[5,8-23]

Focused echocardiography is a goal-directed examination that is used only to answer defined clinical questions and not to detect all possible cardiac pathology. The key is to keep the examination straightforward by evaluating for gross abnormalities and overall cardiac function.[2,24,25] Focused echocardiography is not meant to replace comprehensive echocardiographic examinations; rather, its purpose is to provide clinicians with vital, real-time information when comprehensive echocardiography is unavailable.[24,26]

▶ CLINICAL CONSIDERATIONS

Focused transthoracic echocardiography is an ideal diagnostic tool for detecting life-threatening cardiac conditions in the emergency department. Much of the information obtained from a focused bedside echocardiographic examination could also be obtained by invasive monitoring techniques. Although emergency physicians and critical care physicians routinely use invasive monitoring, it is not practical to use invasive techniques on all patients with potentially life-threatening conditions. Patients who have quickly reversible hemodynamic compromise do not need invasive monitoring. In addition, placement of invasive monitoring devices is time consuming and has complications.

Without bedside echocardiography or invasive monitoring, clinicians would be left to manage critically ill patients with only indirect information about cardiac structure and function. "Classic" physical examination findings and changes in vital signs are often absent and unreliable for making critical diagnoses. An electrocardiogram (ECG) is very helpful in patients with certain cardiovascular problems who have diagnostic findings, but the majority of critically ill patients have nonspecific ECG findings. A chest radiograph may also provide some helpful information, but is just as likely to be nonspecific as well.

In cardiac arrest with pulseless electrical activity (PEA), it is critical to determine whether the patient has true electromechanical dissociation (EMD) with cardiac standstill or pseudo-EMD with mechanical cardiac contractions too weak to generate a palpable blood pressure.[27] Some patients thought to be in cardiac arrest have extreme hypotension. Other patients with PEA have cardiac tamponade, massive pulmonary embolism (PE), or severe left ventricular dysfunction. All of these conditions can be detected with bedside transthoracic echocardiography. Echocardiography can be performed serially during a critical resuscitation as long as the examination itself does not interfere with resuscitative efforts.

A controversial use of focused echocardiography is for patients who are stable and minimally symptomatic. Stable patients presenting with nonspecific symptoms may benefit from a focused echocardiographic examination. Pericardial effusions often cause nonspecific or minimal symptoms until tamponade develops. Focused echocardiography is the most efficient method to evaluate for "silent" pericardial effusion since it is not reasonable to order a comprehensive echocardiographic examination on every patient with such vague complaints in the emergency department. Also, 6% of all patients over 45 years of age have "silent" heart failure.[30] Many patients also have "silent" valvular disease and may benefit from focused echocardiography, even if the only information gained is an estimate of gross chamber size.

Transesophageal echocardiography (TEE) may be used as an alternative or complementary diagnostic tool to transthoracic echocardiography. While transthoracic echocardiography does not require sedation or airway protection, TEE is a more invasive procedure that may necessitate those maneuvers. Nevertheless, although not yet widely used by emergency or acute care physicians, TEE has the capability of obtaining excellent resolution of intracardiac abnormalities with little artifact or ultrasound window difficulty. TEE is portable and can be performed at the bedside and during ongoing cardiopulmonary resuscitation without interruption of chest procedures. Other advantages include that it is reproducible, rapid, and accurate. Disadvantages of TEE are that it is very operator dependent, may not be well tolerated by some patients, and may expose patients to vomiting and aspiration. Limitations of TEE are that it may not visualize the extension of aortic dissection into supra-aortic arteries and that it may have difficulty assessing a small distal portion of the ascending aorta and branches of the aortic arch behind the respiratory tract.[28–31] Table 6-1

contrasts transthoracic echocardiography with various other diagnostic testing and evaluation methods.

► CLINICAL INDICATIONS

Any patient at risk for significant cardiovascular compromise is a candidate for a focused bedside echocardiographic examination. Patients with significant disease have widely varying presentations, from cardiac arrest to vague symptoms of dizziness, shortness of breath, or chest discomfort.[32,33] The challenge is to determine which echocardiographic findings can be readily recognized by noncardiologists with minimal training and which patients need comprehensive echocardiography.

Primary indications for performing focused echocardiography include

- cardiac arrest,
- pericardial effusion,
- massive pulmonary embolism,
- assessment of left ventricular function,
- unexplained hypotension,
- estimation of central venous pressure, and
- external cardiac pacing.

Other indications that require more training and experience with focused echocardiography include

- severe valvular dysfunction,
- proximal aortic dissection, and
- myocardial ischemia.

► CARDIAC ARREST

Bedside echocardiography is invaluable in helping resuscitate patients with PEA. Prior to the 1980s all patients with an organized electrical rhythm but no pulse were thought to have EMD. In the mid-1980s, using arterial catheters and echocardiography, physicians discovered that many patients with apparent EMD have mechanical contractions that are too weak to produce a blood pressure detectable by palpation.[2,3,34–36]

A 1988 study described two very different categories of EMD, those with "true" EMD and those with mechanical cardiac contractions. It observed that those with "true" EMD, or cardiac standstill, have a dismal prognosis, similar to the prognosis for asystole.[2]

It has been reported that 86% of patients with PEA have mechanical cardiac contractions.[36]

Studies have confirmed that palpation of pulses is an unreliable means of assessing cardiac function and blood pressure. One study questioned whether carotid, femoral, or radial pulses correlated with certain blood pressure measurements.[37] They attempted to palpate pulses in 20 hypotensive patients who had arterial lines

	TTE	Clinical Examination	CVP	PA Line	EKG	Chest Radiograph	Arteriography	CT	MRI	Pericardial Window	Thoracotomy
Ease of use	+++	+++	+	+	+++	+++	+	++	+++	+	+
Diagnostic cardiac accuracy	+++	+	+	++	++	++	+++	++	+++	+++	+++
Lack of invasiveness	++	+++	+	+	+++	+++	+	++	++	+	+
Limitations	Aortic anatomy, coronary anatomy, pulmonary anatomy, valvular vegetation	Pulmonary embolism, myocardial ischemia	LVEDP not measured	Invasive pressures only measured	Lack of anatomical findings, nonspecificity for valvular lesions and aortic disease	Chamber size, hemodynamics, location of disease	Dye load, catheterization laboratory availability, valvular anatomy, right and left heart—different procedures	Breath hold, intracardiac anatomy, pressure readings	Breath hold, need for stable patient	Intracardiac anatomy	Invasiveness, need for bypass
Strengths	Repeatable, noninvasiveness, bedside intracardiac anatomy	Valvular, lack of invasiveness	Availability, right heart pressures	Blood sampling, LVEDP accurate measurement	Availability	Pulmonary disease, availability	Coronary anatomy, chamber pressure, aortic disease	Other thoracic/abdominal anatomy, aortic disease	Other thoracic/abdominal anatomy, aortic disease	Avoidance of thoracotomy	Proximal control, repair of cardiac/thoracic lesions

Note. TTE = Transthoracic echocardiography; CVP = central venous pressure; PA = pulmonary artery; EKG = electrocardiogram; CT = computed tomography; MRI = magnetic resonance imaging; LVEDP = left ventricular end-diastolic pressure
0 = None; + = Minimal; ++ = Moderate; +++ = Large.

and invasive blood pressure measurement already established. They found that as systolic blood pressure declined the radial pulse always disappeared before the femoral pulse, which always disappeared before the carotid pulse. Surprisingly, the disappearance of pulses from a specific location did not correlate with an absolute blood pressure but was widely variable; for instance, several patients had palpable carotid pulses with a measured systolic blood pressure between 30 and 60 mmHg. More worrisome was the finding that about 10% of these patients had no palpable carotid pulse with measured systolic blood pressures between 50 and 80 mmHg.[37]

Since carotid pulses are an unreliable means for determining true cardiac arrest, basic life support guidelines put forth by the American Hearth Association no longer recommend that lay people even try to check for a carotid pulse.[38] One study found that health care providers may not be any better than lay people when palpating carotid pulses and questioned the use of carotid pulse checks during cardiopulmonary resuscitation (CPR), even by health care providers.[39] Bedside echocardiography allows clinicians to directly visualize the heart and determine the presence and quality of mechanical cardiac function during a cardiac arrest. If a carotid pulse is absent but echocardiography shows reasonable mechanical cardiac function, then clinicians should proceed with aggressive resuscitation.

Several studies have examined whether bedside echocardiography in PEA could predict the outcome of cardiac arrest resuscitation.[8,21,22,40] A 2001 study reported that 56% of patients presenting to two community hospitals with PEA had cardiac contractions on bedside echocardiography; 26% of those with contractions and 4% (one patient) with cardiac standstill survived to hospital admission.[22] In a multicenter trial from four academic centers, 32% of patients with PEA had mechanical contractions. No patient with cardiac standstill had return of spontaneous circulation (ROSC) and 73% of those with mechanical contractions had ROSC.[21]

The data suggest that when echocardiography shows cardiac standstill it may be reasonable to consider terminating resuscitative efforts although return of mechanical contraction was reported in 4 of 18 patients who initially had cardiac standstill.[41] In current practice, many emergency physicians use echocardiography to confirm cardiac standstill before terminating resuscitation in all cardiac arrests. Beyond predicting the outcome of resuscitation, echocardiography is essential in helping to rapidly identify the cause of the cardiac arrest since PEA is often associated with specific clinical states that may be readily reversed when identified and treated appropriately.[27] The most common causes of PEA are hypovolemia, hypoxia, acidosis, hypo/hyperkalemia, hypoglycemia, hypothermia, drug overdose, cardiac tamponade, tension pneumothorax,

massive myocardial infarction, and massive PE.[34] Hypovolemia, cardiac tamponade, massive PE, and massive myocardial infarction can be detected by bedside echocardiography so that early aggressive management of these abnormalities can then be instituted.[41-44]

The first question to answer using bedside echocardiography is whether the etiology of the arrest is likely to be cardiac or noncardiac. Severe left ventricular dysfunction from massive myocardial infarction, acidosis, drug overdose, or electrolyte abnormality will be apparent. Kaul and colleagues reported using a similar approach to determine whether hypotension had a cardiac or noncardiac etiology. The authors compared 2-D echocardiography to hemodynamic measurements from pulmonary artery catheters and found that in 86% of cases echocardiography correctly determined whether the etiology of shock was cardiac or noncardiac.[45] In addition, studies have shown that emergency physicians can accurately estimate left ventricular function, especially when left ventricular dysfunction is severe.[15,19,46]

Patients in cardiac arrest with PEA as a result of severe hypovolemia will have a small, empty appearing heart on bedside echocardiography.[42] Both the right and left ventricles will be poorly filled and the right ventricle will be almost completely collapsed. The left ventricle will usually be vigorous. The inferior vena cava (IVC) will have a small diameter and its lumen will disappear completely during inspiration (or expiration when positive pressure ventilation is being used). These findings on bedside echocardiography should prompt the clinician to aggressively replace volume and consider the etiology of hypovolemia.

The most straightforward application of bedside echocardiography during cardiac arrest is evaluating for a pericardial effusion.[2,18,47] A pericardial effusion presents as an anechoic stripe surrounding the heart and should be obvious if it is large enough to cause cardiac tamponade. This finding should prompt the clinician to perform an immediate pericardiocentesis using echocardiography guidance (see chapter 20). Pericardiocentesis can be life-saving and the removal of just a small amount of fluid may result in significant improvement in cardiac output.[2,3,5,44]

Massive PE is responsible for about 10% of cardiac arrests in cases where a primary cardiac etiology is clinically suspected.[48,49] The routine use of bedside echocardiography in cardiac arrest may allow immediate detection of massive PE, even in cases where the diagnosis is not clinically suspected.[43,50-54] It is important to immediately recognize that PE is the cause of a cardiac arrest because early thrombolytic therapy has been shown to significantly improve the chance of ROSC. A review of 60 cases of cardiac arrest caused by massive PE found that 81% of patients who received early thrombolysis had ROSC compared with 43% for those who did not receive the therapy.[48]

▶ PERICARDIAL EFFUSION

In 1992, Plummer reported 100% sensitivity for recognizing pericardial effusion in the first 6 years after his group of emergency physicians began screening penetrating trauma patients with echocardiography. More importantly, the use of bedside echocardiography significantly reduced the time to diagnosis and disposition to the operating room from 42.4 minutes to 15.5 minutes while the actual survival improved from 57.1 to 100%.[19] Bedside focused echocardiography is now the standard of care for patients with potential penetrating cardiac injuries.[20,55,56]

Patients at risk for nontraumatic pericardial effusions are more difficult to identify clinically because they usually have nonspecific signs and symptoms. Most patients with a pericardial effusion are stable and have nonspecific symptoms such as dyspnea, chest pain, cough, or fatigue.[57,58] Since cardiac tamponade can develop rapidly, even in those with chronic pericardial effusion, it is prudent to make the diagnosis as early as possible. Patients at risk for a pericardial effusion include those with the following disease processes: idiopathic/viral pericarditis, HIV, hepatitis B, bacterial pericarditis, fungal pericarditis, lupus, rheumatoid arthritis, scleroderma, polyarteritis nodosa, temporal arteritis, early postmyocardial infarction, Dressler syndrome, drug induced (isoniazid, cyclosporine), neoplastic, radiation induced, postcardiac surgery, postcardiac procedure/device, chronic renal failure, hypothyroidism, amyloidosis, aortic dissection, congestive heart failure, and blunt/penetrating chest trauma.[57,59] Effusions associated with neoplastic disease or bacterial, fungal, or HIV infections have a higher risk of progressing to tamponade.[59] Patients who have had recent invasive cardiac procedures, such as coronary angiography and pacemaker or defibrillator placement, are at high risk for pericardial effusion with tamponade.

Any patient with a pericardial effusion is at risk for developing cardiac tamponade, which is a life-threatening condition that occurs when a pericardial effusion causes significant compression of the heart leading to a decrease in cardiac output. When a pericardial effusion develops acutely, tamponade can occur with as little as 150 mL of fluid. Because the parietal pericardium can stretch over time, a chronic effusion can have a volume of more than 1000 mL without causing tamponade. The rate of pericardial fluid accumulation relative to pericardial stretch is the critical factor. The steep rise in the pericardial pressure-volume curve makes tamponade a "last-drop" phenomenon, the last few milliliters of fluid accumulation produce critical cardiac compression and the first milliliters of drainage produce the largest relative decompression.[58,60] Cardiac tamponade presents with hypotension that rapidly progresses to PEA and death if not rapidly diagnosed and treated.[61,62] Echocardiogra-

phy is now the standard means to evaluate for cardiac tamponade[63] and can also be used to guide pericardiocentesis.

One study evaluated bedside echocardiography on 103 patients with unexplained dyspnea and found that 14 had pericardial effusions. Four had large effusions requiring pericardiocentesis and 3 had moderate-sized effusions that were treated conservatively. The authors recommended that emergency department patients with unexplained dyspnea should be evaluated for pericardial effusion.[32] Mandavia and colleagues performed bedside echocardiography on 515 patients presenting to their emergency department with high-risk risk criteria to determine the accuracy of bedside echocardiography performed by emergency physicians to detect pericardial effusions. These criteria consisted of unexplained hypotension or dyspnea, congestive heart failure, cancer, uremia, lupus, or pericarditis. They found 103 pericardial effusions in this high-risk population and determined that bedside echocardiography by emergency physicians was 97.5% accurate.[57]

Most nonhemorrhagic pericardial effusions that cause tamponade are moderate to large (300–600 mL) in size.[58] Therefore, an indication for emergent pericardiocentesis is the finding of a moderate or large effusion in a patient with clinical signs of tamponade. Large pericardial effusions surround the entire heart while small effusions collect first around the more dependent, mobile ventricles.[47] Effusions can be categorized by the maximal width of the echogenic pericardial stripe. A stripe less than 10 mm is small, 10–15 mm is moderate, and greater than 15 mm is large.[32] These are gross measurements and do not correlate perfectly to the volume of the effusion. Also, hemorrhagic effusions can occur outside the setting of trauma and tend to accumulate rapidly and cause tamponade even when they are small.

▶ MASSIVE PULMONARY EMBOLISM

Massive pulmonary embolism (PE) is a condition for which bedside echocardiography is invaluable for making a rapid diagnosis.[51,52,64,65] Echocardiography can also help exclude diagnoses that mimic PE such as pericardial tamponade, pneumothorax, and myocardial infarction.[64] Patients with massive PE often present with significant symptoms or with impending cardiac arrest. Patients who present in extremis require rapid intervention since 70% of patients who die from PE die within the first hour. Early thrombolytic therapy or embolectomy is required and rapid treatment often precludes obtaining time-consuming imaging studies.[66–74] This is a challenging scenario for clinicians because thrombolytic therapy can have significant morbidity and embolectomy requires mobilization of significant resources. Bedside echocardiography can help clinicians quickly confirm or refute the clinical diagnosis of massive PE. The echocardiographic findings in massive PE are not subtle and include massive right ventricular dilatation and right-sided heart failure with a small vigorously contracting left ventricle.[43] In some cases, thrombus can actually be seen in the right atrium or ventricle.

The detection of massive PE by bedside echocardiography should not be confused with using echocardiography to evaluate hemodynamically stable patients suspected of having PE. In stable patients without severe symptoms right-sided heart strain is often subtle and difficult to appreciate on bedside echocardiography. Also, there are many other underlying diseases that cause chronic right-sided heart strain, thus making the diagnosis of acute cor pulmonale in these patients difficult and unreliable.[75]

▶ ASSESSMENT OF LEFT VENTRICULAR FUNCTION

Echocardiography is the preferred first-line test for patients with symptoms or signs consistent with left ventricular dysfunction.[76] Patients who present with nonspecific complaints may have unexpected left ventricular failure. More than half of patients with moderate to severe systolic dysfunction have never been diagnosed with heart failure.[28] Patients with moderate to severe left ventricular dysfunction are at higher risk for complications regardless of their presentation. In addition, when patients present with cardiogenic shock both short- and long-term mortality are associated with the degree of initial left ventricular systolic dysfunction and the degree of mitral regurgitation.[77]

Several studies have demonstrated that noncardiologists can use focused ultrasound in assessment of left ventricular function by estimating left ventricular ejection fraction. One study reported that emergency physicians with prior ultrasound training and 16 hours of additional training could accurately measure left ventricular ejection fraction (LVEF) in hypotensive emergency department patients.[15] All of the echocardiographic examinations were recorded and reviewed by two masked cardiologists. Emergency physicians and cardiologists had 84% overall agreement compared with 88% interobserver agreement between the two cardiologists. The study concluded that bedside echocardiography adds diagnostic value in patients presenting to the emergency department with unexplained hypotension.

Another study reported that emergency physicians with only 3 hours of additional training could accurately estimate left ventricular ejection fraction. They performed a bedside echocardiography on emergency department patients who had a "comprehensive echocardiography" ordered for any reason regardless of hemodynamic status or symptoms. The authors found 86% overall agreement between emergency physicians and cardiologists. Their technique for determining LVEF was restricted to a subjective visual estimate of the change in left ventricular size in diastole versus systole. There was no attempt to clinically correlate these results but the authors suggested that emergency physicians could use bedside echocardiography to differentiate patients with primary pump failure from those with other potential causes of hypotension.[19]

Noncardiologists who use echocardiography to assess left ventricular function should be aware that left ventricular function includes more than just the LVEF. Ejection fraction is largely an assessment of systolic function. Measuring LVEF usually leads to correct interpretation of pathophysiology, especially in cases of heart failure caused by coronary disease and cardiomyopathy. Ejection fraction may not be a good indicator of cardiac output for aortic stenosis, mitral regurgitation, and concentric left ventricular hypertrophy.[78] Diastolic dysfunction is also an important factor in heart failure. Approximately 50% of patients with overt congestive heart failure have diastolic dysfunction without reduced ejection fraction. Determination of diastolic dysfunction requires Doppler measurements.

▶ UNEXPLAINED HYPOTENSION

Unexplained hypotension or shock is a common presentation in the emergency department or critical care setting. The main utility of bedside echocardiography in shock is to allow clinicians to immediately narrow the differential diagnosis and begin early aggressive resuscitation. A simple assessment of global cardiac function and chamber size allows clinicians to assign hypotensive patients to one of four diagnoses: cardiogenic shock from severe left ventricular dysfunction, cardiac tamponade, massive PE, or severe hypovolemia.[47] In addition to assessment of cardiac chamber size and left ventricular function, evaluation of the proximal IVC can be easily used to estimate right atrial filling pressure. Hypovolemia should be considered whenever low (or moderate) right atrial filling pressure is found in combination with a hyperdynamic left ventricle. When hypovolemic shock is suspected from echocardiographic findings, a search for hemorrhagic etiologies may include sonographic examinations for free intraperitoneal fluid and ruptured abdominal aortic aneurysm.[79]

Shock resulting from severe left ventricular dysfunction, cardiac tamponade, or massive PE should be readily apparent on bedside echocardiography.[15,18,19,43,44,46] The finding of moderate or severely reduced left ventricular ejection fraction does not prove that an acute or primary cardiac abnormality is the cause. Clinicians must realize that there are many other factors to consider such as preexisting cardiac disease and the effects of drugs or acidosis on left ventricular function. As with all echocardiographic findings, clinical correlation is required, but the unexpected finding of significant left ventricular dysfunction in any hypotensive patient is always clinically important.

A prospective study analyzed bedside echocardiography to evaluate the left ventricular function of emergency department patients with atraumatic, unexplained hypotension. Seventeen percent of the patients were found to have a hyperdynamic left ventricle. Of those with a hyperdynamic left ventricular, 76% had a final diagnosis of sepsis. The authors concluded that in emergency department patients with atraumatic, unexplained hypotension the finding of a hyperdynamic left ventricle is highly specific for sepsis as the etiology of shock.[15] Extending the bedside ultrasound examination to include assessment for intraperitoneal fluid or abdominal aortic aneurysm is appropriate in some settings.[47] Rose and coinvestigators reported using an undifferentiated hypotensive patient protocol for the use of ultrasound to rapidly evaluate for cardiac tamponade, intraperitoneal blood, and abdominal aortic aneurysm.[79]

▶ ESTIMATION OF CENTRAL VENOUS PRESSURE

Assessment of the size and respiratory variations of the proximal IVC can provide information about central venous pressure (CVP) and fluid status. The IVC can dilate or collapse depending on intraluminal pressure. In general, a large IVC correlates with higher CVP and a small IVC correlates with a lower CVP. There is usually significant respiratory variation in the size of the IVC because inspiration produces negative intrathoracic pressure and draws blood out of the IVC and into the right atrium, causing the IVC to collapse. The reverse occurs during expiration and the IVC expands. Several investigators have attempted to correlate IVC findings with CVP values, which is difficult since absolute IVC size varies between patients and the IVC can completely collapse with inspiration in a normovolemic patient. Although IVC measurements cannot accurately measure CVP values, they can be used to effectively estimate whether CVP is very low or very high.

The proximal IVC is found in the subxiphoid view as it courses posterior to the liver and into the right atrium. It is usually measured about 3–4 cm distal to its junction with the atrium or 2-cm distal to the entry to the hepatic viens.[80–82] It is measured in the AP diameter in the sagittal plane.[80] One study measured the IVC in 27 patients who had pulmonary artery catheters

in-place with right atrial ports and found that in general patients with high right atrial pressure had a larger maximal IVC. There was a stronger correlation between inspiratory collapse of the IVC and CVP. Specifically, the CVP was nearly always >10 mmHg if the IVC did not collapse more than 50% with full inspiration. Patients with low CVP had maximal collapse with low inspiratory pressures and those with higher CVP had a gradual collapse of the IVC that was greatest at high inspiratory pressures.[82] Another study found that 86% of patients with CVP <10 mmHg had IVC collapse >50%, and 89% with CVP ≥10 mmHg had IVC collapse ≤50% with inspiration.[83]

One study found that nearly all trauma patients who presented in shock or later required blood transfusion had an IVC ≤9 mm and those who were stable had IVC >9 mm. The group who presented in shock had a mean hemoglobin level of 9.1 g/dL while the control group had a mean hemoglobin level of 11.3 g/dL.[84] These findings suggested that measurements of IVC may be useful in identifying patients who are in early shock before they develop classic signs of shock. The data also suggested that serial IVC measurements may be useful for monitoring patients with known or suspected blood loss or any other process that may lead to shock.

From a practical standpoint, the initial size and respiratory variation of the IVC is not as helpful (except when at the extremes) as the changes that occur in these parameters in response to a fluid challenge. When a patient presents with undifferentiated hypotension, the initial treatment often involves a fluid challenge. Serial monitoring of the IVC can help the clinician evaluate the effect of this treatment more accurately. In general, if the patient's hemodynamics improve and the IVC changes little on ultrasound, more fluid can be given. When the IVC measurements indicate rapidly increasing fluid pressures, further fluid administration should be limited.

▶ EXTERNAL CARDIAC PACING

Transcutaneous cardiac pacing is a common treatment for hemodynamically unstable bradycardias. Application and use of external pacing devices is simple but assessment of mechanical ventricular capture during pacing can be confusing. If the pacing unit is used for electrocardiographic monitoring, then a pacing filter may allow correct assessment of electrical capture. Even with a filter pacer spikes can drown out the native QRS complexes and give a false impression that there is electrical capture when there is none. An alternative means of assessing the capture is to feel the patients pulse and confirm that pulses correspond to pacer output. However, this can also be difficult especially if pacing causes significant skeletal muscle contractions.[85]

The use of bedside echocardiography to assess pacemaker capture is straightforward and was described in the earliest report of emergency department bedside echocardiography.[4] The utility of echocardiography for determining the capture during external pacing was studied using an animal model and showed that blinded interpreters could identify ventricular capture with good agreement.[86]

Bedside echocardiography can also be used to help guide placement of a temporary transvenous pacemaker wire. Emergency physicians have used echocardiography guidance to correctly place pacer wires into the apex of the right ventricle and confirm ventricular capture with excellent success.[87]

► VALVULAR ABNORMALITIES

Valvular dysfunction and structural abnormalities have not traditionally been a focal part of the emergent echocardiography examination. In select cases of acute hemodynamic compromise, detection of significant valvular abnormalities by echocardiography may be lifesaving. Since the mitral valve is the most straightforward valve to visualize by echocardiography, severe abnormalities of this valve may be apparent. Acute rupture of chordae tendineae or papillary muscles can be seen as a result of myocardial infarction or infective endocarditis.[88] Rupture is more likely to result from an inferior wall myocardial infarction with involvement of the right coronary artery. Acute mitral valve incompetence causes dyspnea, pulmonary edema, and cardiogenic shock. Rupture of the entire papillary muscle usually results in acute severe mitral regurgitation.[89] This process may be suspected in patients presenting with new onset severe pulmonary edema. Rapid diagnosis and emergency surgery is the key to survival for these patients.

Both leaflets of the mitral valve are usually clearly visualized if a good parasternal long axis view can be obtained. In this view, rupture of one of the mitral valve leaflets will usually show a clear flail leaflet if the entire papillary muscle is ruptured. Alternatively, a four-chamber apical view will clearly show both mitral valve leaflets. Color Doppler will demonstrate regurgitant flow in an eccentric distribution opposite in direction to the leaflet with the anatomic defect.[89]

Aortic stenosis is typically seen in the elderly and is caused by degenerative heart disease or calcific aortic stenosis. Critical aortic stenosis can cause angina, syncope, and eventually heart failure. Sudden death from dysrhythmias occurs in 25% of such patients. Patients who present with congestive heart failure should be treated with oxygen and diuretics but nitrates are not well tolerated in patients with severe aortic stenosis as decreasing preload may result in significant hypotension.[90] Recognizing aortic disease on bedside echocardiography may not be as straightforward as detecting mitral abnormalities because movements of the aortic valve leaflets are much more difficult to visualize. Most patients with aortic stenosis will have significant calcifications and thickening of the aortic valve leaflets that may be visualized by echocardiography.

Aortic valve incompetence is an acute process in about 20% of cases and most commonly caused by infective endocarditis or proximal aortic dissection. In acute aortic valve incompetence, left ventricular failure develops rapidly and mortality from pulmonary edema and cardiac arrest is high, even with intensive medical therapy. The key to survival for these patients is rapid recognition of their condition and emergency surgery. Detecting aortic incompetence will require utilization of color Doppler flow across the aortic valve. Significant incompetence should be apparent with subjective visualization of color Doppler.

► AORTIC DISSECTION

Aortic dissection occurs when the intima is violated, allowing blood to enter the media and dissect between the intimal and adventitial layers. Common sites for tear include the ascending aorta and the region of the ligamentum arteriosum. The Stanford classification categorizes aortic dissection as Type A, which involves the ascending aorta; and Type B, which involves only the descending aorta.

Aortic dissection and intramural hematoma may be detected by transthoracic echocardiography on parasternal long, parasternal short, and suprasternal views. A linear echogenic flap, indicative of aortic dissection, may be seen across the aortic lumen anywhere along its length. The ascending aorta can be seen on the parasternal views while the descending aorta is usually seen only in cross section on parasternal views. The aortic arch may be visualized on the suprasternal view in a segment of the population.[28–31] A dissection that extends beyond the thoracic aorta may be detected with abdominal sonography.

TEE provides much better resolution and visualization of aortic dissection than transthoracic echocardiography. Spiral CT, TEE, and magnetic resonance imaging (MRI) have been demonstrated to have comparable sensitivity, and specificity, with accuracy rates approaching 100%.[28–31] One study found that all three modalities approach 100% sensitivity; the specificities for spiral CT, TEE, and MRI were 100, 94, and 94%, respectively.[91]

Important issues to address with aortic dissection include (1) presence of pericardial effusion as a sign of imminent mortality without surgical intervention; (2) presence of ascending aorta involvement without pericardial involvement; (3) evidence of isolated descending aorta involvement; (4) location of the entry site; and (5) evidence of involvement of major branch vessels.[28-31]

▶ MYOCARDIAL ISCHEMIA

The diagnosis of acute myocardia ischemia can be made by echocardiographic findings of wall motion abnormalities. Myocardial function is immediately affected by ischemia and may precede ECG changes. New regional wall motion abnormalities, however, may be difficult to differentiate from old wall motion changes without reviewing prior echocardiograms. Studies have demonstrated that the recognition of regional wall motion abnormalities by echocardiography in patients with acute chest pain is a sensitive predictor for Q-wave myocardial infarction. Sensitivity for acute myocardial infarction generally is high, but specificity remains moderate because of old wall motion abnormalities.[92,93] Resting echocardiography in patients with acute chest pain is not sufficiently sensitive for exclusion of cardiac ischemia.[94,95] In the emergency department, however, the combination of resting echocardiography and cardiac enzyme serum markers may be a promising combination for the stratification of patients at risk for complications within the hospital and on discharge.[96] The identification of echocardiographic abnormalities may expedite admission for stable patients who are being evaluated in an emergency department.

Echocardiography plays an important role in the noninvasive evaluation of patients with known myocardial infarction, including evaluation of its complications such as left ventricular systolic dysfunction, development of ventricular septal defects, left ventricular rupture, and mitral regurgitation.[97] In fact, one study on emergency department patients reported six cases of myocardial rupture with hemopericardium from acute myocardial infarction with early ventricular rupture. As four of these patients met the criteria for emergency thrombolytic therapy, the emergency management was significantly changed by these findings on the focused echocardiogram.[18] Chronic complications such as pericarditis, pericardial effusion, left ventricular aneurysm, and left ventricular thrombus may also be evaluated by echocardiography.

▶ ANATOMIC CONSIDERATIONS

HEART

The heart is a hollow muscular organ, placed between the lungs, and enclosed within the pericardium. It is divided by a septum into two halves, right and left, each half being further subdivided into two cavities, the atrium and the ventricle (Figure 6-1). Blood flows from the right atrium into the right ventricle through the tricus-

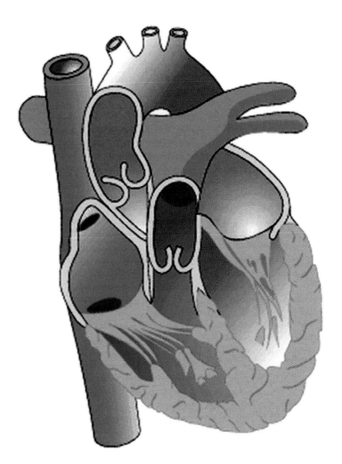

Figure 6-1. Cardiac circulation.

pid valve. From the right ventricle, unoxygenated blood is carried to the lungs through the pulmonary artery. Blood flows from the left atrium into the left ventricle through the mitral valve. From the left ventricle, oxygenated blood is distributed to the body through the aorta. The outflow tract through the aortic valve into the proximal aorta starts anteriorly and revolves posteriorly into the posterior mediastinum next to the esophagus. The aorta is divided into the ascending aorta, the aortic arch, and the descending aorta. The ascending aorta is approximately 5 cm in length; the only branches of the ascending aorta are the coronary arteries. The aortic arch has three branches: the innominate artery, the left common carotid artery, and the left subclavian artery.

The pericardium is composed of two layers, the parietal and visceral layers, which normally oppose each other without any significant fluid accumulation. The pericardium attaches to the superior left atrium and envelopes the proximal aspects of the great vessels (Figure 6-2).

THORACIC CAVITY

The thoracic cavity provides both windows and impediments to the accurate sonographic view of the heart

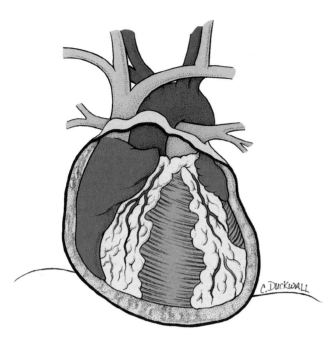

Figure 6-2. Pericardium.

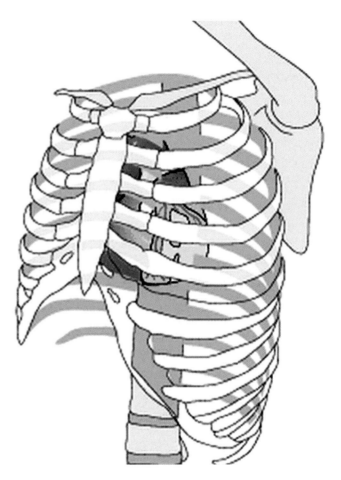

Figure 6-3. Chest cage.

(Figure 6-3). The heart has very few sonographic windows since ribs, the sternum, and the lungs surround it (Figure 6-4). Common windows include the parasternal, apical, subxiphoid, and suprasternal views. The left parasternal interspace allows for small sonographic windows into the mediastinum. The superior aspect of the abdomen also allows for soft tissue windows via the left lobe of the liver. The heart can shift closer to the chest wall in the left decubitus position.

CARDIAC AXES

The heart has a long axis from the right shoulder to the left hip. The transverse view, or short axis of the heart, is rotated 90° from the long axis of the heart (left shoulder to right hip) (Figure 6-5). The apical view, or four-chamber axis, is a coronal image of the heart from its apex to its base. The apex of the heart is usually located at the nipple line in the anterior axillary line. The base of the heart lies in an axis, anterior to posterior, from the parasternal right 2nd intercostal space to the posterior thorax next to the esophagus.

▶ GETTING STARTED

Novice sonologists may find transthoracic echocardiography difficult to learn initially because of the complex anatomy of the heart and difficulty obtaining standard images due to the surrounding air-filled lungs (Figures 6-1 and 6-4). It is important to note that the long axis

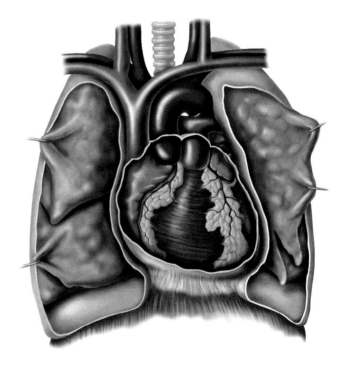

Figure 6-4. Surrounding structures.

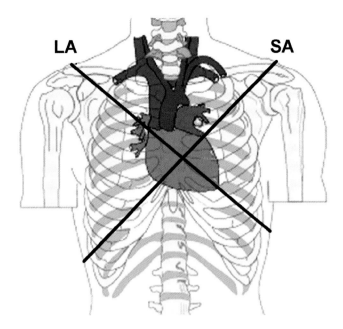

LA   **SA**

Figure 6-5. Cardiac axes. Long axis (LA), short axis (SA).

Transducer Type	Curved linear Array	Flat phased Array
Image on monitor	Sector	Sector
Moving structures capture	Poor	Good
Small window capability	Generally worse	Excellent
Gray scale differentiation of echogenic structures	Good	Poor

of the heart lies diagonal to the long axis of the torso (Figure 6-5). The long axis of the heart is more horizontal in short obese patients and more vertical in tall thin patients. Standard images of the heart are usually obtained from three anatomic locations on and below the chest wall: the subxiphoid window, the parasternal window, and the apical window. The heart lies higher in the chest cavity in obese patients and those who are supine. It lies lower in the chest cavity in thin patients and those who are sitting upright. The apex is found more medially in normal hearts and more laterally in enlarged hearts. Parasternal and apical images may be very difficult to obtain in patients with hyperexpanded lungs.

While most echocardiographers prefer to scan from the patient's left side, many clinicians scan from the patient's right. Cardiac presets should be selected if available on the machine. Patient positioning and ability to cooperate with inspiratory and expiratory maneuvers are critical to obtaining good images. The subxiphoid views are best obtained in the supine position, the parasternal views may be acquired with supine or left lateral decubitus (LLD) positioning and the apical views are usually best obtained in LLD. Windows through intercostal spaces can be improved by positioning the patient's left hand behind their head, which may slightly widen the window. Nearly any change in patient position may improve cardiac windows and the ability to obtain good images. The subxiphoid image is often significantly improved by having the patient take and hold a deep breath, the parasternal and apical views may at times be aided by an expiratory hold.

Having proper equipment and equipment settings is critical to obtaining good images. Using a phased array cardiac probe is better than a curvilinear for echocardiography (Table 6-2). The phased array probe allows imaging between the ribs and is especially important for the parasternal short axis and all apical views. For cardiac transthoracic echocardiographic studies, a probe with median frequencies of 3.5 MHz (2.5–5.0 MHz) should be used. Most modern ultrasound machines allow operators to use presets for each particular type of examination. Using cardiac presets will produce the best results. Also, modern machines give the operator the ability to change the frequency range of the ultrasound probe and activate tissue harmonics with the touch of a button. Testing different frequency ranges and activating tissue harmonics during each examination allow the operator to optimize images.

Overall gain and time-gain compensation are also simple to adjust and can be used to optimize each image. Ideal equipment settings produce images in which the edges of anatomic structures are sharply demarcated and the inside of the cardiac chambers appears black, not grey. It is important for novice sonologists to learn how to obtain images from all three standard anatomic locations and not just the subxiphoid location because on any given patient one location may produce excellent images while the others are less optimal. Every patient has unique anatomy and no one anatomic location allows adequate imaging in all patients.

▶ TECHNIQUE AND NORMAL ULTRASOUND FINDINGS

TRANSTHORACIC ECHOCARDIOGRAPHY

The arrow (right/left indicator) on the monitor is usually oriented to the right side of the image, which is the opposite of abdominal or pelvic imaging and is done automatically via a cardiac preset or manually by toggling the flip image (horizontal) button. The probe indicator, therefore, is oriented to the patient's left for transverse

▶ **TABLE 6-3. TRANSTHORACIC TRANSDUCER ORIENTATION ON THE SUPINE PATIENT**

Ultrasound Preset	Echocardiography	Abdomen/Pelvis
Machine/probe location	To the patient's left	To the patient's right
Monitor indicator	Right side of the image	Left side of the image
Subcostal	Probe marker directed to the patient's left flank	Probe marker directed to the patient's right flank
Apical four-chamber	Probe marker directed to the left side	Probe marker directed to the right side
	Probe aimed to right shoulder	Probe aimed to right shoulder
Parasternal long	Probe marker directed to the patient's right shoulder (10 o'clock)	Probe marker directed to the patient's left hip (4 o'clock)
Parasternal short	Probe marker directed to the patient's left shoulder (2 o'clock)	Probe marker directed to the patient's right hip (8 o'clock)

images. Table 6-3 provides a comparison of imaging techniques for the heart when using an echocardiography preset versus an abdominal/pelvic preset. Regardless of the machine setup, what is most important is to orient the images in a standard fashion on the monitor. This facilitates recognition of the cardiac chambers for the sonologist and for any others who may review the images.

▶ CARDIAC WINDOWS

TRANSTHORACIC

Subxiphoid Four-Chamber View

The subxiphoid view is the most useful view for emergency ultrasound. It usually does not interfere in resuscitative measures such as thoracostomy, CPR, subclavian line insertion, or intubation. It is easily learned, repeated, and performed as part of both the cardiac and trauma ultrasound evaluations.

The subxiphoid view should be performed at the subxiphoid position of the abdomen (Figure 6-6A). The probe should be held at a 15° angle to the chest wall and aimed toward the left shoulder. The probe marker should be aimed toward the patient's left flank (using a cardiac preset). The transducer should be angled up or down depending on the depth of the chest cavity to obtain images of the beating heart. The depth should then be adjusted to visualize the atria at the bottom of the monitor screen. Poor quality initial images may be improved upon by using an appropriate amount of ultrasound gel, using a shallow angle to the chest wall, moving the transducer to the right to use the left lobe of the liver as a window, and moving off the xiphoid and over to the lower intercostal spaces to image the barrel-chested patient with a larger anterior–posterior diameter.

The subxiphoid four-chamber view should be seen as primarily a diagonal view for the ventricles, atria,

pericardium, and the left lobe of the liver (Figure 6-6B and 6-6C). If the transducer is angled at a more acute angle toward the abdomen, the left lobe of the liver, inferior vena cava, and the hepatic veins should be visualized.

Subxiphoid Short-Axis View

The subxiphoid short axis view can be achieved by rotating the ultrasound probe 90° counterclockwise from the four-chamber view (using a cardiac preset) and aiming the probe toward the patient's left arm (Figure 6-7A). This orientation will resemble the parasternal short axis ("doughnut") view of the left ventricle and may provide virtually all of the same information (Figure 6-7B and 6-7C).

Subxiphoid Long-Axis View

The subxiphoid long axis view uses a sagittal body axis and the probe marker can be aimed toward the patient's feet (using a cardiac preset) (Figure 6-8A). This will place the atrium/diaphragm on the left side of the screen as is the standard for abdominal longitudinal imaging. Echocardiographers (who are envisioning the longitudinal view from the patient's left side) often orient this image with the probe marker pointing cephalad and the atrium/diaphragm on the right side of the screen. A sagittal section of the body views the heart, the left lobe of the liver, the IVC, and hepatic veins (Figure 6-8B). This view allows evaluation of the proximal IVC during expiration and inspiration (Figure 6-8C and 6-8D). The anterior–posterior diameter of the proximal IVC usually measures about 1.5–2.0 cm during expiration and collapses with inspiration. Collapse of less than 50% during inspiration indicates elevated right-sided heart pressures.

Parasternal Long-Axis View

The parasternal long axis view can be best obtained by accepting the long axis of the heart to be roughly from the right shoulder to the left hip (Figure 6-5). The

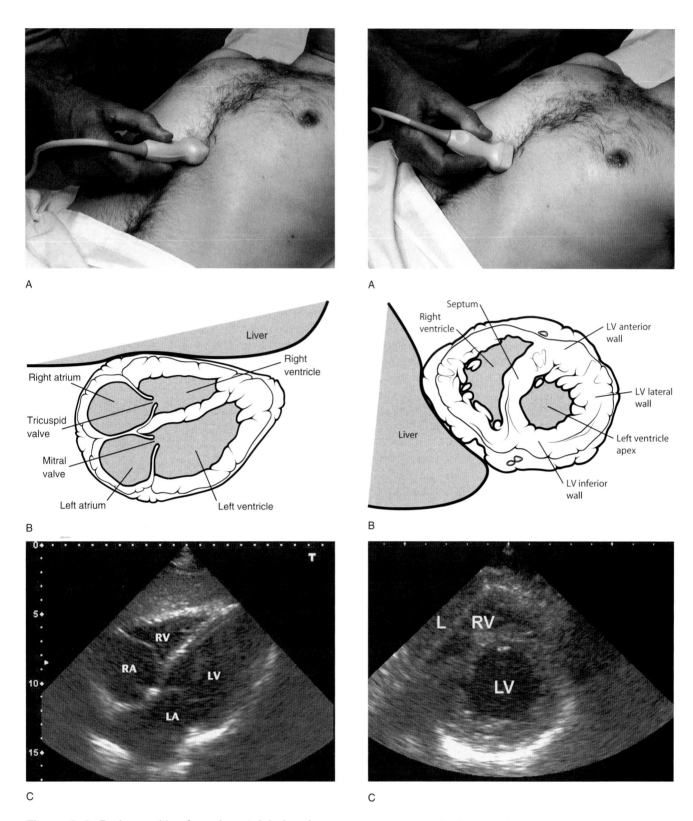

Figure 6-6. Probe position for subcostal 4 chamber view (A). Subcostal four-chamber diagram (B). Subcostal four-chamber normal ultrasound (C). RA = right atrium, RV = right ventricle, LA = left atrium, LV = left ventricle. (Courtesy of Hennepin County Medical Center for (C))

Figure 6-7. Probe position for subcostal short axis view (A). Subcostal short axis diagram (B). Subcostal short axis normal ultrasound (C). L = liver, RV = right ventricle, LV = left ventricle. (Courtesy of James Mateer, MD, for (C))

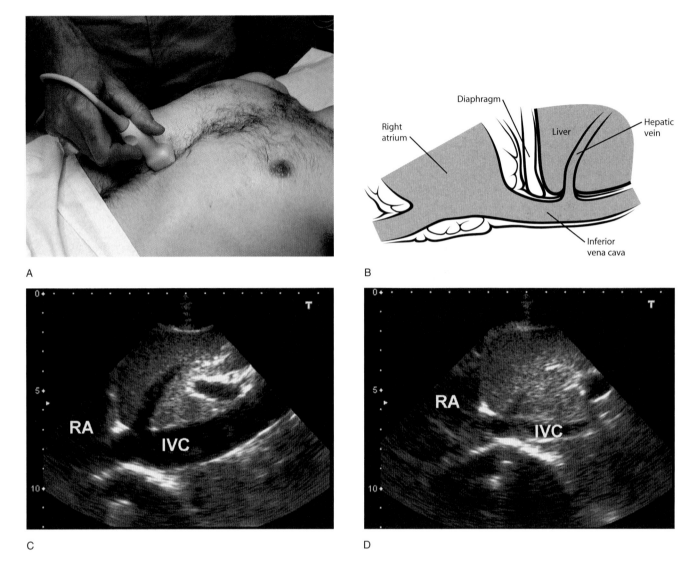

Figure 6-8. Probe position for subcostal long axis view (A). Subcostal long axis diagram (B). Proximal IVC during expiration (C) and inspiration (D). IVC = inferior vena cava, RA = right atrium. (Courtesy of Hennepin County Medical Center for (C,D))

transducer should be placed perpendicular to the chest wall at the 3rd or 4th intercostal space immediately to the left of the sternum with the probe indicator directed toward the right shoulder (using a cardiac preset) (Figure 6-9A). The following structures can be visualized from anterior to posterior on the monitor: right ventricular free wall, right ventricular cavity, interventricular septum, left ventricular cavity, and the posterior left ventricle (Figure 6-9B). On the basal side of the image, the aortic valve with its inflow and outflow tracts, the mitral valve with its inflow and outflow tracts, the left atrium, the posterior pericardium, and possibly the descending aorta should be seen (Figure 6-9C). The probe should be rotated to obtain the best axis to view these structures. Angling and tilting may be needed, but less so than for the short axis view. A reduction in size of the image may be needed

to focus on certain structures or enlargement of the field of view to see the entire left ventricle and left atrium.

Parasternal Short-Axis View

The imaging plane for the parasternal short axis view of the heart stretches from the left shoulder to the right hip (Figure 6-5), and should be obtained in the left 3rd or 4th intercostal space next to the sternum (Figure 6-10A). If the parasternal long axis view has already been obtained, the parasternal short axis views should be obtained by rotating the probe marker 90° clockwise toward the left shoulder (using a cardiac preset). With the probe in this position, several different short axis views can be obtained by sweeping the image from base to apex (Figure 6-10B). Parasternal short axis views can be

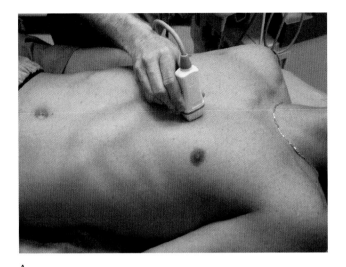

A

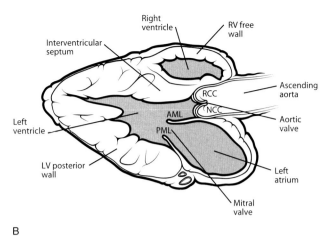

B

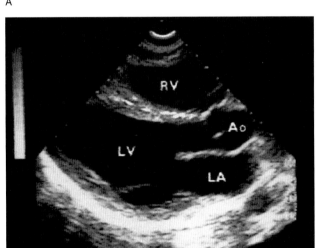

C

Figure 6-9. Probe position for parasternal long-axis view (A). Note: May require left lateral decubitus position. Parasternal long-axis diagram (B). Parasternal long-axis normal ultrasound (C). RV = right ventricle, Ao - aorta, LV = left ventricle, LA = left atrium.

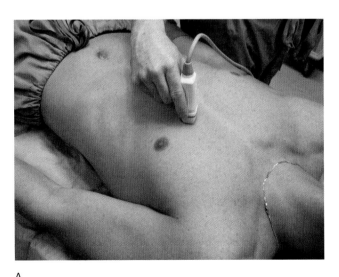

A

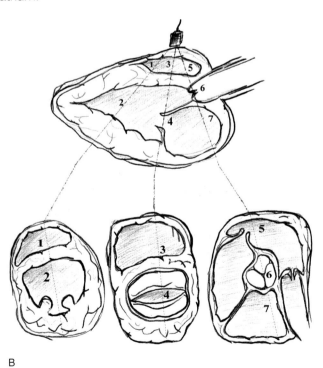

B

Figure 6-10. Probe position for parasternal short-axis view (A). Note: May require left lateral decubitus position. Diagram of short axis views from apex to base (B).

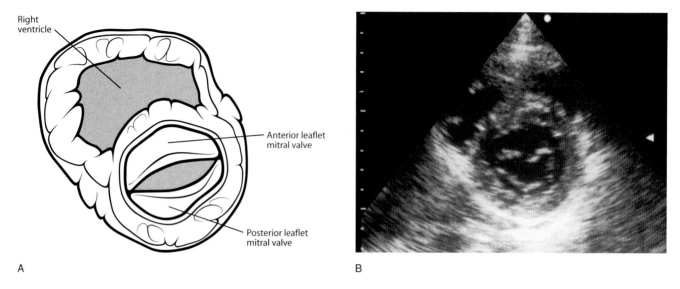

A   B

Figure 6-11. Parasternal short-axis diagram at mitral valve (A). Parasternal short-axis normal ultrasound at mitral valve (B).

obtained at the base of the heart, the level of the mitral valve (Figure 6-11A and 6-11B) the level of the papillary muscles, and at the apex. The short axis view at the level of the papillary muscles is an important view because it allows identification of the different walls of the left ventricle (Figure 6-12A and 6-12B). An ideal short axis view at the base of the heart (Figure 6-13A and 6-13B) visualizes the left atrium, right atrium, tricuspid valve,

right ventricle, and pulmonary valve encircling the aortic valve ("Mercedes Benz sign") in cross section in the middle of the view (Figure 6-14).

Apical Four-Chamber View

The apical 4-chamber view is a coronal view of the heart that images all four chambers in one plane.

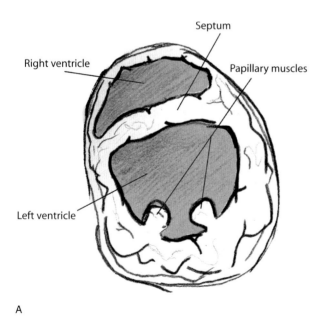

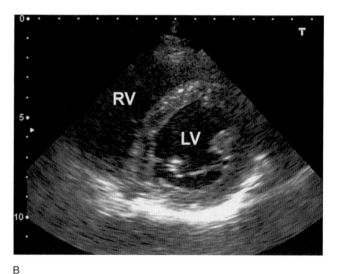

A   B

Figure 6-12. Parasternal short axis diagram at papillary muscles (A). Parasternal short axis normal ultrasound at papillary muscles (B). RV = right ventricle, LV = left ventricle. (B: Courtesy of Hennepin County Medical Center)

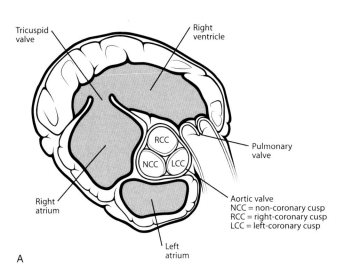

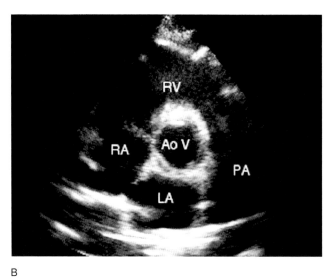

Figure 6-13. Parasternal short axis diagram at aortic valve (A). Parasternal short axis normal ultrasound at aortic valve (B). RV = right ventricular outflow tract, RA = right atrium, LA = left atrium, PA = pulmonary artery, Ao V = aortic valve.

Alterations of this view include the apical two-chamber view, the apical three-chamber view, and the apical five-chamber view. Regardless of the number of chambers, the view is best observed by obtaining the window at the apex of the heart, usually where the point of maximal impulse (PMI) for the heart is located (Figure 6-15A). Alteration of this position may be required to adjust for breast tissue, emphysema, chest deformities, and

other anatomic changes. Whenever possible, the patient should be rotated toward their left side to reduce lung artifact and bring the heart closer to the chest wall. The transducer should be placed at this position, generally in the 5th intercostal space or lower, and aimed toward the right shoulder with the marker directed toward the left lateral chest wall (using a cardiac preset). Some rotation may be needed to allow for all four chambers to be viewed. A rounded, foreshortened heart is usually artifactual. To correct this, the transducer should be aimed in a more anterior direction and/or a lower rib interspace should be used. On this view, the right ventricle with its lateral wall, the interventricular septum (septal wall), the left ventricle with the lateral wall, the two atria, the interatrial septum, and the pulmonary veins should be visualized (Figure 6-15B and 6-15C). This view is advantageous for assessing right ventricular function and the left ventricle for function and presence of blood clots. Doppler studies are often best obtained with apical views as blood flow is parallel to the transducer with this position. Intra-atrial abnormalities, such as myxoma, may be well visualized. When the image sector is swept more anteriorly from the four-chamber view, the left ventricular outflow and aortic valve come into view (five-chamber).

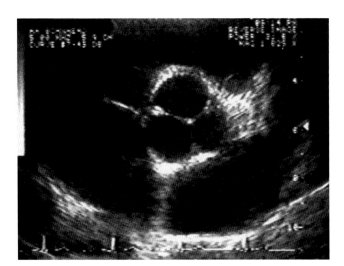

Figure 6-14. Mercedes Benz sign. Parasternal short axis at aortic valve demonstrates closure of all 3 cusps. (Courtesy of Lori Sens and Lori Green, Gulfcoast Ultrasound)

Apical Two-Chamber View

For the apical two-chamber view, the ultrasound probe should be placed in the same orientation as for the apical

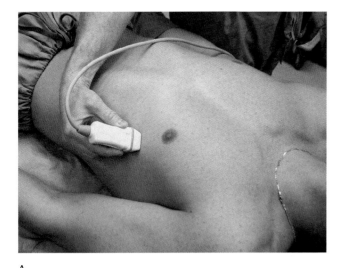

A

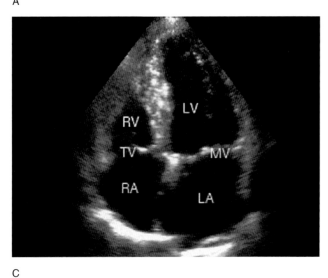

C

Apical 4-Chamber View

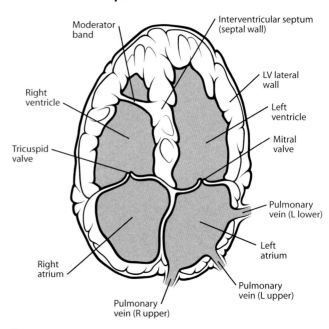

B

Figure 6-15. Probe position for apical 4 chamber view (A). Note: May require left lateral decubitus position with left arm elevated. Apical 4 chamber diagram (B). Apical 4 chamber normal ultrasound (C). RV = right ventricle, LV = left ventricle, MV = mitral valve, LA = left atrium, RA = right atrium, TV = tricuspid valve.

four-chamber view but the transducer should be rotated 90° counterclockwise (using a cardiac preset) until the marker is directed toward the left mid clavicle or head of the patient (Figure 6-16A). This view evaluates anterior and inferior walls, thus complementing the apical four-chamber view of the left ventricle for wall motion and function (Figure 6-16B and 6-16C). Further counterclockwise probe rotation from the two-chamber view

(additional 30°) would create the apical long axis (three-chamber) view.

Suprasternal View

The suprasternal view provides a glimpse of the aortic arch with its three main branches: the brachiocephalic artery, the left carotid artery, and the left subclavian

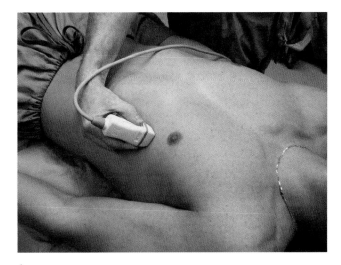

A

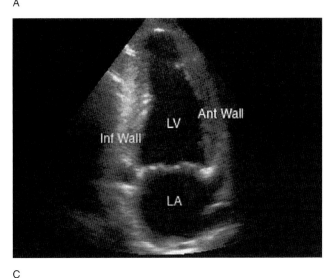

C

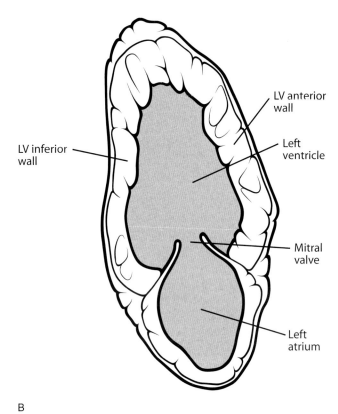

B

Figure 6-16. Probe position for apical two-chamber view (A). Note: May require left lateral decubitus position with left arm elevated. Apical two-chamber diagram (B). Apical two-chamber normal ultrasound (C). LV = left ventricle, LA = left atrium.

artery. The ultrasound probe should be placed in the sternal notch with the transducer marker pointed toward the patient's left shoulder (using a cardiac preset) and probe aimed as far anteriorly as possible (Figure 6-17A). While it is difficult to obtain in many patients, this view may provide a confirmation of aortic aneurysm or dissection in the patient with an optimal window. The right pulmonary artery in cross section can be viewed below the aortic arch. If the transducer is rotated 90° to visualize the aortic arch in cross section, the left pulmonary artery may be seen. Occasionally, the superior vena cava may be viewed lateral to the ascending aorta. The left atrium lies inferior to the pulmonary arteries and, in an optimal window, all four pulmonary veins may be viewed (Figure 6-17B and 6-17C).

▶ MEASUREMENTS

TWO-DIMENSIONAL MEASUREMENT

Chamber dimensions and sizes should be measured at right angles to the long axis of the respective chamber. Measurement of the chamber sizes, wall thickness, and the left ventricular function may be helpful. By measuring the left ventricular dimensions in systole and diastole, one can calculate the ejection fraction manually or by using the ultrasound machine calculation package. Critical to the 2D measurement is the ability to visualize the endocardium and a cine memory in order to scroll to the correct point in the cardiac cycle for measurement. Table 6-4 lists linear dimensions of normal cardiac structures.

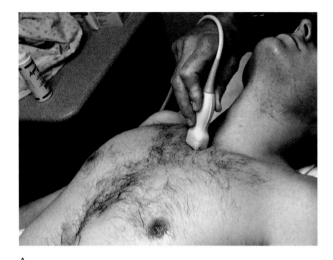

A

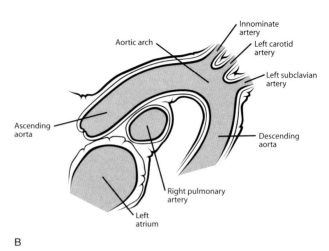

B

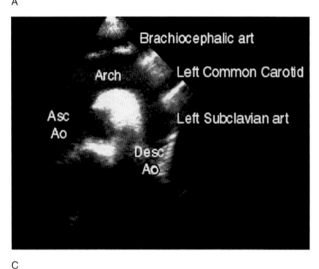

C

Figure 6-17. Probe position for suprasternal view (A). Suprasternal diagram (B). Suprasternal normal ultrasound (C). The branch arteries may be closely approximated as in the diagram or spread apart for some patients as in the ultrasound example. Asc Ao = ascending aorta, Desc Ao = descending aorta.

LEFT VENTRICULAR FUNCTION MEASUREMENT

Several methods exist for the echocardiographic measurement of ejection fraction. These range from observation and fairly simple M-mode measurements to complicated biplane calculations.[98] Many ultrasound software packages have the ability to estimate volume and calculate ejection fraction. This is typically accomplished by border tracing and measurement of cavity length while scanning in an apical four-chamber or apical two-chamber views.

While it may be satisfying to actually calculate a value for ejection fraction, it has been shown that visual estimation of ejection fraction is as good or better than calculated ejection fraction and is much easier to perform.[98–100] This is the most frequent method in clinical use today. With training and practice, noncardiologists may be able to estimate ejection fraction with reasonable accuracy.[15,19] It is important to note that both estimated and calculated ejection fractions are more accurate when the ventricle is regularly shaped and contracts in a symmetric fashion. Wall motion abnormalities and other variations in shape may significantly confound the echocardiographic measurement of ejection fraction.

For those who are more comfortable with a numerical measurement to determine left ventricular function, the EPPS can be determined from the cine review of the mitral valve on a parasternal long axis view. For more discussion, see below: M-Mode Mitral Valve and Left Ventricular Dysfunction.

CENTRAL VENOUS PRESSURE

Right atrial pressures can be estimated by viewing the respiratory change in the diameter of the IVC. Table 6-5 shows common measurements of IVC diameter and change with respiration used to estimate the right atrial pressure. This amounts to a noninvasive CVP measurement and may be helpful in patients with hypotension and uncertain volume status. It is also possible to estimate the end-systolic pulmonary artery pressure (approximates the wedge pressure) by measuring the flow velocity of the tricuspid regurgitant jet and applying it to

▶ TABLE 6-4. NORMAL FINDINGS ON TWO-DIMENSIONAL ECHOCARDIOGRAPHY.

	Range	Range Indexed to BSA	Upper Limit of Normal
Aorta			
Annulus diameter	1.4–2.6 cm	1.3 ± 0.1 cm/m^2	<1.6 cm/m^2
Diameter at leaflet tips	2.2–3.6 cm	1.7 ± 0.2 cm/m^2	<2.1 cm/m^2
Ascending aorta diameter	2.1–3.4 cm	1.5 ± 0.2 cm/m^2	
Arch diameter	2.0–3.6 cm		
Left ventricle			
Short-axis diastole (EDD)	3.5–6.0 cm	2.3–3.1cm/m^2	
Short-axis systole (ESD)	2.1–4.0 cm	1.4–2.1 cm/m^2	
Long-axis diastole	6.3–10.3 cm	4.1–5.7 cm/m^2	
Long-axis systole	4.6–8.4 cm		
End-diastolic volume men	96–157 mL	67 ± 9 mL	
End-diastolic volume women	59–138 mL	61 ± 13 mL	
End-systolic volume men	33–68 mL	27 ± 5mL	
End-systolic volume women	18–65 mL	26 ± 7 mL	
Ejection fraction men	0.59 ± 0.06		
Ejection fraction women	0.59 ± 0.07		
LV – wall thickness end diastole	0.6–1.1 cm		Men ≤1.2 cm Women ≤1.1 cm
LV-mass: men	<294 g	109 ± 20 g/m^2	≤150 g/m^2
LV-mass: women	<194 g	89 ± 15 g/m^2	≤120 g/m^2
Left atrium			
Long-axis AP diameter	2.3–4.5 cm	1.6–2.4 cm/m^2	
Apical four-chamber Medial–lateral diameter	2.5–4.5 cm	1.6–2.4 cm/m^2	
Apical four-chamber Superior-Inferior diameter	3.4–6.1 cm	2.5–3.5 cm/m^2	
Mitral annulus			
End diastole	2.7 ± 0.4 cm		
End systole	2.9 ± 0.3 cm		
Right ventricle			
Wall thickness	0.2–0.5 cm	0.2 ± 0.05 cm/m^2	
Minor dimension	2.2–4.4 cm	1.0–2.8 cm/m^2	
Length diastole	5.5–9.5 cm	3.8–5.3 cm/m^2	
Length systole	4.2–8.1 cm		
Pulmonary artery			
Annulus diameter	1.0–2.2 cm		
Main pulmonary artery	0.9–2.9 cm		
Inferior vena cava			
At right atrial junction diameter	1.2–2.3 cm		

BSA = body surface area; LV = left ventricle; AP = anterior-posterior.
(Adapted from Otto CM and Pearlman AS: *Normal Cardiac Anatomy in Textbook of Clinical Echocardiography*. Philadelphia, Saunders, 1995; p. 35).

▶ TABLE 6-5. INFERIOR VENA CAVA (IVC) ESTIMATES OF RIGHT ATRIAL (RA) PRESSURE

IVC Size, cm	Respiratory Change	RA Pressure, cm
<1.5	Total collapse	0–5
1.5–2.5	>50% collapse	5–10
1.5–2.5	<50% collapse	11–15
>2.5	<50 % collapse	16–20
>2.5	No change	>20

a formula or calculation package. The specifics of this measurement are beyond the scope of the text.

M-MODE

M-mode (motion mode) allows for a one-dimensional tracing of structures over time. M-mode can record motion of structures faster than human vision and record subtle changes. Measurements of valve diameters, wall motion, wall thickness, and stroke volume are possible.

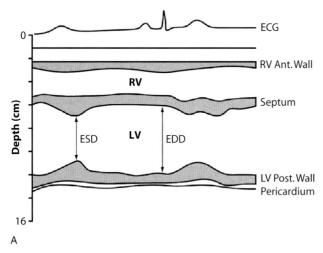

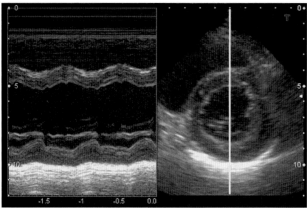

A

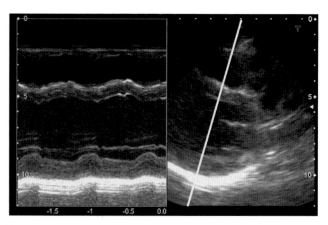

B

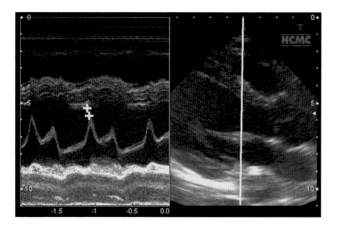

C

Figure 6-18. M-Mode diagram of left ventricle (A). Split screen M-Mode ultrasound from parasternal long-axis view (B). Split screen M-Mode ultrasound from parasternal short-axis view (C). White line indicates approximate position of M-Mode cursor for LV measurements. RV = right ventricle, LV = left ventricle, ESD = end systolic diameter, EDD = end diastolic diameter. (Courtesy of Hennepin County Medical Center for (B,C))

There are several uses of M-mode tracing but the most common in emergency ultrasound is the tracing through the left ventricle for measurement of left ventricular size and function and to confirm the presence of a pericardial effusion.

Figure 6-19. Split screen M-Mode ultrasound at mitral valve level. White line indicates approximate position of M-Mode cursor for recording anterior mitral valve leaflet. Measurement cursors are positioned for EPSS which equals 6 mm in this example. (Courtesy of Hennepin County Medical Center)

M-MODE LEFT VENTRICLE

This is usually performed perpendicular to the long axis of the left ventricle in the parasternal long or short axis at the level of the tips of the mitral valve leaflets (Figure 6-18A–C). This tracing cuts through the right ventricle, interventricular septum, left ventricle anterior wall, left ventricle posterior wall, and posterior pericardium. The end systolic diameter (ESD) is measured at the smallest dimensions of the septum and posterior wall. The end diastolic diameter (EDD) is measured just prior to ventricular thickening and contraction. An EDD measurement >6.0 cm is consistent with LV dilation. These measurements can also be used in formulas to calculate left ventricular fractional shortening and ejection fraction.

M-MODE MITRAL VALVE AND LEFT VENTRICULAR DYSFUNCTION

An M-mode tracing at the mitral valve level in the parasternal long axis shows the right ventricular free wall, interventricular septum, the mitral valve leaflets, the posterior left ventricular wall, and the pericardium. An M-mode tracing through the anterior leaflet of the mitral valve produces a double peak pattern (Figure 6-19).

The first peak is the E point and is caused by passive left ventricular filling. The second peak is the A point and is caused by atrial contraction. This double peak pattern is evidence of sinus rhythm. The distance between this E point and the left ventricular (LV) septal wall is measured as the E-point septal separation (EPSS). A large EPSS (in the absence of mitral stenosis) reflects left ventricular systolic dysfunction, left ventricular dilatation, or aortic regurgitation. An EPSS value greater than 8–10 mm is considered abnormal. The cause of the EPSS increase in these conditions is fairly simple: LV systolic dysfunction limits flow velocity, so maximum valve opening is reduced, LV dilatation increases the distance between the open valve and septum; and significant aortic regurgitation produces backflow that pushes the mitral valve away from the septum.

DOPPLER MEASUREMENTS

The use of the Doppler principle in ultrasound depends on the measurement of frequency shifts from moving red blood cells within cardiac structures. The measured velocity of the red blood cells depends on the transducer frequency, the speed of red blood cells in vessels, and the angle between the beam and the direction of flow. The sampling beam should be positioned as parallel to flow as possible.

Laminar flow is similar to that inside a tube, with a leading edge of fast flow and slow flow along the walls. Pressure differences drive blood across the vessel or in the heart. With turbulent flow, blood is swirling, moving in all directions but is moving forward. At stenoses, the flow is faster than at narrower points because the volume of blood moving across the stenosis must be the same

as in other areas of the heart. Doppler measurements are taken in different windows to measure flows from different chambers and vessels.

COLOR DOPPLER FLOW

Color Doppler flow is a representation of blood flow, usually as red or blue, in regards to the direction from the transducer. Conventionally, red flow is toward the transducer and blue flow is away from the transducer (Figure 6-20A). It should be noted that the colors red and blue do not necessarily signify arterial or venous flow or vessels. In addition, degrees of velocity are mapped as shades of red and blue. Shades of orange, green, or yellow may represent degrees of velocity, variance, or turbulence (Figure 6-20B).

▶ COMMON AND EMERGENT ABNORMALITIES

CARDIAC TAMPONADE

Cardiac tamponade is not dependent on the amount of fluid in the pericardial sac but on the rate of fluid accumulation within the pericardial sac (Figure 6-21).[101] Emergent echocardiographic findings of cardiac tamponade include a pericardial effusion, right atrial collapse during ventricular systole, right ventricular diastolic collapse (Figures 6-22 and 6-23), and lack of respiratory variation in the IVC and hepatic veins.[101] Left atrial or left ventricular collapse may occur in localized left-sided compression or in severe pulmonary hypertension.

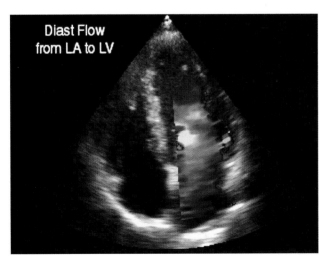

A

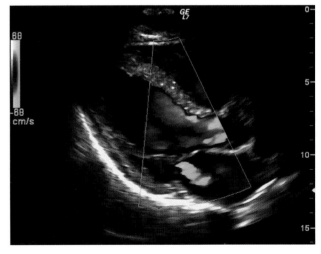

B

Figure 6-20. Color Doppler flow through left ventricle, apical four-chamber view - conventional color key (A). Flow during diastole is toward the transducer and is coded red in this example. Color Doppler flow on parasternal long-axis view - variance mode color key (B). Shades of green have been added to indicate areas of turbulence. (Courtesy of GE Medical for (B))

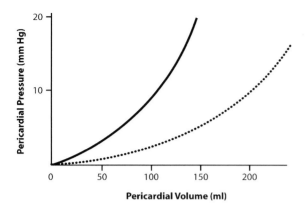

Figure 6-21. Pericardial P/V curve with acute (solid line) vs. chronic effusion (dotted line).

PERICARDIAL EFFUSION

Pericardial effusion is typically characterized by an anechoic fluid collection between the parietal pericardium and the visceral pericardium (Figures 6-24A and 6-24B, 6-25). For all practical purposes, the visceral pericardium is not visualized by transthoracic echocardiography. However, the combined interface of the parietal and visceral pericardium is echogenic.

On transthoracic echocardiography, pericardial effusions may be judged as small or large. Small pericar-

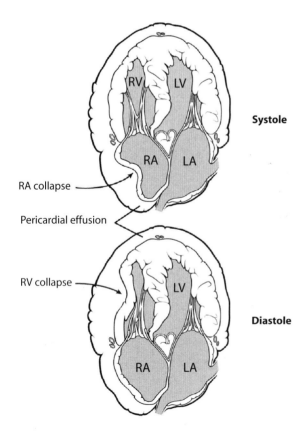

Figure 6-22. Physiology of cardiac tamponade.

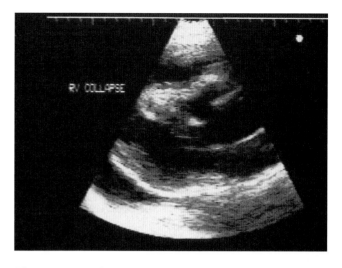

Figure 6-23. Cardiac tamponade. Parasternal long-axis view with diastolic collapse of right ventricle. (Courtesy of James Mateer, MD)

dial effusions are seen as an anechoic space less than 1 cm thick and are often localized, usually between the posterior pericardium and left ventricular epicardium. Large effusions are seen as an anechoic space greater than 1 cm thick, and are usually completely surrounding the heart. In patients with larger effusions, the heart may swing freely within the pericardial sac (Figure 6-26).

Pericardial volumes of up to 50 mL may be normal; however, pathologic fluid collections, if slow in progression, may accumulate hundreds of milliliters. Pericardial fluid is usually anechoic, but exudative effusions, such as pus, malignant effusions, and blood mixed with fibrin material, may be echogenic (Figure 6-27). Pericardial fluid collections can be complicated by gas-forming infections or by gas-causing tamponade (pneumopericardium).

MYOCARDIAL ISCHEMIA

Abnormal wall motion and abnormal ventricular emptying or relaxation characterizes left ventricular dysfunction (Figure 6-28). Wall motion is graded as hypokinesis (reduced ventricular wall thickening and motion), akinesis (absent wall thickening and motion), and dyskinesis (paradoxical motion of the wall—outward movement of the wall during systole).[92,102] Assessment of wall thickening requires ultrasound visualization of the myocardium and endocardium, which can be significantly limited for the typical emergency or critically ill patient. Wall motion may be characterized by gross ventricular wall dysfunction or segmental wall motion defects that usually follow the distribution of coronary blood perfusion (Figure 6-29A). Multiple views of the left ventricle and a knowledge of the coronary vascular anatomy are

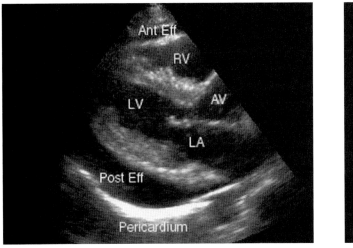

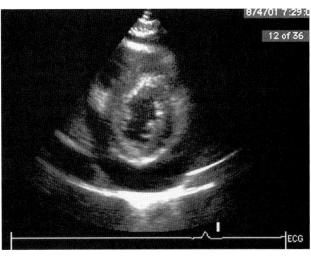

A

B

Figure 6-24. Pericardial effusion on parasternal long-axis view (A) and parasternal short-axis view (B). RV = right ventricle, LV = left ventricle, AV = aortic valve, LA = left atrium.

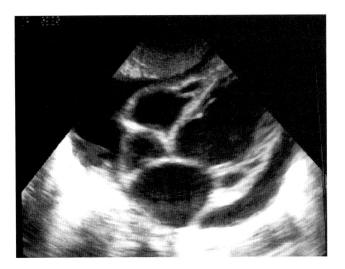

Figure 6-25. Chronic pericardial effusion (Subcostal four-chamber).

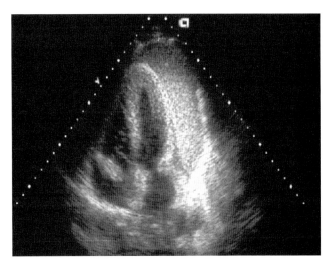

Figure 6-27. Exudative pericardial effusion (apical four-chamber view).

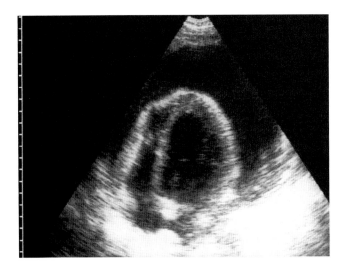

Figure 6-26. Large effusion – apical view. (Courtesy of James Mateer, MD)

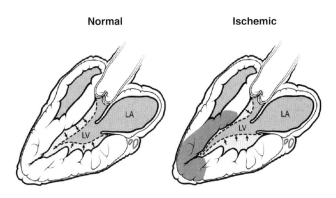

Figure 6-28. Wall motion abnormality.

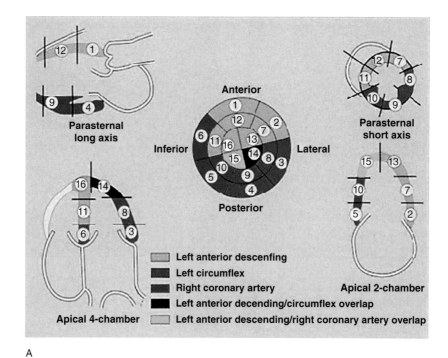

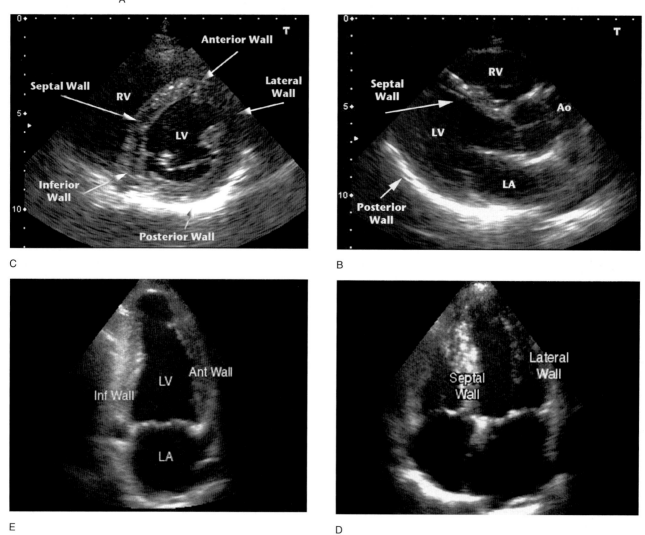

Figure 6-29. Left ventricular wall segments (A). Center 'bullseye" represents LV viewed from apex. Wall segments are color and number coded for regional coronary vasculature. Corresponding ultrasound images of LV wall segments in parasternal long-axis view (B), parasternal short-axis view (C), apical four-chamber view (D), apical two-chamber view (E). RV = right ventricle, LV = left ventricle, Ao = aorta, LA = left atrium. (Courtesy of Hennepin County Medical Center for (B,C))

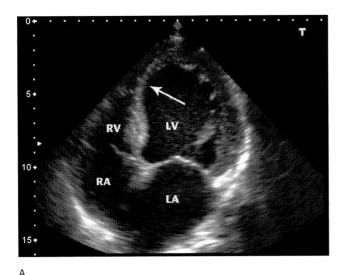

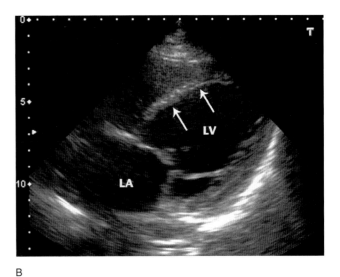

A

B

Figure 6-30. Chronic left ventricular infarction. Apical four-chamber view (A) demonstrates thinning and increased echogenicity of the apical septum (arrow) with increased size of LV and LA chambers. Subcostal four-chamber view (B) shows chronic thinning of the entire inferior septum (arrows). RV = right ventricle, RA = right atrium, LV = left ventricle, LA = left atrium. (Courtesy of Hennepin County Medical Center)

required if the goal is to determine the region affected and correlate findings with the EKG (Figure 6-29B–E).

Echocardiography can detect acute ischemic changes with diastolic dysfunction, increased left ventricular diastolic filling, decreased left ventricular diastolic compliance, and reduced left ventricular diastolic compliance. As the ischemia transforms to transmural infarction, there is impaired systolic thickening, reduction in endocardial motion, and dyssynchronous contraction of myocardial segments. Left ventricular chamber size increases with reduction in systolic ejection fraction. Ultrasound findings of acute left ventricular ischemia or infarction typically include wall motion abnormalities, usually regional in the distribution of a coronary artery or its branch, but without evidence of chronic thinning or scarring of the wall (Figure 6-28).

Ultrasound findings of chronic left ventricular infarction include a dilated left ventricle, global wall motion abnormalities with thinning of the ventricular wall (<7 mm or 30% less than the adjacent normal wall) and increased echogenicity of the segment due to fibrotic changes. (Figure 6-30A and 6-30B). Chronic left ventricular dysfunction will lead to a dilated cardiomyopathy and an immobile aortic root (Figure 6-31). The left atrium may be dilated and there may be thrombus at the apex.

Right ventricular dysfunction or dilatation may be the only sign of severe pulmonary disease, pericardial disease, or right-sided ischemia. The right ventricle is a thin and narrow chamber that is generally two thirds of the size of the left ventricle. While a dilated right ventricle may be seen in any view, the four-chamber apical view may be particularly useful.

MASSIVE PULMONARY EMBOLISM

While direct visualization of a thrombus may occasionally be seen in the right heart, most echocardiographically detectable changes are indirect indices of right heart strain caused by pumping against a fixed blood clot in the lung. These changes include right ventricular dilatation, right ventricular hypokinesis, tricuspid regurgitation, and abnormal septal motion.

The normal right ventricular end diastolic diameter is 21 ± 1 mm in a parasternal long axis view. Abnormal values have been described as being greater than 25–30 mm. The normal right to left ventricle ratio, obtained in

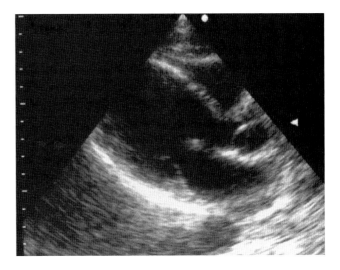

Figure 6-31. Dilated left ventricle in parasternal long-axis view.

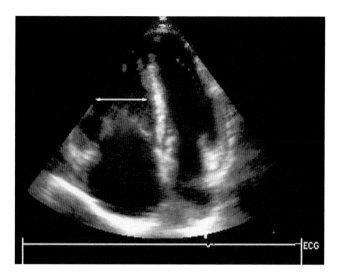

Figure 6-32. RV enlargement. Apical four-chamber transverse diameter exceeds 2.5 cm.

the apical four-chamber view, is less than 0.5. Abnormal ratios vary by author but have been described as being greater than 0.5 or as high as greater than 1 (Figure 6-32). With massive PE the right ventricle will be round in shape and larger than the left ventricle (Figure 6-33).

Tricuspid regurgitation may occur when pulmonary artery pressures exceed right ventricular end diastolic (right atrial) pressures. Measurement of tricuspid regurgitation requires spectral Doppler velocity measurement and is usually obtained on the apical four-chamber view. While many healthy persons have a trivial degree of

tricuspid regurgitation, up to 90% of patients with PE will have measurable tricuspid regurgitation.[103] Normal pulmonary artery systolic pressure is approximately 25 mmHg in a healthy person, corresponding to a regurgitant jet of less than 2 m/s. Over 3 m/s would correspond to a pulmonary artery pressure of 46 mmHg. Studies using cutoff values for diagnosis of PE typically cite velocities over 2.5–2.7 m/s as being elevated.

In addition to right-sided heart strain, a blood clot in the lung may cause decreased venous return to the left heart. This may result in decreased left ventricular end diastolic diameter as well as "paradoxical septal motion." The normal interventricular septum relaxes outward (toward the right ventricle) in diastole. With increased right end diastolic pressures and decreased left-sided pressures, abnormal motion of the septum in diastole may be visualized. While this septal deviation toward the left ventricle (also described as "septal flattening") may also be observed in systole, its presence is more pronounced in diastole and is especially prominent in the acute phase of massive PE.[104]

All of the indirect indicators of right-sided heart strain may occur in conditions other than PE. These conditions include right ventricular infarct, emphysema, and primary pulmonary hypertension. It is worthwhile noting that the acutely strained right-sided heart rarely has the muscle mass to elevate pulmonary artery pressure into an extremely high range and values well over 40 mmHg should suggest a chronic elevation.[103] An increase in muscle mass on measurement of the right ventricular free wall may also indicate a more chronic etiology for right ventricular strain as opposed to a thin, acutely

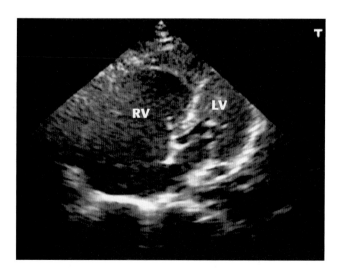

Figure 6-33. Massive pulmonary embolism. Apical view (centered over RV apex) shows severely decompensated right ventricle that is round in shape and much larger than the left ventricle. RV = right ventricle, LV = left ventricle. (Courtesy of Hennepin County Medical Center)

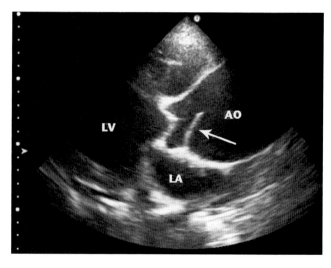

Figure 6-34. Ascending aortic aneurysm with dissection. Parasternal long-axis view shows dilated aortic root and proximal flap (arrow). Ao = aorta, LV = left ventricle, LA = left atrium. (Courtesy of Hennepin County Medical Center)

dilated right ventricle. The normal right ventricular free wall is 2.4 ± 0.5 mm, and is generally considered hypertrophied at measurements of 5 mm and greater.[105]

PROXIMAL AORTIC DISSECTION

On transthoracic echocardiography, patients with a proximal thoracic aortic dissection often have a dilated aortic root (<3.8 cm), which is easily visualized on the parasternal long axis view. An intimal flap can sometimes be seen within the dilated aortic root (Figure 6-34). The descending aorta may also be seen on the parasternal long axis view in cross section posterior to the mitral valve. The arch of the aorta may be seen with transthoracic echocardiography using a suprasternal window in a minority of patients but is more easily visualized when

dilated. A dissection within the aortic arch or descending thoracic aorta may be seen in this view (Figure 6-35A and 6-35B). In addition to the linear flap, aortic dissection is characterized on echocardiography as having two lumens, true and false, with different flow patterns. This may be best demonstrated using transesophageal views (Figure 6-36A and 6-36B).

ASYSTOLE

Asystole is seen as a lack of myocardial contraction on echocardiography. Pooling of blood may be seen and echogenic clots may form with onset of asystole. As severe hypokinesis progresses toward asystole, there is progressive decreased left ventricular diastolic and systolic volumes associated with rising left ventricular

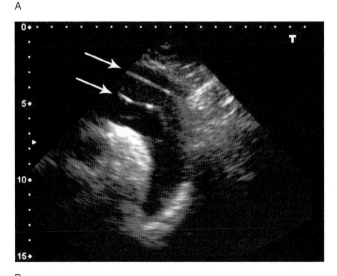

A

B

Figure 6-35. Type A aortic dissection diagram (A). Suprasternal ultrasound view of the aortic arch (B). The imaging plane crosses the intimal flap in two locations (arrows). (Courtesy of Hennepin County Medical Center for (B))

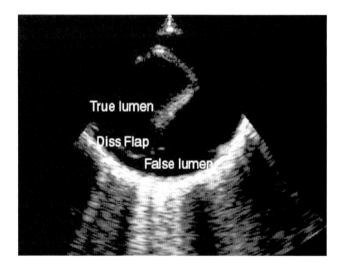

A

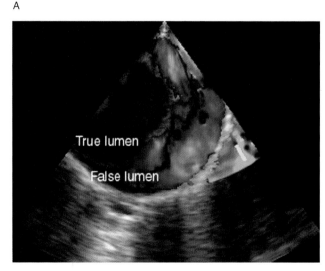

B

Figure 6-36. TEE transverse view of an aortic dissection with flap (A). TEE aortic dissection, color Doppler with true-and-false lumens (B).

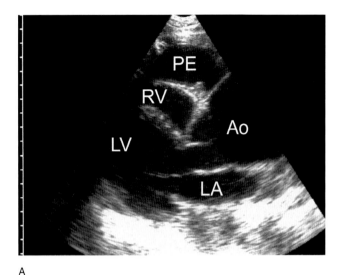

A

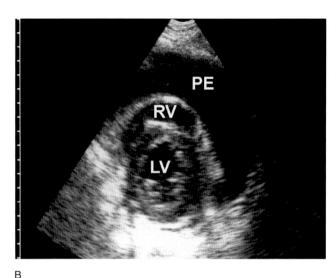

B

Figure 6-37. Aortic aneurism. Parasternal long-axis view shows a 6-cm aneurysm in the ascending aorta (A). The pericardial fluid collected anteriorly. The enlarged aorta may be pushing the LV against the posterior pericardial sac. This is best seen on the parasternal short axis view (B). No intimal flap was found on TEE. Ao = Aorta, LA = left atrium, LV = left ventricle, RV = right ventricle, PE = pericardial effusion. (Courtesy of James Mateer, MD)

pressures. Ventricular wall thickness progressively increases until the heart becomes motionless.[106] Movement of the valves can be seen just with positive pressure ventilation and should not be taken for spontaneous circulation in the absence of myocardial contraction.

▶ COMMON VARIANTS AND SELECTED ABNORMALITIES

ASCENDING AORTIC ANEURYSM

Dilation of the ascending aorta over 1.5 times the normal segment may reflect an aneurysmal change (Figure 6-37A and B). A true aneurysm of the ascending aorta involves all layers of the vessel wall. A false aneurysm, or pseudoaneurysm, involves a penetration of the intima and media layers only. Most thoracic aneurysms are fusiform but may be saccular. Concomitant aortic dissection may occur as well.

On echocardiography, the aorta is usually measured at several locations: aortic annulus, aortic leaflet tip, ascending aorta, aortic arch, and descending aorta. The length and levels of dilatation should be noted. As with the abdominal aorta, if the thoracic aorta diameter is measured at 5–6 cm, then the patient should be referred to a cardiothoracic surgery consultant.

The role of transthoracic echocardiography is limited as the aortic arch and descending aorta cannot be fully visualized because of the depth of the aorta in many views. There is also difficulty in viewing the endothelium and poor windows due to intervening bone and air. TEE,

CT, and MRI are similar in accuracy for the detection and evaluation of aortic aneurysm.

THROMBUS

While a thrombus may be detected in any cardiac chamber, slow-moving chambers or lower pressures chambers are at greater risk for developing a thrombus. A thrombus may be hyperechoic, isoechoic, and even hypoechoic in appearance (Figure 6-38). It is usually laminated, with the layers paralleling the chamber wall. A

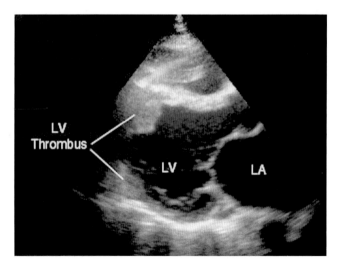

Figure 6-38. A left ventricular thrombus is located near the apex (parasternal long-axis view). LV = left ventricle, LA = left atrium.

thrombus is typically homogeneous with irregular borders, and may fill in the apex of a ventricle or attach itself to a chamber wall or valves of the atria. Near-field or time-gain compensation may have to be adjusted to visualize suspected areas. A thrombus may make differentiating the pericardial layers difficult.

High-frequency transducers that utilize cardiac scanning windows close to the cardiac chamber in question provide the best imaging. While transesophageal transducers are required for thrombus detection in atria, transthoracic scanning is adequate for thrombus detection within the ventricles in many cases. If color Doppler is available, the swirling vortices of flow may indicate the presence of a thrombus. Normal structures, such as the left atrial appendages, right atrial Chiari network, and right ventricular moderator bands must be distinguished from thrombus.

VEGETATIONS

Findings of irregularities on valvular surfaces should prompt further investigation and consultation for more definitive diagnosis (Figures 6-39 and 6-40). Vegetations may be echogenic or isoechoic and have an irregular appearance. Vegetations may be seen on any valve leaflet or part of the apparatus. Laminated or pedunculated attachments to the leaflet of the valve should prompt suspicion. In general, they do not restrict valvular motion but some valve leaflets may not coapt together correctly. Typical appearance of normal valves includes smooth echogenic leaflets. All suspected cases should be referred for transesophageal imaging and cardiology consultation.

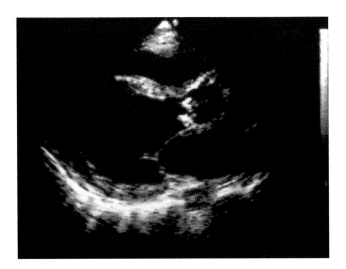

Figure 6-39. Endocarditis. Parasternal long-axis view reveals echogenic mobile vegetations on the aortic valve leaflets. (Courtesy of Lori Sens and Lori Green, Gulfcoast Ultrasound)

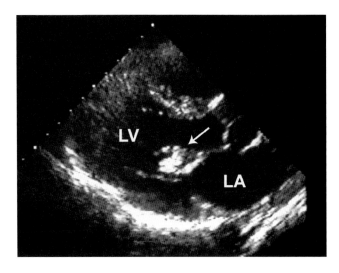

Figure 6-40. Endocarditis. Parasternal long-axis view with echogenic mobile vegetations on the mitral valve leaflets (arrow). LV = left ventricle, LA = left atrium. (Courtesy of Lori Sens and Lori Green, Gulfcoast Ultrasound)

VALVULAR ABNORMALITIES

Valvular abnormalities may present as an incidental finding and should be recognized for appropriate referral (Figure 6-41A and B). Most hemodynamically significant valvular abnormalities will eventually cause cardiac chamber enlargement and this may lead the sonologist to the diagnosis. In the setting of acute myocardial infarction, a new onset murmur can be caused by mitral regurgitation associated with papillary muscle dysfunction or rupture. This may be recognized on ultrasound as prolapse of the mitral valve leaflets or by abnormal color flow Doppler of the mitral valve (Figure 6-42). Another consideration is acute ventricular septal defect that may be seen with color flow imaging.

Tricuspid and pulmonary valve abnormalities usually are not emergencies unless large masses or clots are obstructing the valves. In acute ischemic or traumatic events, the mitral valve may provide a clue to injury. Aortic valve involvement may be associated with ascending aortic abnormalities.

VENTRICULAR HYPERTROPHY

Normal left ventricular wall thickness is 0.6–1.2 cm measured at end diastole. Left ventricular hypertrophy may be concentric (Figure 6-43) or asymmetric (Figure 6-44).

MYXOMA

Myxomas, which are uncommon benign fibrous tumors, are usually attached to a septal wall. Myxomas are

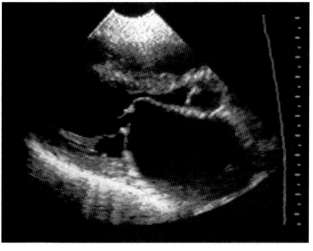

A

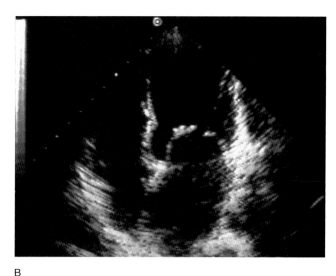

B

Figure 6-41. Mitral stenosis. Parasternal long-axis view (A) shows the typical features: LA enlargement, ballooning of the valve and a "hockey stick" appearance of the anterior leaflet. Apical four-chamber example (B) of this condition. (Courtesy of Lori Sens and Lori Green, Gulfcoast Ultrasound)

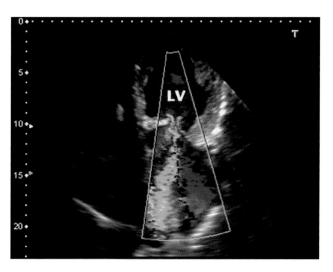

Figure 6-42. Mitral insufficiency. A shortened apical view with color Doppler demonstrates severe mitral regurgitation with turbulent flow. LV = left ventricle. (Courtesy of Hennepin County Medical Center)

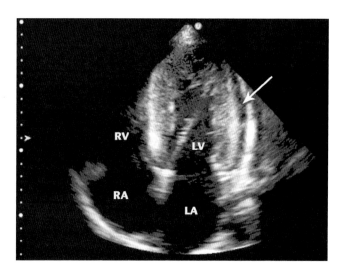

Figure 6-43. Concentric hypertrophy. Apical four-chamber view demonstrates symmetrical thickening of the left ventricular wall. A small pericardial effusion is noted adjacent to the left ventricle (arrow). LA = left atrium, LV = left ventricle, RV = right ventricle, RA = right atrium. (Courtesy of Hennepin County Medical Center)

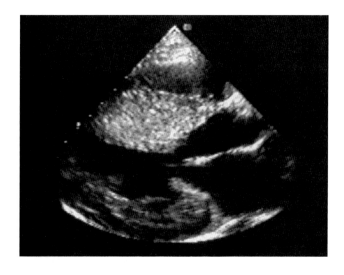

Figure 6-44. Assymetric septal hypertrophy. A thickened, echogenic LV septum is noted in PSL view in a patient with this condition (also known as IHSS). (Courtesy of Lori Sens and Lori Green, Gulfcoast Ultrasound)

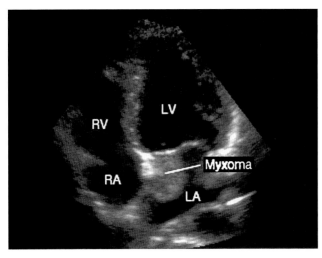

A

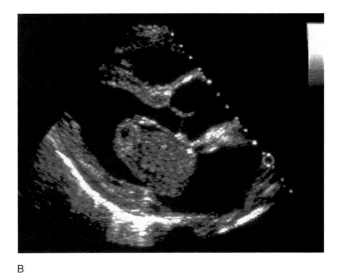

B

Figure 6-45. Left atrial myxoma shown on apical four-chamber view (A). Left atrial myxoma shown on a parasternal long-axis view (B). The mass was mobile and prolapsing into the LV on the real-time exam. (Courtesy of Lori Sens and Lori Green, Gulfcoast Ultrasound)

usually echogenic, globular, and smooth. They are pedunculated with a stalk on one wall that may or may not be visualized. They are usually seen attached to an atrial wall, most often the left atrium (Figure 6-45A and 6-45B).

▶ PITFALLS

1. **Contraindications.** No contraindications exist for transthoracic echocardiography unless its use is interfering with life-saving procedures and treatments.
2. **Inability to obtain adequate views.** Some patients cannot be imaged well by transthoracic echocardiography. These include patients with subcutaneous emphysema, pneumopericardium, large anterior–posterior girth, and chest wall deformities. Suggestions for improving image acquisition include maintaining transducer contact with the chest wall, use of an adequate amount of conduction gel, use of adjacent cardiac windows, and angling, rotating, and tilting the transducer, as necessary. The patient may be turned in the left lateral decubitus position to bring the heart closer to the anterior chest wall.

   a. The subxiphoid window is a mainstay of the emergency cardiac ultrasound examination during resuscitation of a critically ill patient. Suggestions for improving image acquisition for this view include ensuring the transducer is at a shallow angle to the plane of the body (15° in general) and moving the transducer to the patient's right in the subxiphoid space instead of the more intuitive left side. This helps to avoid the air-filled stomach and uses the left lobe of the liver as a soft-tissue window. Also, asking the patient to take a deep inspiration or, if the patient is intubated, providing a large tidal volume will help push the heart toward the subxiphoid space.

   b. The parasternal view is limited by retrosternal air or altered anatomy. Moving the transducer to the left, and then up and down along the anterior–posterior axis may help with obtaining a better view.

   c. The apical view may be improved by changing the angle and aiming the transducer toward the head or right elbow instead of the right shoulder.

3. **Reversed orientation.** Proper imaging requires knowledge of the orientation of the transducer. Reverse orientation may lead the sonologist to mistaken ventricular hypertrophy for normal and vice versa. For example, a dilated right ventricle is an important clue for massive PE, but may be falsely identified as normal if a normal left ventricle is viewed on the reversed side of the monitor screen. When ventricle sizes are similar, the right ventricle can be identified on apical four-chamber view by recognizing that the tricuspid valve is positioned closer to the apex than the mitral valve.

4. **Fluid versus blood clot or fat.** Fluid (serous pericardial fluid, or defibrinated blood) will appear as anechoic. However, a blood clot may

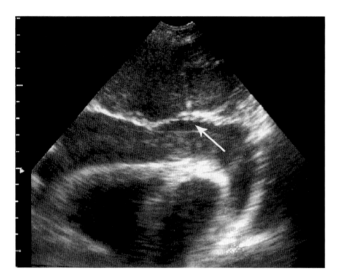

Figure 6-46. Hemopericardium. Echogenic clotted blood with a thin stripe of liquid blood above (arrow) is shown in this subcostal view.

be echogenic initially (Figure 6-46). The borders of clot usually have a thin anechoic stripe. Viewing other windows may assist with identifying free fluid in other aspects of the pericardium. Fat is commonly located in the anterior precordial space. In some patients this appears hypoechoic and can be mistaken for fluid or hematoma. Clues to identification are mildly echogenic septations characteristic of fat and the lack of any dependent pooling of fluid within the posterior pericardial space.

5. **Gain issues.** Gain should be adjusted to allow the posterior aspect of the heart to have the highest time-gain compensation. Cardiac chambers should be anechoic and cardiac structures should be echogenic.

6. **Depth.** Depth should be adjusted to visualize posterior to the cardiac structure in question. The focus, if adjustable, should be placed at the structure of interest. Too much magnification can alter proper interpretation and too shallow depth can minimize pathologic findings. A large pericardial effusion may occasionally be missed by a novice sonologist if the depth is not adequate to capture the entire heart in view and the large fluid stripe between the right ventricular wall and diaphragm in the subxiphoid view is mistaken for the right ventricle.

7. **Dynamic range.** Many machines used for emergency ultrasound applications are preset for abdominal applications; this includes the dynamic range setting. In cardiac ultrasound, the image is more black and white. The dynamic range should be lower than the settings used in abdominal or pelvic imaging.

▶ CASE STUDIES

CASE 1

Patient Presentation

A 64-year-old woman presented to the emergency department by ambulance in severe respiratory distress. A nebulized albuterol treatment was in progress. She told paramedics that her shortness of breath had become progressively worse over the last several hours. She denied chest pain and any history of cardiac or pulmonary disease. The paramedics communicated that her respiratory distress was worsening.

On physical examination, her respiratory rate was 50–60 breaths per minute and she was using all accessory muscles. She could only speak in two or three word sentences due to her dyspnea. Her blood pressure was 161/101 mmHg; heart rate, 136 beats per minute; and oxygen saturation 94% despite receiving 100% supplemental oxygen by nonrebreather mask. Her temperature was normal. Auscultation of her chest revealed diffuse expiratory wheezes, decreased aeration, and a prolonged expiratory phase. There were no crackles appreciated. Cardiovascular examination revealed tachycardia without murmurs and strong, equal peripheral pulses. Neck examination was without any noticeable jugular venous distention. Lower extremity edema was absent. The remainder of her examination was unremarkable.

Management Course

Two minutes after arrival, a bedside echocardiogram was performed and interpreted by the emergency physician. Notable findings were a dilated left ventricle with obvious severe left ventricular failure and a relatively small right ventricle (Figure 6-47A). The nebulization treatment was stopped and she was given high-flow oxygen and sublingual nitroglycerin. The patient received an intravenous bolus of furosemide and an intravenous nitroglycerin infusion was started. By the time her portable chest radiograph was available for viewing (Figure 6-47B) about 15 minutes after arrival, the patient was markedly improved. The chest radiograph confirmed the diagnosis of acute pulmonary edema. An ECG showed sinus tachycardia with nonspecific changes. She was admitted to the cardiac ICU and eventually diagnosed with severe diffuse ischemic cardiomyopathy.

Commentary

Bedside echocardiography was an important tool in the evaluation of this patient's undifferentiated respiratory distress. The course of treatment delivered to this critically ill patient in the emergency department was significantly altered by the information provided by bedside echocardiography. Even though the patient could

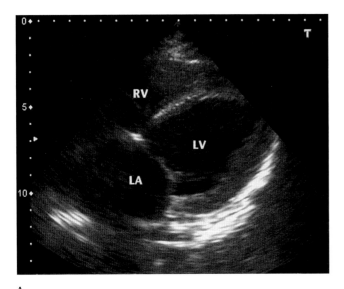

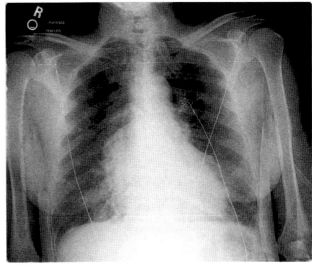

A   B

Figure 6-47. Case 1: Subcostal four-chamber ultrasound view. (A). Portable chest radiograph (B). (Courtesy of Hennepin County Medical Center)

not tolerate lying flat, subxiphoid probe positioning proved adequate visualization of her left ventricular dysfunction. This vital piece of information would not have been detectable by any other diagnostic modality within 2 minutes of the patient's arrival.

CASE 2

Patient Presentation

A 52-year-old man presented to the emergency department with vague, nonradiating chest pain for the past 2–3 hours that was gradual in onset over about 30 minutes. The patient had not experienced any significant shortness of breath, nausea, or palpitations. He acknowledged a history of inconsistently controlled hypertension over the past 20 years and a 40 pack-year history of smoking cigarettes.

On physical examination, blood pressure was noted at 182/100 mmHg; heart rate, 87 beats per minute; respiratory rate, 15 breaths per minute; and oxygen saturation 98% on room air. The patient was afebrile. Head, neck, pulmonary, abdominal, and back examinations were unremarkable. Cardiovascular examination revealed normal heart sounds without murmurs. Normal and equal peripheral pulses were palpable in the upper and lower extremities.

Management Course

The patient was given an aspirin and sublingual nitroglycerin without improvement. Morphine sulfate provided some relief. His ECG showed a normal sinus rhythm and nonspecific ST changes. Chest radiograph

was negative for pneumothorax and showed a normal appearing mediastinum. Laboratory studies, including the initial cardiac enzyme, were unremarkable. The patient was considered to have nonspecific, but concerning chest pain and plans were made for hospital admission, serial cardiac enzymes, cardiac monitoring, and further cardiac workup. As part of a routine chest pain evaluation the emergency physician performed bedside echocardiography and noted a dilated aortic root with a diameter of 4.2 cm (Figure 6-48). Contrast-enhanced CT of the thoracic aorta confirmed suspicions of a proximal aortic dissection. Cardiovascular surgery was contacted and performed a timely repair without incident.

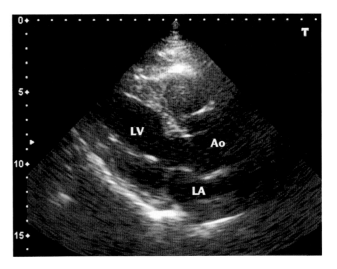

Figure 6-48. Case 2: Parasternal long-axis ultrasound view. (Courtesy of Hennepin County Medical Center)

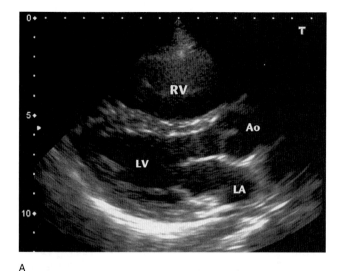

A

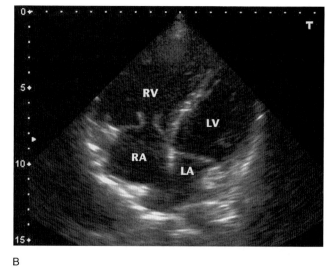

B

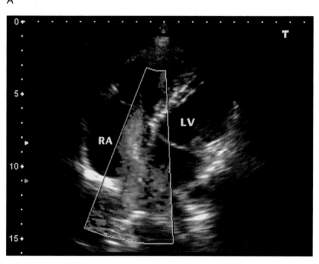

C

Figure 6-49. Case 3: Parasternal long-axis ultrasound view (A). Apical four-chamber ultrasound view (B). Color Doppler activated (C). (Courtesy of Hennepin County Medical Center)

Commentary

Case 2 exemplified the utility of routine bedside echocardiography by emergency physicians during the evaluation of nonspecific chest pain. This patient's aortic dissection may have caused a myocardial infarction, aortic valve failure, cardiac tamponade, or death had it not been identified in the emergency department. Patients with aortic dissection often present without the classic red flags. Bedside echocardiography performed by emergency physicians can provide essential information to help expedite the disposition.

CASE 3

Patient Presentation

A 21-year-old woman presented to the emergency department with 3 days of cough, sore throat, and chest pain. She had mild dyspnea on exertion while working in a restaurant. The chest pain was sharp, bilateral, and increased with coughing. Further review of systems was negative. She denied any past medical history. Oral contraceptives were her only medication. She smoked one to two cigarettes per day.

On physical examination, blood pressure was 110/67 mmHg; heart rate, 96 beats per minute; respiratory rate, 20 breaths per minute; temperature, 97°F; and oxygen saturation 97% on room air. The patient was in no distress. Head, neck, pulmonary, abdominal, and back examinations were unremarkable. There was no murmur appreciated on the initial cardiac examination.

Management Course

Laboratory and imaging studies ensued, with particular concern for possible PE. ECG showed a normal sinus rhythm at 78 beats per minute with a small R wave in lead V_1. Initial cardiac enzymes and a D-dimer were in the normal range. The patient's chest radiograph was unremarkable. The tentative diagnosis was chest wall pain with a viral upper respiratory infection. Bedside echocardiography by the emergency physician showed a markedly enlarged right ventricle on the parasternal long axis view (Figure 6-49A). The apical four-chamber view revealed a dilated right side and an obvious large atrial-septal defect (Figure 6-49B). Color Doppler showed significant left-to-right flow through the defect (Figure 6-49C). The patient was admitted to the cardiology service and had a comprehensive echocardiographic study that was consistent with the emergency physician's findings. She underwent elective surgical repair of the atrial septal defect via thoracotomy and recovered well.

Commentary

This case demonstrated a common finding of right-sided chamber enlargement and a rare incidental finding of an atrial septal defect. The right-sided enlargement was straightforward to detect and apparent on two different views. Right-sided enlargement can be caused by PE, chronic pulmonary disease, and structural heart defects. If only the right-sided enlargement had been detected, it would have prompted further testing and the correct diagnosis would have eventually been made.

▶ ACKNOWLEDGMENTS

The authors acknowledge the contributions of Vivek S. Tayal, Christopher L. Moore, and Geoffery A. Rose, who authored this chapter in the first edition. The authors also thank Ben Dolan and Anne Olson for their contributions to this chapter.

REFERENCES

1. Cheitlin MD, Armstrong WF, Aurigemma GP, et al.: ACC/AHA/ASE 2003 guideline update for the clinical application of echocardiography: Summary article: A report of the American College of Cardiology/American Heart Association Task Force on Practice Guidelines (ACC/AHA/ASE Committee to Update the 1997 Guidelines for the Clinical Application of Echocardiography). *Circulation* 108:1146–1162, 2003.
2. Mayron R, Gaudio FE, Plummer D, Asinger R, Elsperger J: Echocardiography performed by emergency physicians: Impact on diagnosis and therapy. *Ann Emerg Med* 17:150–154, 1988.
3. Jehle D, Davis E, Evans T, et al.: Emergency department sonography by emergency physicians. *Am J Emerg Med* 7:605–611, 1989.
4. Plummer D: Principles of emergency ultrasound and echocardiography. *Ann Emerg Med* 18:1291–1297, 1989.
5. Mazurek B, Jehle D, Martin M: Emergency department echocardiography in the diagnosis and therapy of cardiac tamponade. *J Emerg Med* 9:27–31, 1991.
6. Heller MB, Verdile VP: Ultrasonography in emergency medicine. *Emerg Med Clin North Am* 10:27–46, 1992.
7. Turturro MA: Emergency echocardiography. *Emerg Med Clin North Am* 10:47–57, 1992.
8. Blaivas M, Fox JC: Outcome in cardiac arrest patients found to have cardiac standstill on the bedside emergency department echocardiogram. *Acad Emerg Med* 8:616–621, 2001.
9. Brunette DD: Twelve years of emergency medicine at Hennepin County Medical Center. Changing critical care experience. *Minn Med* 82:42–48, 1999.
10. Davis DP, Campbell CJ, Poste JC, Ma G: The association between operator confidence and accuracy of ultrasonography performed by novice emergency physicians. *J Emerg Med* 29:259–264, 2005.
11. Doostan DK, Steffenson SL, Snoey ER: Cerebral and coronary air embolism: an intradepartmental suicide attempt. *J Emerg Med* 25:29–34, 2003.
12. Durham B: Emergency medicine physicians saving time with ultrasound. *Am J Emerg Med* 14:309–313, 1996.
13. Jones AE, Craddock PA, Tayal VS, Kline JA: Diagnostic accuracy of left ventricular function for identifying sepsis among emergency department patients with nontraumatic symptomatic undifferentiated hypotension. *Shock* 24:513–517, 2005.
14. Jones AE, Tayal VS, Kline JA: Focused training of emergency medicine residents in goal-directed echocardiography: A prospective study. *Acad Emerg Med* 10:1054–1058, 2003.
15. Moore CL, Rose GA, Tayal VS, Sullivan DM, Arrowood JA, Kline JA: Determination of left ventricular function by emergency physician echocardiography of hypotensive patients. *Acad Emerg Med* 9:186–193, 2002.
16. Niendorff DF, Rassias AJ, Palac R, Beach ML, Costa S, Greenberg M: Rapid cardiac ultrasound of inpatients suffering PEA arrest performed by nonexpert sonographers. *Resuscitation* 67:81–87, 2005.
17. Plummer D, Brunette D, Asinger R, Ruiz E: Emergency department echocardiography improves outcome in penetrating cardiac injury. *Ann Emerg Med* 21:709–712, 1992.
18. Plummer D, Dick C, Ruiz E, Clinton J, Brunette D: Emergency department two-dimensional echocardiography in the diagnosis of nontraumatic cardiac rupture. *Ann Emerg Med* 23:1333–1342, 1994.
19. Randazzo MR, Snoey ER, Levitt MA, Binder K: Accuracy of emergency physician assessment of left ventricular ejection fraction and central venous pressure using echocardiography. *Acad Emerg Med* 10:973–977, 2003.
20. Rozycki GS, Feliciano DV, Ochsner MG, et al.: The role of ultrasound in patients with possible penetrating cardiac wounds: A prospective multicenter study. *J Trauma* 46:543–551; discussion 51–52, 1999.
21. Salen P, Melniker L, Chooljian C, et al.: Does the presence or absence of sonographically identified cardiac activity predict resuscitation outcomes of cardiac arrest patients? *Am J Emerg Med* 23:459–462, 2005.
22. Salen P, O'Connor R, Sierzenski P, et al.: Can cardiac sonography and capnography be used independently and in combination to predict resuscitation outcomes? *Acad Emerg Med* 8:610–615, 2001.
23. Schiavone WA, Ghumrawi BK, Catalano DR, et al.: The

use of echocardiography in the emergency management of nonpenetrating traumatic cardiac rupture. *Ann Emerg Med* 20:1248–1250, 1991.

24. Plummer D: Diagnostic ultrasonography in the emergency department. *Ann Emerg Med* 22:592–594, 1993.

25. Plummer D: Whose turf is it, anyway? Diagnostic ultrasonography in the emergency department. *Acad Emerg Med* 7:186–187, 2000.

26. Heller MB: Emergency ultrasound: Echoes of the future. *Ann Emerg Med* 23:1353–1354, 1994.

27. Guidelines 2000 for Cardiopulmonary Resuscitation and Emergency Cardiovascular Care. Part 6: advanced cardiovascular life support: Section 7: Algorithm approach to ACLS emergencies: Section 7A: Principles and practice of ACLS. The American Heart Association in collaboration with the International Liaison Committee on Resuscitation. *Circulation* 102:I136–I139, 2000.

28. Flachskampf FA, Daniel WG: Aortic Dissection. *Card Clinics* 18:807–817, 2000.

29. Dmowski AT, Carey MT: Aortic Dissection. *Am J Emerg Med* 17:372–178, 1999.

30. Pretre R, Segesser LK: Aortic Dissection. *Lancet* 349:1461–1464, 1997.

31. Desanctis RW, Doroghazi RM, Austen WG, et al.: Aortic Dissection. *NEJM* 317:1060–1065, 1987.

32. Blaivas M: Incidence of pericardial effusion in patients presenting to the emergency department with unexplained dyspnea. *Acad Emerg Med* 8:1143–1146, 2001.

33. Mandavia DP, Aragona J, Chan L, Chan D, Henderson SO: Ultrasound training for emergency physicians—A prospective study. *Acad Emerg Med* 7:1008–1014, 2000.

34. 2005 American Heart Association Guidelines for Cardiopulmonary Resuscitation and Emergency Cardiovascular Care. *Circulation* 112:IV1–IV203, 2005.

35. Berryman CR: Electromechanical dissociation with directly measurable arterial blood pressure (Abstract). *Ann Emerg Med* 15:625, 1986.

36. Bocka JJ, Overton DT, Hauser A: Electromechanical dissociation in human beings: An echocardiographic evaluation. *Ann Emerg Med* 17:450–452, 1988.

37. Deakin CD, Low JL: Accuracy of the advanced trauma life support guidelines for predicting systolic blood pressure using carotid, femoral, and radial pulses: observational study. *BMJ* (Clinical research ed) 321:673–674, 2000.

38. Cummins RO, Hazinski MF: The most important changes in the international ECC and CPR guidelines 2000. *Circulation* 102:I371–I376, 2000.

39. Lapostolle F, Le Toumelin P, Agostinucci JM, Catineau J, Adnet F: Basic cardiac life support providers checking the carotid pulse: Performance, degree of conviction, and influencing factors. *Acad Emerg Med* 11:878–880, 2004.

40. Sanders AB, Kern KB, Berg RA: Searching for a predictive rule for terminating cardiopulmonary resuscitation. *Acad Emerg Med* 8:654–657, 2001.

41. Varriale P, Maldonado JM: Echocardiographic observations during in hospital cardiopulmonary resuscitation. *Crit Care Med* 25:1717–1720, 1997.

42. Hendrickson RG, Dean AJ, Costantino TG: A novel use of ultrasound in pulseless electrical activity: The diagnosis of an acute abdominal aortic aneurysm rupture. *J Emerg Med* 21:141–144, 2001.

43. MacCarthy P, Worrall A, McCarthy G, Davies J: The use of transthoracic echocardiography to guide thrombolytic therapy during cardiac arrest due to massive pulmonary embolism. *Emerg Med J* 19:178–179, 2002.

44. Tayal VS, Kline JA: Emergency echocardiography to detect pericardial effusion in patients in PEA and near-PEA states. *Resuscitation* 59:315–318, 2003.

45. Kaul S, Stratienko AA, Pollock SG, Marieb MA, Keller MW, Sabia PJ: Value of two-dimensional echocardiography for determining the basis of hemodynamic compromise in critically ill patients: A prospective study. *Echocardiogr* 7:598–606, 1994.

46. Pershad J, Myers S, Plouman C, et al.: Bedside limited echocardiography by the emergency physician is accurate during evaluation of the critically ill patient. *Pediatrics* 114:e667–e671, 2004.

47. Plummer D, Heegaard W, Dries D, Reardon R, Pippert G, Frascone RJ: Ultrasound in HEMS: Its role in differentiating shock states. *Air Med J* 22:33–36, 2003.

48. Kurkciyan I, Meron G, Sterz F, et al.: Pulmonary embolism as a cause of cardiac arrest: Presentation and outcome. *Arch Intern Med* 160:1529–1535, 2000.

49. Silfvast T: Cause of death in unsuccessful prehospital resuscitation. *J Intern Med* 229:331–335, 1991.

50. Frazee BW, Snoey ER: Diagnostic role of ED ultrasound in deep venous thrombosis and pulmonary embolism. *Am J Emerg Med* 17:271–278, 1999.

51. Johnson ME, Furlong R, Schrank K: Diagnostic use of emergency department echocardiogram in massive pulmonary emboli. *Ann Emerg Med* 21:760–763, 1992.

52. Karavidas A, Matsakas E, Lazaros G, Panou F, Foukarakis M, Zacharoulis A: Emergency bedside echocardiography as a tool for early detection and clinical decision making in cases of suspected pulmonary embolism—A case report. *Angiology* 51:1021–1025, 2000.

53. Madan A, Schwartz C: Echocardiographic visualization of acute pulmonary embolus and thrombolysis in the ED. *Am J Emerg Med* 22:294–300, 2004.

54. Bottiger BW, Bohrer H, Bach A, Motsch J, Martin E: Bolus injection of thrombolytic agents during cardiopulmonary resuscitation for massive pulmonary embolism. *Resuscitation* 28:45–54, 1994.

55. Moscati R, Reardon R: Clinical application of the FAST exam. In: Jehle D, Heller MB, eds. *Ultrasonography in Trauma: The FAST Exam*. Dallas: American College of Emergency Physicians; 39–60, 2003.

56. Thourani VH, Feliciano DV, Cooper WA, et al.: Penetrating cardiac trauma at an urban trauma center: A 22-year perspective. *Am Surgeon* 65:811–816; discussion 7–8, 1999.

57. Mandavia DP, Hoffner RJ, Mahaney K, Henderson SO: Bedside echocardiography by emergency physicians. *Ann Emerg Med* 38:377–382, 2001.

58. Spodick DH: Acute cardiac tamponade. *N Engl J Med* 349:684–690, 2003.

59. LeWinter M, Samer K: Pericardial disease. In: Braunwald E, ed. *Braunwauld's Heart Disease*. Philadelphia: Elsevier, 1757–1780, 2005.

60. Spodick DH: Pathophysiology of cardiac tamponade. *Chest* 113:1372–1378, 1998.

61. Cooper JP, Oliver RM, Currie P, Walker JM, Swanton RH: How do the clinical findings in patients with pericardial

effusions influence the success of aspiration? *Br Heart J* 73:351–354, 1995.

62. Feldman J: Cardiac ultrasound in the ED. *Ann Emerg Med* 18:230–231, 1989.

63. American College of Emergency Physicians. ACEP emergency ultrasound guidelines-2001. *Ann Emerg Med* 38:470–481, 2001.

64. Kucher N, Goldhaber SZ: Management of massive pulmonary embolism. *Circulation* 112:e28–e32, 2005.

65. Tayama E, Ouchida M, Teshima H, et al.: Treatment of acute massive/submassive pulmonary embolism. *Circ J* 66:479–483, 2002.

66. Konstantinides S: Thrombolysis in submassive pulmonary embolism? Yes. *J Thromb Haemost* 1:1127–1129, 2003.

67. Konstantinides S: Should thrombolytic therapy be used in patients with pulmonary embolism? *Am J Cardiovasc Drugs* 4:69–74, 2004.

68. Konstantinides S: Pulmonary embolism: Impact of right ventricular dysfunction. *Curr Opin Cardiol* 20:496–501, 2005.

69. Konstantinides S: Diagnosis and therapy of pulmonary embolism. *VASA Zeitschrift fur Gefasskrankheiten* 35:135–146, 2006.

70. Konstantinides S, Geibel A, Heusel G, Heinrich F, Kasper W: Heparin plus alteplase compared with heparin alone in patients with submassive pulmonary embolism. *N Engl J Med* 347:1143–1150, 2002.

71. Konstantinides S, Geibel A, Kasper W: Submassive and massive pulmonary embolism: A target for thrombolytic therapy? *Thrombosis Haemostasis* 82(Suppl. 1):104–108, 1999.

72. Konstantinides S, Hasenfuss G: [Acute cor pulmonale in pulmonary embolism. An important prognostic factor and a critical parameter for the choice of a therapeutic strategy]. *Der Internist* 45:1155–1162, 2004.

73. Konstantinides S, Tiede N, Geibel A, Olschewski M, Just H, Kasper W: Comparison of alteplase versus heparin for resolution of major pulmonary embolism. *Am J Cardiol* 82:966–970, 1998.

74. Sadeghi A, Brevetti GR, Kim S, et al.: Acute massive pulmonary embolism: Role of the cardiac surgeon. *Texas Heart Institute Journal*/from the Texas Heart Institute of St, 32:430–433, 2005.

75. Jackson RE, Rudoni RR, Hauser AM, Pascual RG, Hussey ME: Prospective evaluation of two-dimensional transthoracic echocardiography in emergency department patients with suspected pulmonary embolism. *Acad Emerg Med* 7:994–998, 2000.

76. Armstrong WF: Echocardiography. In: Braunwald E, ed. *Braunwald's Heart Disease*. Philadelphia, PA: Elevier; 2005:187–203.

77. Picard MH, Davidoff R, Sleeper LA, et al.: Echocardiographic predictors of survival and response to early revascularization in cardiogenic shock. *Circulation* 107:279–284, 2003.

78. Carabello BA: Evolution of the study of left ventricular function: Everything old is new again. *Circulation* 105:2701–2703, 2002.

79. Rose JS, Bair AE, Mandavia D, Kinser DJ: The UHP ultrasound protocol: A novel ultrasound approach to the empiric evaluation of the undifferentiated hypotensive patient. *Am J Emerg Med* 19:299–302, 2001.

80. Lyon M, Blaivas M, Brannam L: Sonographic measurement of the inferior vena cava as a marker of blood loss. *Am J Emerg Med* 23:45–50, 2005.

81. Natori H, Tamaki S, Kira S: Ultrasonographic evaluation of ventilatory effect on inferior vena caval configuration. *Am Rev Respiratory Dis* 120:421–427, 1979.

82. Simonson JS, Schiller NB: Sonospirometry: A new method for noninvasive estimation of mean right atrial pressure based on two-dimensional echographic measurements of the inferior vena cava during measured inspiration. *J Am Coll Cardiol* 11:557–564, 1988.

83. Kircher BJ, Himelman RB, Schiller NB: Noninvasive estimation of right atrial pressure from the inspiratory collapse of the inferior vena cava. *Am J Cardiol* 66:493–496, 1990.

84. Yanagawa Y, Nishi K, Sakamoto T, Okada Y: Early diagnosis of hypovolemic shock by sonographic measurement of inferior vena cava in trauma patients. *J Trauma* 58:825–829, 2005.

85. Ettin D, Cook T: Using ultrasound to determine external pacer capture. *J Emerg Med* 17:1007–1009, 1999.

86. Holger JS, Minnigan HJ, Lamon RP, Gornick CC: The utility of ultrasound to determine ventricular capture in external cardiac pacing. *Am J Emerg Med* 19:134–136, 2001. *Am J Emerg Med* 23:197–198, 2005.

87. Aguilera PA, Durham BA, Riley DA: Emergency transvenous cardiac pacing placement using ultrasound guidance. *Ann Emerg Med* 36:224–227, 2000.

88. Bonow R, Braunwald E: Valvular heart disease. In: Braunwald E, ed. *Braunwald's Heart Disease*. Philadelphia, PA: Elsevier; 2005:1553–1620.

89. Feigenbaum H, Armstrong WF, Ryan T: Mitral valve disease. In: Feigenbaum H, Armstrong WF, Ryan T, eds. *Feigenbaum's Echocardiography*. Philadelphia, PA: Lippincott Williams & Wilkins; 2005:306–351.

90. Cline D: Valvular emergencies. In: Tintinalli J, ed. *Emergency Medicine: A Comprehensive Study Guide*. 6th ed. New York: McGraw-Hill; 2003:373–378.

91. Sommer T, Fehske W, Holzknecht N: Aortic dissection: A comparative study of diagnosis with spiral CT, multiplanar transesophageal echocardiography and MR imaging. *Radiology*, 199:347–352, 1996.

92. Horowitz RS, Morganroth J, Parrotto C, Chen CC, Soffer J, Pauletto FJ: Immediate diagnosis of acute myocardial infarction by two-dimensional echocardiography. *Circulation* 65:323–329, 1982.

93. Sabia P, Afrookteh A, Touchstone DA, Keller MW, Esquivel L, Kaul S: Value of regional wall motion abnormality in the emergency room diagnosis of acute myocardial infarction. A prospective study using two-dimensional echocardiography. *Circulation* 84:I85–I92, 1991.

94. Levitt MA, Promes SB, Bullock S, et al.: Combined cardiac marker approach with adjunct two-dimensional echocardiography to diagnose acute myocardial infarction in the emergency department. *Ann Emerg Med* 27:1–7, 1996.

95. Muttreja MR, Mohler ER, III: Clinical use of ischemic markers and echocardiography in the emergency department. *Echocardiography* 16:187–192, 1999.

96. Mohler ER, III, Ryan T, Segar DS, et al.: Clinical utility of

troponin T levels and echocardiography in the emergency department. *Am Heart J* 135:253–260, 1998.

97. Reardon MJ, Carr CL, Diamond A, et al.: Ischemic left ventricular free wall rupture: Prediction, diagnosis, and treatment. *Ann Thoracic Surgery* 64:1509–1513, 1997.

98. Mueller X, Stauffer JC, Jaussi A, Goy JJ, Kappenberger L: Subjective visual echocardiographic estimate of left ventricular ejection fraction as an alternative to conventional echocardiographic methods: Comparison with contrast angiography. *Clin Cardiol,* 14:898–902, 1991.

99. Amico AF, Lichtenberg GS, Reisner SA, Stone CK, Schwartz RG, Meltzer RS: Superiority of visual versus computerized echocardiographic estimation of radionuclide left ventricular ejection fraction. *Am Heart J,* 118:1259–1265, 1989.

100. Stamm RB, Carabello BA, Mayers DL, Martin RP: Two-dimensional echocardiographic measurement of left ventricular ejection fraction: Prospective analysis of what constitutes an adequate determination. *Am Heart J* 104:136–144, 1982.

101. Tsang TS, Oh JK, Seward JB: Diagnosis and management of cardiac tamponade in the era of echocardiography. *Clin Cardiol* 22:446–452, 1999.

102. Oh JK, Miller FA, Shub C, Reeder GS, Tajik AJ: Evaluation of acute chest pain syndromes by two-dimensional echocardiography: Its potential application in the selection of patients for acute reperfusion therapy. *Mayo Clinic Proc* 62:59–66, 1987.

103. Come PC: Echocardiographic recognition of pulmonary arterial disease and determination of its cause. *Am J Med* 84:384–394, 1988.

104. Jardin F, Dubourg O, Gueret P, Delorme G, Bourdarias JP: Quantitative two-dimensional echocardiography in massive pulmonary embolism: Emphasis on ventricular interdependence and leftward septal displacement. *J Am Coll Cardiol* 10:1201–1206, 1987.

105. Stein J: Opinions regarding the diagnosis and management of venous thromboembolic disease. ACCP Consensus Committee on Pulmonary Embolism. *Chest* 109:233–237, 1996.

CHAPTER 7

Abdominal Aortic Aneurysm

Robert F. Reardon, Thomas Cook, and Dave Plummer

Aneurysm of the abdominal aorta is a relatively common disease in patients over 50 years of age.[1-3] Rupture of an abdominal aortic aneurysm (AAA) has a high mortality and causes as many as 30,000 deaths per year in the United States, which is more than AIDS or prostate cancer.[4] It is one of the least-known killers in American society.[4]

More than 100 years ago, William Osler said, "There is no disease more conducive to clinical humility than aneurysm of the aorta." This remains true today, as the diagnosis of ruptured AAA continues to confound clinicians. Misdiagnosis of ruptured AAA is common because many patients have not had a previously asymptomatic AAA formally diagnosed; they also may present with nonspecific complaints and have normal vital signs.[5-7] Mortality due to AAA is decreased if the diagnosis is made prior to rupture or if the diagnosis is made rapidly after rupture of AAA.[8-13]

The availability of bedside ultrasound in the emergency department (ED) has allowed emergency physicians to change their approach to patients at risk for a ruptured AAA. A screening bedside ultrasound examination can now be obtained on patients over 50 years of age who present with pain in the abdomen, back, flank, or groin, and on those who present with dizziness, syncope, unexplained hypotension, or car-

diac arrest.[2,14] This practice is analogous to the immediate acquisition of an electrocardiogram for all patients with possible myocardial infarction. In this capacity, ultrasound clearly can save lives, making this application one of the indisputable benefits of emergency bedside ultrasound.[8,9,13,15]

▶ CLINICAL CONSIDERATIONS

Abdominal aortic aneurysm occurs in 2–5% of the population over 50 years of age and about 10% of men over 65 years of age who have risk factors for vascular disease.[16-22] The prevalence is even higher in patients with first-degree relatives who have an AAA and those with peripheral vascular disease.[4,23] AAA is about four times more prevalent in men than in women.[24-26] The prevalence has been steadily rising in both men and women over the past several decades, so despite advances in diagnostic imaging and surgical techniques there has been essentially no change in the number of patients presenting with ruptured AAA.[27-31]

The risk of AAA rupture is directly related to the largest diameter of the aneurysm and increases dramatically in those greater than 5 cm. Estimates of rupture risk are as follows: less than 2% per year for aneurysms smaller than 4 cm, 1–5% per year for those 4–5 cm, 3–15% per year for those 5–6 cm, 10–20% per year for those 6–7 cm, and 20–50% per year for those larger than 7 cm.[32–37] Other factors such as continued smoking, uncontrolled hypertension, and emphysema increase the risk of rupture.[38,39] Also, women have a higher risk for rupture than men with the same-size aneurysm.[32,40–42] Current guidelines for elective treatment of AAA suggest operative repair of aneurysms 5.5 cm or larger in the "average" patient.[43] Of course, each patient's situation is unique and requires an analysis of the risks and benefits prior to elective surgery.[4]

Most patients with an AAA are asymptomatic until rupture occurs. The overall mortality for ruptured AAA is roughly 80%. About 60% die prior to receiving any medical care and 40–50% of those who have emergent operative repair die.[18,44–49] Rapid diagnosis and early surgical management has been shown to decrease mortality.[10–13] Unfortunately, 30–60% of patients with a ruptured AAA may be initially misdiagnosed.[6,44,50,51] Delayed or misdiagnosis occurs because the symptoms may mimic other common conditions such as renal colic, diverticulitis, gastrointestinal hemorrhage, sepsis, or acute coronary syndrome. The "classic triad" of abdominal or back pain, hypotension, and a palpable abdominal mass is not usually present.[52] Patients do not usually know that they have an aneurysm, and many have normal vital signs and initially appear well.[6,18,47,51–53]

Emergency physicians routinely manage a large number of patients over 50 years of age who have symptoms that could be consistent with a ruptured AAA. Most of these patients do not have a ruptured AAA, but those who do must be diagnosed rapidly. Even when an aneurysm is suspected, physical examination findings are not reliable for excluding or confirming the diagnosis.[6,18,47,51–55] Therefore, clinicians need an accurate diagnostic screening test that can be effectively used on a large number of patients. The diagnostic test must be rapid and easy to obtain so that clinicians will have a low threshold for using it. The only diagnostic test that fits this description is bedside ultrasound performed by the clinician who is already caring for the patient.[50] Laboratory tests are unhelpful and plain radiographs are unreliable; the two essentially have no place in the diagnostic evaluation for an acute AAA. Computed tomography is very accurate for detecting AAA but it exposes patients to ionizing radiation and is very expensive. Furthermore, unstable patients may be difficult to resuscitate in the CT suite. The use of bedside ultrasound performed by clinicians has been extensively studied and is nearly 100% accurate for detecting or excluding AAA.[5,7,56–59]

In 1989, the first report on the use of bedside ultrasound by emergency physicians to rapidly diagnose ruptured AAA was published.[60] Two prospective studies reported that emergency physicians with limited training could diagnose AAA with sensitivity and specificity

approaching 100%.[57,61] In 2000, a study analyzed 68 patients over 50 years of age presenting to an ED with symptoms worrisome for a ruptured AAA.[56] Bedside ultrasound was performed by emergency physicians who had attended a 3-day emergency ultrasound training course but had no prior experience performing or interpreting sonograms. They detected 26 AAAs and had 100% sensitivity and 100% specificity compared with gold standard diagnostic testing. They concluded that relative novice sonologists can perform aortic ultrasound examinations accurately. In 2003, a prospective study analyzed 114 patients presenting to an ED with symptoms suggestive of ruptured AAA.[7] Bedside ultrasound examinations were performed by emergency physicians and senior emergency medicine residents. The investigators diagnosed AAA in 29 patients, had 100% sensitivity, and 98% specificity compared to confirmatory testing, and concluded that emergency physicians could use bedside ultrasound to diagnose or exclude AAA. A 2005 study evaluated 238 patients who presented to an ED with symptoms concerning for ruptured AAA.[5] Ultrasound examinations were performed by 3rd-year emergency medicine residents who had been trained following guidelines of the American College of Emergency Physicians.[62] They diagnosed 36 aortic "abnormalities" and were 100% sensitive and 100% specific for this endpoint compared to gold standard diagnostic testing. They correctly measured the AAA diameter in 34 of 36 patients and incorrectly measured 2 AAAs but recognized dissection in one case and intraluminal clot in the other. The investigators concluded that appropriately trained emergency medicine residents can accurately determine the presence of AAA.

A 1998 study conducted by Plummer and coworkers dramatically demonstrated the need for emergency bedside ultrasound.[13] They reviewed the medical records of 50 consecutive patients presenting to their ED with a ruptured AAA. Twenty-five patients who had an immediate bedside ultrasound examination had an average time to diagnosis of 5.4 minutes and a median time to disposition for operative intervention of 12 minutes. Twenty-five patients who did not receive an immediate bedside ultrasound examination had an average time to diagnosis of 83 minutes and a median time to disposition for operative intervention of 90 minutes. Their most important finding was that those patients who received an early bedside ultrasound examination had a 40% mortality compared to a 72% mortality for those patients who did not receive a bedside ultrasound examination.

Although ultrasound is operator dependent and the quality of the examination may be influenced by the expertise of the sonologist, bedside aortic ultrasound can achieve 100% accuracy with brief training.[56,63] There is not much interobserver variability, even in inexperienced hands.[56] Ultrasonography is inadequate to demonstrate the presence of extraluminal retroperitoneal blood associated with rupture, which is found with a sensitivity less than 5%.[64] However, in the appropriate clinical setting, a large AAA should be considered ruptured until proven otherwise.[52,65]

▶ CLINICAL INDICATIONS

The main indication for bedside aortic ultrasound examination is to rapidly identify patients with a ruptured AAA. Aneurysmal disease of the abdominal aorta is a silent process until the time of rupture. Patients with signs or symptoms that could be attributable to a ruptured AAA should undergo an immediate bedside ultrasound examination. Patients with a ruptured AAA have widely varying presentations. Reasonable indications for bedside aortic ultrasound examination include all patients over 50 years of age with the following signs or symptoms:

- The classic presentation of ruptured AAA
- Any pain consistent with ruptured AAA
- Unexplained hypotension, dizziness, or syncope
- Cardiac arrest

It is certainly preferable to diagnose AAA prior to rupture since early recognition and repair carries a much lower mortality. In 2005, the U.S. Preventive Services Task Force (USPSTF) published recommendations that endorsed the one-time screening for abdominal aortic aneurysm (AAA) by ultrasonography in men aged 65–75 who had any history of tobacco use. It has been demonstrated that screening for AAA and surgical repair of large AAAs (5.5 cm or more) in men aged 65–75 with a history of tobacco use (current or former smokers) led to decreased AAA-specific mortality.[8]

▶ CLASSIC PRESENTATION OF RUPTURED AAA

The "classic" presentation of a ruptured AAA is the triad of abdominal, back, or flank pain; a palpable abdominal mass; and hypotension. This "classic" presentation may be found in less than 25% of cases.[6,47,50,51,53] Pain is the most consistent part of the triad and is present in more than 80% of those seeking medical attention.[6,51,53] Palpation of an abdominal mass on physical examination is an unreliable finding. One study reported that a palpable mass was noted in only 18% of 329 patients presenting with a ruptured AAA.[53] In addition, many thin patients with an apparent pulsatile abdominal mass have a normal abdominal aorta.[54] Finally, hypotension is not universally present with ruptured AAA. Most aneurysms rupture into the retroperitoneum, resulting in a transient tamponade effect; thus, 30–50% of patients have a normal blood pressure at the time of presentation with ruptured AAA.[6,18,51−53,66]

▶ PAIN CONSISTENT WITH RUPTURED AAA

Pain is the most common reason for patients with a ruptured AAA to seek medical care. Most patients complain of pain in the abdomen, back, or flank. Studies have found that about 80% of ruptured AAA patients have abdominal pain, about 60% have back or flank pain, and 22% have groin pain at the time of presentation.[6,51] In another study of 329 cases of ruptured AAA, it was found that 49% had abdominal pain and 36% had back pain at the time of presentation.[53] Clinicians should be aware that patients often present with referred pain to the scrotum, buttocks, thighs, shoulders, chest, or other locations.[2] Many patients with ruptured AAA are misdiagnosed with renal colic, diverticulitis, or musculoskeletal pain.[50] When patients present with nonspecific pain and stable vital signs, it is common to miss or delay the diagnosis. In these difficult patients it is imperative to rapidly diagnose a ruptured AAA because those who develop hypotension prior to surgery have a higher mortality.[10,13,18,67] No patient with a known or suspected AAA rupture should be considered stable regardless of initial vital signs.[52]

▶ UNEXPLAINED HYPOTENSION, DIZZINESS, OR SYNCOPE

Hypotension is present in 50% or more of patients presenting with ruptured AAA.[6,18,51−53,66] Altered mental status secondary to hypotension can make it difficult to obtain a history of abdominal, back, or flank pain. Therefore, patients may present with unexplained hypotension and no other clues of a ruptured AAA. Many of these patients are misdiagnosed with gastrointestinal hemorrhage, sepsis, or myocardial infarction.[6,50,51,53] Both hypotension and altered mental status prior to surgery are independent predictors of mortality from a ruptured AAA.[18,67,68] A review of 231 cases of ruptured AAA presenting to the Mayo Clinic found 62% mortality when preoperative hypotension occurred.[18] Rose and colleagues developed a protocol for screening all ED patients who present with undifferentiated hypotension.[69] They described their success, using an empiric ultrasound examination to screen for pericardial effusion, free intraperitoneal fluid, and AAA. They pointed out that this approach is especially valuable when clinical history is limited or unknown and suggested that it should be a routine part of evaluation of patients with unexplained hypotension.

Relative hypotension, orthostatic hypotension, dizziness, or syncope may be precursors to overt hypotension and are indications for aortic ultrasound. Relative hypotension occurs in patients with baseline hypertension who have a decrease in blood pressure level but still have values that are within the "normal" range. These patients may present with altered mental status, vague weakness, dizziness, or syncope. It is imperative to have a high suspicion for ruptured AAA in such patients. A study that reviewed the records of 23 patients with a ruptured AAA found that 61% were initially misdiagnosed.[51] Only 13% of patients had overt hypotension (systolic blood pressure less than 90 mm Hg) but 26% had syncope and 48% had an initial systolic blood pressure less than 110 mm Hg or orthostatic hypotension.

► CARDIAC ARREST

Cardiac arrest is a fairly common presentation in patients with ruptured AAA.[18] Clinicians should recognize that patients with pulseless electrical activity may be in a state of severe hypotension that could possibly be reversible if the cause is rapidly identified and aggressively treated.[70] A case report described a patient with pulseless electrical activity in whom emergency physicians used bedside ultrasound to immediately identify mechanical cardiac activity despite lack of pulses.[71] This finding led to aggressive resuscitation and a search for potential hemorrhage. They then used bedside ultrasound to detect a large AAA, allowing the patient to proceed directly to the operating room for surgical repair. They concluded that patients presenting with PEA who are found to have mechanical cardiac activity should have immediate ultrasound imaging of their aorta.

Some physicians argue that patients who have sustained cardiac arrest from a ruptured AAA have a miniscule chance of survival and that surgical repair is a waste of resources, but this view is not supported by current data.[67] One study found that preoperative cardiac arrest occurred in 24% of patients with ruptured AAA, but 28% of those survived operative repair.[18]

► SCREENING FOR AAA IN HIGH-RISK ASYMPTOMATIC PATIENTS

Ultrasound screening for AAA and its impact on mortality has been extensively studied.[16,72–76] A 2005 evidence-based systematic review of population-based screening for AAA concluded that selective screening for AAA significantly improves AAA-related mortality. When the study extrapolated the findings to the entire U.S. population of men aged 65–74 years it estimated that 11,392 AAA deaths could be prevented over a 5-year period.[9] A study analyzing the cost-effectiveness of a "quick-screen" program for AAA found that the cost-effectiveness ratio (cost per life saved) was lower than the cost of breast cancer screening. It also noted that the average time to perform a limited screening examination of the abdominal aorta was 4 minutes and the accuracy was 100%.[58] Properly trained emergency physicians can perform limited AAA screening examinations with 100% sensitivity.[7,56] There is also evidence that internal medicine and surgery residents can learn to perform accurate AAA screening examinations with little training.[77,78]

Kent and colleagues provided a review of the utility of AAA screening and a consensus statement that was supported by the Society for Vascular Surgery, the American Association of Vascular Surgery, and the Society for Vascular Medicine and Biology.[4] They analyzed the cost-effectiveness of screening men over 60 years of age and found it to be similar to screening mammography for breast cancer. On the basis of the results of six prospective randomized studies, they recommended ultrasound screening for AAA in all men aged 60–85 years, women aged 60–85 years with cardiovascular risk factors, and men and women older than 50 years with a family history of AAA.[16,25,72,74,76,79–81] They also recommended that patients found to have an AAA 3–4 cm in diameter have an annual follow-up ultrasound examination, those with an AAA 4–4.5 cm have a follow-up examination every 6 months, and those with an AAA greater than 4.5 cm be referred to a vascular surgeon.

► ANATOMICAL CONSIDERATIONS

The abdominal aorta is entirely a retroperitoneal structure. It begins at the aortic hiatus of the diaphragm at approximately the 12th thoracic vertebrae and courses anterior to the spine before bifurcating into the common iliac arteries. The inferior vena cava (IVC) courses to the right of the abdominal aorta and may be confused for the abdominal aorta by novice sonologists. The psoas muscle and kidney are posterior-lateral to the abdominal aorta on the left side. The left lobe of the liver is located anterior to the proximal abdominal aorta and acts as the primary acoustic window for this area of the vessel. More caudal, the aorta is posterior to the transverse colon, the pancreas, and proximal duodenum. The distal duodenum crosses over the abdominal aorta distal to the superior mesenteric artery. Other areas of the small bowel lie anterior to the abdominal aorta as it courses distally to its bifurcation at approximately the 2nd lumbar vertebrae (or umbilicus). Components of the gastrointestinal system may contain air that can block visualization of the abdominal aorta and its vascular branches.

artery; the right renal artery courses under the IVC. The paired gonadal arteries (testicular and ovarian) come off the anterior wall distal to the renal vessels. The inferior mesenteric artery comes off the anterior wall 2 to 3 cm proximal to the iliac bifurcation and supplies blood to the lower gastrointestinal tract. Both the gonadal vessels and inferior mesenteric artery are usually difficult to visualize by ultrasound and rarely contribute to evaluation and management of the patient.

▶ GETTING STARTED

The bedside scenario when performing an ultrasound examination of the aorta can vary from a calm physician's office to a resuscitation bay crowded with medical personnel working together to provide simultaneous components of patient care. There are a variety of protocols that clinicians may adopt to complete an examination; however, an abbreviated examination of the aorta is usually easy to complete in less than 1 or 2 minutes. Ideally, the entire length of the abdominal aorta from the diaphragm to the bifurcation should be evaluated in both the longitudinal and transverse planes.

Most patients are examined in the supine position, but the patient can be placed into the right or left decubital positions if excessive bowel gas is present. Bowel gas is the most common cause for inability to view the abdominal aorta; by placing the patient in either decubitus position, bowel gas may be displaced from the aorta.

Since there are no ribs or other bony structures overlying the abdominal aorta, a variety of probes can be used for the examination, ranging from curvilinear transducers with large footprints to small phased array probes typically designed for echocardiography. Most examiners use abdominal "presets" for the examination. Focal zones and frequency may need to be augmented to accommodate the patient's body habitus. Appropriate patient draping and room light are often dictated by the bedside scenario as well.

The examination begins with the machine placed at the patient's right side. A liberal amount of gel should be placed in the area from the xiphoid process to the umbilicus. By convention the abdominal aorta is imaged in the longitudinal (sagittal) plane by pointing the probe marker dot toward the patient's head and in the transverse (axial) plane by pointing the probe marker dot toward the patient's right side. The vast majority of imaging of the abdominal aorta is done on the anterior surface along the patient's midline (Figure 7-2). The critical portion of the abdominal aorta examination (just above the bifurcation) is accomplished in the transverse orientation with the probe indicator pointed toward the patient's right side.

A curved array transducer is typically used to examine the aorta. Frequency selection should be based

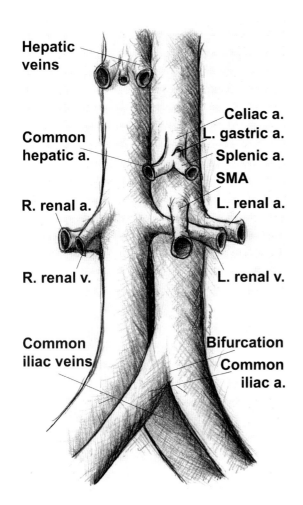

Figure 7-1. Branches of the abdominal aorta and inferior vena cava. SMA = superior mesenteric artery.

The abdominal aorta is 10–20 cm in length in adults with a maximum external diameter that is normally less than 3.0 cm (2.1 cm for men over 55 years and 1.8 cm for women over 55 years). It tapers to approximately 1.5 cm at the bifurcation, but it can be less than 1.0 cm in diameter in smaller adults. The first large branch of the abdominal aorta is the celiac trunk (Figure 7-1). It comes off the anterior wall of the abdominal aorta approximately 1–2 cm below the level of the diaphragm and courses anteriorly for 1–2 cm before splitting into the common hepatic and splenic arteries. The splenic artery courses to the left and follows the superior border of the pancreas before entering the spleen. The common hepatic artery courses to the right and supplies blood to the liver, stomach, pancreas, and duodenum. The superior mesenteric artery arises from the anterior wall of the aorta approximately 1 to 2 cm distal from the celiac trunk and courses caudally to supply blood to the small bowel. Both renal arteries come off the lateral wall of the abdominal aorta, just distal to the superior mesenteric

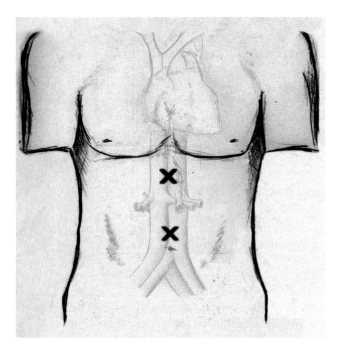

Figure 7-2. Ultrasound probe positions for imaging the abdominal aorta. The length of the aorta can be imaged using sweeping views from these probe positions. This can avoid potential interference from gas in the transverse colon.

on body habitus to achieve the best balance of resolution and penetration. An average-sized adult is usually scanned at approximately 3.5 MHz. A lower frequency should be selected for greater penetration in patients with a large body habitus. Smaller or thinner adults may be scanned at resolutions as high as 5 MHz. Standard two-dimensional gray scale imaging is adequate; additional features such as color Doppler and power Doppler are not required but can facilitate differentiation of the abdominal aorta from other structures. A sufficient depth should be selected at the beginning of the examination until the abdominal aorta is identified. Upon visualizing the aorta, the sonologist should adjust the depth, focal zone, and frequency to optimize the image.

Although not required for all examinations of the abdominal aorta, identification of landmark structures including arterial branches, venous structures, and other abdominal organs can ensure that an adequate segment of the aorta has been imaged. Visualization of this entire length of abdominal aorta is required to exclude AAA. Should its diameter be adequately visualized and appear normal over this length, then a ruptured AAA can be excluded with an essentially 100% negative predictive value.

There are two primary obstacles to obtaining adequate images of the abdominal aorta: bowel gas and obesity. Bowel gas may force the examiner to move the probe slightly to either side of the midline to acquire

views. Another option is to press firmly in order to compress the bowel with the transducer and move bowel gas away from the area of interest. This may require several minutes of pressure on the abdominal surface with the transducer.

Strategies to overcome obesity include using firm pressure to decrease the distance from the skin-transducer interface to the target organ and rolling the patient in a left lateral decubitus position to swing the pannus away from the midline. Firm pressure on the transducer will allow visualization of the aorta in nearly all patients. Iatrogenic rupture of an AAA by firm pressure during physical examination or an ultrasound examination has not been reported.[52]

► TECHNIQUE AND NORMAL ULTRASOUND FINDINGS

If time permits for a complete examination of the abdominal aorta, the transducer initially should be placed just caudal to the xiphoid process (Figures 7-3 and 7-4). In the transverse plane, an excellent point of reference is the spine. It appears as a posteriorly oriented concave structure that is highly reflective (hyperechoic) and casts a shadow. The abdominal aorta is easily found immediately anterior and slightly to the left of the spine. It is pulsatile and round to ovular in shape. This usually makes it easy to differentiate from the IVC, which is thin-walled, varies in size with respiration, and is often flattened by minimal pressure from the transducer. This view also provides an opportunity to angle the transducer beam into the frontal plane (i.e., toward the head) in order to acquire a subcostal view of the heart. Superficial to the most proximal abdominal aorta will be the

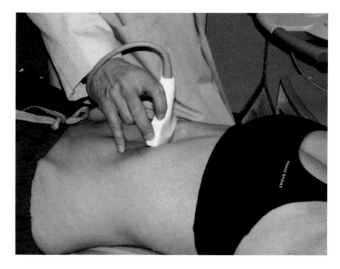

Figure 7-3. Initial transducer position for complete imaging of the abdominal aorta–transverse with indicator to the patient's right.

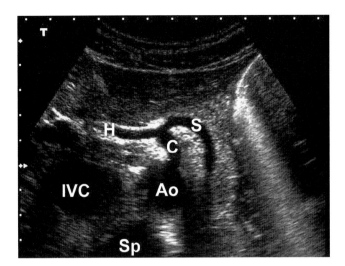

Figure 7-4. Transverse view of the upper aorta (at the level of the celiac trunk). By using a large convex probe in a thin patient, the relative positions of the anatomical landmarks can be visualized. The liver serves as an acoustic window to the structures below. The aorta and IVC are immediately above the spine. H = hepatic artery, S = splenic artery, C = celiac artery, IVC = inferior vena cava, Ao = aorta, Sp = spine.

subcutaneous tissue and left lobe of the liver. It is important to note that the left lobe of the liver acts as the acoustic window for imaging the proximal portion of the abdominal aorta.

As the transducer is moved more caudal, branches of the abdominal aorta come into view starting with the celiac trunk and then the superior mesenteric artery. The latter is in close proximity to several other vascular structures in the transverse plane (Figure 7-5A). The left renal vein courses under the superior mesenteric artery and over the abdominal aorta joining the IVC. The splenic vein crosses over the superior mesenteric artery along the body of the pancreas before joining the superior mesenteric vein to create the portal vein in the liver. One or both renal arteries and veins may be seen just inferior to the take-off of the superior mesenteric artery (SMA) coursing posterior-lateral to the kidneys. When the renal arteries are not visible, involvement of an aneurysm with these branch vessels can be predicted on the basis of proximity to the SMA. The renal arteries are likely to be involved if the aneurysm is within 2 cm of the branching point for the SMA.

Since the distal abdominal aorta is the most common location of an AAA, sonologists may opt to examine the distal aorta first in the unstable patient. The distal aorta is best viewed by placing the transducer just superior to the umbilicus in the transverse plane (Figure 7-2). However, there is much to be said for starting in the epigastric region every time and take the additional seconds to orient to the anatomy as the sonologist proceeds distally. The distal transverse view often demonstrates only the abdominal aorta and spine posterior as the IVC may be collapsed because of compression from the transducer (Figure 7-5B). Anterior–posterior (AP) diameter from outer wall to outer wall in transverse section provides the most accurate measurement of the external diameter of the abdominal aorta. In contrast, measurement of the longitudinal dimension may cause a "cylinder

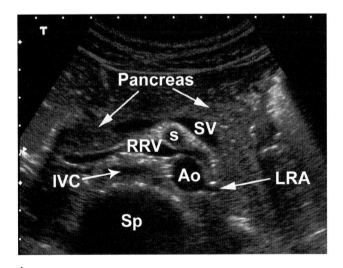

A

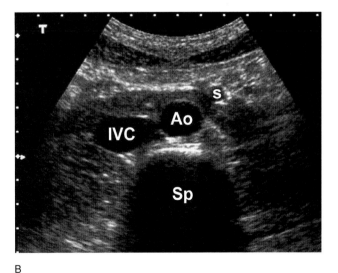

B

Figure 7-5. (a) Transverse view of the middle portion of the abdominal aorta (at a level just below the branching point for the SMA). RRV = right renal vein, s = superior mesenteric artery (SMA), SV = splenic vein, IVC = inferior vena cava, Ao = aorta, LRA = left renal artery, Sp = spine. (b) Transverse view of the distal abdominal aorta (at a level above the bifurcation). IVC = inferior vena cava, Ao = aorta, s = superior mesenteric vein (or artery). Sp = spine.

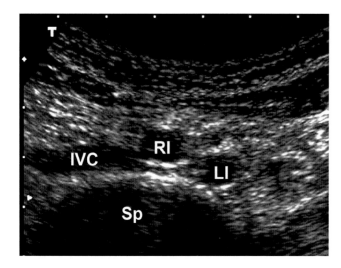

Figure 7-6. Transverse view of the bifurcation of the abdominal aorta. IVC = inferior vena cava, RI = right iliac artery, LI = left iliac artery, Sp = spine.

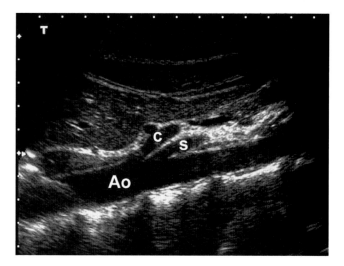

Figure 7-8. Longitudinal view of the abdominal aorta. The celiac artery (C) is the first vessel to branch off the aorta. The superior mesenteric artery (S) is immediately below the celiac artery and courses parallel to the aorta (Ao).

tangent" error (described in Pitfalls section). If a careful measurement is required, then the freeze frame option on the ultrasound machine should be used along with the caliper measurement software. In some patients, the bifurcation of the aorta can be seen, and iliac arteries followed to exclude iliac artery aneurysm if suspected (Figure 7-6).

In the longitudinal plane at the xiphoid process (Figures 7-7 and 7-8), the examiner can angle the ultrasound beam from right to left to image the proximal IVC and abdominal aorta. Some sonologists utilize a "sniff" test to help with differentiation of these structures as well. By having the patient quickly sniff, a sudden drop in thoracic pressure is created that pulls blood from the IVC into the thorax and causes the structure

to collapse. This technique fails with fluid overload and increased central venous pressure, in which the IVC is dilated and may not collapse at all. In addition, the IVC is often seen directly entering the right atrium of the heart (Figure 7-9), while the abdominal aorta will demonstrate the celiac trunk and superior mesenteric artery exiting from its anterior surface. The splenic vein and left renal vein may be seen in their short axes above and below the superior mesenteric artery, respectively, and the left renal vein may be seen coursing under the IVC.

A final option for ultrasound imaging of the aorta is the coronal view. The transducer is placed in the right

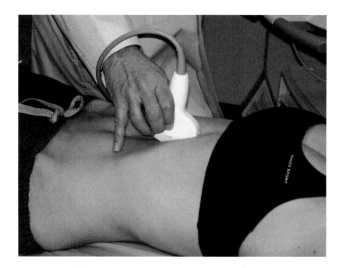

Figure 7-7. Transducer position for longitudinal views of the aorta—indicator is cephalad.

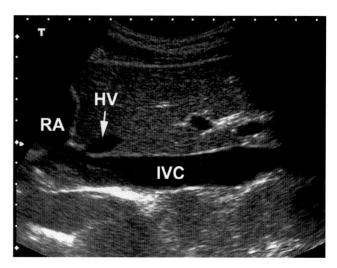

Figure 7-9. Longitudinal view of the inferior vena cava (IVC). RA = right atrium, HV = hepatic vein.

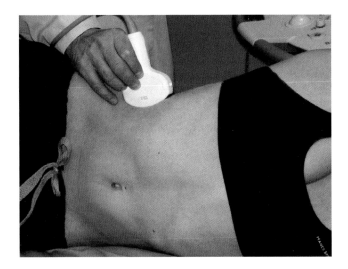

Figure 7-10. Transducer position for coronal views of the aorta—indicator is cephalad.

anterior axillary line and, using the hepatic acoustic window, the aorta imaged in the coronal plane. The examination should be initiated with the image display at maximum depth. This will yield an image with the inferior vena cava toward the top of the screen and the aorta lying deeper (Figures 7-10 and 7-11).

► COMMON ABNORMALITIES

ABDOMINAL AORTIC ANEURYSM

The primary abnormality is aneurysmal enlargement of the abdominal aorta. This is most frequently seen in the

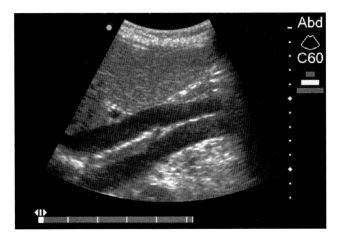

Figure 7-11. Coronal view of the aorta. The IVC is above the aorta in this right coronal view. Both renal arteries are seen branching off the aorta at a 45° angle (forming an arrowhead appearance in the mid aorta). The renal arteries are not routinely visualized in this view (Courtesy of James Mateer, MD).

transverse view as an aorta greater than 3.0 cm in diameter (Figure 7-12). Aneurysmal dilation is usually fusiform, resulting in a uniform concentric enlargement of the circumference (Figure 7-13). Localized outpouching of a segment of the aortic wall results in the more unusual saccular aneurysm formation (Figure 7-14). Aneurysmal dilatation is most often confined to the infrarenal aorta and usually terminates proximal to the bifurcation. Contiguous thoracoabdominal aneurysm occurs in a minority of cases (2%) and involves the thoracic aorta in addition to the abdominal aorta, including the segment involving the celiac, superior mesenteric, and renal arteries. The iliac arteries are involved in some patients with AAA (Figure 7-15A), and occasionally, iliac artery aneurysms occur in an isolated fashion. More than 90% of AAAs occur in the distal abdominal aorta, inferior to the renal arteries. An AAA may rarely be detected only in the proximal abdominal aorta (Figure 7-15B).

INTRALUMINAL THROMBUS

With increasing diameter, the laminar flow rate decreases at the periphery, resulting in blood stagnation and thrombus formation. This intraluminal thrombus is well visualized on ultrasound and is more common anteriorly and laterally but may be circumferential (Figure 7-12). Thrombus is found in both ruptured and unruptured AAAs. It is not an indication of rupture or dissection, and is not a false lumen.

HEMOPERITONEUM

Rupture into the peritoneal cavity may present with acute hemoperitoneum that may be visualized with the right intercostal oblique window of the FAST examination (Figure 7-16) or other windows.

► COMMON VARIANTS AND OTHER ABNORMALITIES

TORTUOSITY OF THE AORTA

Variations of the position and size of vessels are common. The aorta often becomes tortuous with age. This can cause difficulty with following the course of the vessel and finding the correct plane for transverse and longitudinal views (Figure 7-17).

CONTAINED AORTIC RUPTURE

A contained rupture of an AAA is not commonly diagnosed with ultrasound. When present, it may be seen as

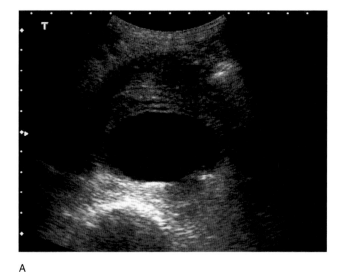

A

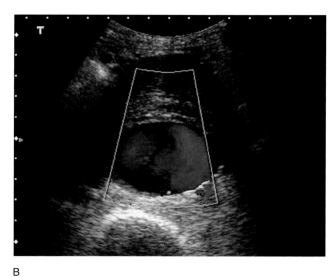

B

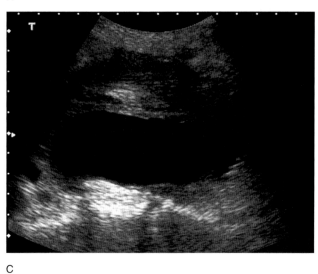

C

Figure 7-12. AAA. This fusiform aneurism demonstrates a thickened wall secondary to mural thrombus. Transverse view (A). Color Doppler confirms this is a vascular structure (B). Longitudinal view (C).

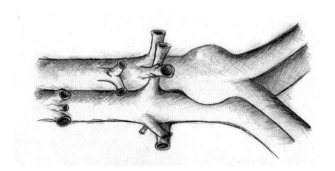

Figure 7-13. Fusiform Aneurism.

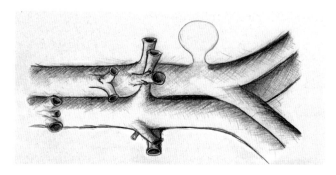

Figure 7-14. Saccular aneurysm (uncommon).

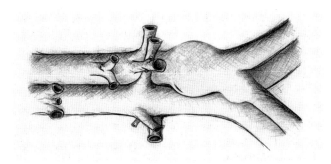

A

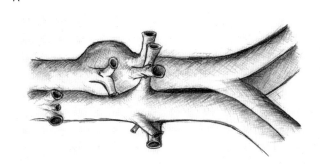

B

Figure 7-15. (a) Iliac artery aneurism. A fusiform AAA with extension into the right common iliac artery is illustrated. (b) Isolated proximal AAA (uncommon).

a hypoechoic mixed density area (from contained hemorrhage and hematoma) surrounding the aorta (Figure 7-18).

HYDRONEPHROSIS

A large AAA can cause secondary complications by compressing surrounding structures. Compression of

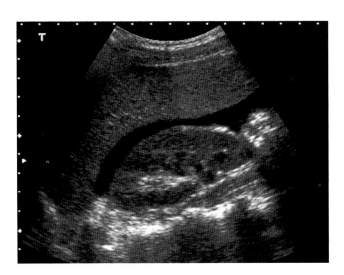

Figure 7-16. Coronal view of the right kidney demonstrates free intraperitoneal fluid.

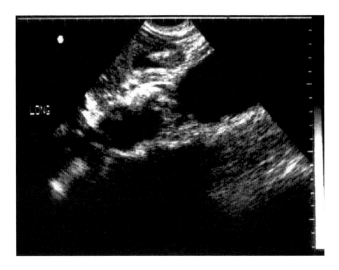

Figure 7-17. Longitudinal view of an AAA. The normal distal tapering of the aorta is reversed. The echogenic area within the aorta is not a clot, but is the sidewall of the vessel due to tortuosity. (Courtesy of James Mateer, MD)

the left ureter can lead to hydronephrosis and eventually to a perinephric urinoma from calyceal rupture (Figure 7-19).

ACUTE ABDOMINAL AORTIC DISSECTION

This disease entity may be confused with ruptured AAA and can occur with or without a coexisting aneurysm. Only 2%–4% of patients with an aortic dissection experience it in the abdominal aorta. The presenting symptoms are similar to those seen in ruptured AAA. Sonologists may even find aortic dilation in the presence of a dissection and mistakenly diagnose a small AAA. Care should be taken to examine for a flap in the lumen (Figure 7-20). Utilizing color Doppler will occasionally show flow in only one portion of the abdominal aorta in transverse orientation. Even if the flap cannot be well visualized, this finding should raise the suspicion for a dissection.

AORTOVENOUS FISTULA

Formation of an aortovenous fistula occurs when an AAA ruptures into an adjacent vein; the left renal vein or the inferior vena cava are most often involved. Because these aneurysms are usually large (11–13 cm on average), a pulsatile mass can often be palpated on physical examination. The presenting symptoms are similar to those seen in AAA rupture. An ultrasound examination demonstrating a large AAA, along with a CT scan documenting a retroaortic left renal vein and an IVP

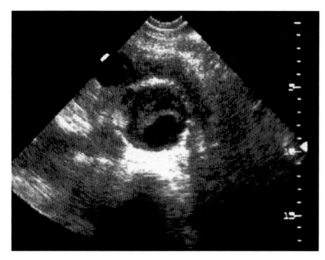

A

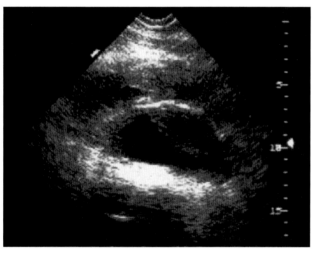

B

Figure 7-18. Contained rupture of an AAA: Transverse view reveals an AAA with mural thrombus (A). Wrapping around the anterior aorta is a hypoechoic mixed density area (from contained hemorrhage and hematoma). Longitudinal view of the same patient (B). (Courtesy of James Mateer, MD)

showing absence of left renal filling, may help confirm the diagnosis.

▶ PITFALLS

1. **Contraindication.** The only absolute contraindication to performing this ultrasound examination of the abdominal aorta is if it delays clearly indicated, immediate surgical intervention.

2. **Overreliance on examination.** The finding of an enlarged aorta alone is not sufficient to diag-

nose rupture of the abdominal aorta. There are no reliable ultrasound findings of retroperitoneal hematoma associated with the most common form of AAA rupture. The finding of AAA accompanied by other clinical manifestations, such as acute hemodynamic compromise, strongly suggests the diagnosis of AAA rupture. When hemodynamically stable, contained rupture may be diagnosed by definitive imaging prior to surgical intervention.

3. **Patient factors limiting imaging.** Obesity and bowel gas always render ultrasound imaging more difficult. Failure to determine the involvement of the major branches of the aorta makes operative planning more difficult for the surgeon. When bowel gas or other technical factors prevent a complete systematic real-time scan through all tissue planes, these limitations should be identified and documented. Such limitations may mandate further evaluation by alternative methods, as clinically indicated.[82]

4. **Errors in imaging.** Two common errors in imaging should be avoided. First, the physician must take care not to inadvertently sweep the plane of the beam into a right parasagittal plane, which may result in a long-axis view of the inferior vena cava (Figure 7-21). The inferior vena cava here is thin walled and easily compressed, and can be mistaken for the abdominal aorta. The examiner can avoid this error by visualizing the aorta and IVC in the transverse plane, or when in longitudinal plane by visualizing the celiac trunk and superior mesenteric artery at the proximal abdominal aorta (Figure 7-22). The second error may result from the "cylinder tangent" effect (Figure 7-23). Limited window accessibility may result in a situation in which the plane of the beam enters the cylinder of the aorta at a tangent and display an incorrect AP diameter. This is not an artifact error but an operator error. The aorta should be measured in both sagittal and transverse planes to avoid this error.

5. **A small aneurysm does not preclude rupture.** A patient with symptoms and signs consistent with acute AAA and an aortic diameter greater than 3.0 cm should have this diagnosis (or alternative vascular catastrophes) fully investigated.

6. **Large para-aortic nodes may be confused for AAA.** Large para-aortic nodes usually occur anterior to the aorta, but may be posterior, displacing the aorta away from the vertebral body. They can be distinguished by an irregular nodular shape, which is identifiable in realtime. If color flow Doppler is utilized, the nodes will not demonstrate luminal flow.

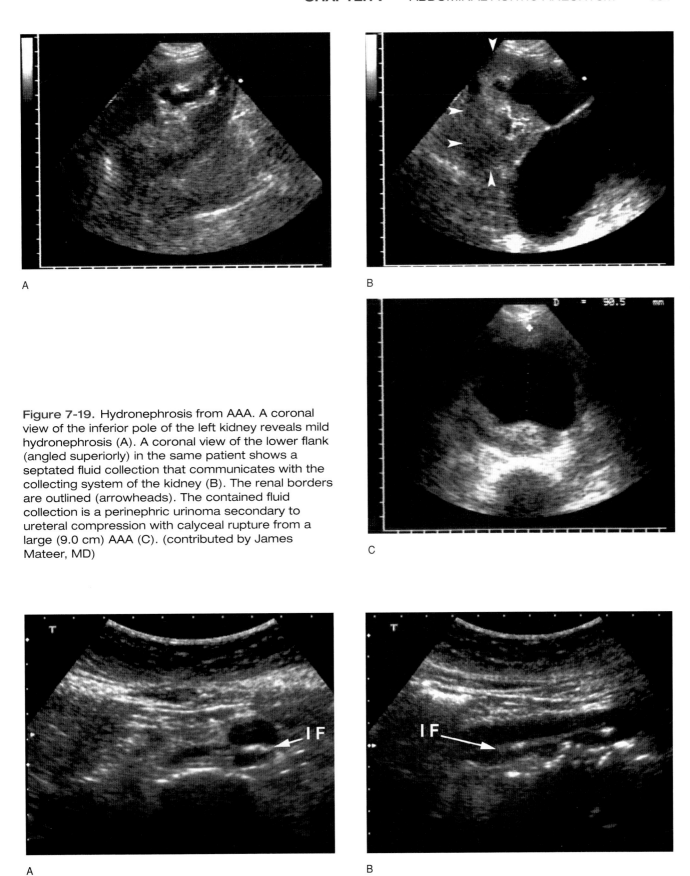

Figure 7-19. Hydronephrosis from AAA. A coronal view of the inferior pole of the left kidney reveals mild hydronephrosis (A). A coronal view of the lower flank (angled superiorly) in the same patient shows a septated fluid collection that communicates with the collecting system of the kidney (B). The renal borders are outlined (arrowheads). The contained fluid collection is a perinephric urinoma secondary to ureteral compression with calyceal rupture from a large (9.0 cm) AAA (C). (contributed by James Mateer, MD)

Figure 7-20. Acute abdominal aortic dissection. Transverse (A) and longitudinal views (B) showing intimal flap (IF).

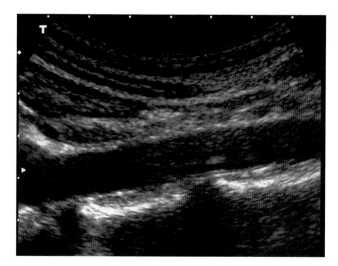

Figure 7-21. Long-axis view of the IVC. Note the thinner walls compared to the aorta, and the lack of branching vessels.

▶ CASE STUDIES

CASE 1

Patient Presentation

A 65-year-old man presented to the ED after a witnessed syncopal episode. Upon awaking in the morning, the patient complained of feeling weak and constipated. The patient had a history of well-controlled hypertension.

On physical examination, the patient was awake, alert, and oriented. His blood pressure was 110/50 mmHg; pulse, 100 beats per minute; respirations, 18 per minute; temperature, 98.9°F. He appeared pale and

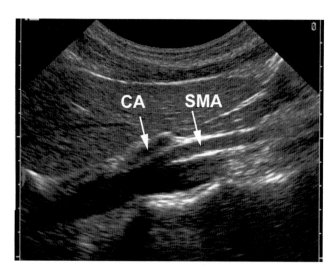

Figure 7-22. Long-axis view of the Aorta. The upper abdominal aorta shows characteristic thick echogenic walls and anterior branching vessels. CA = celiac artery, SMA = superior mesenteric artery.

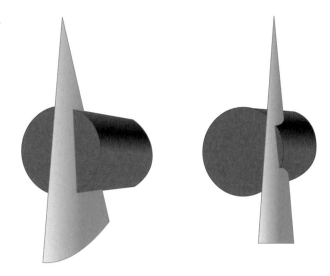

Figure 7-23. The cylinder tangent effect. A longitudinal beam slice through the center of the vessel will show the maximum diameter, while an off center slice will show a reduced diameter.

slightly diaphoretic. His lungs were clear to auscultation, neck veins flat, and abdomen soft and nontender with no peripheral edema. The remainder of his physical examination was unremarkable.

Management Course

On arrival, two large bore IVs were established in the upper extremities while the primary examination was simultaneously performed. As part of his secondary survey, a rapid cardiac view by the subcostal window revealed a hyperdynamic heart. Repositioning of the transducer immediately revealed an enlarged abdominal aorta with an AP diameter of 7.2 cm (Figure 7-24). There was no free intraperitoneal fluid. Surgical consultation was initiated.

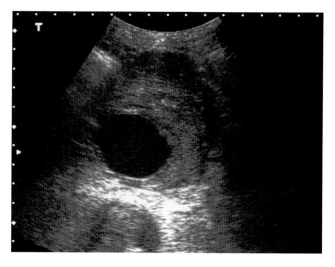

Figure 7-24. Case 1. AAA 7.2 cm. Transverse view.

Reassessment revealed a decline in blood pressure to 80/50 mmHg. No other diagnostic maneuvers were employed and the patient was transported directly to the operating room for exploratory laparotomy. Operative findings included a rupturing 7.4 cm AAA that was successfully grafted.

Commentary

Case 1 was an example of a patient presenting to the ED with hemodynamic alteration from a rupturing AAA. This type of syncope followed by near-normalization of vital signs with subsequent decline in perfusion parameters is one of the most common presentations for ruptured AAA. This patient exemplifies an unstable hemodynamic profile that requires limited diagnostic evaluation and rapid surgical intervention. It is important to note that the same ultrasound examination was used to demonstrate marked global hyperkinesis of the heart, essentially excluding left ventricular failure as a cause of gradual hemodynamic decline. This was performed before performing either an electrocardiogram or a chest radiograph.

CASE 2

Patient Presentation

A 74-year-old man presented to the ED at 2 a.m., complaining of left "hernia" pain. The patient said that he had been diagnosed with a left inguinal hernia more than 10 years earlier and he had decided against surgical repair because it did not cause him pain. He said that he began having left groin pain last night after supper and it had gradually worsened. He denied any other medical history.

On physical examination, the patient was awake and alert and was in no distress. His blood pressure was 160/80 mm Hg; pulse rate, 85 beats per min; respirations, 20 per minute; temperature, 99.0°F. He had a left inguinal hernia that was moderately tender to palpation. The hernia sac was firm and protruded into his scrotum about 3–4 cm and could not be reduced on examination. His abdomen was mildly obese and nontender. The remainder of his examination was unremarkable.

Management Course

An IV line was established and the patient was given 50 micrograms of IV fentanyl with good relief of his pain. A second attempt to reduce the hernia was unsuccessful. Basic laboratory tests, including a urinalysis, were unremarkable and a plain radiograph revealed no signs of bowel obstruction. The on-call surgeon was consulted because the patient was thought to have an incarcerated inguinal hernia. While awaiting surgical consultation the patient became diaphoretic and dizzy, his blood pressure dropped to 100/60 mm Hg, and he began complaining of left flank pain. A bedside ultrasound examination was performed in the ED and he was noted to have an 8 cm AAA (Figure 7-25). The surgeon was called again and informed of the new information. The patient had an additional large bore IV placed and was aggressively resuscitated and taken to the operating room within 20 minutes. Despite these efforts, he died on the operating table.

Commentary

This case demonstrated a complex presentation of a ruptured AAA. The patient's longstanding inguinal hernia convinced both the patient and the emergency physician

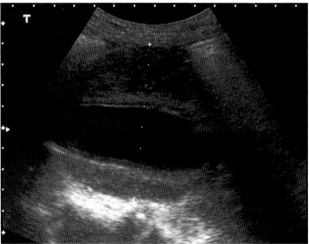

A   B

Figure 7-25. Case 2. AAA 8 cm. Transverse (A) and longitudinal (B) views.

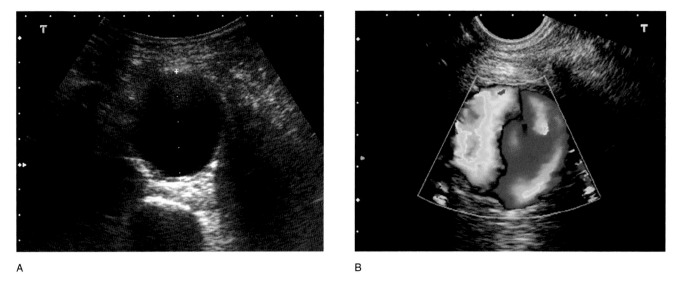

A   B

Figure 7-26. Case 3. AAA 4.2 cm. Transverse (A) and color Doppler transverse views (B).

that the etiology of his pain was the hernia. It is common to delay or miss the diagnosis of ruptured AAA because referred pain to the groin, back, or flank is thought to be caused by another diagnosis. In this case the physician did not initially consider the diagnosis of ruptured AAA because of the patient's confusing symptoms and normal vital signs.

CASE 3

Patient Presentation

An emergency physician was giving his 62-year-old father a tour of his ED. While showing off for his father, he performed a bedside abdominal aortic ultrasound examination on his father and was surprised to discover a 4.2-cm AAA (Figure 7-26). His father had a history of smoking, but was asymptomatic and had no other medical history or risk factors.

Management Course

The AAA was monitored every 6 months with serial ultrasound examinations. Two years after it was initially discovered, the AAA measured 5.2 cm in AP diameter. The patient was referred to a surgeon who advised that he delay elective repair until the AAA became 5.5 cm. The patient saw another surgeon for a second opinion and was advised to have the AAA repaired as soon as possible. The second surgeon also recommended having an open repair rather than an angiographic stent because he was otherwise healthy and a good surgical candidate. The patient had an open repair and placement of a Gortex graft without complications and had an uneventful

recovery. He was able to play golf just a few months later and continues to be asymptomatic.

Commentary

This case demonstrated the importance of screening asymptomatic patients who are at risk for AAA. Men over 60 years of age who have ever smoked are at higher risk for AAA (up to 10%). There are over 50,000 elective AAA repairs per year in the United States, with a very low surgical mortality rate. Conversely, the mortality rate after AAA rupture is 80%.

▶ ACKNOWLEDGMENT

The authors would like to thank Ben Dolan and Scott Joing, MD, for their contributions to this chapter.

REFERENCES

1. Collin JAL, Walton J, et al.: Oxford screening program for abdominal aortic aneurysm in men aged 65 to 74 years. *Lancet* 2:613–615, 1988.
2. Phelan MP, Emerman CL: Focused aortic ultrasound to evaluate the prevalence of abdominal aortic aneurysm in ED patients with high-risk symptoms. *Am J Emerg Med* 24:227–229, 2006.
3. Scott RA, Ashton HA, Kay DN: Routine ultrasound screening in management of abdominal aortic aneurysm. *Br Med J* 296:1709–1710, 1988.
4. Kent KC, Zwolak RM, Jaff MR, et al.: Screening for abdominal aortic aneurysm: A consensus statement. *J Vasc Surg* 39:267–269, 2004.

5. Costantino TG, Bruno EC, Handly N, Dean AJ: Accuracy of emergency medicine ultrasound in the evaluation of abdominal aortic aneurysm. *J Emerg Med* 29:455–460, 2005.

6. Marston WA, Ahlquist R, Johnson G, Jr., Meyer AA. Misdiagnosis of ruptured abdominal aortic aneurysms. *J Vasc Surg* 16:17–22, 1992.

7. Tayal VS, Graf CD, Gibbs MA: Prospective study of accuracy and outcome of emergency ultrasound for abdominal aortic aneurysm over two years. *Acad Emerg Med* 10:867–871, 2003.

8. Screening for abdominal aortic aneurysm: Recommendation statement. *Ann Intern Med* 142:198–202, 2005.

9. Fleming C, Whitlock EP, Beil TL, Lederle FA: Screening for abdominal aortic aneurysm: A best-evidence systematic review for the U.S. Preventive Services Task Force. *Ann Intern Med* 142:203–211, 2005.

10. Hans SS, Huang RR: Results of 101 ruptured abdominal aortic aneurysm repairs from a single surgical practice. *Arch Surg* 138:898–901, 2003.

11. Harris LM, Faggioli GL, Fiedler R, Curl GR, Ricotta JJ: Ruptured abdominal aortic aneurysms: Factors affecting mortality rates. *J Vasc Surg* 14:812–818; discussion 9–20, 1991.

12. Hoffman M, Avellone JC, Plecha FR, et al.: Operation for ruptured abdominal aortic aneurysms: A community-wide experience. *Surgery* 91:597–602, 1982.

13. Plummer D, Clinton J, Matthew B: Emergency department ultrasound improves time to diagnosis and survival of abdominal aortic aneurysm. *Acad Emerg Med* 5:417, 1998.

14. Physicians ACoE: Clinical policy: Critical issues for the initial intervention and management of patients presenting with a chief complaint of nontraumatic acute abdominal pain. *Ann Emerg Med* 36:406–415, 2000.

15. Miller J, Miller J: Small ruptured abdominal aneurysm diagnosed by emergency physician ultrasound. *Am J Emerg Med* 17:174–175, 1999.

16. Ashton HA, Buxton MJ, Day NE, et al.: The Multicentre Aneurysm Screening Study (MASS) into the effect of abdominal aortic aneurysm screening on mortality in men: A randomised controlled trial. *Lancet* 360:1531–1539, 2002.

17. Boll AP, Verbeek AL, van de Lisdonk EH, van der Vliet JA: High prevalence of abdominal aortic aneurysm in a primary care screening programme. *Br J Surg* 85:1090–1094, 1998.

18. Gloviczki P, Pairolero PC, Mucha P, Jr., et al.: Ruptured abdominal aortic aneurysms: Repair should not be denied. *J Vasc Surg* 15:851–857, 1992.

19. Lederle FA: Ultrasonographic screening for abdominal aortic aneurysms. *Ann Intern Med* 139:516–522, 2003.

20. Lederle FA, Johnson GR, Wilson SE, et al.: The aneurysm detection and management study screening program: Validation cohort and final results. Aneurysm Detection and Management Veterans Affairs Cooperative Study Investigators. *Arch Intern Med* 160:1425–1430, 2000.

21. Smith FC, Grimshaw GM, Paterson IS, Shearman CP, Hamer JD: Ultrasonographic screening for abdominal aortic aneurysm in an urban community. *Br J Surg* 80:1406–1409, 1993.

22. Vohra R, Reid D, Groome J, Abdool-Carrim AT, Pollock JG: Long-term survival in patients undergoing resection of abdominal aortic aneurysm. *Ann Vasc Surg* 4:460–465, 1990.

23. Webster MW, Ferrell RE, St Jean PL, Majumder PP, Fogel SR, Steed DL: Ultrasound screening of first-degree relatives of patients with an abdominal aortic aneurysm. *J Vasc Surg* 13:9–13; discussion-4, 1991.

24. Lederle FA, Johnson GR, Wilson SE: Abdominal aortic aneurysm in women. *J Vasc Surg* 34:122–126, 2001.

25. Scott RA, Bridgewater SG, Ashton HA: Randomized clinical trial of screening for abdominal aortic aneurysm in women. *Br J Surg* 89:283–285, 2002.

26. Singh K, Bonaa KH, Jacobsen BK, Bjork L, Solberg S: Prevalence of and risk factors for abdominal aortic aneurysms in a population-based study: The Tromso Study. *Am J Epidemiol* 154:236–244, 2001.

27. Acosta S, Ogren M, Bengtsson H, Bergqvist D, Lindblad B, Zdanowski Z: Increasing incidence of ruptured abdominal aortic aneurysm: A population-based study. *J Vasc Surg* 44:237–243, 2006.

28. Best VA, Price JF, Fowkes FG: Persistent increase in the incidence of abdominal aortic aneurysm in Scotland, 1981–2000. *Br J Surg* 90:1510–1515, 2003.

29. Bickerstaff LK, Hollier LH, Van Peenen HJ, Melton LJ, III, Pairolero PC, Cherry KJ: Abdominal aortic aneurysms: The changing natural history. *J Vasc Surg* 1:6–12, 1984.

30. Heller JA, Weinberg A, Arons R, et al.: Two decades of abdominal aortic aneurysm repair: Have we made any progress? *J Vasc Surg* 32:1091–100, 2000.

31. Melton LJ, III, Bickerstaff LK, Hollier LH, et al: Changing incidence of abdominal aortic aneurysms: A population-based study. *Am J Epidemiol* 120:379–386, 1984.

32. Brown LC, Powell JT: Risk factors for aneurysm rupture in patients kept under ultrasound surveillance. UK Small Aneurysm Trial Participants. *Ann Surg* 230:289–296, 1999.

33. Jones A, Cahill D, Gardham R: Outcome in patients with a large abdominal aortic aneurysm considered unfit for surgery. *Br J Surg* 85:1382–1384, 1998.

34. Lederle FA, Johnson GR, Wilson SE, et al.: Rupture rate of large abdominal aortic aneurysms in patients refusing or unfit for elective repair. *JAMA* 287:2968–2972, 2002.

35. Nevitt MP, Ballard DJ, Hallett JW, Jr.: Prognosis of abdominal aortic aneurysms. A population-based study. *N Engl J Med* 321:1009–1014, 1989.

36. Reed WW, Hallett JW, Jr., Damiano MA, Ballard DJ: Learning from the last ultrasound. A population-based study of patients with abdominal aortic aneurysm. *Arch Intern Med* 157:2064–2068, 1997.

37. Scott RA, Tisi PV, Ashton HA, Allen DR: Abdominal aortic aneurysm rupture rates: A 7-year follow-up of the entire abdominal aortic aneurysm population detected by screening. *J Vasc Surg* 28:124–128, 1998.

38. Cronenwett JL, Sargent SK, Wall MH, et al.: Variables that affect the expansion rate and outcome of small abdominal aortic aneurysms. *J Vasc Surg* 11:260–268; discussion 8–9, 1990.

39. Strachan DP: Predictors of death from aortic aneurysm among middle-aged men: The Whitehall study. *Br J Surg* 78:401–404, 1991.

40. Brown PM, Sobolev B, Zelt DT: Selective management of abdominal aortic aneurysms smaller than 5.0 cm in a prospective sizing program with gender-specific analysis. *J Vasc Surg* 38:762–765, 2003.

41. Evans SM, Adam DJ, Bradbury AW: The influence of gender on outcome after ruptured abdominal aortic aneurysm. *J Vasc Surg* 32:258–262, 2000.

42. Powell JT, Brown LC: The natural history of abdominal aortic aneurysms and their risk of rupture. *Acta Chir Belg* 101:11–16, 2001.

43. Brewster DC, Cronenwett JL, Hallett JW, Jr., Johnston KW, Krupski WC, Matsumura JS: Guidelines for the treatment of abdominal aortic aneurysms. Report of a subcommittee of the Joint Council of the American Association for Vascular Surgery and Society for Vascular Surgery. *J Vasc Surg* 37:1106–1117, 2003.

44. Akkersdijk GJ, van Bockel JH: Ruptured abdominal aortic aneurysm: Initial misdiagnosis and the effect on treatment. *Eur J Surg* 164:29–34, 1998.

45. Bown MJ, Sutton AJ, Bell PR, Sayers RD: A meta-analysis of 50 years of ruptured abdominal aortic aneurysm repair. *Br J Surg* 89:714–730, 2002.

46. Ingoldby CJ, Wujanto R, Mitchell JE: Impact of vascular surgery on community mortality from ruptured aortic aneurysms. *Br J Surg* 73:551–553, 1986.

47. Kiell CS, Ernst CB: Advances in management of abdominal aortic aneurysm. *Adv Surg* 26:73–98, 1993.

48. Magee TR, Galland RB, Collin J, et al.: A prospective survey of patients presenting with abdominal aortic aneurysm. *Eur J Vasc Endovasc Surg* 13:403–406, 1997.

49. Tambyraja AL, Murie JA, Chalmers RT: Outcome and survival of patients aged 65 years and younger after abdominal aortic aneurysm rupture. *World J Surg* 29:1245–1247, 2005.

50. Clinical policy: Critical issues for the initial evaluation and management of patients presenting with a chief complaint of nontraumatic acute abdominal pain. *Ann Emerg Med* 36:406–415, 2000.

51. Lederle FA, Parenti CM, Chute EP: Ruptured abdominal aortic aneurysm: The internist as diagnostician. *Am J Med* 96:163–167, 1994.

52. Bessen H: Abdominal aortic aneurysm. In: Marx J, ed. *Rosen's Emergency Medicine: Concepts and Clinical Practice.* 6th ed. Philadelphia, PA: Mosby Elsevier, 2006:1330–1341.

53. Rose J, Civil I, Koelmeyer T, Haydock D, Adams D: Ruptured abdominal aortic aneurysms: Clinical presentation in Auckland 1993–1997. *ANZ J Surg* 71:341–344, 2001.

54. Fink HA, Lederle FA, Roth CS, Bowles CA, Nelson DB, Haas MA: The accuracy of physical examination to detect abdominal aortic aneurysm. *Arch Intern Med* 160:833–836, 2000.

55. Lederle FA, Simel DL: The rational clinical examination. Does this patient have abdominal aortic aneurysm? *JAMA* 281:77–82, 1999.

56. Kuhn M, Bonnin RL, Davey MJ, Rowland JL, Langlois SL: Emergency department ultrasound scanning for abdominal aortic aneurysm: Accessible, accurate, and advantageous. *Ann Emerg Med* 36:219–223, 2000.

57. Lanoix R, Leak LV, Gaeta T, Gernsheimer JR: A preliminary evaluation of emergency ultrasound in the setting of an emergency medicine training program. *Am J Emerg Med* 18:41–45, 2000.

58. Lee TY, Korn P, Heller JA, et al.: The cost-effectiveness of a "quick-screen" program for abdominal aortic aneurysms. *Surgery* 132:399–407, 2002.

59. Salen P, Melanson S, Buro D: ED screening to identify abdominal aortic aneurysms in asymptomatic geriatric patients. *Am J Emerg Med* 21:133–135, 2003.

60. Jehle D, Davis E, Evans T, et al.: Emergency department sonography by emergency physicians. *Am J Emerg Med* 7:605–611, 1989.

61. Schlager D, Lazzareschi G, Whitten D, Sanders AB: A prospective study of ultrasonography in the ED by emergency physicians. *Am J Emerg Med* 12:185–189, 1994.

62. American College of Emergency Physicians. ACEP emergency ultrasound guidelines-2001. *Ann Emerg Med* 38:470–481, 2001.

63. LaRoy LL, Cormier PJ, Matalon TA, Patel SK, Turner DA, Silver B: Imaging of abdominal aortic aneurysms. *AJR Am J Roentgenol* 152:785–792, 1989.

64. Shuman WP, Hastrup W, Jr., Kohler TR, et al.: Suspected leaking abdominal aortic aneurysm: Use of sonography in the emergency room. *Radiology* 168:117–119, 1988.

65. Chandler JJ: The Einstein sign: The clinical picture of acute cholecystitis caused by ruptured abdominal aortic aneurysm. *N Engl J Med* 310:1538, 1984.

66. Ernst CB: Abdominal aortic aneurysm. *N Engl J Med* 328:1167–1172, 1993.

67. Kniemeyer HW, Kessler T, Reber PU, Ris HB, Hakki H, Widmer MK: Treatment of ruptured abdominal aortic aneurysm, a permanent challenge or a waste of resources? Prediction of outcome using a multi-organ-dysfunction score. *Eur J Vasc Endovasc Surg* 19:190–196, 2000.

68. Shackleton CR, Schechter MT, Bianco R, Hildebrand HD: Preoperative predictors of mortality risk in ruptured abdominal aortic aneurysm. *J Vasc Surg* 6:583–589, 1987.

69. Rose JS, Bair AE, Mandavia D, Kinser DJ: The UHP ultrasound protocol: A novel ultrasound approach to the empiric evaluation of the undifferentiated hypotensive patient. *Am J Emerg Med* 19:299–302, 2001.

70. 2005 American Heart Association guidelines for cardiopulmonary resuscitation and emergency cardiovascular care. *Circulation* 112:IV1–203, 2005.

71. Hendrickson RG, Dean AJ, Costantino TG. A novel use of ultrasound in pulseless electrical activity: The diagnosis of an acute abdominal aortic aneurysm rupture. *J Emerg Med* 21:141–144, 2001.

72. Lawrence-Brown MM, Norman PE, Jamrozik K, et al.: Initial results of ultrasound screening for aneurysm of the abdominal aorta in Western Australia: Relevance for endoluminal treatment of aneurysm disease. *Cardiovasc Surg* 9:234–240, 2001.

73. Lederle FA, Johnson GR, Wilson SE, et al.: Prevalence and associations of abdominal aortic aneurysm detected through screening. Aneurysm Detection and Management (ADAM) Veterans Affairs Cooperative Study Group. *Ann Intern Med* 126:441–449, 1997.

74. Lindholt JS, Juul S, Fasting H, Henneberg EW: Hospital costs and benefits of screening for abdominal aortic aneurysms. Results from a randomised population screening trial. *Eur J Vasc Endovasc Surg* 23:55–60, 2002.

75. Norman PE, Jamrozik K, Lawrence-Brown MM, et al.: Population based randomised controlled trial on impact of screening on mortality from abdominal aortic aneurysm. *BMJ* 329:1259, 2004.

76. Scott RA, Wilson NM, Ashton HA, Kay DN: Influence of screening on the incidence of ruptured abdominal aortic aneurysm: 5-year results of a randomized controlled study. *Br J Surg* 82:1066–1070, 1995.

77. Bailey RP, Ault M, Greengold NL, Rosendahl T, Cossman D: Ultrasonography performed by primary care residents for abdominal aortic aneurysm screening. *J Gen Intern Med* 16:845–849, 2001.

78. Lin PH, Bush RL, McCoy SA, et al.: A prospective study of a hand-held ultrasound device in abdominal aortic aneurysm evaluation. *Am J Surg* 186:455–459, 2003.

79. Heather BP, Poskitt KR, Earnshaw JJ, Whyman M, Shaw E: Population screening reduces mortality rate from aortic aneurysm in men. *Br J Surg* 87:750–753, 2000.

80. Irvine CD, Shaw E, Poskitt KR, Whyman MR, Earnshaw JJ, Heather BP: A comparison of the mortality rate after elective repair of aortic aneurysms detected either by screening or incidentally. *Eur J Vasc Endovasc Surg* 20:374–378, 2000.

81. Wilmink TB, Quick CR, Hubbard CS, Day NE: The influence of screening on the incidence of ruptured abdominal aortic aneurysms. *J Vasc Surg* 30:203–208, 1999.

82. Emergency ultrasound imaging criteria compendium. American College of Emergency Physicians. *Ann Emerg Med* 48:487–510, 2006.

83. Lyon M, Brannam L, Ciamillo L, Blaivas M: False positive abdominal aortic aneurysm on bedside emergency ultrasound. *J Emerg Med* 26:193–196, 2004.

CHAPTER 8

Hepatobiliary

Daniel Theodoro

The prevalence of hepatobiliary disease in the emergency and acute care settings is high. Ultrasound allows for accurate diagnosis in a large number of these cases. Emergency physicians who can effectively perform ultrasound benefit enormously from the ability to make rapid bedside diagnoses, especially in undifferentiated cases of vague abdominal pain.

▶ CLINICAL CONSIDERATIONS

The primary tools in the evaluation of acute hepatobiliary disease are ultrasound, hepatobiliary iminodiacetic acid scintigraphy (commonly referred to as HIDA scan or cholescintigraphy), computed tomography (CT), and endoscopic retrograde cholangiopancreatography (ERCP). Prior to the late 1980s and early 1990s, several imaging modalities were in use to diagnose hepatobiliary disease, such as oral and intravenous cholangiography. These methods took an extraordinary amount of time, required consumption or injection of potentially harmful contrast agents, and exposed the patient to radiation.[1] Ultrasound largely replaced these imaging modalities in the 1980s. Ultrasound has the highest sensitivity for detecting the presence of gallstones while HIDA has a reported higher sensitivity for detecting the presence of acute cholecystitis.[2] Data derived solely from a set of emergency department patients, however, suggest that emergency ultrasound of the gallbladder may prove as useful for the detection of acute cholecystitis as HIDA.[3,4] Although CT also has a role in the evaluation of patients with suspected hepatobiliary disease, its application is limited by its inability to detect 25% of gallstones. CT may play a greater role when other causes of abdominal pain are also being considered in the work-up of abdominal pain.[5,6] Ultrasound also has the added advantage of not exposing the patient to ionizing radiation. ERCP has its own unique risks, including pancreatitis and even death, and the test consumes a great deal of time and resources.

▶ CLINICAL INDICATIONS

The clinical indications for performing emergency bedside hepatobiliary ultrasound by clinicians include

- gallstones and biliary colic,
- acute cholecystitis,
- jaundice and biliary duct dilatation,
- abdominal sepsis,
- ascites, and
- hepatic abnormalities.

▶ GALLSTONES AND BILIARY COLIC

Emergency physicians expect to see biliary pathology in up to a third of all abdominal pain cases they encounter.[7] The classic presentation of biliary colic portrays an obese woman of child-bearing age with recurrent colicky pain in the right upper quadrant shortly after the consumption of a fatty meal. While gallstones are more prevalent in young, multiparous women than in young men, the ratio balances out with advancing age.[8] In older patients, the pain does not wax and wane after meals but is constant and occurs mostly at night at predictable hours, lasting for an average of 1–5 hours.[9] Physiologic studies conducted on patients while they were undergoing cholecystectomy concluded that a majority of patients with cholelithiasis will experience epigastric discomfort or dyspepsia with mechanical stimulation of the gallbladder. In fact, some feel that symptoms tend not to migrate to the right upper quadrant until the inflamed gallbladder irritates the peritoneum.[10–12] Patients who experience right-sided pain may present complaining of right flank pain, shoulder pain, or chest pain.[13] The resolution of symptoms in the setting of a clear history, absence of fever, and general improvement of the patient may cinch the diagnosis of biliary colic and preclude the necessity to image the gallbladder; however, most patients who present to the emergency department are symptomatic for some time. In these cases, emergency ultrasound can expedite the diagnosis and focus the clinician's effort and use of resources.[7,14] An algorithm that demonstrates how focused ultrasound can be utilized for decision making in patients with possible biliary colic is outlined (Figure 8-1).

Several studies demonstrate that emergency physicians with adequate experience acquire and interpret ultrasound images with skill similar to traditional imaging providers, especially when detecting gallstones.[15,16] In the hands of emergency physicians, the sensitivity and specificity for detecting gallstones (86–96% and 88–97%, respectively) resembled the pooled sensitivities and specificities in data gathered from imaging specialists (84% and 99%, respectively). One particular advantage to the emergency physician is increased efficiency.[17] On average, emergency physicians take 10 minutes to conduct a focused examination of the gallbladder. This expedient and accurate information has been shown to effectively decrease emergency department length of stay and influence emergency physician's probabilistic judgments especially when diagnosing diseases that are not readily apparent by the clinical presentation.[7,17] Since the differential diagnosis for upper abdominal pain can include many different etiologies, emergency ultrasound of the gallbladder can streamline the number of diagnoses the emergency physician must consider when evaluating and treating the patient, especially

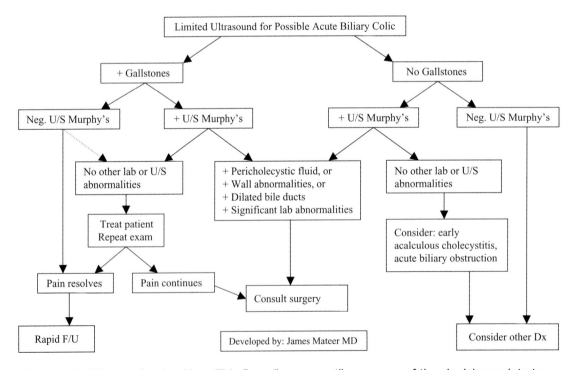

Figure 8-1. Biliary colic algorithm. This flow diagram outlines some of the decision points to consider for patient disposition based on clinical parameters and ultrasound findings. (Courtesy of James Mateer, MD)

when the presenting symptoms are consistent with biliary colic.

The clinician must take caution, however, when interpreting the findings of gallstones in a patient with atypical symptoms. Clolelithiasis is a prevalent disease and a majority of patients are asymptomatic. Although it may be convenient to attribute a patient's symptoms to biliary disease, the astute clinician will always remember that biliary colic remains a clinical diagnosis and not a sonographic diagnosis.

ACUTE CHOLECYSTITIS

The diagnosis of acute cholecystitis cannot be made by any constellation of physical examination or laboratory findings. The patient may present with right upper quadrant pain, fever, and a leukocytosis. In the emergency department, however, these findings are not present in a majority of cases. The lack of clinical sensitivity makes the firm diagnosis of acute cholecystitis heavily dependent on imaging studies.[18,19] This becomes particularly problematic for the emergency physician when one considers that, in the United States, more patients require cholecystectomy (both elective and emergent) than appendectomy.[20]

In general, ultrasound is thought to have a 94% sensitivity and 84% specificity in identifying cases of acute cholecystitis.[2] Focused emergency ultrasound performed by emergency physicians is reported to have a 91% sensitivity and a 66% specificity (of note, over two thirds of the emergency physicians in this study had no formal training). Ninety-five percent to 99% of patients with acute cholecystitis have gallstones.[21] The sonographic Murphy's sign (pain elicited by pressing over the fundus of the gallbladder with an ultrasound probe) may be present in 98.8% of cases but is not by itself specific for cholecystitis. The sensitivity of the sonographic Murphy's sign for cholecystitis was 75% for emergency physicians performing the test at the bedside compared to 45% for the formal ultrasound examination.[16–22] Nevertheless, the sonographic Murphy's sign helps localize the source of the abdominal pain and when clearly positive, along with an ultrasound that is positive for gallstones, suggests that the patient has at least a diagnosis of biliary colic (Figure 8-1). Although no single ultrasound finding predicts cholecystitis with sufficient accuracy for definitive diagnosis, studies have shown that a combination of positive findings increases the accuracy of ultrasound for this diagnosis. A combination of gallstones and a sonographic Murphy's sign had a positive predictive value of 92.2%, whereas a combination of gallstones and gallbladder wall thickening had a positive predictive value of 95.2% for cholecystitis.[21]

In general, the emergency physician can rely on the presence of gallstones and a thickened gallbladder wall in conjunction with the clinical presentation and laboratory findings to identify cases with a high probability of acute cholecystitis that will need further intervention.

JAUNDICE AND BILIARY DUCT DILATATION

In a patient with jaundice who presents to the emergency department, the emergency physician must decide whether the patient's hyperbilirubinemia is caused by a physical obstruction of the biliary tree or another disease process. Ultrasound is useful for detecting dilatation of intrahepatic ducts or the common hepatic and bile ducts.[23] Ultrasound is less sensitive at defining the exact etiology of obstruction, which may include a pancreatic head tumor, ampullary carcinoma, common bile duct stone, or bile duct compression from another cancer.[24] Once an obstructive process is detected, the next concern is whether the patient is presenting with clinical signs of cholangitis (fever, leukocytosis), which may precipitate the need for urgent ductal decompression (surgery, ERCP, transhepatic stenting). While ultrasound may detect dilated extra- or intrahepatic ducts and assist in the general management of these cases, other modalities such as CT and ERCP are usually utilized to direct diagnosis and treatment.

ABDOMINAL SEPSIS

Early goal-directed therapy in patients with sepsis is known to decrease patient mortality.[25] A majority of these patients tend to be elderly and often do not have a clear source of infection.[26] In cases of abdominal sepsis in the elderly, approximately 25% are due to cholecystitis and cholangitis.[27] Emergency ultrasound can serve as a prompt adjunct in potentially detecting the source of sepsis in critically ill patients when the etiology is not readily apparent.[28]

ASCITES

Detection of ascitic fluid is a useful diagnostic procedure when evaluating the patient with abdominal distention without signs of intestinal obstruction. On physical examination, the sensitivity of an abdominal fluid wave is low. In the emergency and acute care settings, determining whether a patient has ascites may influence initial management and disposition. For example, in a patient with abdominal pain or fever, the presence of ascites would require the clinician to consider the possibility of bacterial peritonitis.

► HEPATIC ABNORMALITIES

Patients may present to the emergency department with a substantial number of hepatic abnormalities, such as liver mass or metastases, abscess, or hepatomegaly. Although it may be helpful for the clinician to have an understanding of the sonographic appearance of these conditions, the specific differentiation of these conditions lies outside the routine scope of practice for the clinician in the emergent setting.

► ANATOMICAL CONSIDERATIONS

A variety of solid and hollow organs are located in the right upper quadrant of the abdomen. The predominant organ is the liver, bordered superiorly by the diaphragm and coronary/triangular ligament confluence (Figure 8-2), inferomedially by the duodenum and head of pancreas, and inferiorly by the gallbladder, hepatic flexure of the ascending colon, and superior pole of right kidney. The gastric fundus is located posterolateral to the

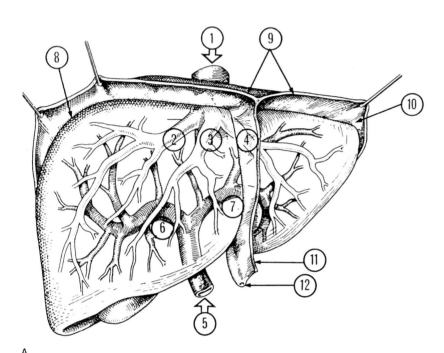

A

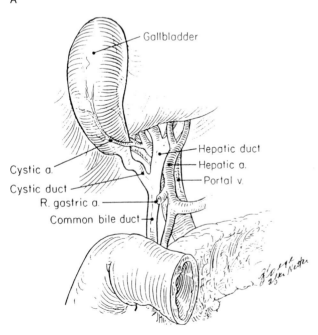

B

Figure 8-2. (A) Surgical anatomy of the liver: (1) inferior vena cava; (2) right hepatic vein; (3) middle hepatic vein; (4) left hepatic vein; (5) portal vein; (6) right branch portal vein; (7) left branch portal vein; (8) right triangular ligament; (9) coronary ligament; (10) left triangular liment; (11) falciform ligamen; (12) ligamentum teres. (Reproduced from Feliciano et al. *Trauma,* 3rd ed. Norwalk, CT: Appleton Lange, 1996:489.) (B) Normal anatomy. The diagram depicts the relationships in the porta hepatis. The triangle of Calot is bordered by the edge of the liver, the cystic duct, and the hepatic duct. (Reproduced from Schwartz et al. *Principles of Surgery,* 6th ed. New York: McGraw-Hill, 1994:1368.)

left hepatic lobe. The liver is divided (Figure 8-2) into right and left lobes by the major lobar fissure, which contains the middle hepatic vein and extends from the gallbladder fossa anteriorly to the inferior vena cava posteriorly. The right lobe is divided into anteromedial and posterolateral segments by the right hepatic vein, and the left lobe is divided into anterior and posterior segments by the left hepatic vein. After draining the liver of venous blood, all hepatic veins converge on the inferior vena cava posteriorly, just inferior to the atriocaval junction. The main portal vein courses from the intestinal venous drainage arcades, through the lesser omentum to the hepatic hilum, where it bifurcates into right and left branches and enters the liver (Figure 8-2A). The hepatic artery courses toward the hepatic hilum in the lesser omentum, occupying a position anterior to the main portal vein (Figure 8-2B). At the hilum, it divides into right and left branches and enters the liver parenchyma.

The biliary system begins with the intrahepatic right and left hepatic ducts, which course toward the hilum, uniting to form the extrahepatic common hepatic duct. After exiting the hilum, the common hepatic duct is joined by the cystic duct (from the gallbladder) to form the common bile duct, which courses anterior to the main portal vein, and usually to the right of the hepatic artery (Figure 8-2B) in the lesser omentum before entering the duodenum. It is important to remember the anatomical relationships of the hepatic artery, common bile duct, and main portal vein as they traverse the lesser omentum in the region of the hepatic hilum to form the main portal triad since this will aid in identification and differentiation during sonographic evaluation. Within the liver, branches of the main portal vein, proper hepatic artery, and biliary tree follow parallel pathways of distribution to the liver parenchyma in bundles known as lesser portal triads. Hepatic venous tributaries do not follow this system.

The gallbladder is divided into a fundus, body, and neck (Figure 8-2B). The fundus may project below the inferior hepatic margin, illustrating the anatomic basis for a "sonographic Murphy's sign" (a point of maximal tenderness elicited by compressing the gallbladder with the ultrasound probe). The body is contiguous with the inferior surface of the liver and narrows at the neck. The neck often contains spiral valves known as Spiral Valves of Heister that are occasionally misdiagnosed as impacted stones. The neck is continuous with the cystic duct, which empties into the common hepatic duct to create the common bile duct.

▶ GETTING STARTED

Patient positioning and respiratory maneuvers play an important role in the hepatobiliary ultrasound examination. The patient's body habitus will dictate which transducer is best; in difficult cases, adjustments to the probe

frequency, gain, focus point, and harmonic settings can make the difference between an indeterminate and successful ultrasound examination.

When the patient's gallbladder lies inferior enough to the lowest rib, the patient can be scanned in the recumbent position. However, this tends to be the exception rather than the rule. The ribs overlie the gallbladder and interfere with direct visualization in most cases. To improve the chance of success, the patient should be positioned in the left lateral decubitus position (Figure 8-3A). The liver tends to shift due to gravity, which provides a better "acoustic window" and, in effect, pulls the gallbladder out from underneath the acoustic interference of the ribs. Occasionally, the patient must roll past the left lateral decubitus position to an almost prone position with the probe "underneath" the patient's abdomen, but this is quite rare. If the left lateral decubitus position is insufficient, then the patient should be asked to take and hold a deep breath. This maneuver fills the lungs, flattening the diaphragm and shifting the gallbladder down. When the common bile duct is measured, the same maneuvers can assist in bringing key structures into view.

For the abdominal ultrasound examination, there is no absolute "correct probe." Most patients require a medium to low transducer frequency (2–5 MHz) to view the gallbladder. A phased array transducer can be helpful when there is no option but to image between ribs. However, a curvilinear transducer typically suffices in most cases. Initially, positioning the probe sagittally (probe indicator toward the patient's head) just inferior to the right costal margin may help locate the gallbladder. Probe positioning after localization should focus on obtaining standard images that are most familiar to consultants and fellow sonologists. Color Doppler can be used to confirm that the cystic structure is not a vessel. Since there is great variability in anatomy, probe position can vary between a cross-sectional and sagittal position.

Adjusting the depth, focus point(s), and gain optimizes most images in the emergency department. These knobs or buttons vary from machine to machine. The depth should be adjusted so that the gallbladder fills at least two thirds of the screen. The focus point(s) should be focused at the structures of interest.[29] The gain, akin to brightness on a computer monitor, should not be set too high or low because image quality may be distorted. Some machines are currently equipped with tissue harmonic imaging (THI), which may help identify smaller stones typically not visualized without harmonics.[30]

▶ TECHNIQUE AND NORMAL ULTRASOUND FINDINGS

A low- to medium-frequency ultrasound transducer will suffice for most typical examinations; however, if other options exist that may be of more benefit, the sonologist

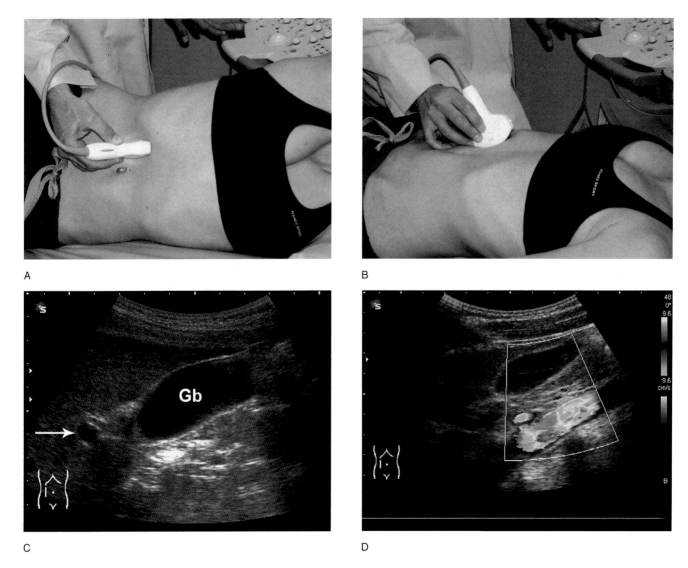

A

B

C

D

Figure 8-3. Longitudinal views of the gallbladder. Initial probe position with patient in lateral decubitus (A) and supine positions (B). Gallbladder imaging is often facilited with a deep inspiratory hold. Probe is angled cephalad under the rib margins. Corresponding ultrasound image (C) with main portal vein indicated (arrow). Color Doppler may assist in delineating large vascular structures (D). Gb = gallbladder. (Courtesy of James Mateer, MD).

must be willing to adapt and use them. This may include the use of a linear transducer for a very anterior gallbladder in a thin patient. The goal is to answer a focused question that enhances the diagnostic workup or therapeutic disposition.

EVALUATION OF THE GALLBLADDER AND COMMON BILE DUCT

Four components are necessary to complete the evaluation of the gallbladder in cases of suspected biliary colic and acute cholecystitis. First, the gallbladder should be viewed in at least two planes to minimize the chance of missing an inconspicuous finding. Second, the gallbladder should be traced from the fundus to the neck carefully examining for small stones impacted in the neck. Third, the anterior gallbladder wall should be measured at its clearest point, which is usually in the mid-portion of the ultrasound beam emanating from the transducer. If focal wall thickening is encountered, several measurements should be made, one of which includes the focally thickened area. Fourth, the common bile duct should be measured and traced as far medially as possible if dilated.

A sagittal approach will initially locate the gallbladder (Figure 8-3B). Placing the probe under the right costal margin at about the mid-clavicular line with the probe marker directed toward the patient's head, the sonologist can sweep the right upper quadrant until an image of the gallbladder is obtained (Figure 8-3C). This will usually be a transverse or oblique cut through the fundus. Having the patient take and hold a deep breath may be very helpful if the gallbladder is not readily identified. Color and power Doppler aid in delineating large vascular structures. The gallbladder should have no Doppler signal and is typically the most anterior cystic structure in the abdomen (Figure 8-3D). Conversely, identifying the main portal vein also helps identify the gallbladder. Typically, the main portal vein connects to the gallbladder via a thick fibrous band known as the main lobar fissure. Occasionally locating the main portal vein and following the main lobar fissure is the only way to locate an obscure gallbladder.

The next step is to obtain a longitudinal profile of the gallbladder by gently sweeping the ultrasound beam, keeping other three-dimensional aspects of the beam's orientation constant. Thus, a three-dimensional mental image of the gallbladder in long axis is built out of multiple two-dimensional images. The gallbladder neck should be interrogated whenever possible. Having the patient take a deep breath will help the sonologist identify the neck leading into the main portal triad. One of the most difficult skills for the novice sonologist to master is the technique of converting transverse or long-axis sections into longitudinal or short-axis cuts, respectively. To change planes, the transducer should be moved slowly, keeping some element of the gallbladder in view. This is the time to adjust the patient's position or perform respiratory maneuvers if the gallbladder is not initially visualized. Short-axis views should be obtained after the longitudinal images (Figure 8-4). These views assist with clarifying whether shadowing is from stones inside the gallbladder or from adjacent bowel gas outside the gallbladder. If imaging remains difficult after patient

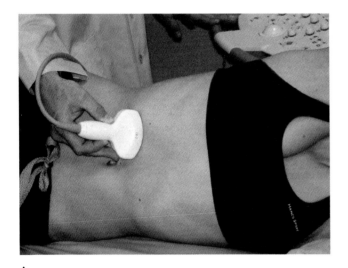

A

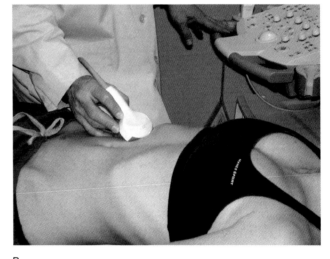

B

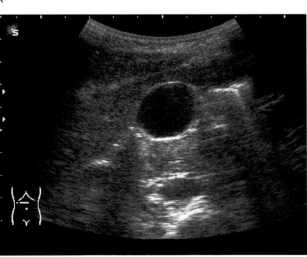

C

Figure 8-4. Transverse views of the gallbladder. Initial probe position with patient in lateral decubitus (A) and supine positions (B). Note the deep inspiration used and cephalad angulation of the probe to view under rib margins. Corresponding ultrasound image (C). Shadowing is from adjacent bowel gas outside the gallbladder. (Courtesy of James Mateer, MD)

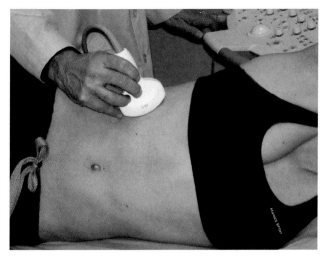

A

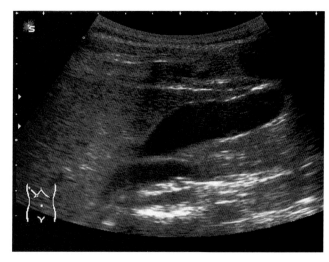

B

Figure 8-5. Intercostal views of the gallbladder. Initial probe position with patient in lateral decubitus (A). Initial imaging plane is aligned parallel to the ribs. Corresponding ultrasound image (B). A small segment of the portal vein is seen below the neck of the gallbladder. (Courtesy of James Mateer, MD)

positioning and deep inspiratory efforts, consider intercostal views (Figure 8-5). These views are helpful when the gallbladder is positioned under the ribs and/or the patient is unable to take a deep breath.

The gallbladder should be scanned for the presence or absence of gallstones, determination of wall thickness, and for the presence or absence of pericholecystic fluid. An accurate measurement of wall thickness is made on the anterior wall that is perpendicular to the imaging plane (greater than 3 mm being abnormal). If gallstones are detected, the patient should be rolled or elevated into various positions in an attempt to document movement of the gallstones. If a stone or stones do not respond to gravity by rolling "downhill" with body position change, then they may be impacted in the gallbladder neck. Alternatively, the sonologist may be dealing with a calcified polyp or sessile mass. If clinically applicable, the probe should be used to compress the gallbladder in an attempt to elicit a "sonographic Murphy's sign."

Identification of the portal vein in the longitudinal axis aids in finding the main portal triad (Figure 8-6A). The portal vein will have bright echogenic walls compared with the hepatic veins. It can usually be visualized coursing toward the porta hepatis. The main portal triad is made up of the main portal vein, hepatic artery, and the common bile duct. By rotating the probe 90 degrees (counterclockwise) from a longitudinal orientation, a transverse image of the portal vein with the associated common bile duct (anterior/lateral) and hepatic artery (anterior/medial) may be visualized (Figure 8-6B). This is the classic "Mickey Mouse sign." It is advantageous to use color or power Doppler to identify vascular structures. The portal vein and hepatic artery will usually give off color Doppler signals while the remaining common bile duct will not (Figure 8-6C,D). Measurement of the common bile duct is made from inner wall to inner wall; normal is in general less than 7 mm thick.[31–33] Tissue harmonics may also help delineate the common bile duct. However, tissue harmonics increases the measured thickness of walls and must be used with caution. The site of common bile duct obstruction from stones is often near its termination close to the pancreatic head. This area may be visualized in a thin patient with little interfering gas (Figure 8-7). It will be difficult to visualize this point in the majority of patients.

EVALUATION OF ACUTE JAUNDICE AND BILIARY OBSTRUCTION

No gallbladder examination is complete without evaluation of the bile ducts. The initial step of this examination technique is to locate the main portal triad, which can be accomplished in two ways. The first method uses the portal vein as a landmark and is described above. The second method involves tracing more peripheral branches of the portal venous system as they course centrally toward the hilum. Their echogenic walls and their normal enlargement can identify portal venous branches as they course centrally toward the hilum to join the main portal vein in the main portal triad. They are clearly distinguished from the hepatic venous system, with its thin, hypoechoic walls and enlargement as it converges on the inferior vena cava posteriorly (Figure 8-8). Without the presence of biliary tract disease, they are rarely visible within the hepatic parenchyma. Color Doppler helps differentiate between the portal and biliary trees by

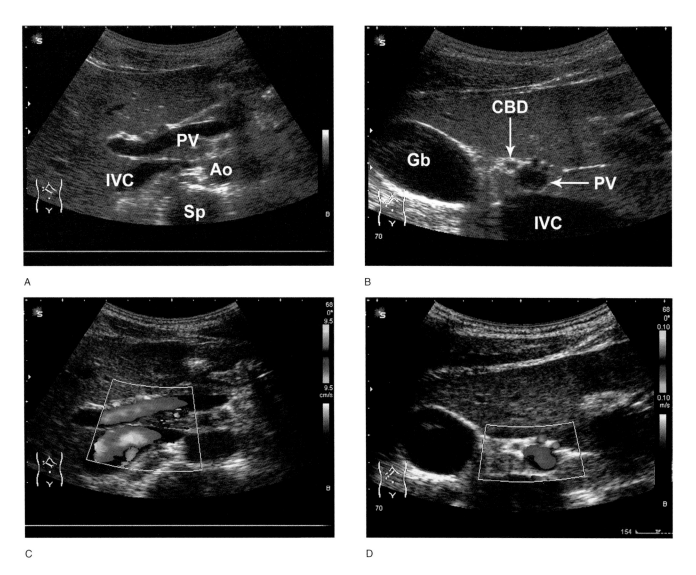

Figure 8-6. Portal vein and normal common bile duct. Longitudinal view of the portal vein (A). Transverse view of the portal vein (B). Corresponding color Doppler images (C,D). Patient has a duplicated hepatic artery. IVC = inferior vena cava, PV = portal vein, Ao = aorta, Sp = spine, GB = gallbladder, CBD = common bile duct. (Courtesy of James Mateer, MD)

demonstrating flow within the former. (Figure 8-6). Once the main portal triad has been identified, examination and measurement of the common duct are performed. The duct is usually normal if the transverse diameter, in millimeters, is less than one tenth of the patient's age. However, after cholecystectomy, the common bile duct may normally range up to 1 cm in all age groups.

The most convenient method for intrahepatic duct evaluation involves transverse imaging of the left lobe of the liver. Intrahepatic ducts run in the transverse plane in this location, allowing longitudinal images of the ducts to be obtained by orienting the ultrasound beam axis transversely. Longitudinal imaging of the ducts allows easier detection and evaluation of abnormalities in the intrahepatic system. While it was once thought that any

visualization of the intrahepatic ducts was abnormal, this may not be the case with modern equipment and the greatly improved resolution it delivers.

▶ COMMON AND EMERGENT ABNORMALITIES

GALLBLADDER DISEASE

Emergency physicians will most commonly use ultrasound to detect gallstones and acute cholecystitis. Gallstones typically appear as echogenic foci with acoustic shadowing beneath the gallstone. They can range in size from that of a golf ball to the size of sand particles

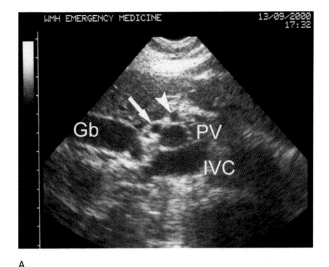

A

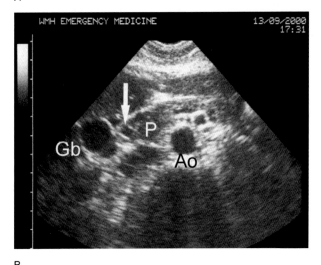

B

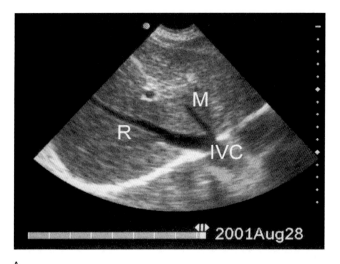

A

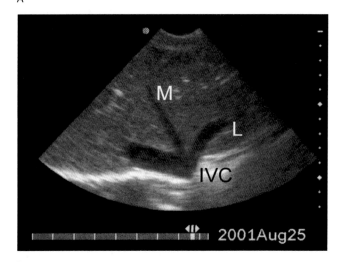

B

Figure 8-7. (a) Short-axis view of the portal vein (PV), with the associated common bile duct (anterior/lateral)[arrow] and hepatic artery (anterior/medial) [arrowhead]. The relative positions of the gallbladder (Gb) and inferior vena cava (IVC) are noted. (b) Transverse view of the upper abdomen. The position of the the common bile duct (arrow) near its termination by the pancreatic head (P) is noted along with the relative positions of the gallbladder (Gb) and aorta (Ao). (Courtesy of James Mateer, MD)

Figure 8-8. (a) Transverse view of the upper portion of the liver. The hepatic venous system, with its thin, hypoechoic walls and enlargement as it converges on the inferior vena cava (IVC) posteriorly is noted. The right hepatic vein (R) and a portion of the middle hepatic vein (M) are seen in this view. (b) Transverse/oblique view of the upper liver demonstrating the junction of the inferior vena cava (IVC) with the the the middle hepatic vein (M) and left hepatic vein (L). (Courtesy of James Mateer, MD)

(Figures 8-9, 8-10, and 8-11), but over two thirds will be greater than 5 mm in diameter.[34] The shadow is produced by ultrasound waves that are strongly reflected off of the gallstone. Shadowing may not be present if the gallstone diameter is less than 4 mm depending on the transducer being used and its frequency and resolution. Unless the gallstone is impacted in the neck of the gallbladder, gallstones will layer in the most dependent region of the gallbladder and will move with patient positional changes. This is important, as non-

shadowing stones may, otherwise, be difficult to distinguish from echogenic nonshadowing cholesterol polyps (Figure 8-12).

In patients with cholelithiasis and the appropriate clinical presentation, additional sonographic findings consistent with cholecystitis may include one or more of the following: wall thickness greater than 4 mm (Figure 8-13), pericholecystic fluid, and the presence of a sonographic Murphy's sign. Ninety-two percent of

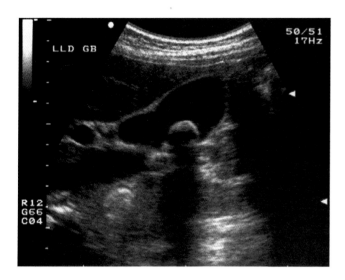

Figure 8-9. Longitudinal view of the gallbladder demonstrating a large solitary stone with prominent posterior acoustic shadowing. (Courtesy of Lori Sens, Gulfcoast Ultrasound)

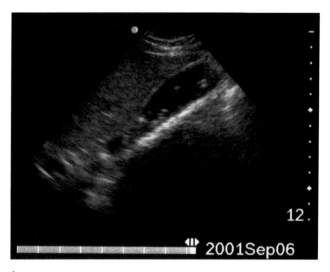

A

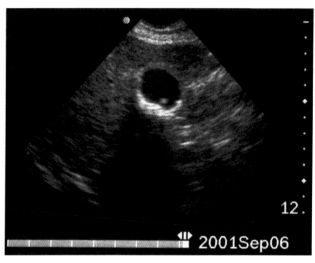

B

patients with cholecystitis will have a thickened gallbladder wall > 3 mm. However, gallbladder wall thickening can occur in a variety of conditions such as pancreatitis, ascites, and alcoholic hepatitis; although sensitive for acute cholecystitis, gallbladder wall thickening cannot be considered pathognomonic.[35,36] The mean gallbladder measurement in patients with acute cholecystitis is typically 9 mm. For cases of chronic cholecystitis the mean measurement is 5 mm. Measurements between 3 and 5 mm are recognized as being abnormal but lack

Figure 8-11. (a) Longitudinal view of the gallbladder shows multiple polyps suspended inside the wall. The dense posterior shadowing is from multiple tiny stones (sand-like) layering along the posterior wall of the gallbladder. This is best appreciated in the transverse view. (b) Transverse view. The posterior layering of the sand-like stones and the source of the shadowing is best appreciated in this view. (Courtesy of James Mateer, MD)

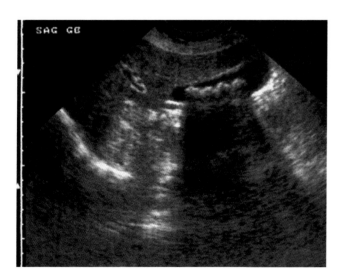

Figure 8-10. Longitudinal view of the gallbladder demonstrating multiple moderate-sized stones resembling "peas in a pod" also with prominent posterior acoustic shadowing. (Courtesy of Lori Sens and Lori Green, Gulfcoast Ultrasound)

diagnostic certainty. The sonographic Murphy's sign is considered positive when the point of maximal tenderness elicited by pressure from the ultrasound probe occurs over the sonographically identified gallbladder. Further more, transducer pressure not directly over the gallbladder should elicit much less or no pain. Pericholecystic fluid is a less common finding, but when present it is quite specific for cholecystitis.[37] The size of the gallbladder is not sensitive enough to rely on. Of note, no single sonographic sign is sensitive enough to make the

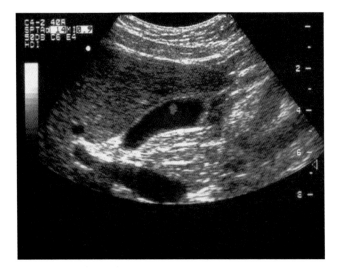

Figure 8-12. Longitudinal view of the gallbladder with solitary small polyp attached to the anterior wall. There was no shadowing and no movement with patient positioning. (Courtesy of Lori Sens and Lori Green, Gulfcoast Ultrasound)

diagnosis of acute cholecystitis and a small percentage of patients may present with no sonographic evidence of disease.[21] Physicians must consider the clinical presentation of the patient and may need adjunctive testing or a high clinical suspicion to definitively diagnose these cases.

Complications include gangrenous and hemorrhagic cholecystitis. When organisms that produce gas are involved, emphysematous changes in the gallbladder wall may be seen. In cases of hemorrhagic cholecystitis, internal echoes caused by bleeding represent sloughing of the gallbladder mucosa. The wall of the gallbladder will be enlarged and have a striated appearance in these cases (Figure 8-14).[38]

Finally, the WES sign (wall echo shadow) is commonly seen in gallstone-filled gallbladders. This occurs when the gallbladder is contracted around many stones with most of the bile emptied. The WES sign consists of an anterior echogenic line arising from the near wall of the gallbladder, an intervening anechoic stripe generated from bile when present, and a posterior brightly echogenic line representing stone material followed by a prominent posterior acoustic shadow (Figure 8-15).

JAUNDICE AND BILIARY OBSTRUCTION

Biliary obstruction, regardless of underlying etiology, is often initially detected by demonstrating dilated biliary ducts on ultrasound. Dilated extrahepatic ducts will appear as an enlarged, anechoic tubular structure (with echogenic walls) in the main portal triad, anterior to and following the course of the main portal vein. This is referred to as the parallel channel sign (Figure 8-16). Dilatation of the extrahepatic ducts implies obstruction of the common bile duct. Common causes of extrahepatic obstruction include choledocholithiasis

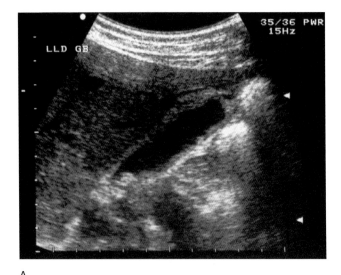

A

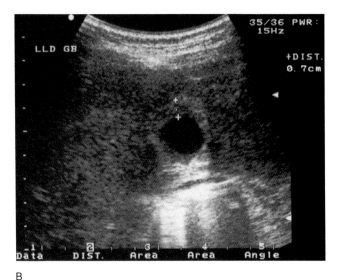

B

Figure 8-13. (a) Longitudinal view of a gallbladder with abnormal thickening of the wall. The bright echoes and shadowing below the gallbladder are from gas within the colon. (b) Transverse view. Wall thickness measures 7 mm. This patient was diagnosed with chronic cholecystitis. (Courtesy of Lori Sens, Gulfcoast Ultrasound)

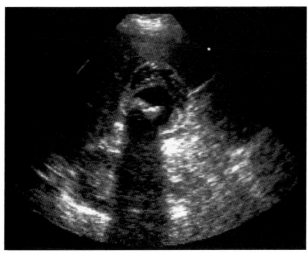

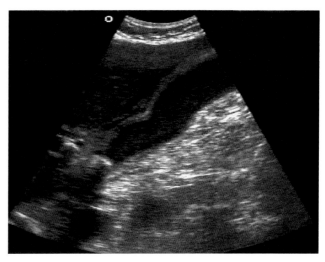

A   B

Figure 8-14. (a) Transverse view of the gallbladder shows marked thickening of the anterior wall and associated edema separating the layers of the wall. Cholelithiasis with shadowing is obvious. This patient was diagnosed with acute cholecystitis. (b) Hemorrhagic cholecystitis. Internal echoes caused by bleeding from sloughing of the gallbladder mucosa. The wall of the gallbladder is thickened and may have a striated appearance. Note the shadowing stone lodged in the gallbladder neck.

(Figure 8-17), pancreatic masses, and strictures. Left untreated, an extrahepatic obstruction will eventually also lead to dilatation of the intrahepatic ducts. Dilated intrahepatic ducts appear as anechoic tubules with echogenic walls coursing through the hepatic parenchyma. Morphologically, they are described as "antler signs" (Figure 8-18). Dilatation of the intrahepatic ducts alone

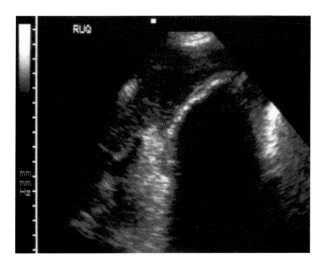

Figure 8-15. The WES sign (wall echo shadow). Note the superficial echogenic line arising from the near wall of the gallbladder, an intervening anechoic stripe generated from bile when present, and a posterior brightly echogenic line representing stone material, followed by a prominent posterior acoustic shadow. (Courtesy of James Mateer, MD)

suggests an obstructive process within the common hepatic duct or more proximal. Causes of primary intrahepatic obstruction may include inflammatory conditions (Figure 8-19), intrahepatic masses, or biliary duct cancer. Although ultrasound is sensitive in detecting ductal dilation, it may be less accurate for detecting the underlying cause of the obstruction. For example, ultrasound has a sensitivity of 15–55% for detecting common duct stones.[39] The precise etiology is often determined by other modalities such as CT or ERCP.

Common causes of nonobstructive jaundice are hepatitis and cirrhosis. Sonographically, hepatitis usually appears as a relatively decreased parenchymal echogenicity secondary to the increased fluid content of the tissue.[40] The diaphragm and portal vessel walls are not involved in the edema, and remain brightly echogenic. Their relative "accentuated brightness" is the classic finding associated with acute hepatitis but this ultrasound finding is often not obvious. As inflammation becomes more chronic, and cirrhosis develops, the liver size decreases, parenchymal echogenicity and surface irregularity increase, and intrahepatic anatomy becomes distorted (Figure 8-20).[41]

ASCITES

In patients presenting with abdominal distention, ultrasound can quickly differentiate between dilated gas filled loops of bowel and a patient with ascites (Figure 8-20). The ultrasound technique for detecting ascites

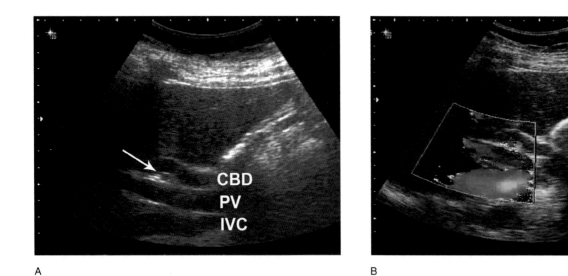

A

B

Figure 8-16. Dilated CBD (A) above the portal vein with the hepatic artery (arrow) between the two ("olive sandwich" appearance). Including the IVC below, the 3 tubular structures are also known as the "parallel channel sign." Color Doppler (B) distinguishes structures with flow (portal vein and hepatic artery) from those without flow (dilated CBD). CBD = common bile duct, PV = portal vein, IVC = inferior vena cava.

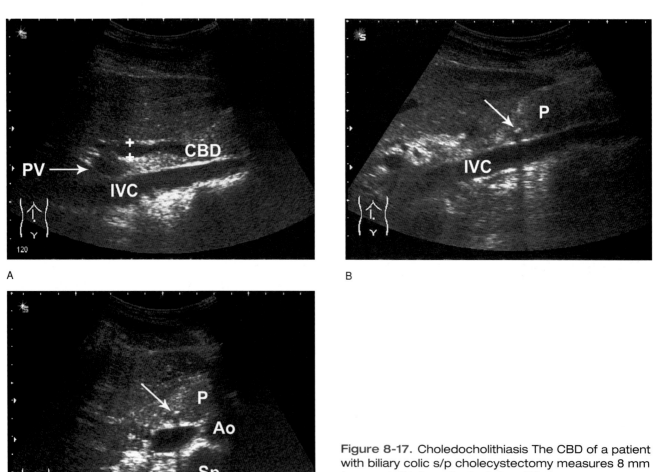

A

B

C

Figure 8-17. Choledocholithiasis The CBD of a patient with biliary colic s/p cholecystectomy measures 8 mm (cursors) (A). Longitudinal view (B) shows pancreas above IVC with a 4-mm stone (arrow) lodged in the distal common bile duct (CBD). Transverse view (C) confirms. CBD = common bile duct, PV = portal vein, IVC = inferior vena cava, P = pancreas, Ao = aorta, Sp = spine. (Courtesy of James Mateer, MD)

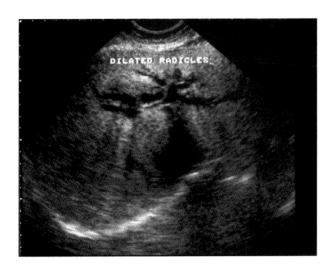

Figure 8-18. Antler signs. Transverse view of the liver. Dilated intrahepatic ducts appear as irregular anechoic tubules coursing through the hepatic parenchyma. (Courtesy of Lori Sens and Lori Green, Gulfcoast Ultrasound)

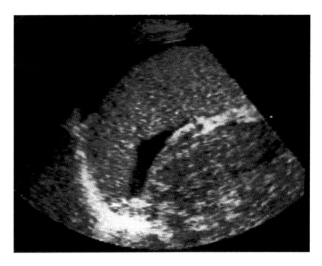

Figure 8-20. Cirrhosis of the liver. This oblique view of the right lobe demonstrates the findings of contracted size, increased echogenicity, and irregular texture of the liver. There is surrounding echo-free ascites.

is similar to that used in the FAST examination. The clinician should carefully note the echo characteristics of any intraperitoneal fluid detected. Large free floating echogenic particles may indicate clotted blood while multiple small free floating particles may indicate spilled abdominal contents and/or peritonitis

(Figure 8-21). Most frequently the fluid is consistently anechoic. It is difficult to discern the etiology of ascites by ultrasound.[42] Though the incidence of complications during paracentesis is 3%, ultrasound can assist in successfully sampling fluid collection for analysis.[43,44]

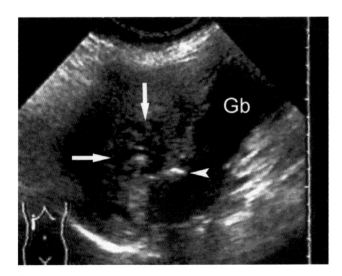

A

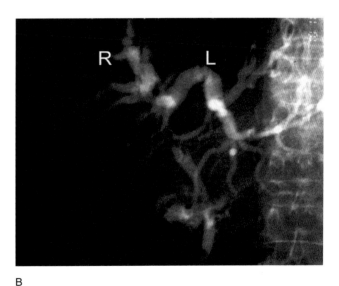

B

Figure 8-19. (a) Mirizzi syndrome. Longitudinal view of the gallbladder (Gb) reveals massive enlargement (Hydrops) and evidence of dilated intrahepatic ducts (arrows). At laparotomy, a large stone was found in the gallbladder neck area (arrowhead) with surrounding inflammation resulting in common hepatic duct obstruction. This is an unusual cause of intrahepatic obstruction. (b) ERCP radiograph of the same patient demonstrates dilatation of the right (R) and left (L) hepatic ducts. (Courtesy of James Mateer, MD)

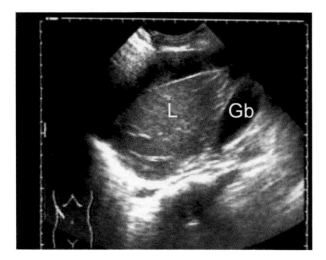

Figure 8-21. Coronal view of the right lobe of the liver (L) and gallbladder (Gb) shows echogenic ascites fluid with strand-like projections on the liver surface. The patient was diagnosed with bacterial peritonitis. (Courtesy of James Mateer, MD)

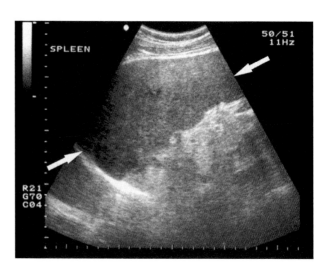

Figure 8-23. Long-axis view of the spleen measures more than 17 cm. Calipers should be placed on the longest length from the diaphragm to the spleen tip (arrows). (Courtesy of Lori Sens, Gulfcoast Ultrasound)

HEPATOMEGALY AND SPLENOMEGALY

Ultrasound is an ideal bedside tool for detection of hepatomegaly. If the liver parenchyma of the right lobe extends to or beyond the inferior pole of the right kidney, hepatic enlargement is probable (Figure 8-22). Alternatively, a longitudinal scan can be obtained at the mid-hepatic line, and the liver is measured from the dome (diaphragm) to the inferior margin. Enlargement is considered to be a measurement greater than 12.8 cm.[21] Since enlargement of the left lobe of the liver and

splenomegaly can be confused on physical examination, the ultrasound evaluation for possible hepatomegaly should be completed with long-axis views of the spleen. Splenomegaly is confirmed when the length measured in long axis exceeds 12–14 cm (Figure 8-23).

► COMMON VARIANTS AND SELECTED ABNORMALITIES

A number of variants may be noted with respect to the gallbladder. Mucosal indentations may produce septations of the lumen (Figure 8-24), which can be mistaken

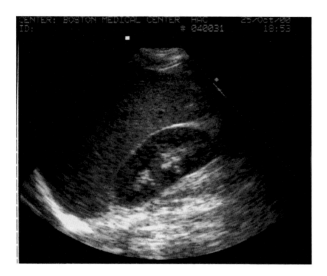

Figure 8-22. Longitudinal view of the liver and kidney shows possible hepatomegaly. The liver parenchyma of the right lobe extends to or beyond the inferior pole of the right kidney.

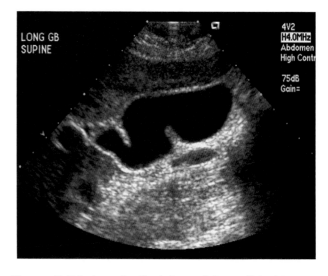

Figure 8-24. Longitudinal view of the gallbladder demonstrates nonshadowing mucosal folds on the mid-posterior wall and the anterior neck areas. (Courtesy of James Mateer, MD, Waukesha Memorial Hospital)

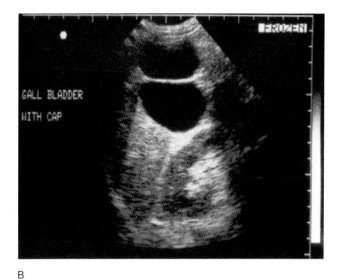

A

B

Figure 8-25. (a) Phyrigian cap. Longitudinal view demonstrates a folded gallbladder at the fundus. (b) Transverse views of the same patient create the illusion of a double gallbladder in this plane. (Courtesy of James Mateer, MD)

for gallstones, although shadowing does not usually occur. Folds of the fundus may produce a Phrygian cap (Figure 8-25). Agenesis of the gallbladder has an incidence of less than 0.05%. Intrahepatic gallbladder, secondary to abnormal developmental migration of the gallbladder bud, should always be considered if not found in its typical location. Duplicated gallbladder occurs with an incidence of 0.02%. Biliary sludge may be detected as a dependent layer of variable nonshadowing echogenicity in the gallbladder (Figure 8-26). Although the sequelae of sludge are largely unknown, it is frequently detected in states associated with biliary stasis, such as limited oral intake.[45] Tumefactive sludge is nonlayering, thickened, polypoid sludge that can be mistaken for a gallbladder wall tumor (Figure 8-27). A contracted gallbladder, commonly occuring in the postprandial patient, may be difficult to detect, and may demonstrate a nonpathologically thickened wall (Figure 8-28).

Riedel's lobe of the liver is a thin projection of otherwise normal hepatic tissue extending from the right lobe inferiorly toward the iliac crest (Figure 8-29). If not recognized, this could be mistaken for hepatomegaly.

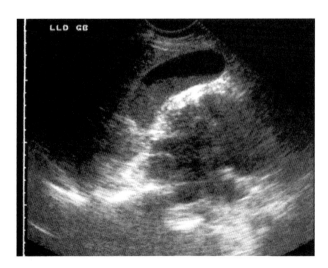

Figure 8-26. Biliary sludge is demonstrated as a dependent layer of nonshadowing mid-level echoes in this long-axis view of the gallbladder. (Courtesy of Lori Sens and Lori Green, Gulfcoast Ultrasound)

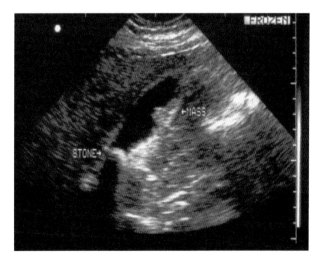

Figure 8-27. Tumefactive sludge. Dense polypoid sludge can be mistaken for a gallbladder wall tumor (<MASS). The patient also has a stone impacted in the Gb neck (STONE>). (Courtesy of James Mateer, MD)

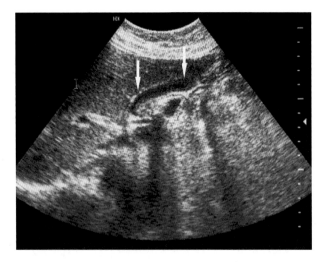

Figure 8-28. Contracted gallbladder. Can be difficult to detect (arrows), and may demonstrate a nonpathologically thickened wall. (Courtesy of Lori Sens, Gulfcoast Ultrasound)

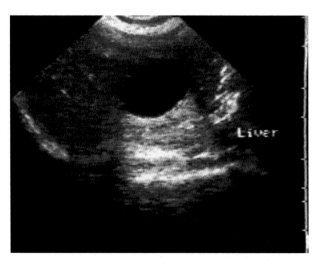

Figure 8-30. Liver cyst. Sharp margins, no internal echoes, and increased "through transmission" are demonstrated in this simple cyst of the right lobe of the liver. (Courtesy of Lori Sens and Lori Green, Gulfcoast Ultrasound)

Simple hepatic cysts are often an incidental finding. Their features include sharp margins, no internal echoes, and increased "through transmission" (Figure 8-30).[46] Hepatic abscesses, although an uncommon finding, are worthy of mention. Ultrasonographic features include thickened, poorly defined walls surrounding fluid of variable echogenicity, which is dependent on the nature of the internal pus (Figure 8-31).[47]

Intrinsic and metastatic tumors of the liver produce variable echo patterns, depending on histology and secondary tumor necrosis and hemorrhage.[48] They can exhibit smooth, well-defined, or irregular borders, and can

be of increased or decreased echogenicity relative to the general hepatic tissue. Necrosis produces areas of decreased echogenicity, whereas hemorrhage can create foci of increased or decreased echogenicity depending on the age and degeneration of blood. Common benign tumors include hemangiomas, with well-defined margins and a hyperechoic appearance (Figure 8-32), and hepatic adenomas, with well-defined margins and variable echogenicity (Figure 8-33). Common sources of metastatic lesions include colon, breast, and pancreas (Figure 8-34).[49]

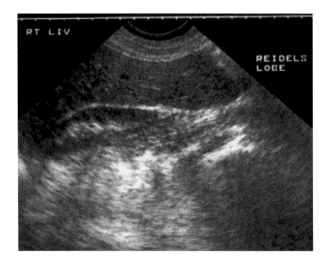

Figure 8-29. Reidel's Lobe. Longitudinal view of the abdomen at the anterior axillary line, centered over the kidney. A projection of normal hepatic tissue extends from the right lobe inferiorly toward the iliac crest. (Courtesy of Lori Sens, Gulfcoast Ultrasound)

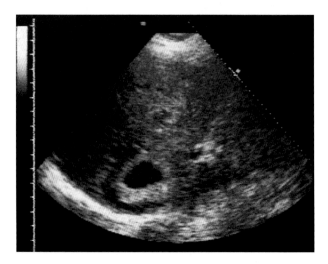

Figure 8-31. Liver abcess. An oblique view of the right lobe shows a fluid-filled cavity with thickened, poorly defined walls.

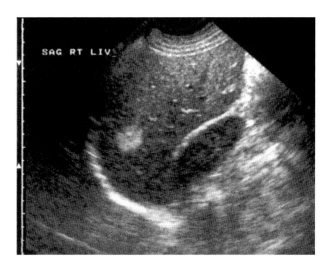

Figure 8-32. Hemangioma. Longitudinal view of the right lobe of the liver demonstrates the typical appearance. (Courtesy of Lori Sens and Lori Green, Gulfcoast Ultrasound)

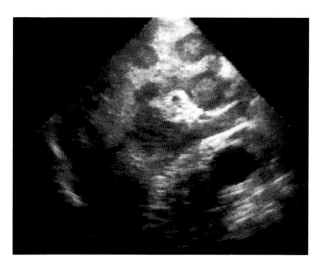

Figure 8-34. Metastatic tumors. Longitudinal view of the right lobe shows numerous target lesions. A cyst is also present within the lower pole of the kidney. (Courtesy of Lori Sens and Lori Green, Gulfcoast Ultrasound)

▶ PITFALLS

1. **Misidentifying the gallbladder.** Oblique sections through the inferior vena cava and the duodenum can be mistaken for the gallbladder. This pitfall can be avoided by ensuring the main lobar fissure connects the assumed gallbladder to the main portal triad. Another method involves using Doppler color flow. The gallbladder is typically the most anterior cystic structure and will not demonstrate Doppler color flow. Bowel can easily take on the appearance of a gallbladder,

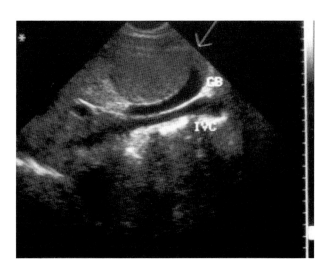

Figure 8-33. Hepatic adenoma. A hypoechoic mass (arrow) is seen compressing the gallbladder (GB) in this long-axis view. (Courtesy of Lori Sens and Lori Green, Gulfcoast Ultrasound)

especially if it contains both fluid and solids. Observing such a segment of bowel will typically result in visualization of peristaltic movement.

2. **Inadequate visualization of the gallbladder and biliary system.** Intestinal gas can interfere with complete imaging of the gallbladder and biliary system. The patient should be positioned in the left lateral decubitus to prone positions. If time permits, having the patient drink water may encourage gas to move and improve visualization.

3. **Confusion with shadowing.** A common error after detecting shadowing is making the diagnosis of a small gallstone impacted in the gallbladder neck without actually visualizing a gallstone. Causes of shadowing in the region of the gallbladder neck include the spiral valves of Heister (Figure 8-35), fat in the porta, duodenal gas, and edge artifacts from the gallbladder wall/fluid interface. A gallstone must be directly visualized before making this diagnosis. When a solitary gallstone is lodged in the neck of the gallbladder, however, it can be easily missed (Figure 8-36). A persistent clean shadow behind a rounded bright echo that is present from several viewing angles should be identified. Tissue harmonics may be exceedingly useful in detecting such small stones due to improve contrast resolution. A gallbladder packed with stones and containing little or no liquid bile may be confusing because of dense shadowing in the area that must be differentiated from shadowing caused by bowel gas (Figure 8-37).

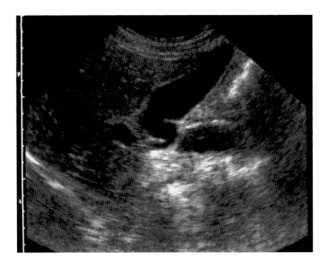

Figure 8-35. Hartman's pouch. Long-axis view of the Gb neck (Hartman's pouch) demonstrates the spiral valves of Heister. (Courtesy of Lori Sens and Lori Green, Gulfcoast Ultrasound)

4. **Misdiagnosing cholelithiasis and cholecystitis.** Cholesterol polyps and mucosal folds can be mistaken for gallstones. Bowel loops filled with echogenic material just under the gallbladder are a frequent finding and can appear to protrude into the gallbladder lumen. Making sure that any potential stone is actually within the gallbladder lumen will decrease the possibility of misinterpretation. Gallstones can be missed when they are small or when the entire gallbladder is not visualized because of intestinal gas or large mucosal folds. A thickened gallbladder wall is a nonspecific finding, and may be consistent with cholecystitis, hepatitis, ascites, hypoalbuminemia, and systemic volume overload states (Figure 8-38). The entire clinical picture should always be considered. In 2% of cases, cholecystitis may be diagnosed with the absence of gallstones (acalculous cholecystitis), which typically occur in patients who are chronically debilitated, diabetic, immunocompromised, on hyperalimentation, or recovering from a recent traumatic injury.

5. **Misdiagnosing dilated intrahepatic ducts.** Intrahepatic branches of the portal vein may be mistaken for dilated intrahepatic ducts as both have echogenic walls and become larger as they confluence toward the hepatic hilum. Color or power Doppler can help identify the vascular structures more precisely. Bile ducts do not demonstrate flow.

6. **Misdiagnosing ascites.** On ultrasound, ascites can be confused with hemoperitoneum, and vice versa. This can occur between simple transudative ascites and fresh blood (both typically echo free) and between complex exudative fluid and partially clotted blood (both with varying degrees of echogenicity). Clinical correlation, along with fluid sampling, should be used to make the correct diagnosis.

7. **Cystic Duct stone.** Stones in the cystic duct may be difficult to identify as the gallbladder may appear free of stones. A stone lodged in the cystic duct can appear in a different plane from the

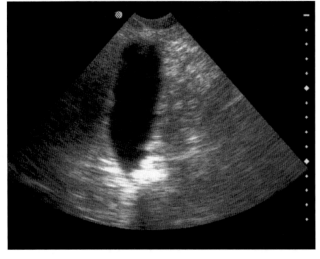
A

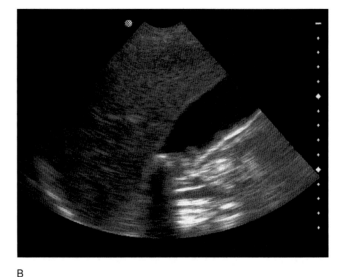
B

Figure 8-36. (a) Longitudinal view with the probe positioned at the tip of the Gb. Cholelithiasis is not obvious. (b) Intercostal oblique view of the same patient. Impacted stone in the Gb neck and prominent shadowing are more obvious in this view. (Courtesy of James Mateer, MD)

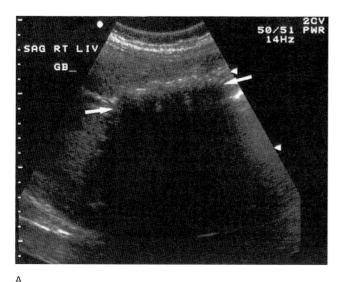
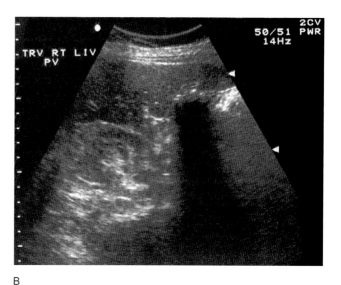

A

B

Figure 8-37. (a) Packed gallbladder. Longitudinal view of the Gb (arrows) shows dense shadowing from a collapsed Gb filled with stones. (b) Transverse views of the same patient clarify that the shadowing emanates from the GB fossa. (Courtesy of Lori Sens, Gulfcoast Ultrasound)

gallbladder and may be mistaken for bowel gas not associated with the gallbladder even by experienced sonographers. Any bright echo in vicinity of the gallbladder should be investigated, at least until peristalsis is seen.

8. **Common bile duct stones.** Common bile duct stones can be exceedingly difficult to identify, especially if they are not highly echogenic (Figure 8-17). Many common bile duct stones are not seen at all and the only indication is dilation of the duct. Complicating this further is the fact that the common bile duct may not be dilated with all stones, especially if only partial duct obstruction exists or the obstruction has occurred recently.

9. **Misdiagnosis of Biliary Colic.** In the United States, at least 20% of women and 8% of men over 40 years of age have been found to have gallstones at autopsy. It is estimated that

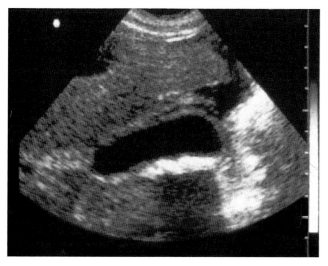
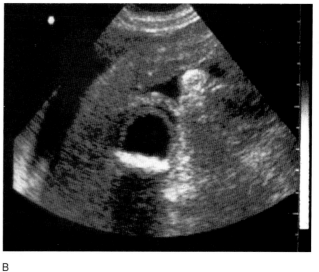

A

B

Figure 8-38. (a) Long-axis view of the GB shows typical ultrasound signs of cholecystitis: stones, a thickened wall, and pericholecystic fluid. (b) Transverse views of the same patient demonstrate ascites as the cause for wall thickening. The patient did not have cholecystitis on further clinical evaluation. (Courtesy of James Mateer, MD)

20 million persons in the United States have gallstones and at any given time, the vast majority are asymptomatic.[50] When a patient presents with abdominal pain that is atypical and is found to have gallstones on ultrasound, the astute clinician would exercise caution when attributing the symptoms to gallbladder disease. Biliary colic remains a clinical diagnosis and not a sonographic diagnosis.

▶ CASE STUDIES

CASE 1

Patient Presentation

A 64-year-old man was brought to the emergency department with complaints of epigastric pain, nausea, and vomiting. He had not tolerated food for the previous 48 hours because of dyspepsia. He noted a low-grade fever but no chills. The patient denied any chest pain, shortness of breath, or cough. He had no surgical history. He denied hematemesis or melena. He occasionally drank alcoholic beverages.

Vital signs revealed a temperature of 37.8°C; blood pressure, 118/58 mmHg; pulse, 119 beats per minute; respiratory rate, 18 breaths per minute. He appeared in moderate distress but nontoxic. There was no evidence of scleral icterus, the lungs were clear, and he did not exhibit costovertebral angle tenderness. The abdomen was tender in the epigastrium and right upper quadrant without guarding, and there were no pulsatile masses. Stool was guaiac negative.

Management Course

An ECG, chest radiograph, and urinalysis were normal. The white blood cell count was 13,400/μL. Lipase and chemistry profile were normal as were the liver transaminases. After administration of analgesics and intravenous fluids, he continued to complain of pain and dyspepsia. A focused emergency ultrasound examination of the right upper quadrant revealed a large gallstone, sludge, and a thickened anterior gallbladder wall. The patient was immediately given intravenous antibiotics; later in the day, he was taken to the operating room for laparoscopic cholecystectomy.

Commentary

Epidemiological and physiologic studies have not corroborated the stereotypical history and physical examination findings for cholecystitis. The ratio of biliary disease in men and women evens out later in life. Epigastric complaints occur as frequently as right upper quadrant complaints. The threshold for performing ultrasound on such patients in the emergency setting should be low to make an expeditious diagnosis.

CASE 2

Patient Presentation

An 88-year-old woman was brought to the emergency department by ambulance. When the family arrived, they noted she had become increasingly confused and somnolent over the past 2 days because of "fatigue." She was completely unresponsive and appeared short of breath. Vital signs revealed a temperature of 39.1°C; blood pressure, 78/52 mmHg; pulse, 128 beats per minute; and respirations, 28 breaths per minute; pulse oximetry, 90% on room air. She was minimally responsive and moaned occasionally with her eyes closed. Her lung examination revealed bibasilar crackles; heart rhythm was regular, but tachycardic; and her extremities were cool. Abdominal examination revealed diffuse tenderness. The patient was noted to be jaundiced.

Management Course

The patient was intubated for airway support. Intravenous fluids and pressors were initiated with good response. ECG and chest radiograph were normal. Urinalysis was normal. Further laboratory data revealed a white blood cell count of 14,000/μL, a normal lipase, a total bilirubin of 14 with a direct component of 9, and an ALT and AST that doubled. Lactate returned at 3.8. A focused ultrasound examination revealed multiple small gallstones in the gallbladder, a thickened anterior gallbladder wall, and a common bile duct that measured 1.2 cm. A diagnosis of cholangitis was made. The patient underwent ERCP and sphincterotomy with removal of two gallstones.

Commentary

Biliary pathology accounts for 25% of all suspected abdominal sepsis sources in the elderly. Focused emergency ultrasound can quickly identify a source of infection and expedite therapy. In addition, focused emergency ultrasound of the biliary tree can readily differentiate between obstructive and nonobstructive causes of jaundice and direct management between medical and surgical treatments.

CASE 3

Patient Presentation

A 42-year-old man presented to the emergency department complaining of abdominal distention that began 20 hours before arrival. He admitted to chronic alcohol abuse and stated that he required "abdominal drainage" for a similar complaint in the past. He also complained of shortness of breath and vomited frequently. Prior records indicated a history of spontaneous bacterial peritonitis that required inpatient admission as well as a history of appendectomy when he was 14 years old.

Vital signs revealed a temperature of 37.3°C; blood pressure, 110/74 mmHg; pulse, 102 beats per minute; respirations, 18 breaths per minute. The patient appeared in mild discomfort, but nontoxic. There was no evidence of jaundice, heart sounds were normal, and lungs had rales at the bases bilaterally. His abdomen was distended and diffusely tender without rebound or guarding. There was also minimal edema in the lower extremities.

Management Course

ECG and chest radiograph were normal. White blood cell count was 9,800/μL. Basic chemistries and lipase were normal. The AST and ALT were 100 and 125 respectively, and bilirubin was normal. The presumptive diagnosis of a recurrence of spontaneous bacterial peritonitis was made and the admitting physician prepared for a paracentesis. Prior to the procedure, a focused ultrasound examination of the right upper quadrant was performed that revealed no evidence of ascites. The ultrasound probe was moved to the left lower quadrant where the paracentesis would have been performed and no pockets of free fluid were identified. An acute abdominal series revealed evidence of early small bowel obstruction later confirmed by CT. The patient was taken to the operating room for lysis of adhesions likely from prior appendectomy.

Commentary

Ascites may be difficult to detect on physical examination. In cases where the physician has a suspicion for ascites, focused bedside ultrasound provides a quick and efficient way to make the diagnosis. If ascites is present, ultrasound can identify a deep pocket easily drained for diagnostic or therapeutic purposes. If no ascites is visible, then the physician should look for other sources of abdominal distention such as a bowel obstruction.

REFERENCES

1. Matolo N, Stadainik R, McGahan J: Comparison of ultrasonography, computerized tomography, and radionuclide imaging in the diagnosis of acute and chronic cholecystitis. *Am J Surg* 144:676–681, 1982.
2. Shea JA, Berlin JA, Escarce JJ, et al.: Revised estimates of diagnostic test sensitivity and specificity in suspected biliary tract disease. 10.1001/archinte.154.22.2573. *Arch Intern Med* 154:2573–2581, 1994.
3. Justice AC, Covinsky KE, Berlin JA: Assessing the generalizability of prognostic information. *Ann Intern Med* 130:515–524, 1999.
4. Blaivas M, D: Utility of cholescintigraphy as an adjunct to emergency bedside ultrasonographic evaluation of cholecystitis. *Ann Emerg Med* 40:A 268, 2002.
5. Bennett GL, Balthazar EJ: Ultrasound and CT evaluation of emergent gallbladder pathology. *Radiol Clin North Am* 41:1203–1216, 2003.
6. Harvey RT, Miller WT, Jr.: Acute biliary disease: Initial CT and follow-up US versus initial US and follow-up CT. *Radiology* 213:831–836, 1999.
7. Bassler D, Snoey ER, Kim J: Goal-directed abdominal ultrasonography: Impact on real-time decision making in the emergency department. *J Emerg Med* 24:375–378, 2003.
8. Friedman GD: Natural history of asymptomatic and symptomatic gallstones. *Am J Surg* 165:399–404, 1993.
9. Traverso L: Clinical manfiestations and the impact of gallstone disease. *Am J Surg* 163:405–409, 1993.
10. Zollinger R: Observations following distension of the gallbladder and common duct in man. *Proc Soc Exp Biol Med* 30:1260–1261, 1933.
11. Zollinger R: Localization of pain following faradic stimulation of the common bile duct. *Proc Soc Exp Biol Med* 35:267–268, 1936.
12. Gallbladder Survey Committee OC, ACS: 28,621 cholecystectomies in Ohio. *Am J Surg* 119:714–717, 1970.
13. Diehl AK, Sugarek NJ, Todd KH. Clinical evaluation for gallstone disease: Usefulness of symptoms and signs in diagnosis. *Am J Med* 89:29–33, 1990.
14. Jehle D, Davis E, Evans T, et al.: Emergency department sonography by emergency physicians. *Am J Emerg Med* 7:605–611, 1989.
15. Schlager D, Lazzareschi G, Whitten D, Sanders AB: A prospective study of ultrasonography in the ED by emergency physicians. *Am J Emerg Med* 12:185–189, 1994.
16. Kendall JL, Shimp RJ: Performance and interpretation of focused right upper quadrant ultrasound by emergency physicians. *J Emerg Med* 21:7–13, 2001.
17. Blaivas M, Harwood RA, Lambert MJ: Decreasing length of stay with emergency ultrasound examination of the gallbladder. *Acad Emerg Med* 6:1020–1023, 1999.
18. Trowbridge RL, Rutkowski NK, Shojania KG: Does This patient have acute cholecystitis? 10.1001/jama.289.1.80. *JAMA* 289:80–86, 2003.
19. Singer AJ, McCracken G, Henry MC, Thode J, Henry C, Cabahug CJ: Correlation among clinical, laboratory, and hepatobiliary scanning findings in patients with suspected acute cholecystitis. *Ann Emerg Med* 28:267–272, 1996.
20. DeFrances CP, MN: 2004 National hospital discharge survey. In advance data from vital and health statistics. Hyattsville, MD: National Center for Health Statistics, 2006.
21. Ralls P, Colletti P, Lapin S, et al.: Real-time sonography in suspected acute cholecystitis. Prospective evaluation of primary and secondary signs. *Radiology* 155:767–771, 1985.
22. Bree RL: Further observations on the usefulness of the sonographic Murphy sign in the evaluation of suspected acute cholecystitis. *J Clin Ultrasound* 23:169–172, 1995.
23. Abboud P, Malet P, Berlin J, et al.: Predictors of common bile duct stones prior to cholecystectomy: A meta-analysis. *Gastrointestinal Endoscopy* 44:450–457, 1996.

24. Haubek A, Pedersen J, Burcharth F, Gammelgaard J, Hancke S, Willumsen L: Dynamic sonography in the evaluation of jaundice. *Am J Roentgenol* 136:1071–1074, 1981.

25. Rivers E, Nguyen B, Havstad S, et al.: The Early Goal-Directed Therapy Collaborative Group: Early Goal-Directed Therapy in the Treatment of Severe Sepsis and Septic Shock. *N Engl J Med* 345:1368–1377, 2001.

26. Martin G, Mannino D, Moss M: The effect of age on the development and outcome of adult sepsis. *Crit Care Med* 34:15–21, 2006.

27. Podnos YD, Jimenez JC, Wilson SE: Intra-abdominal sepsis in elderly persons. *Clin Infect Dis* 35:62–68. Epub 2002 Jun 2007, 2002.

28. Cobden I, Venables CW, Lendrum R, James OFW: Gallstones presenting as mental and physical debility in the elderly. *Lancet* 323:1062–1064, 1984.

29. AIUM Official Statement: 3D Technology. November 12, 2005 [cited; Available from: http://www.aium.org/publications/statements/'statementSelected.asp?statement=23.

30. Choudhry S, Gorman B, Charboneau JW, et al.: Comparison of tissue harmonic imaging with conventional US in abdominal disease. *Radiographics* 20:1127–1135, 2000.

31. Cooperberg P: High-resolution real-time ultrasound in the evaluation of the normal and obstructed biliary tract. *Radiology* 129:477–480, 1978.

32. Koenigsberg M, Wiener S, Walzer A: The accuracy of sonography in the differential diagnosis of obstructive jaundice: A comparison with cholangiography. *Radiology* 133:157–165, 1979.

33. Ortega D, Burns PN, Hope Simpson D, Wilson SR: Tissue harmonic imaging: Is it a benefit for bile duct sonography? *Am J Roentgenol* 176:653–659, 2001.

34. Jensen K, Jorgensen T: Incidence of gallstones in a Danish population. *Gastroenterology* 100:790–794, 1991.

35. Sanders RC: The significance of sonographic gallbladder wall thickening. *J Clin Ultrasound* 8:143–146, 1980.

36. Laing F, Federle M, Jeffrey R, Brown T: Ultrasonic evaluation of patients with acute right upper quadrant pain. *Radiology* 140:449–455, 1981.

37. Elyaderani MK: Accuracy of cholecystosonography with pathologic correlation. *W V Med J* 80:111–115, 1984.

38. Teefey S, Baron R, Bigler S: Sonography of the gallbladder: Significance of striated (layered) thickening of the gallbladder wall. *Am J Roentgenol* 156:945–947, 1991.

39. Laing FC, Jeffrey RB: Choledocholithiasis and cystic duct obstruction: Difficult ultrasonographic diagnosis. *Radiology* 146:475–479, 1983.

40. Kurtz AB, Rubin CS, Cooper HS, et al.: Ultrasound findings in hepatitis. *Radiology* 136:717–723, 1980.

41. Taylor KJ, Gorelick FS, Rosenfield AT, et al.: Ultrasonography of alcoholic liver disease with histological correlation. *Radiology* 141:157–161, 1981.

42. Edell S, Gefter W: Ultrasonic differentiation of types of ascitic fluid. *Am. J. Roentgenol.* 133:111–114, 1979.

43. Mallory A, Schaefer JW: Complications of diagnostic paracentesis in patients with liver disease. *JAMA* 239:628–630, 1978.

44. Blaivas M: Emergency diagnostic paracentesis to determine intraperitoneal fluid identity discovered on bedside ultrasound of unstable patients. *J Emerg Med* 29:461–465, 2005.

45. Angelico M, De Santis A, Capocaccia L: Biliary sludge: A critical update. *J Clin Gastroenterol* 12(6):656–662, 1990.

46. Weaver RM, Goldstein HM, Green B, et al.: Gray scale ultrasonographic evaluation of hepatic cystic disease. *Am J Roentgenol* 130:849–852, 1978.

47. Kuligowska E, Connors SK, Shapiro JH: Liver abscess: Sonography in diagnosis and treatment. *Am J Roentgenol* 138:253–257, 1982.

48. Green B, Bree RL, Goldstein HM, et al.: Gray scale ultrasound evaluation of hepatic neoplasms: Patterns and correlations. *Radiology* 124:203–208, 1977.

49. Viscomi G, Gonzalez R, Taylor K: Histopathological correlation of ultrasound appearances of liver metastases. *J Clin Gastroenterol* 3:395, 1981.

50. Johnston DE, Kaplan MM: Medical progress: Pathogenesis and treatment of gallstones. *N Engl J Med* 328:412–415, 1993.

CHAPTER 9

General Surgery Applications

Masaaki Ogata

Over the past 25 years, abdominal sonography has become increasingly utilized as a diagnostic tool for surveying hepatobiliary, vascular, urologic, or gynecologic disorders. With progress in the resolution of scanning devices, abdominal sonography has also been used for the evaluation of various acute gastrointestinal abnormalities. The operator-dependent nature of ultrasonography, however, may limit the application of the examination in the emergency setting. In the United States, ultrasonography has been a domain of radiology and, subsequently, the application of the examination for the acute abdomen in the emergency department has been somewhat limited. In most hospitals, the difficulty in providing 24 hour service by expert sonographers has been a major factor in preventing ultrasonography from becoming a primary imaging modality in the emergency or acute care setting. It is quite important, however, to utilize the advantages of ultrasonography to improve patient evaluation in the emergency or acute care setting.

▶ CLINICAL CONSIDERATIONS

The evaluation of acute abdominal disorders begins with a careful history and physical examination. When required, the clinical findings may be supplemented by laboratory tests or conventional plain radiographs. Plain radiography may show some significant findings, such as pneumoperitoneum and bowel dilatation, but unsatisfactorily, it shows nonspecific findings in a significant number of patients. The development of high-resolution computed tomography (CT) and ultrasonography has greatly facilitated the identification of pathology in many patients with an acute abdomen.

CT scanning is an excellent imaging modality to evaluate not only intraperitoneal disorders but also retroperitoneal abnormalities. CT scanning has a greater specificity than plain radiography but has not been used as a routine screening tool for the acute abdomen because it is expensive and not immediately available in many hospitals. Both plain radiography and CT are noninvasive, but are contraindicated in pregnant patients.

In contrast, sonography does not expose patients to ionizing radiation and is noninvasive, readily available, repeatable at the bedside, and less expensive than CT scan. It has been accepted as a useful imaging modality for hepatobiliary, cardiovascular, urologic, or gynecologic disorders. In addition, recent studies have shown that sonography is applicable and may be accurate for acute gastrointestinal disorders such as acute appendicitis, acute colonic diverticulitis, intussusception, and bowel obstruction. It is also beneficial for patients who are hemodynamically unstable, who have unreliable physical examination findings due to drug intoxication or central nervous system disorders, or who have unexplained shock symptoms and an equivocal physical examination. Abdominal sonography, however, has some disadvantages, such as difficulty in visualizing intraperitoneal or retroperitoneal abnormalities in patients who are obese, or who have excessive bowel gas.

The operator-dependent nature of ultrasonography has been identified as a factor influencing the reliability of emergency ultrasound performed by nonradiologist physicians. Indeed, the clinical applications and results of emergency ultrasound are influenced by the clinical experience, skill, and interest of the sonologist. In several European countries and Japan, however, bedside ultrasound performed by nonradiologist physicians has been accepted as a rapid and useful screening tool for evaluating the acute abdomen as well as for abdominal trauma. Physicians who are well trained to perform emergency ultrasound will significantly improve patient evaluation, initial treatment, selection of further diagnostic modalities, and timely consultation of surgeons or gastrointestinal specialists.

▶ CLINICAL INDICATIONS

In a general surgical setting, the clinical indications for applying an emergency ultrasound examination are

- acute abdominal pain,
- peritonitis,
- abdominal distension or mass, and
- unexplained shock or sepsis.

All patients who have been diagnosed with an acute abdomen on the basis of clinical findings are candidates for the examination. The common etiologies of acute abdomen are

1. hemorrhage,
2. gastrointestinal perforation,
3. bowel obstruction,
4. inflammatory disorder, and
5. circulatory impairment.

▶ HEMORRHAGE

Active intraperitoneal or gastrointestinal bleeding is a life-threatening etiology for which rapid diagnosis and treatment are required. If patients are hemodynamically unstable, adequate resuscitation is the first priority. Rapid assessment for the approximate site of hemorrhage (intraperitoneal or gastrointestinal) should be made on the basis of clinical findings. The use of sonography for patients with massive hematemesis is limited in the emergency setting because they should be referred for emergency endoscopy. Patients who are hemodynamically unstable without gastrointestinal bleeding should be urgently examined for intraperitoneal hemorrhage. In this setting, abdominal sonography is very useful and reliable for the evaluation of intraperitoneal hemorrhage. It can be utilized during the resuscitation of the unstable patient in the emergency setting, whereas other imaging modalities, such as CT and angiography, require hemodynamic stability of patients.

INTRAPERITONEAL HEMORRHAGE

Since intraperitoneal hemorrhage may be severe enough to produce hypovolemic shock, the rapid detection of free peritoneal fluid is essential for patients who are suspected of having intraperitoneal hemorrhage on the basis of their clinical findings. For this purpose, the focused assessment with sonography for free intraperitoneal fluid is beneficial as in cases of abdominal trauma. As described in Chapter 5, sonography has been recognized as a rapid, sensitive, and specific diagnostic modality for detecting free peritoneal fluid in many clinical studies.[1,2] Appropriately trained, nonradiologist clinicians, such as emergency physicians or surgeons, can accurately perform and interpret abdominal sonography for free intraperitoneal fluid in cases of acute abdomen as well as abdominal trauma. On the other hand, plain radiographs are insensitive and inappropriate for the early recognition of intraperitoneal hemorrhage since radiographic signs for the accumulation of peritoneal fluid, such as widening of the paracolic gutter or a "dog's ear" appearance, require a large amount of peritoneal fluid. CT scanning is unavailable for immediate use in some emergency departments and inappropriate for hemodynamically unstable patients. However, it is very useful in detecting intraperitoneal hemorrhage and retroperitoneal hematoma

In making a decision for surgical exploration, it is important to detect the presence and the amount of intraperitoneal hemorrhage even if primary lesions are not identified. As abdominal sonography can be used to estimate not only the amount but also the rate of intraperitoneal hemorrhage through serial examinations, it will supplement clinical findings in evaluating whether the hemorrhage is active or not.

Common sites where free intraperitoneal fluid accumulates are Morison's pouch, the rectovesical pouch, the pouch of Douglas, and bilateral subphrenic spaces. A small amount of free intraperitoneal fluid may be seen only between bowel loops. A large amount of free intraperitoneal fluid can be seen above the bowels, located adjacent to the anterior peritoneum. On sonographic images, hemoperitoneum appears anechoic with coarse internal echoes as the blood is clotted. Bloody or purulent ascites or peritoneal fluid containing intestinal contents also may be shown as having similar images.[1,2] It is not very difficult, however, to differentiate hemoperitoneum from ascites on the basis of a careful history and physical examination. If required, paracentesis (guided by ultrasound) can be applied for the definite diagnosis of hemoperitoneum.

The pathology causing intraperitoneal hemorrhage can be evaluated with abdominal sonography. While CT remains the gold standard for detecting specific intra-abdominal pathology, it is beneficial to utilize bedside ultrasound for this purpose, especially with unstable patients. Common causes of intraperitoneal hemorrhage are rupture of a hepatoma, aortic aneurysm, ectopic pregnancy, or ovarian bleeding. Abdominal sonography can be performed as a rapid screening tool for detecting such specific lesions as hepatoma and abdominal aortic aneurysm. Early recognition of these etiologies is beneficial for selecting further examinations and making a strategy for treatment that is either immediate surgery or interventional radiology. In young female patients who present with hypotensive shock and associated lower abdominal pain, gynecological disorders, such as rupture of an ectopic pregnancy or ovarian bleeding unrelated to pregnancy, should be always taken into consideration. Although transabdominal sonography may demonstrate only nonspecific findings, massive hemorrhage warrants immediate surgical treatment.

GASTROINTESTINAL HEMORRHAGE

Patients with an upper gastrointestinal hemorrhage generally present with various degrees of hematemesis or melena. However, some may present with only complaints of epigastric pain or with unexplained shock. Primary causes of upper gastrointestinal hemorrhage are duodenal ulcer, gastric ulcer, hemorrhagic gastritis, esophageal or gastric varices, and Mallory–Weiss syndrome. Patients suspected of having massive gastrointestinal hemorrhage should be referred for emergency endoscopy, which makes it possible to identify the bleeding source in up to 90% of cases of upper gastrointestinal hemorrhage. In contrast, other diagnostic modalities, such as plain radiography, sonography, and CT, and gastrointestinal contrast studies do not contribute to the diagnosis of acute gastrointestinal hemorrhage. When appropriate, emergency ultrasound may be used to detect adjunct findings such as liver cirrhosis and splenomegaly. Abnormalities of the gastroduodenal wall occasionally may be shown with sonography in cases of gastric cancer, peptic ulcer, or acute gastric mucosal lesion.[3,4]

In cases of massive lower gastrointestinal hemorrhage, direct endoscopic evaluation may be disturbed by a large amount of blood and stool in the colon. Furthermore, at times, the causes of lower gastrointestinal hemorrhage originate in the small bowel. For these reasons, emergency angiography or scintigraphy is reserved for patients in whom colonoscopy is unsuccessful in locating the bleeding source. Abdominal sonography can be used as a screening tool to evaluate intra-abdominal abnormalities suggesting a bleeding source (e.g., colon cancer, ischemic colitis) and its adjunct findings (e.g., liver cirrhosis, bowel obstruction or abscess formation).

► GASTROINTESTINAL PERFORATION

Gastrointestinal perforations are serious disorders requiring rapid diagnosis and treatment. Since they may be severe enough to produce septic or hypovolemic shock, rapid decision-making for urgent laparotomy is crucially important. The initial diagnosis is generally made on the basis of clinical symptoms and signs of peritonitis and then supplemented by plain radiography demonstrating pneumoperitoneum. Plain radiographs, however, may not always show pneumoperitoneum in cases of gastrointestinal perforation, and are useless in detecting underlying etiologies. The incidence of pneumoperitoneum appreciated on conventional radiographs was reported as 80–90% in cases of gastroduodenal perforation but only 20–30% and 30–50%, respectively, in cases of small bowel and large bowel perforation.[5,6] Moreover, in the elderly, signs of peritonitis on physical examination may be obscured and laboratory tests may show a normal white blood cell count. These clinical and radiographic features may cloud the diagnosis of gastrointestinal perforation in elderly patients. Consequently, any delay in making a decision for urgent laparotomy may lead to further deterioration in the clinical status of the patients, especially in cases of large bowel perforation. To avoid such delay in the diagnosis and treatment, therefore, conventional plain radiography should be supplemented with other diagnostic modalities, which include CT, sonography, contrast studies, and endoscopy. CT is much sensitive for demonstrating not only pneumoperitoneum but also ectopic gas in the retroperitoneal space. CT has been reported to demonstrate a very small pneumoperitoneum that was not appreciated on conventional plain radiographs.[7]

Abdominal sonography is not as sensitive as plain radiography for demonstrating pneumoperitoneum. It may be valuable, however, in complementing plain radiographs by rapidly identifying pneumoperitoneum in the supine patient.[8–12] Subphrenic free air can be identified as an echogenic line with posterior reverberation artifacts on the ventral surface of the liver. It should be discriminated from gas in the gastrointestinal lumen or the lung to avoid a false diagnosis. Hyperventilation may interfere with the examination for visualization of free air. Hepatodiaphragmatic interposition of the colon also may cause subphrenic gas echoes.

As for the underlying pathology, bedside ultrasound can be applied for the evaluation of specific lesions. It may detect a primary lesion, such as colon cancer, acute colonic diverticulitis, or an acute duodenal ulcer, and secondary abnormalities, such as free peritoneal fluid, a localized abscess, or paralytic ileus. Upper gastrointestinal perforation is not very difficult to diagnose on the basis of clinical and radiographic findings. If required, emergency endoscopy can be adopted for identifying gastroduodenal lesions. Therefore, it is not essential to detect images of a peptic ulcer or gastric cancer by sonography or CT. As a screening tool available at bedside, however, abdominal sonography may occasionally demonstrate a duodenal ulcer or gastric cancer as hypoechoic wall thickening.[3,4]

The strategies for treatment of a peptic ulcer, which is the leading cause of upper gastrointestinal perforation, have been changed in recent years. Nonoperative treatments using anti-ulcerative agents have been successful in selected patients with a perforated duodenal ulcer. This new option in treating perforated peptic ulcers may influence the use of diagnostic modalities. A patient with a perforated duodenal ulcer can be a candidate for nonoperative treatments when signs of peritonitis are localized in the right upper quadrant. In this setting, consequently, pneumoperitoneum itself is not considered to be an absolute indication for immediate surgery. Serial examinations with sonography can be used as follow-up studies to evaluate the accumulation of peritoneal fluid or occurrence of any other abnormalities when nonoperative treatments are adopted for a perforated duodenal ulcer.

On sonographic images of gastrointestinal perforation, free intraperitoneal fluid often contains gray level echoes inside an anechoic space in the pelvis or Morison's pouch, or adjacent to intestinal loops. The image is regarded as showing turbulent, purulent, or feculent peritoneal fluid. Gas echoes may be occasionally identified as echogenic spots inside an anechoic space. Although the nature of peritoneal fluid cannot be ascertained strictly on ultrasound, such sonographic images can be helpful in making a decision for surgical intervention when pneumoperitoneum is not identified.

▶ BOWEL OBSTRUCTION

Bowel obstruction is a common etiology of acute abdomen. The clinical picture of a patient with bowel obstruction varies depending on location, form, etiology, and degree of the obstruction. Thus, strategies for treatment should be carefully determined on the basis of clinical findings, laboratory tests, and imaging methods. Generally, plain radiography is conventionally used as an initial imaging method when bowel obstruction is considered. It serves to confirm the distribution of gaseous dilated bowel and the approximate site of obstruction. However, it is widely known that plain radiography cannot reliably differentiate strangu-

lation from simple obstruction and is useless to demonstrate causative lesions for bowel obstruction.[13,14]

For years, the application of sonography for bowel obstruction has been regarded as inappropriate and unreliable because of the significant artifact arising from gastrointestinal gas. This misconception has prevented not only radiologists but also surgeons and emergency physicians from utilizing sonography for the evaluation of bowel obstruction. With progress in the resolution of scanning devices, however, abdominal sonography has become more popular for the evaluation of gastrointestinal diseases.[15-17] Ultrasound's role in recognizing fluid-filled distended bowel was reported in the literature during the latter half of 1970s.[18,19] Fleischer and coworkers first introduced sonographic patterns of distended, fluid-filled bowel both in vivo and in vitro in 1979.[18] Since the latter half of 1980s, abdominal sonography has gained increasing popularity for the evaluation of bowel obstruction in Japan and Germany. Some studies have shown the usefulness of abdominal sonography for demonstrating a radiograph-negative small bowel obstruction, and for differentiating between a small bowel obstruction and a paralytic ileus.[20-23] In the 1990s, the use of sonography for the differentiation between strangulation and simple small bowel obstruction was reported.[24-26] Ogata and colleagues introduced the usefulness of sonography in identifying radiograph-negative large bowel obstruction, and Ogata and Mateer prospectively demonstrated that initial bedside ultrasound was as sensitive as, and more specific than, plain radiographs for the diagnosis of bowel obstruction in an emergency department setting.[27,28]

The pathophysiological appearances of bowel obstruction are characterized primarily by the accumulation of fluid and electrolytes in the gastrointestinal tract proximal to the obstruction.[29] Along with further progression of bowel obstruction, the bowel loops become distended with accumulated fluid in the lumen. In addition, the bowel wall may be thickened with interstitial edema, and free fluid may accumulate in the peritoneal cavity. Taking these features into consideration, abdominal sonography as well as CT may be appropriate and applicable to the diagnosis of bowel obstruction because it is superior to plain radiography in visualizing accumulated fluid. Furthermore, real-time sonography can provide a dynamic view of intestinal peristalsis, which is not recognized with CT. These advantages of real-time sonography have made a revolutionary progress in the diagnosis of bowel obstruction, especially in the early recognition of strangulation small bowel obstruction.

Strangulation small bowel obstruction involves compromise of blood supply to the strangulated loop of bowel and requires early surgical intervention. A number of clinical studies have shown that it is difficult to recognize the early stages of strangulation because of lack of reliable criteria.[13] Difficulty in making the early diagnosis of strangulation has resulted in a recommendation of early surgical intervention. While this strategy seems logical in reducing delays in surgical repair, it increases the number of surgical cases for nonstrangulated obstruction that could have been relieved without operative therapy. On the other hand, in order to safely elect nonoperative treatment, the exclusion of strangulation is essential. Ogata and associates reported that abdominal sonography was useful in revealing the presence of strangulation that was not suspected by clinical judgment. Abdominal sonography was also useful for excluding the presence of strangulation in patients with simple obstruction who were clinically suspected of having strangulation.[24] According to their report, the sensitivity and specificity of sonography for strangulation were 90% and 92%, respectively, in the study using 231 patients with small bowel obstruction by adhesions. The use of sonography to differentiate strangulation from simple obstruction may permit earlier operative intervention for strangulation and allow wider use of nonoperative management for simple small bowel obstruction.

When abdominal sonography is applied for the evaluation of bowel obstruction, it is clinically important to analyze the following points in each case:

1. To identify the evidence of mechanical bowel obstruction
2. To locate the level of obstruction
3. To differentiate strangulation from simple obstruction
4. To evaluate the etiology of bowel obstruction
5. To estimate the severity of bowel obstruction
6. To survey the whole abdomen for other abnormalities

MECHANICAL BOWEL OBSTRUCTION VERSUS ILEUS

The clinical manifestations of a mechanical bowel obstruction depend on the level of the obstruction (proximal or distal small bowel or large bowel) and the blood supply to the affected loop of bowel (simple or strangulated obstruction). The evidence of a mechanical bowel obstruction is confirmed by demonstrating a distinct point of transition between dilated proximal bowel and collapsed distal bowel with an imaging modality such as plain radiography, sonography, or CT. In contrast, the diagnosis of ileus is based on the absence of such a distinct point of transition along with a clinical presentation consistent with ileus. Abdominal sonography, as well as plain radiography and CT, can be used for the differentiation of a mechanical bowel obstruction versus an ileus.[20,28,30] In the early stage of ileus, slightly dilated small bowel loops (less than 25 mm wide in diameter) are often recognized on ultrasound. Gas echoes,

which are more dominant than fluid collection inside the bowel, are featured in the sonographic images of ileus. Also, other abnormalities suggesting the primary etiology of ileus may be shown on ultrasound. In the advanced stage of ileus, real-time sonography may occasionally show fluid-filled, dilated bowel loops without peristaltic activity.

SMALL BOWEL OBSTRUCTION VERSUS LARGE BOWEL OBSTRUCTION

Initially, abdominal sonography was used in suggesting the diagnosis of small bowel obstruction in patients with atypical plain radiographs, such as a "pseudotumor" appearance or a totally "gasless" abdomen, and also in demonstrating an intussusception in patients with an abdominal mass suspected of the entity. Recent studies have suggested, however, that real-time bedside ultrasound can be used as an initial imaging method for the evaluation of small bowel obstruction.[21,23,25] According to the report by Ogata and associates, gastrointestinal gas interfered with ultrasound examinations in only 3 of 231 patients with small bowel obstruction by adhesions.[24]

As for patients clinically suspected of having a large bowel obstruction, plain radiographs are routinely used as the initial imaging modality as it serves to confirm the diagnosis and locate the obstruction in the majority of the cases. However, plain radiographs may show an isolated small bowel dilatation but no gaseous colonic dilatation in approximately 15% of patients with large bowel obstruction.[14,27] In such cases, it is difficult to differentiate a large bowel obstruction from a small bowel obstruction on plain radiographs alone. The use of sonography for the diagnosis of large bowel obstruction has not yet been fully evaluated because of the belief that accumulated gas in the colon interferes with the examination. Indeed, it is difficult to evaluate the gaseous distended colon with sonography. In cases of large bowel obstruction, however, abdominal sonography often reveals dilated colon as filled with dense spot echoes, which seem to represent feculent, liquid contents including small bubbles of gas. According to the study by Ogata and associates, abdominal sonography provided a diagnosis of large bowel obstruction in 33 of 39 patients with this condition, and proved useful in detecting radiograph-negative colonic dilatation that was occasionally seen in patients with large bowel obstruction proximal to the splenic flexure.[27]

STRANGULATION VERSUS SIMPLE OBSTRUCTION

Strangulated small bowel obstruction is most commonly caused by adhesive bands. The strangulated, closed loop may be occasionally shown as a "pseudotumor" appearance on plain radiographs. Numerous studies have shown the value and effectiveness of sonography in demonstrating the closed loop filled with fluid. Real-time sonography also can provide a dynamic view of peristalsis in the obstructed loops.

The sonographic criteria for simple small bowel obstruction include the presence of dilated small bowel proximal to collapsed small bowel or ascending colon, and the presence of peristaltic activity in the entire dilated proximal small bowel. The peristaltic activity is appreciated as peristalsis of the bowel wall or to-and-fro movements of spot echoes inside the fluid-filled dilated small bowel. The criteria for early strangulation include (1) the presence of an akinetic dilated loop, (2) the presence of peristaltic activity in dilated small bowel proximal to the akinetic loop, and (3) rapid accumulation of peritoneal fluid after the onset of obstruction. An established strangulation is recognized by asymmetric wall thickening (more than 3 mm) with increased echogenicity in the akinetic loop, or a large amount of peritoneal fluid containing scattered spot echoes indicating bloody ascites. Although the presence of peritoneal fluid is not specific for strangulation, the quantitative evaluation of peritoneal fluid will be helpful in differentiating strangulation from simple obstruction.

SPECIFIC ETIOLOGIES OF OBSTRUCTION

Abdominal sonography offers the advantage of providing additional information about specific etiologies of obstruction that is not obtained with plain radiographs. Although adhesions obstructing the small bowel cannot be visualized, sonography can image the specific etiologies of small bowel obstruction, which include cecal carcinoma, intussusception, external hernias, inflammatory bowel diseases (tuberculosis, Crohn's disease, or radiation enteritis), small bowel tumors, afferent loop obstruction following Billroth II gastrectomy, and gallstone ileus. Except intussusception and incarceration of external hernia, the specific etiologies are relatively rare but should be considered.

Intussusception is a common etiology of bowel obstruction in children but relatively rare in adults, accounting for only about 5% of all intussusception cases and 1–3% of adult patients with bowel obstruction. Unlike in children, the causative lesion can be identified in more than 80% of adult patients. The most common cause is a polypoid tumor of the small bowel. Ileocolic intussusception is the most common form (more than 70%), followed by enteroenteric and colocolic intussusception. Plain radiographs rarely define the intussusception as a mass of soft tissue density, and show no evidence of bowel obstruction in the acute stage. In contrast, abdominal sonography can present the characteristic appearances of intussusception. The cross-sectional image is well known as the "multiple concentric ring sign" or "target sign."[31,32] The multilaminar structure also can be demonstrated in the long-axis planes. It is very rare, however, to demonstrate the causative lesion itself (i.e., tumor or diverticulum) with sonography. The sonographic appearance of bowel obstruction may not yet be established when the diagnosis of intussusception is obtained.

Incarceration, which is a common complication of external hernias, produces a bowel obstruction and impairs the blood supply to the entrapped bowel segment. Among the common external hernias including external inguinal hernia, internal inguinal hernia, femoral hernia, and abdominal incisional hernia, incarceration occurs most frequently in cases of femoral hernia. The common hernia content is small bowel. The diagnosis is not difficult to make on the basis of a careful physical examination in most cases. If physical examination findings are equivocal, abdominal sonography can be used to demonstrate an incarcerated hernia, showing an entrapped bowel segment in the abdominal wall. On the other hand, obturator hernia is a rare entity among the external hernias, and hardly noticed as a mass because it is located deep in the femoral region. It is usually diagnosed as a small bowel obstruction by clinical symptoms, physical examination, and plain radiographs. However, abdominal sonography can demonstrate an entrapped small bowel segment medial to the femoral artery and vein, and posterior to the pectineus muscle in the femoral region.

As for the etiologies of large bowel obstruction, obstructing colon carcinoma, which is by far the most common cause of large bowel obstruction, may be detected as an irregular-shaped hypoechoic mass with echogenic core inside or a localized circular wall thickening. Intraluminal tumor obstructing the lumen may be occasionally demonstrated with sonography. Ogata and associates reported that sonography demonstrated the obstructing lesion in 14 of 35 patients with primary or metastatic colorectal carcinoma.[27] Even when the obstructing lesion is not visualized, detecting the associated lesions such as metastatic liver tumors would be useful in making the diagnosis. In volvulus of the sigmoid colon, however, sonography shows only vast gas echoes that spread beneath the abdominal wall because the twisted and obstructed colon loop is markedly distended with excessive gas. Plain radiography is diagnostic of this entity by presenting the classic "coffee bean" sign. In volvulus of the entire small bowel, a rare entity in the Western countries, sonography may show fluid-filled, dilated loops with mural thickening and peritoneal fluid. Peristaltic activity dwindles as the intestinal infarction progresses.

▶ INFLAMMATORY DISORDER

Various kinds of inflammatory disorders are included in the etiologies of acute abdomen. Abdominal sonography can be used for evaluating the site, extent, or severity of the inflammatory disorder by visualizing interstitial edema or hemorrhage, and peritoneal fluid. Segmental wall thickening of the bowel may be demonstrated in inflammatory gastrointestinal disorders such as appendicitis, diverticulitis, infectious enterocolitis, ischemic colitis, or Crohn's disease.[17] Also, wall thickening of the gallbladder can show the severity of acute cholecystitis, and the echogenicity of the pancreas can vary according to the degree of interstitial edema or hemorrhage in acute pancreatitis.

ACUTE APPENDICITIS

Acute appendicitis is the most common cause of the acute abdomen in Western countries. The diagnosis is straightforward in most patients who present with typical clinical symptoms and signs. It is not uncommon, however, to face difficulties in making a diagnosis of appendicitis in patients who have an equivocal presentation. Conventional radiographs present nonspecific findings, such as regional bowel dilatation, in most cases of acute appendicitis. The most specific finding on plain radiographs is the presence of a calcified appendicolith, which is noted in about 10% of adults with appendicitis.

On the other hand, abdominal sonography has been increasingly used for the diagnosis of acute appendicitis and, consequently, is considered to be useful for (1) direct visualization of the inflamed appendix, (2) assessment for the degree of inflammatory changes, (3) identification of abscess formation or free peritoneal fluid, (4) differentiation from other acute abdominal disorders, and (5) application to pregnant patients.

Since Puylaert reported that high-resolution ultrasound with a graded compression technique was successful in visualizing the abnormal appendix in a high percentage of cases, many physicians have adopted the technique and confirmed the high diagnostic accuracy of the technique for acute appendicitis.[33–38] The sensitivity and specificity of graded compression sonography in experienced hands were reported to be 76–90% and 90–98%, respectively, in prospective studies. In the United States, abdominal CT scan is commonly utilized for evaluating patients with possible appendicitis; its accuracy for confirming or ruling out appendicitis has been reported to be 93–98%.

The accuracy of sonography is examiner-dependent. Practically, inexperienced sonographers will face difficulties in obtaining such a high accuracy in the diagnosis of acute appendicitis.[39,40] The most important reason for a false-negative study is overlooking the inflamed appendix. Dilated bowel loops due to an associated ileus may obscure the appendix. Optimal images may not be obtained because of the inability to achieve adequate compression of the right lower quadrant. This is caused by severe pain or marked obesity. False-negative studies may also occur in patients with retrocecal or perforated appendicitis. A false-positive diagnosis can be made if a normal appendix is mistaken for an inflamed one or if a terminal ileum is confused with an enlarged inflamed appendix. With adequate training and enough experience, however, nonradiologist physicians can obtain an acceptable accuracy rate in comparison with experienced radiologists.[41–44]

Sonography is more sensitive for the detection of an appendicolith than plain radiographs, and has been reported as detecting intraluminal fecaliths in up to 30% of cases. In general, a normal appendix (about 6 mm or smaller) can rarely be visualized by graded compression sonography although some investigators have reported that in the majority of patients a normal appendix can be identified with modern equipment in experienced hands.[44,46]

Acute appendicitis may present in various stages at the time of diagnosis: catarrhal, phlegmonous, gangrenous, or perforated accompanying pericecal abscess or purulent peritonitis. Abdominal sonography can be used to evaluate the pathologic severity of acute appendicitis by delineating the layer structure of thickened appendiceal wall. In cases of catarrhal or phlegmonous appendicitis, a swollen appendix maintains the mural lamination. In contrast, focal loss of the layer structure is often observed in patients with gangrenous appendicitis. A pericecal abscess can be demonstrated as fluid collection with a thick, noncompressible wall. With a pericecal abscess secondary to perforated appendicitis, it may be quite difficult to identify the gangrenous appendix itself. Even if an inflamed appendix is not detected, identifying an abscess or free peritoneal fluid in the pelvis or the pericecal region can be valuable for surgeons to make a decision for urgent exploration. On the other hand, it is still controversial whether surgical intervention or conservative treatment with antibiotics should be adopted in the early stage of appendicitis. In general, sonographic findings should be correlated with both clinical and laboratory findings to determine an indication for surgery.

Acute appendicitis in pregnant women can be rather difficult to diagnose because of the deviated location of the appendix and equivocal presentation. Abdominal sonography can be applied for the evaluation of appendicitis in pregnant patients. In this setting, it is important to take the deviated location of the appendix into consideration.

Sonography is also useful for establishing an alternative diagnosis in patients examined with suspicion of appendicitis. The spectrum of differential diagnoses includes mesenteric lymphadenitis (particularly in children), right-sided adnexal pathology in young women, enterocolitis, diverticulitis, Crohn's disease, cholecystitis, and colon cancer.

ACUTE COLONIC DIVERTICULITIS

The prevalence of colonic diverticulosis increases with age. Acute colonic diverticulitis is a relatively common etiology of the acute abdomen in elderly patients, although approximately 80–90% of all diverticula remain asymptomatic for life. The rectosigmoid colon is the most frequently involved segment in acute colonic diverticulitis. Diverticulitis in the ascending colon and cecum is less frequently involved, but seen in younger patients. It is occasionally misdiagnosed as acute appendicitis since it is accompanied with the symptoms or signs similar to the entity.

Plain radiographs are of little value in obtaining direct findings of acute diverticulitis, but may demonstrate pneumoperitoneum or ileus in complicated cases. The use of contrast barium enema for demonstrating the extent of the disease is limited to the cases of clinically mild diverticulitis because it is hazardous in cases of possible colonic perforation. Water-soluble contrast enema is safe and available in complicated cases, although the quality of images is inferior to barium contrast enema.

Abdominal sonography can be applied for the initial evaluation of possible diverticulitis. Both the sensitivity and specificity of sonography for this etiology was reported as greater than 80% when the examination was performed by experienced sonographers.[47,48] Abdominal sonography may reveal additional findings such as pericolonic abscess or free peritoneal fluid in complicated cases. CT is more optimal in demonstrating not only colonic diverticula but also extracolonic complications including pericolonic or pelvic abscess, free perforation, or colovesical fistula.

ACUTE PANCREATITIS

Acute pancreatitis is defined as an inflammation of the pancreas associated with typical abdominal complaints and elevated serum and urinary pancreatic enzymes, and may be classified according to the clinical pictures, etiologic factors, or pathologic changes. The clinical course ranges from a mild, benign process to a severe, fulminant process that may lead to fatal outcomes. The two most common etiologic factors are alcoholism and biliary stone disease, although up to 10–30% of patients with acute pancreatitis may present without a history of either.

The pathologic forms are classified generally as edematous and necrotizing pancreatitis. Edematous pancreatitis is characterized by interstitial edema and mild pancreatic and peripancreatic inflammation, and accounts for 80–85% of cases. The mortality rate is less than 2%. Necrotizing pancreatitis is characterized by interstitial hemorrhage, fat necrosis, extensive extrapancreatic infiltration, and suppuration. Bacterial infection occurs in up to 40% of patients with necrotizing pancreatitis and is gradually manifested within several weeks after the onset of pancreatitis. On the whole, necrotizing pancreatitis is a far more severe form of acute pancreatitis that often requires hemodynamic support and mechanical ventilation, and leads to severe complications and mortality rates of 10–40%.[49,50] Although it is clinically important to distinguish patients with either edematous or necrotizing pancreatitis in terms of therapy and prognosis, it is rather difficult at the early stage of their clinical course. Quantitative assays of serum pancreatic enzymes may be useful for the diagnosis of acute pancreatitis, but the degree of the enzymes does not correlate with the severity of the disease. Plain radiographs may show nonspecific findings such as the "sentinel loop sign," "colon cut-off sign," or a generalized ileus, but are of little use in evaluating acute pancreatitis.

Direct imaging of the pancreas with CT or sonography may provide morphologic information to establish the diagnosis of pancreatitis and its complications.[50–52] In general, CT is clearly superior to sonography in demonstrating complex extrapancreatic involvement as well as contour irregularities or focal changes in the pancreas. Ultrasound examinations are frequently disturbed by excessive gastrointestinal gas caused by an accompanying ileus, especially in cases of severe pancreatitis. Therefore, the main role of emergency ultrasound is to evaluate the biliary tree for gallstone disease as a remediable cause. Sonographic diagnosis of choledocholithiasis or significant dilatation of the common bile duct may obviate the need for invasive diagnostic procedures.

Abdominal sonography can also be used for the initial survey of acute pancreatitis. The echogenicity of the pancreas generally decreases in acute pancreatitis as a result of interstitial edema. In some patients, the echogenicity is normal or increased. Cotton and coworkers noted that the echogenicity of the pancreas compared to the liver was increased in 16% and normal in 32% of patients with acute pancreatitis.[51] The variability may be caused by pancreatic hemorrhage, necrosis, or fat saponification. Enlargement of the pancreas in acute pancreatitis is also variable, and significant individual variations are recognized in pancreatic dimensions. Therefore, enlargement is of limited value for the diagnosis of acute pancreatitis. Clinically important findings obtained with sonography are peripancreatic fluid collections or echogenic pancreatic masses, which suggest the progress of necrotizing pancreatitis. Such sonographic findings should be confirmed with both contrast and noncontrast CT for the definitive diagnosis.

Extrapancreatic fluid collections are most commonly detected in the superior recess of the lesser sac and the anterior pararenal space. Fluid collections are generally visualized as anechoic or hypoechoic images on ultrasound. CT is more advantageous in locating fluid collections to specific anatomic compartments. It is difficult, however, to distinguish pancreatic abscess from uninfected necrosis or fluid collections, although pancreatic abscess are often associated with extensive, ill-defined multicompartmental changes. CT-guided fine-needle aspiration is used to make an early diagnosis of pancreatic abscess.

On the other hand, acute peripancreatic fluid collections resolve with conservative therapy in 70–90% of the cases. The remaining fluid collections persist long enough (at least 6 weeks) to develop a fibrous wall, and then are called pancreatic pseudocysts. Pseudocysts may develop in association with chronic pancreatitis, or after pancreatic surgery or trauma. Uncomplicated small pseudocysts (smaller than 6 cm) may allow persistent observation, but larger pseudocysts should be drained by surgical, endoscopic, or percutaneous means to reduce the risk of complications, which include secondary infection, rupture, and hemorrhage.[49,50] Serial examinations with CT or sonography can document the gradual development of pseudocysts. The advantage of sonography is lower cost for follow-up studies. On sonographic images, pancreatic pseudocysts are generally visualized as cystic masses of various sizes, which are well defined by adjacent organs and a visible capsule. However, small well-defined cystic masses should be examined with color Doppler scanning to exclude a pancreatic pseudoaneurysm, which may occasionally develop 2–3 weeks after the onset of severe pancreatitis.

ACUTE CHOLECYSTITIS

Since acute cholecystitis may lead to serious complications such as sepsis, pericholecystic abscess, or bilious peritonitis secondary to gallbladder perforation, immediate surgery is often required. Therefore, it is critically important to make a rapid and accurate diagnosis of acute cholecystitis and to determine the indication for surgical intervention. Abdominal sonography is a rapid and reliable technique for establishing or excluding the diagnosis of acute cholecystitis, even though sonographic findings should be always correlated with clinical and laboratory findings (see also Chapter 8).

There are three important indirect signs to establish the diagnosis of acute cholecystitis.[53,54] Gallstones are the prime etiologic factor since approximately 90% of cases with acute cholecystitis develop as a complication of cholelithiasis. The identification of impacted stones in the gallbladder neck or cystic duct is highly specific for acute calculous cholecystitis, although sonography may be unable to detect a small impacted gallstone in a few cases of calculous cholecystitis. Biliary sludge along with the absence of gallstones in the expanded gallbladder can be identified in cases of acalculous cholecystitis. The most specific sign of acute cholecystitis is the "sonographic Murphy's sign," which corresponds to the spot of maximum tenderness directly over the gallbladder (Murphy's sign is elicited with focal tenderness over the gallbladder with inspiratory arrest). According to the report by Ralls and associates, 99% of patients with acute cholecystitis had calculi and a positive sonographic Murphy's sign.[54] In cases of acalculous cholecystitis, however, focal tenderness over the gallbladder may be difficult to obtain.

Thickening of the gallbladder wall to more than 3 mm is another sign for acute cholecystitis, although it is not specific as long as the wall maintains a distinct trilaminar structure with a hypoechoic band surrounded by two hyperechoic lines. Irregular sonolucent layers in the gallbladder wall may be indicative of more advanced cholecystitis. The presence of asymmetric thickening of the gallbladder wall or intraluminal membranes parallel to the gallbladder wall may be identified in patients with acute gangrenous cholecystitis. Localized pericholecystic fluid collection may be caused by gallbladder perforation and abscess formation. The site of perforation may occasionally be visualized as a defect in the gallbladder wall. These sonographic findings can be indicative of the need for immediate surgery.

▶ CIRCULATORY IMPAIRMENT

Another relatively common and clinically important entity is ischemic bowel disease, which can be lethal if not promptly diagnosed and appropriately treated by surgical exploration or interventional radiology. Embolism of the superior mesenteric artery and ischemic colitis are the most commonly encountered events in the emergency department.

EMBOLISM OF THE SUPERIOR MESENTERIC ARTERY

Acute mesenteric ischemia is notoriously difficult to diagnose early in its clinical course, and subsequently often results in delayed surgical intervention in a number of cases. Patients with this entity present with sudden onset of abdominal pain, diarrhea, or vomiting. However, the symptoms are nonspecific and there may be a striking disparity between the severity of symptoms and the lack of direct physical findings. Progressive signs of shock may be apparent in the initial stage. Therefore, it is clinically important to suspect an embolism of the superior mesenteric artery (SMA) when elderly patients with mitral valve disorders or atrial fibrillation present with nonspecific abdominal symptoms.

Routine abdominal sonography do not provide specific findings in cases of an SMA embolism. In the initial stage, fluid-filled dilatation of the small bowel is minimal. Peritoneal fluid and mural thickening in the small bowel without peristaltic activity are nonspecific, but suggest the possibility of acute mesenteric ischemia. Compared with strangulation small bowel obstruction, dilatation of the small bowel is not recognized as significant. In the advanced stages, a large amount of peritoneal fluid can be demonstrated. Color Doppler can be used to demonstrate an occlusion of the main trunk of the SMA.[55] However, it is not so easy to confirm the etiology by the examination because excessive gastrointestinal gas caused by an accompanying ileus disturbs the examinations.

Contrast and noncontrast CT can demonstrate decreased enhancement in the vascular territories of the SMA, and may directly demonstrate an occluding thrombus within the SMA, pneumatosis of the bowel wall, or gas in the portal vein in conjunction with peritoneal fluid, bowel wall thickening, or dilatation of fluid-filled loops of the small bowel. When the disease is suspected, immediate angiography should be applied for the definite diagnosis of SMA embolism.

ISCHEMIC COLITIS

Ischemic colitis is characterized by the abrupt onset of crampy abdominal pain and diarrhea that often contains blood. Since the clinical features are nonspecific and few symptoms may be present initially, it is especially important to consider this entity in elderly patients. Unlike small bowel ischemia, most cases of colonic ischemia are not associated with a visible arterial occlusion. The pathophysiology is believed to relate to decreased perfusion of the colon wall due to peripheral vasoconstriction (e.g., in cardiac failure), sepsis, or hypovolemia. Age-related atherosclerotic disease is a predisposing factor. The effects range from reversible mucosal ischemia to transmural infarction. Strictures and stenoses can follow the resolution of conservatively managed cases.

Abdominal sonography may suggest ischemic colitis by demonstrating segmental wall thickening of the affected colon. Colonoscopy and contrast studies remain the primary methods to evaluate patients with clinically suspected ischemic colitis. The most common site of involvement is the distal colon within the vascular territory of the inferior mesenteric artery. The proximal colon to the splenic flexure area (the so-called "watershed zone") may be involved. As routine sonography cannot reliably differentiate inflammatory changes from ischemic changes, color Doppler should be applied for the differentiation between colonic diverticulitis and ischemic colitis.[56] Mural blood flow is diminished in the affected

segment of ischemic colitis. Both routine sonography and color Doppler scanning can be used for a follow-up study of ischemic colitis. In cases of reversible mucosal ischemia, wall thickening is gradually reduced approximately in 1 week. In cases of transmural infarction, sonography may show rapid accumulation of peritoneal fluid. CT can be used for the same purpose and is more sensitive for complications such as perforation or abscess formation.

▶ ANATOMIC CONSIDERATIONS

FREE PERITONEAL FLUID

The site of accumulation of peritoneal fluid, which is discussed in Chapter 5, is dependent on the position of the patient and the etiology that causes free fluid to accumulate. In the supine patient, peritoneal fluid in the pelvis or Morison's pouch is most easily detected by sonography.

STOMACH

The gastric antrum is generally located posterocaudally to the left lobe of the liver. The proximal stomach is usually difficult to delineate because of the significant artifact arising from gas in the stomach. When filled with liquid contents, the proximal stomach can be identified medially to the splenic hilum with left intercostal or coronal scanning.

DUODENUM

The duodenal bulb is located medially to the gallbladder, posterior to the liver, and anterior to the pancreatic head. The inferior vena cava is another landmark located posterior to the duodenal C-loop.

SMALL BOWEL

Normal small bowel loops are generally recognized as a tubular structure with peristalsis. However, the sonographic images of the small bowel vary depending on the nature and volume of the intestinal contents.

LARGE BOWEL

The ascending colon is easily demonstrated anterior to the right kidney in the right flank. The transverse colon can be identified caudally to the gastric antrum in a sagittal plane. The descending colon can be demonstrated anterior to the lower pole of the left kidney in the left flank. The sigmoid colon may be difficult to examine. The rectum can be demonstrated posterior to the uterus or prostate. The normal colonic wall thickness is up to 3 mm.

APPENDIX VERMIFORMIS

The position of the appendix is highly variable. The most common position is caudal to the cecum and terminal ileum, followed by a retrocecal position. Other less common positions are deep within the pelvis, lateral to the cecum, and mesocecal. The psoas muscle and the external iliac artery and vein are important anatomic landmarks when searching for the appendix.

PANCREAS

The pancreas is easily located by its vascular landmarks. In transverse planes, the pancreas lies posterocaudal to the left lobe of the liver and cross over the aorta and the inferior vena cava. The splenic vein is a useful landmark for identifying the pancreas as it runs along the posterior surface of the pancreas. In sagittal planes, the pancreatic body is located posterior to the gastric antrum and the left lobe of the liver, and anterior to the splenic vein and the superior mesenteric artery. The pancreatic head lies anterior to the inferior vena cava and caudal to the portal vein. The pancreatic duct runs along the length of the gland, and is best imaged in the pancreatic body. With modern ultrasound equipment, the duct can be frequently visualized as a tubular structure with reflective walls with maximum diameter up to 2 mm. The anteroposterior diameters of the head and body are, in general, less than 3 and 2 cm, respectively. Wide normal variations are noted in pancreatic dimensions, and tend to decrease with age. The normal pancreas is homogeneous with the echogenicity greater than or equal to the adjacent liver.

▶ GETTING STARTED

In the emergency and acute care setting, a rapid, focused inspection and systematic survey of the entire abdomen are required for obtaining useful information. Among a number of factors that influence the accuracy of emergency ultrasound, the most critical is the sonologist's experience, which includes not only the technique of scanning but also the knowledge of the clinical and pathologic findings in acute abdominal disorders.

Positioning of the patient during the emergency ultrasound examination is important for obtaining optimal images. A patient is generally placed in the supine position. To avoid interference by gas echoes, they may be placed in the semi-lateral, lateral, or semi-erect positions.

Oblique or coronal planes are more frequently used than sagittal or transverse planes, especially in patients who have a bowel obstruction or ileus. The standard examination is performed using a sweeping motion with a 3.5 MHz probe. A higher-frequency (greater than 7 MHz) probe should be used for delineating the laminar structure of the appendix, intestinal wall, or specific lesions of the abdominal wall.

Focused assessment with sonography is recommended according to the purposes, situations, and various levels of examiners. An unnecessary, time-consuming examination for obtaining unfocused findings should be avoided so as not to delay patient treatment. Inexperienced sonologists should begin with the survey for free intraperitoneal fluid, and then proceed to the focused assessment for gallstone-related disorders, hydronephrosis, dilated small bowel, or large abdominal tumors. Peritoneal fluid is the first priority to evaluate in cases of acute abdomen as well as trauma, since the presence, amount, and location of accumulated intraperitoneal fluid are correlated with the etiology or severity of acute abdominal disorders.

▶ TECHNIQUE AND NORMAL ULTRASOUND FINDINGS

FOCUSED EXAMINATION FOR THE ACUTE ABDOMEN

When presented with an acute abdomen, a rapid inspection for free intraperitoneal fluid should be performed in a manner similar to the FAST examination (see also Chapter 5). The right intercostal and coronal views should be used to examine for free intraperitoneal fluid in Morison's pouch and the right subphrenic space. From these views, the right kidney and the right lobe of the liver can be inspected briefly. The left intercostal and left coronal views should be used to examine for free intraperitoneal fluid in the left subphrenic space and the splenorenal recess. From these views, the spleen and the left kidney can be inspected briefly. Then, the pelvic (sagittal and transverse) views should be used to examine for free intraperitoneal fluid in the pelvis. From these views, the bladder and the prostate or uterus can be inspected briefly. Next, a focused inspection for acute abdominal disorders should be performed in a systematic fashion. The areas to be examined first should be determined according to the clinical findings, but the entire abdomen should be surveyed to exclude less suspicious disorders in the differential diagnosis. Subphrenic free air is best visualized on the ventral surface of the liver with right intercostal scanning. The patient may be placed in the semi-lateral position elevating the right flank.

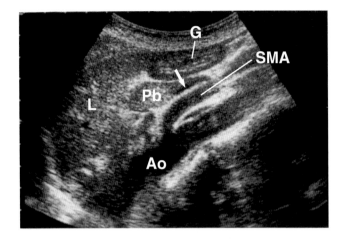

A

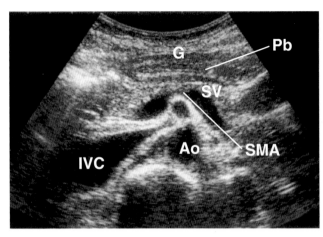

B

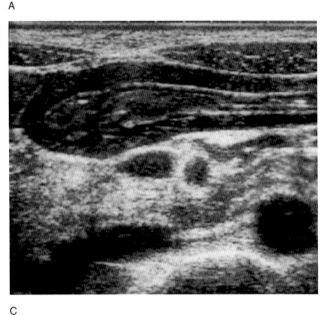

C

Figure 9-1. Normal gastric antrum. (A) In an epigastric sagittal plane, the cross section of antrum (G) is visualized anterior to the pancreatic body (Pb) and caudal to the left lobe of the liver (L). The pancreatic body is located anterior and cephalad to the splenic vein (arrow) and the superior mesenteric artery (SMA). (B) In a transverse plane, the gastric antrum is demonstrated anterior to the pancreatic body. (C) Five-layer structure of the gastric wall is demonstrated in a transverse scanning with a high-frequency probe. Ao = aorta, IVC = inferior vena cava, SV = splenic vein.

EPIGASTRIC REGION

In scanning the epigastric region, the gastric antrum can be demonstrated anterior to the pancreatic body and caudal to the left lobe of the liver (Figure 9-1). Intricate details of the structure of the gastric wall can be demonstrated using a high-frequency probe. The duodenal bulb may be visualized between the gallbladder and the gastric antrum. It is difficult to clearly visualize the duodenal C-loop except when it is dilated with accumulated fluid (Figure 9-2). It may be visualized anterior to the inferior vena cava in a coronal or oblique plane from the right anterior flank.

BOWEL OBSTRUCTION

For cases of possible bowel obstruction, the examination begins from scanning the ascending colon and the hepatic flexure in the right flank. The hepatic flexure is viewed at the ventral side of the right kidney, and then the longitudinal views of the ascending colon are obtained by positioning the probe caudally in the mid- to posterior axillary line. A sequence of gas echoes separated with the haustra folds can be seen inside the hypoechoic wall (Figure 9-3). When a distended ascending colon is identified, the scanning proceeds to the left flank to inspect the descending colon. The approximate site of obstruction can be evaluated on the basis of whether or not the descending colon is distended. When an ascending colon is not distended, the ileocecal region should be carefully examined to guard against overlooking collapsed ileal loops or specific lesions. The scanning then proceeds to survey the degree of dilatation, peristaltic activities, wall thickening, or specific lesions in the small bowel loops, and peritoneal fluid between the loops. When appropriate, a high-frequency probe may be used to demonstrate the layer structure of

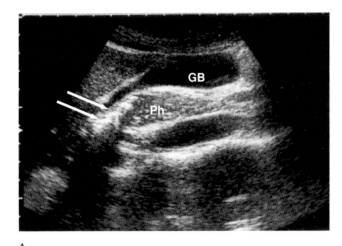

A

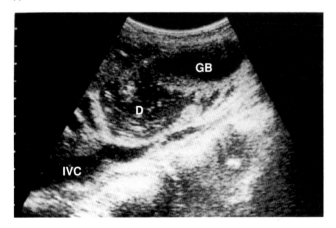

B

Figure 9-2. Duodenum. Longitudinal views. (A) A normal proximal duodenum (arrows) is visualized between the gallbladder (GB) and the pancreatic head (Ph). The posterior wall of the duodenum is usually impossible to demonstrate because of the gas in the lumen. (B) A slightly dilated duodenal C-loop (D) is visualized anterolateral to the inferior vena cava (IVC) and posterior to the gallbladder.

the bowel wall (Figure 9-4). Real-time sonography may demonstrate peristaltic activity as peristalsis of the bowel wall or to-and-fro movements of intestinal contents. Akinesis of the loop can be established with observation for several minutes or serial observations in order to avoid overlooking intermittent peristaltic activity.

APPENDICITIS

For cases of possible appendicitis, the standard examination with a 3.5 or 3.75 MHz probe is initially performed to survey the anatomic orientation in the right lower quadrant. The psoas muscle and the external iliac artery and vein are important landmarks when searching for the

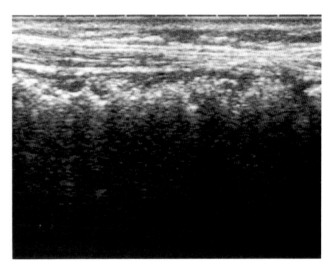

Figure 9-3. Normal ascending colon. A sequence of gas echoes separated with the Haustra folds is seen inside the hypoechoic wall.

appendix (Figure 9-5). A graded-compression technique with a high-frequency probe is usually applied when searching for an inflamed appendix. Gentle, progressive application and withdrawal of pressure is important not to elicit peritoneal irritation for the patient. Graded compression can express all overlying fluid or gas from normal bowel to visualize the inflamed noncompressible appendix. The terminal ileum can be recognized as crossing over the psoas muscle to the cecum. Just caudal to this area is the cecal tip. To locate a tip of the appendix, a careful inspection with graded-compression technique should be done to the point of maximal abdominal tenderness.

PANCREATITIS

For cases of possible pancreatitis, it may be difficult to obtain optimal sonographic images of the pancreas because of the significant artifacts arising from gastrointestinal gas. To avoid such interference, the semi-erect position can be adopted to visualize the pancreatic head and body. In this position, gas in the stomach rises to the fundus and the left lobe of the liver often provide an acoustic window for imaging the pancreas and the lesser sac. The standard planes are sagittal and transverse along the vascular landmarks (Figure 9-1A and 9-6). The tail of the pancreas can be best visualized with a coronal view in a right posterior oblique position. The spleen is used as an acoustic window in this position. The anterior pararenal space is best imaged through a coronal flank approach.

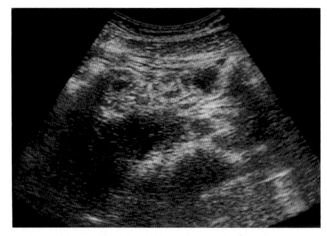

A

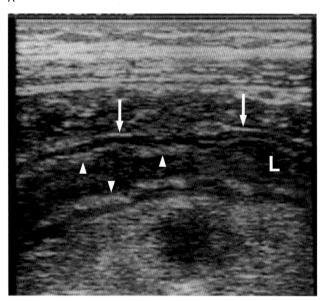

B

Figure 9-4. Normal small bowel loop. (A) No unified images of the small bowel are obtained with routine sonography using a 3.5 MHz probe. (B) Wall structure of the small bowel is demonstrated with a high-frequency probe. The lumen (L) is bounded by the broad hyperechoic mucosal layer (arrowheads), and then surrounded by the hypoechoic muscular layer, which is bounded externally by the fine, hyperechoic reflection from the serosa (arrows).

▶ COMMON ABNORMALITIES

FREE PERITONEAL FLUID

Free peritoneal fluid is delineated as an anechoic stripe with sharp edges (Figure 9-7). Intraperitoneal hemorrhage, bloody or purulent ascites, or peritoneal fluid containing intestinal contents may be shown as having gray level echoes inside.

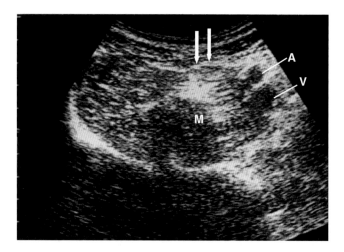

Figure 9-5. Transverse ultrasonogram of the right lower quadrant. The psoas muscle (M) and external iliac artery (A) and vein (V) are important anatomic landmarks for the appendix. The terminal ileum (arrows) crosses over the psoas muscle to the cecum.

PNEUMOPERITONEUM

Subphrenic free air can be identified as an echogenic line with posterior reverberation artifacts on the ventral surface of the liver, separated from gas echoes in the gastrointestinal lumen at the caudal side and those in the lung at the cephalic side (Figure 9-8).

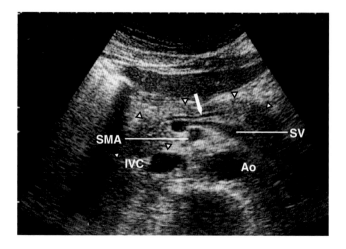

Figure 9-6. Normal pancreas. In a transverse plane the pancreas (arrowheads) lies caudal to the left lobe of the liver and crosses over the aorta (Ao) and the inferior vena cava (IVC). The splenic vein (SV) runs along the posterior surface of the pancreas. The pancreatic duct (arrow) is visualized as a tubular structure with reflective walls. SMA = superior mesenteric artery.

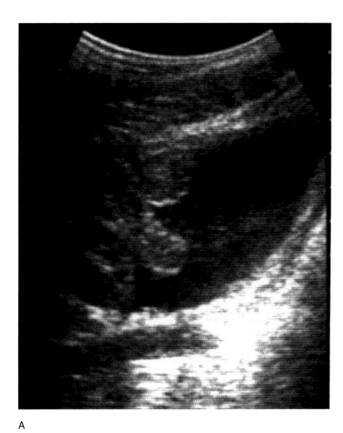

A

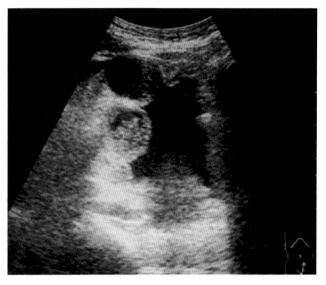

B

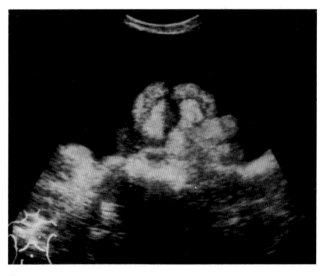

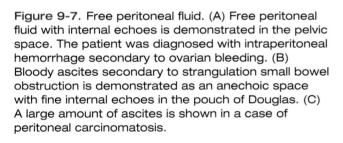

C

Figure 9-7. Free peritoneal fluid. (A) Free peritoneal fluid with internal echoes is demonstrated in the pelvic space. The patient was diagnosed with intraperitoneal hemorrhage secondary to ovarian bleeding. (B) Bloody ascites secondary to strangulation small bowel obstruction is demonstrated as an anechoic space with fine internal echoes in the pouch of Douglas. (C) A large amount of ascites is shown in a case of peritoneal carcinomatosis.

Gas in the abscess or free peritoneal fluid may be occasionally recognized as echogenic spots inside the anechoic or hypoechoic fluid (Figure 9-9).

SMALL BOWEL OBSTRUCTION

In cases of small bowel obstruction, dilated small bowel proximal to collapsed small bowel or ascending colon can be identified (Figure 9-10). Dilated small bowel is usually visualized as fluid-filled dilated loops with the maximal diameter greater than 25 mm (usually greater than 30 mm) at the time of diagnosis of small bowel obstruction. In the early stage of distal small bowel obstruction, no dilated loops may be observed in the proximal jejunum. The sonographic images of dilated loops vary depending on the degree of distension and the nature of intestinal contents (Figure 9-11). The well-known "keyboard sign" is not essential for the diagnosis of small bowel obstruction. The sonographic appearance of Kerckring's folds varies depending on scanning planes and intestinal contents, and they are rarely visualized in the distal ileum.[17] The criterion for simple obstruction is the presence of peristaltic activity in the entire dilated proximal small bowel (Figure 9-12).

STRANGULATION OBSTRUCTION

A strangulated loop is demonstrated as an akinetic dilated small bowel loop with real-time sonography (Figure 9-13A, B). In contrast, peristaltic activity can be recognized in the dilated small bowel proximal to the

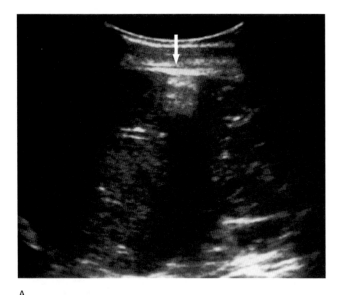

A

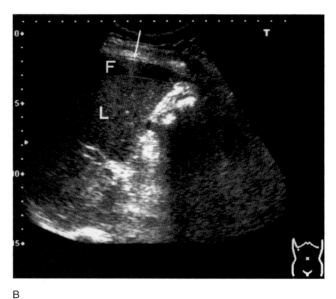

B

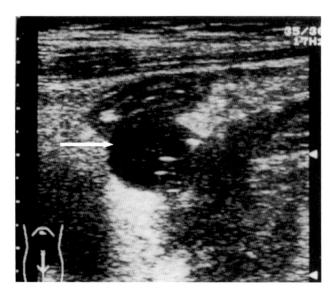

C

Figure 9-8. Pneumoperitoneum. (A) Subphrenic free air (arrow) is recognized at the ventral side of the liver in a case of perforated duodenal ulcer. (B) A small collection of free air (arrow) within the peritoneal fluid (F) is recognized in the subphrenic space. (C) Longitudinal epigastric view. A perforated duodenal ulcer is delineated as penetrating gas echoes (arrow) in the thickened wall of the duodenal bulb with echogenic lumen. D = duodenal bulb, L = liver, Ao = aorta

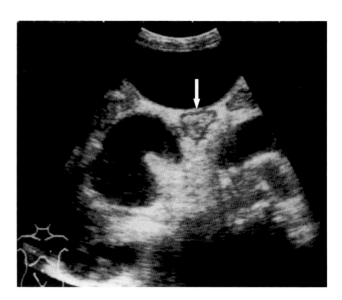

Figure 9-9. Gas echoes in an abscess. Gas in a paracolonic abscess is demonstrated as echogenic spots inside the hypoechoic fluid (arrow) in a case of perforated colonic diverticulitis.

Figure 9-10. Mechanical small bowel obstruction. Both dilated small bowel and a collapsed one (arrow) are demonstrated in the right lower abdomen.

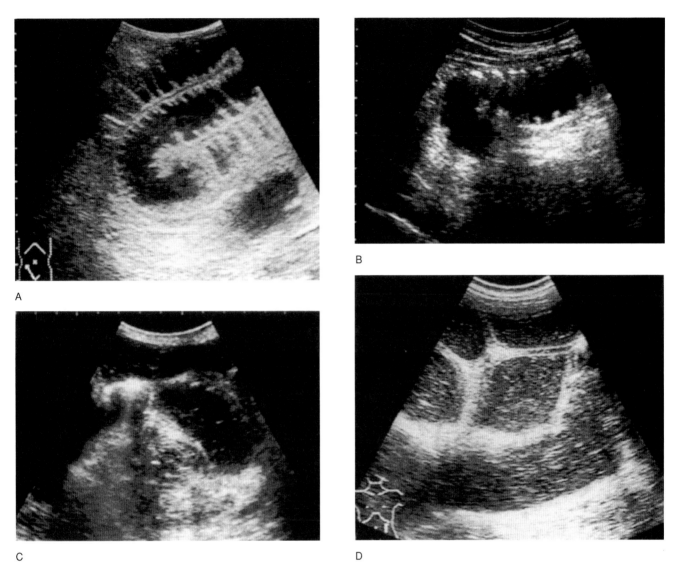

Figure 9-11. Varied sonographic images of dilated small bowel. (A) The "keyboard sign" is characteristic of fluid-filled, dilated jejunum. (B) The sonographic image of small bubbles of gas entrapped between the Kerckring's folds inside dilated small bowel loops is similar to the "string of beads sign" on plain radiographs. (C) In mild or early stages of small bowel obstruction, gas echoes may be more dominant than anechoic fluid in the dilated loops. (D) Dilated small bowel may be filled with spot echoes when intestinal contents become more feculent.

akinetic loop. Peritoneal fluid can be demonstrated in most cases and rapidly accumulates after the onset of obstruction. In cases of an established strangulation, real-time sonography may demonstrate wall thickening with increased echogenicity and flattened folds within the akinetic loop, and/or a large amount of peritoneal fluid (Figure 9-13C).

LARGE BOWEL OBSTRUCTION

In cases of large bowel obstruction, the dilated colon proximal to the obstruction is usually delineated as filled with dense spot echoes around the periphery of the abdomen (Figure 9-14A), whereas the dilated small bowel loops are located more centrally. Haustral indentations may be visualized as widely spaced in the dilated ascending colon. Real-time sonography can occasionally reveal to-and-fro movements of the intestinal contents through the ileocecal valve when the valve is incompetent (Figure 9-14B). In cases of large bowel obstruction distal to the splenic flexure, however, sonography may show a dilated colon simply as wide gas echoes around the periphery of the abdomen (Figure 9-14C).

The criterion for large bowel obstruction is the presence of dilated colon proximal to normal or collapsed

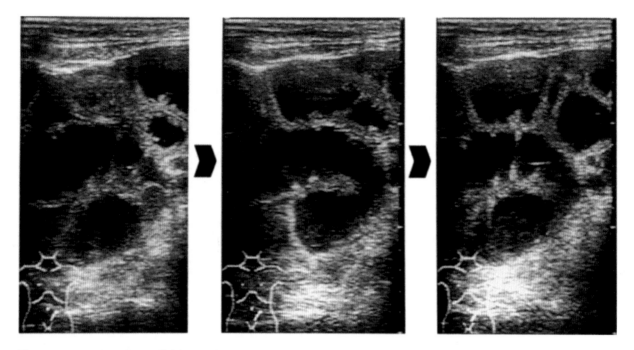

Figure 9-12. Simple small bowel obstruction. Selected images from real-time sonography reveal intermittently increased peristaltic activity of the entire dilated small bowel proximal to the obstruction.

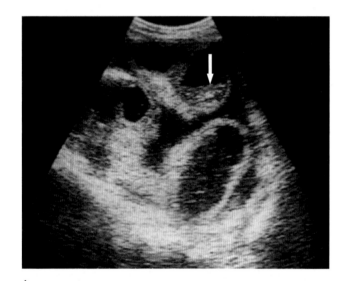

A

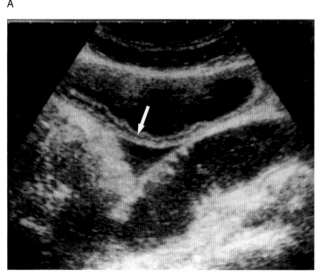

B

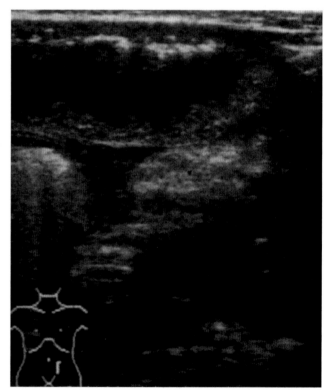

C

Figure 9-13. Strangulation small bowel obstruction. (A) Real-time sonography reveals an akinetic dilated loop accompanied by a large amount of peritoneal fluid in the cul-de-sac. Inside the akinetic loop, spot echoes are demonstrated as deposited like sludge (arrow). (B) Submucosal edema caused by mild strangulation is demonstrated as a hypoechoic layer (arrow) of the wall. (C) In a case of established strangulation with hemorrhagic necrosis, wall thickening with increased echogenicity and flattened folds is visualized within the akinetic loop (7.5 MHz).

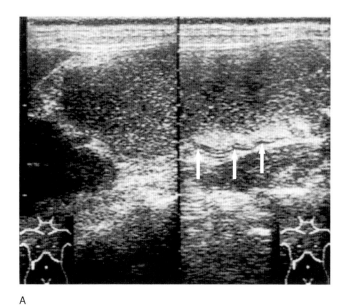

A

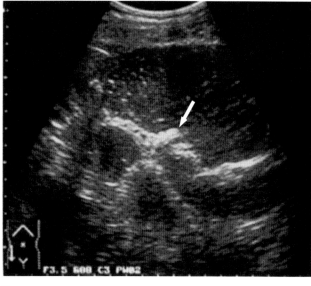

B

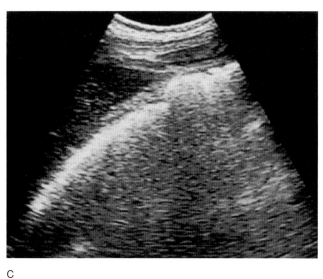

C

Figure 9-14. Dilated ascending colon. (A) A dilated ascending colon filled with feculent, liquid contents is delineated as filled with dense spot echoes. Haustral indentations (arrows) may be visualized in the dilated ascending colon. (B) To-and-fro movements of the internal spot echoes through the ileocecal valve (arrow) are occasionally identified with real-time sonography. (C) A dilated ascending colon with excessive gas inside is recognized as wide gas echoes around the periphery of the abdomen.

large bowel. Ascending colon and descending colon are the initial checkpoints for the sonographic evaluation of large bowel obstruction. The site of obstruction can be estimated on the basis of distribution of the dilated colon (greater than 50 mm for the ascending colon). Clinically, it is unnecessary to strictly define the accurate site or cause of obstruction with sonography because water-soluble contrast enema demonstrates the degree and level of obstruction and helps to clarify its cause.

SPECIFIC ETIOLOGIES OF BOWEL OBSTRUCTION

Intussusception

The cross-sectional image of intussusception is known as the "multiple concentric ring sign" or "target sign"

(Figure 9-15A). Multilaminar structure may be demonstrated with scanning along the long axis of the intussusception (Figure 9-15B).

Incarcerated Hernia

An incarcerated small bowel segment can be demonstrated as entrapped within the hernia sac in the abdominal wall (Figure 9-16). An incarcerated obturator hernia is delineated posterior to the pectineus muscle in the femoral region. In contrast, an incarcerated femoral hernia is located in the subcutaneous space anterior to the muscle.

Afferent Loop Obstruction

Afferent loop obstruction after a Billroth II gastrojejunostomy may result from adhesions or recurrent carcinoma.

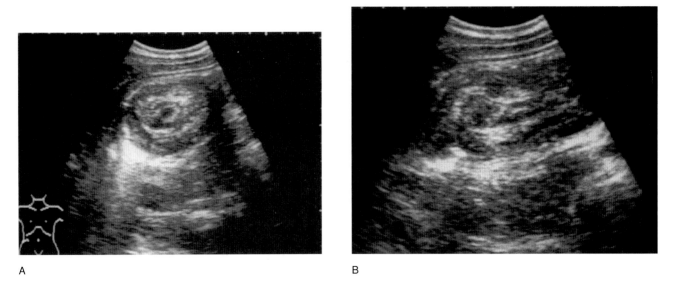

A

B

Figure 9-15. Ileocolic intussusception in an adult patient. (A) A cross-sectional image of intussusception is demonstrated as a "multiple concentric ring sign." (B) Multiple layer structure of intussusception in the long axis plane is demonstrated.

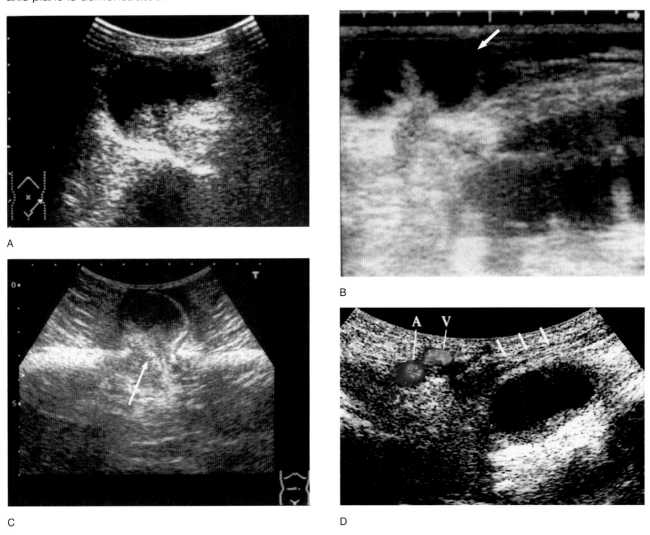

A

B

C

D

Figure 9-16. Incarcerated hernia. (A) An incarcerated femoral hernia is demonstrated as a small bowel segment herniated through the femoral canal. (B) In an incarcerated incisional hernia, a small bowel segment (arrow) is demonstrated as herniated through a small orifice in the abdominal wall. Dilated small bowel loops proximal to the incarceration are also shown in the peritoneal cavity. (C) In an umbilical hernia, a herniated small bowel segment is demonstrated within the fluid space in the hernia sac. The segment was softly strangulated at the hernia orifice (arrow) formed by defect of the fascia, and was easily reduced by manipulation in the case. (D) An incarcerated obturator hernia is demonstrated deep in the femoral region. It locates posterior to the pectineus muscle (arrows) and medial to the femoral artery (A) and vein (V).

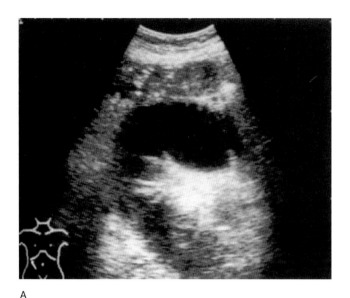
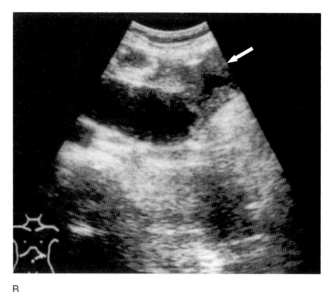

A

B

Figure 9-17. Afferent loop obstruction. (A) Dilated duodenal C-loop and (B) dilated jejunum proximal to the anastomosis are demonstrated in a case of recurrent carcinoma (arrow) at the site of anastomosis.

Abdominal sonography can show a dilated duodenum and jejunum proximal to the anastomosis (Figure 9-17). The diagnosis of afferent loop obstruction can be made on the basis of the sonographic features and the clinical findings consistent with acute pancreatitis in patients with a prior history of a Billroth II gastrectomy.

Gallstone Ileus

Gallstone ileus is a rare complication of acute cholecystitis. The sonographic features diagnostic of gallstone ileus include pneumobilia, small bowel obstruc-

tion, and a large calculus (average diameter greater than 3 cm) obstructing the small bowel (Figure 9-18A). The most common site of impaction is the ileocecal valve. Biliary-enteric fistula may be suggested by gas echoes inside the intra- or extrahepatic biliary tree (Figure 9-18B).

Small Bowel Tumor

It is rare for a small bowel tumor to cause a bowel obstruction. Malignant small bowel tumor, such as metastatic carcinoma, malignant lymphoma or leiomyosarcoma,

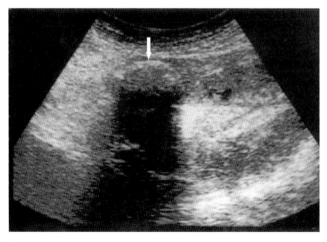
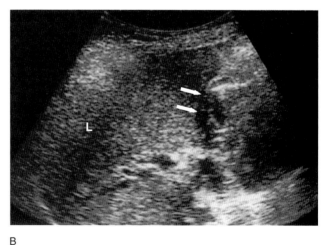

A

B

Figure 9-18. Gallstone ileus. (A) The impacted gallstone (arrow) obstructing the small bowel is directly visualized with a prominent acoustic shadow inside the dilated small bowel. (B) Gas echoes in the atrophic gallbladder (arrows) are recognized as showing the presence of a biliary-enteric fistula between the gallbladder and the duodenum (or less commonly the stomach, jejunum). L = liver.

may occasionally be identified by sonography (Figure 9-19).

Inflammatory Bowel Disease

Segmental wall thickening of the small bowel may be identified in cases of inflammatory bowel disease such as intestinal tuberculosis, Crohn's disease, or radiation enteritis (Figure 9-20).

Colon Cancer

Colorectal cancer is by far the most common cause of large bowel obstruction, and may be detected as an irregular-shaped hypoechoic mass with echogenic core inside (Figure 9-21A) or a localized circular wall thickening (Figure 9-21B and C). Intraluminal tumor obstructing the lumen may occasionally be demonstrated (Figure 9-21D).

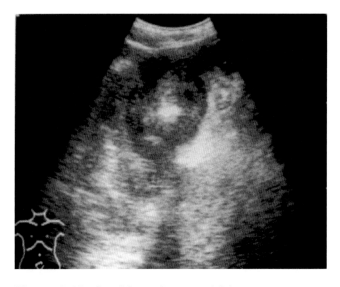

Figure 9-19. Small bowel tumor. A leiomyosarcoma causing a small bowel obstruction is recognized as an oval-shaped mass with a mosaic image.

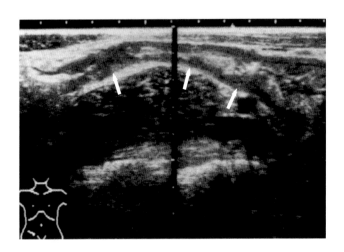

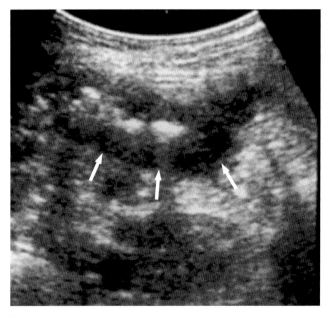

B

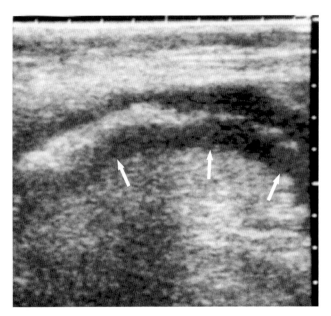

C

Figure 9-20. Inflammatory bowel diseases. A segmental wall thickening (arrows indicate posterior wall) of the small bowel is demonstrated in cases of (A) intestinal tuberculosis (7.5 MHz), (B) Crohn's disease (3.5 MHz), or (C) radiation enteritis (3.5 MHz).

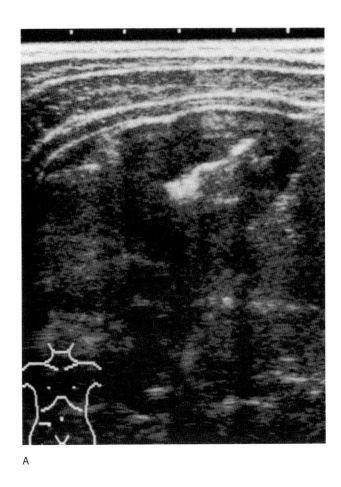

A

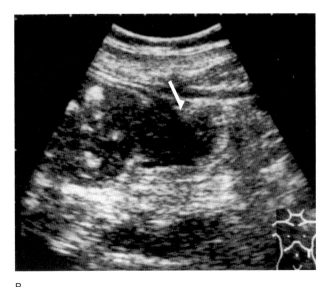

B

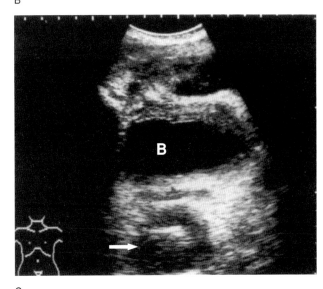

C

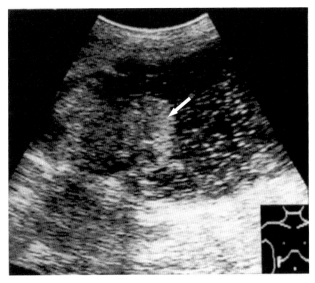

D

Figure 9-21. Colon carcinoma. (A) A colon cancer is often demonstrated as an irregular-shaped hypoechoic mass with an echogenic core inside, which is called the "pseudokidney sign" (7.5 MHz). (B) An obstructing colon cancer (arrow) is demonstrated as a circular wall thickening at the site of obstruction, where dilated colon filled with dense spot echoes is tapering (3.5 MHz). (C) Circular wall thickening of the rectum (arrow) is demonstrated in a case of recurrent gastric carcinoma (3.5 MHz). (D) Occasionally, a prominent tumor (arrow) obstructing the lumen may be demonstrated (3.5 MHz). B = urinary bladder.

Ileus

In the early stage of an ileus, slightly dilated small bowel loops (less than 25 mm wide in diameter) may be recognized on ultrasound. Gas echoes are more dominant than fluid collection inside the bowel (Figure 9-22).

Acute Appendicitis

Demonstration of a swollen, noncompressible appendix greater than 6 mm in diameter is the prime sonographic criterion for the diagnosis of acute appendicitis. The typical appearance of an inflamed appendix is a tubular structure with one blind end (Figure 9-23A and B). Maximal outer diameter ranges from 7 to 16 mm. Sonography may also demonstrate an appendicolith with acoustic shadowing (Figure 9-23C). The presence of

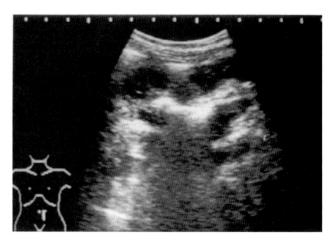

Figure 9-22. Ileus. Slightly dilated small bowel is demonstrated in a case of peritonitis secondary to perforated appendicitis.

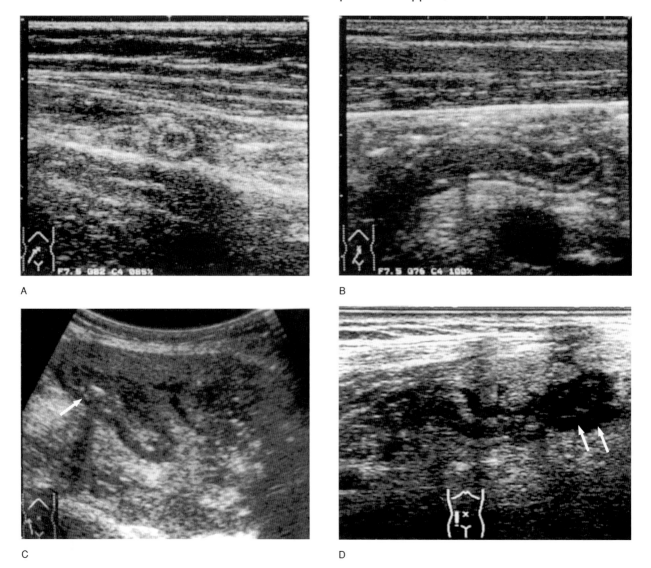

A

B

C

D

Figure 9-23. Acute appendicitis. A noncompressible, inflamed appendix is shown in (A) a cross-sectional view (7.5 MHz), and (B) a longitudinal section (7.5 MHz). Mural lamination of the swollen appendix is maintained in the early stages of acute appendicitis. (C) An appendicolith (arrow) with acoustic shadowing is demonstrated (5 MHz). (D) A focal loss of mural lamination in the appendiceal tip (arrows) is demonstrated as a result of gangrene (9 MHz).

appendicolith is always indicative of acute appendicitis in patients with acute right lower quadrant abdominal pain.

In cases of catarrhal or phlegmonous appendicitis, a swollen appendix maintains the layer structure of the wall. In cases of gangrenous appendicitis, a progressive loss of mural lamination and organ contours can be demonstrated as a result of gangrene (Figure 9-23D). With progression of the inflammation, the inflamed appendix or pericecal abscess may be often observed as surrounded by reflective fatty tissue that represents the mesentery or omentum. Atony of the terminal ileum may be seen as well as swelling of the cecal wall. A pericecal abscess can be demonstrated as fluid collection with a thick, noncompressible wall (Figure 9-24). Free peritoneal fluid in the pelvis is another common finding.

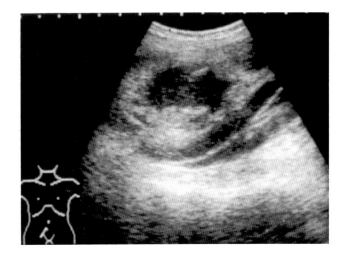

Figure 9-24. Pericecal abscess. A pericecal abscess secondary to perforated appendicitis is demonstrated as a hypoechoic fluid collection with a thick, noncompressible wall.

Acute Colonic Diverticulitis

On ultrasound, acute diverticulitis is shown as hypoechoic wall thickening (5–18 mm in thickness) of the affected segment (Figure 9-25A). Graded compression over the site of tenderness is a simple method of localizing any inflammatory mass. Diverticulum may be demonstrated as a focal, hypoechoic prominence with a hyperechoic fecalith or gas echoes inside, although it is not always identified in all cases of acute colonic diverticulitis (Figure 9-25B). Pericolonic abscess or purulent peritoneal fluid may be recognized in cases of complicated diverticulitis (Figure 9-9).

Acute Pancreatitis/Pancreatic Pseudocyst

Diffuse swelling of the pancreas is often recognized in cases of acute edematous pancreatitis. Decreased echogenicity of the pancreas represents interstitial edema (Figure 9-26A). In cases of severe pancreatitis, peripancreatic fluid collections or echogenic pancreatic masses may be demonstrated (Figure 9-26B and C). Pancreatic pseudocysts are generally visualized as

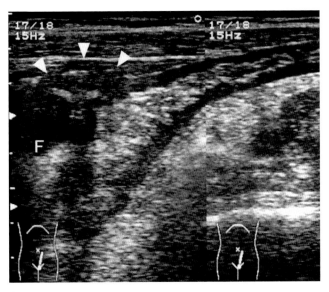

A

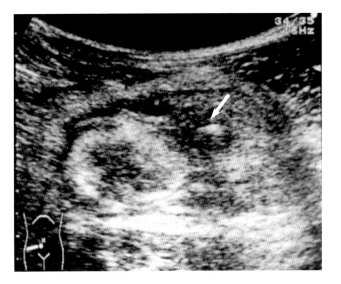

B

Figure 9-25. Acute colonic diverticulitis. (A) In a case of perforated diverticulitis of the sigmoid colon, a focal, hypoechoic prominence (arrowheads) with gas echoes inside is visualized along the thickened intestinal wall. Paracolonic fluid collection (F) is also visualized adjacent to the hypoechoic lesion (7.5 MHz). (B) In a case of diverticulitis of the ascending colon, a solitary diverticulum (arrow) within the thickened wall is demonstrated at the maximum point of tenderness (7.5 MHz).

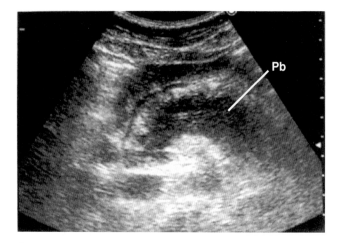

A

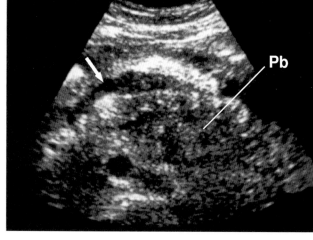

B

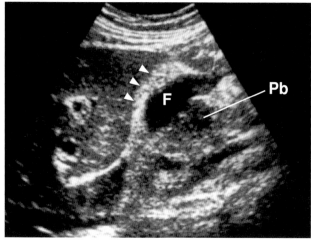

C

Figure 9-26. Acute pancreatitis. (A) Transverse view of the upper abdomen. Diffuse, homogeneous swelling of the pancreatic body (Pb) with decreased echogenicity is demonstrated in a case of acute edematous pancreatitis. (B) Transverse view of the upper abdomen. In a case of acute necrotizing pancreatitis the pancreatic body is visualized as a heterogenous mass with an unclear border. Hypoechoic inflammatory exudate (arrow) is demonstrated anterior to the pancreatic body. (C) Peripancreatic fluid collection (F) is demonstrated between the hypoechoic pancreatic body and reflective fatty tissue (arrows).

well-defined cystic masses in which sludge-like echoes may be identified (Figure 9-27).

Acute Cholecystitis

Irregular sonolucent layers in the gallbladder wall are indicative of serious cholecystitis (Figure 9-28A). The presence of asymmetric thickening of the gallbladder wall or intraluminal membranes parallel to the gallbladder wall can be identified in patients with acute gangrenous cholecystitis. Pericholecystic fluid collection can be caused by gallbladder perforation or abscess formation (Figure 9-28B).

Acute Mesenteric Ischemia

Wall thickening of the small bowel associated with a significant amount of peritoneal fluid is nonspecific but suggestive of acute mesenteric ischemia as well as peritonitis and peritoneal carcinomatosis (Figure 9-29).

Ischemic Colitis

In cases of ischemic colitis, hypoechoic wall thickening is often demonstrated in the affected segment especially from the splenic flexure to the rectosigmoid junction (Figure 9-30).

► COMMON VARIANTS AND OTHER ABNORMALITIES

Common normal variants that may be erroneously identified as free peritoneal fluid are discussed in Chapter 5. Fluid in the stomach when examining the perisplenic views and fluid in a collapsed bladder or an ovarian cyst when examining the pelvic views may be erroneously identified as free intraperitoneal fluid. Also, premenopausal women can occasionally have a small amount of free fluid in the pouch of Douglas.

Collapsed small bowel can be visualized similarly to a swollen appendix vermiformis, leading to a

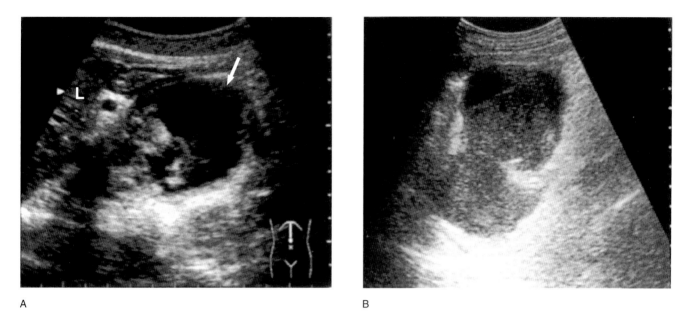

A   B

Figure 9-27. Pancreatic pseudocyst. (A) A well-defined cystic mass (arrow) is demonstrated posterior to the gastric antrum. (B) An irregular-shaped cystic mass filled with spot echoes is demonstrated medial to the splenic hilum in a case of infected pseudocyst. L = liver.

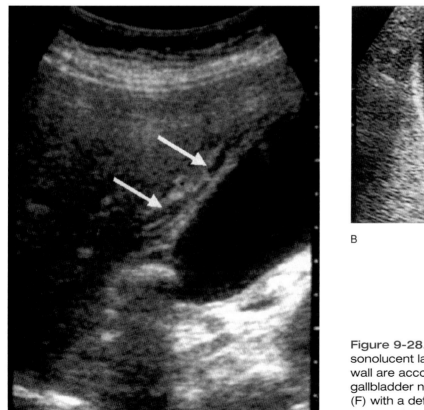

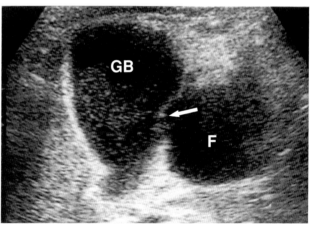

B

Figure 9-28. Acute cholecystitis. (A) Irregular sonolucent layers (arrows) in the swollen gallbladder wall are accompanied by an impacted stone in the gallbladder neck. (B) Pericholecystic fluid collection (F) with a defect (arrow) in the gallbladder wall, which represents a gallbladder perforation, is directly visualized with sonography. GB = gallbladder.

A

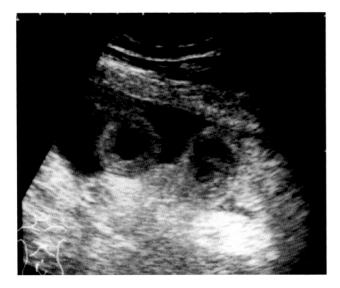

Figure 9-29. Acute mesenteric ischemia. Slightly dilated small bowel with wall thickening and peritoneal fluid are nonspecific but suggestive of acute mesenteric ischemia.

false-positive diagnosis of acute appendicitis (Figure 9-31). Peristaltic activity is not observed in the appendix, while it should be recognized in the small bowel.

GASTRIC OUTLET OBSTRUCTION

Gastric outlet obstruction may be demonstrated with emergency ultrasound (Figure 9-32). It can be caused

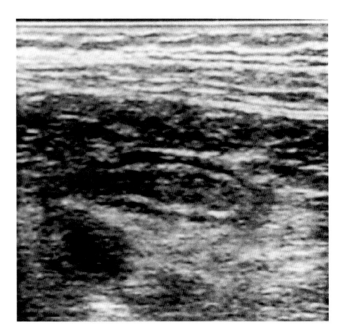

Figure 9-31. Normal collapsed ileum. A normal ileum may be misdiagnosed as a swollen appendix vermiformis (7.5 MHz). Peristaltic activity is recognized in the normal small bowel, while it is not observed in the appendix.

by a variety of lesions including gastric cancer, peptic ulcer, and pancreatic cancer. To confirm the diagnosis, endoscopy and contrast studies are usually applied after decompression of the distended stomach.

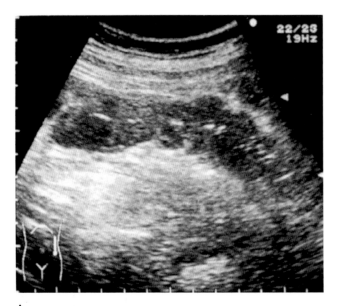

A

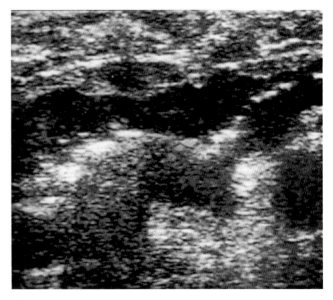

B

Figure 9-30. Ischemic colitis. (A) Hypoechoic wall thickening is delineated in the descending colon (3.5 MHz). (B) An irregular contour of the wall of the affected segment with decreased echogenicity is visualized in the advanced stage of ischemic colitis (7.5 MHz).

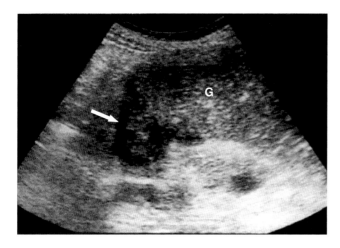

Figure 9-32. Gastric outlet obstruction. Distended stomach (G) filled with spot echoes is demonstrated proximal to the circular, hypoechoic wall thickening (arrow) in the pylorus, which represents a gastric cancer.

TORSION OF THE PEDICLE OF OVARIAN TUMOR

Ovarian torsion rarely occurs in patients without ovarian tumors or enlarged cysts. The clinical symptoms and physical findings may be confused with appendicitis, salpingitis, or gastroenteritis. The sonographic findings may be nonspecific and demonstrate a complex or cystic-appearing mass accompanied by free fluid in the pouch of Douglas (Figure 9-33). With a hemorrhagic infarction, the ovarian tumor may be hyperechoic.

RECTUS SHEATH HEMATOMA

Acute or subacute hematoma in the rectus sheath, generally confined to the upper or lower quadrant, can occasionally be experienced without trauma in a patient who has bleeding diathesis or after strenuous physical exertion. It is not always easy to differentiate rectus sheath hematoma from intra-abdominal pathology because most patients with the hematoma present with significant abdominal swelling and tenderness. Without suspicion of this pathologic entity, a nontherapeutic laparotomy might be performed for an acute abdomen when conservative treatment or percutaneous drainage is indicated. Abdominal sonography is useful in this clinical situation by demonstrating the hematoma within the abdominal wall (Figure 9-34).

ACUTE ENTEROCOLITIS

Imaging modalities have seldom been used in cases of acute enterocolitis. Recently, sonography has been

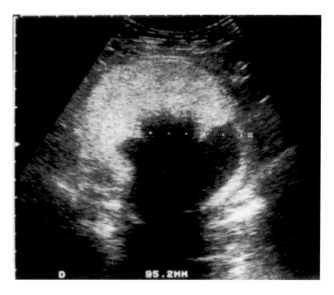

Figure 9-33. Torsion of the pedicle of an ovarian tumor. A solid and cystic tumor is demonstrated in the pouch of Douglas. The dense central shadowing suggests calcified components. The mixed components may represent a Desmoid tumor. Significant tenderness on the tumor suggests possible torsion of the pedicle. Color Doppler may be helpful if available.

increasingly applied for infectious enterocolitis. Only slightly dilated bowel loops with normal wall thickness and increased peristalsis can be obtained with sonography in cases of mild enterocolitis. Mural thickening of the terminal ileum and colon accompanied with enlarged mesenteric lymph nodes may be identified in more severe cases (Figure 9-35).

▶ PITFALLS

1. **Contraindication.** For cases of acute abdomen, there is no absolute contraindication to performing the emergency ultrasound examination. A rapid ultrasound examination can be applied even while the resuscitation efforts are performed on patients in shock.

2. **Overreliance on the emergency ultrasound examination.** A pitfall is the overreliance of an initial negative ultrasound examination in caring for patients with acute abdomen. Each examination is a single data point in the overall clinical picture. As the clinical symptoms and findings change, serial ultrasound examinations should be applied to evaluate any changes of sonographic findings. If the ultrasound examination presents equivocal findings, abdominal CT, other radiographic procedures using contrast media or

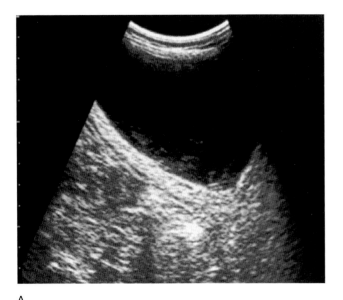

A

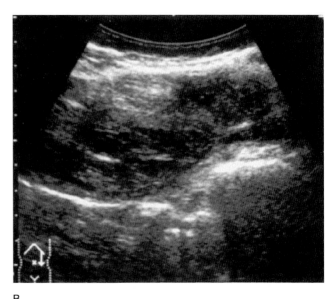

B

Figure 9-34. Rectus sheath hematoma. (A) Sonography shows a large hematoma as a circumscribed fluid collection within the abdominal wall. (B) In the early stage a rectus sheath hematoma may be shown as a heterogeneous image.

endoscopy should be utilized for the further evaluation.

3. **Limitations of the emergency ultrasound examination.** Limitations include difficulty in imaging patients who are morbidly obese or have an immense amount of gastrointestinal gas. Various artifacts may interfere with the examination in obtaining optimal images. Also, it may be difficult to determine the nature of free intraperitoneal fluid. If clinically required, an ultrasound-guided paracentesis of the fluid can be applied to clarify the issue. Another limitation is that ultrasound is an operator-dependent examination for both obtaining and interpreting the images.

4. **Limitations associated with pregnancy.** In pregnant patients, the distortion of usual landmarks caused by the presence of a gravid uterus can complicate the identification of an inflamed appendix. Interpreting sonographic images of extra-uterine vasculature may be difficult for inexperienced sonographers. Nonobstructive dilatation of the renal collecting system may occur after 6 weeks in a normal pregnancy.

5. **Technical difficulties with the emergency ultrasound examination.** Many clinicians will not have enough experience initially to confidently apply sonography for the diagnosis of gastrointestinal disorders such as bowel obstruction, acute appendicitis, or acute diverticulitis. Significant tenderness, peritoneal irritability, or hyperventilation can interfere with the examination.

6. **Etiologies undetected by sonography.** Certain etiologies that can cause an acute abdomen may not be detected initially by the emergency ultrasound examination. These include perforation of a vesical bladder or gastrointestinal tract, embolism of the SMA, colonic volvulus, and gastrointestinal hemorrhage. Color Doppler can potentially be used to evaluate the blood flow through the SMA in a patient suspected to have an SMA embolism (Figure 9-36).

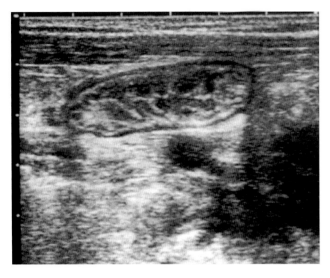

Figure 9-35. Infectious enterocolitis. Mural thickening of the ileum is regarded as reflective of inflammatory changes in the intestinal wall (7.5 MHz).

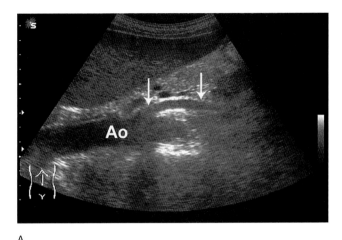
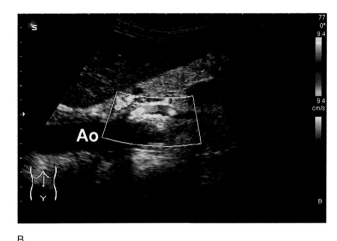

A   B

Figure 9-36. Application of color Doppler ultrasound technique. (A) Longitudinal view of the aorta (Ao) and superior mesenteric artery (arrows). (B) A color Doppler ultrasound of the same area shows blood flow through the SMA on longitudinal view. (Courtesy of James Mateer, MD)

► CASE STUDIES

CASE 1

Patient Presentation

A 68-year-old man presented to the emergency department with complaints of intermittent epigastric pain, nausea, and vomiting. He felt the sudden onset of pain prior to dinner. The pain increased intermittently and was accompanied by emesis of bilious fluid. He denied hematemesis, abdominal distention, and constipation. He had a bowel movement earlier in the day. He had a medical history of gastrectomy for gastric cancer and cholecystectomy for gallstone disease.

On physical examination, his blood pressure was 160/90 mmHg; pulse, 82 beats per minute; respirations, 16 per minute; temperature 37.1°C. His head, neck, pulmonary, and cardiovascular examinations were unremarkable. His abdomen was soft and flat but had moderate tenderness to palpation and rebound tenderness in the epigastric region. No muscle guarding was appreciated. On rectal examination, his stool was guaiac negative.

Management Course

While his plain radiographs showed no apparent subphrenic free air, they revealed dilated small bowel with multiple air-fluid levels. His urinalysis was normal. Laboratory tests revealed an elevated serum glucose level (171 mg/dL) and leukocytosis (WBC 10,300/μL). His serum CPK, amylase, and liver enzymes were within normal range. An emergency ultrasound examination revealed dilated loops of small bowel with peristaltic activity in the entire abdomen and collapsed loops localized in the right lower quadrant (Figure 9-37A). The maximal diameter of visualized dilated loops was 34 mm. A small amount of peritoneal fluid was also identified between the dilated loops. No evidence of hepatobiliary disorders, splenomegaly, or pancreatitis was found.

The patient was admitted with the diagnosis of small bowel obstruction by adhesions and treated conservatively with nasogastric tube decompression and intravenous fluids. Although his symptoms were relieved after the nasogastric tube decompression, sonographic appearances of small bowel obstruction were slightly progressive. Three days after admission, a long intestinal tube was inserted for decompression of dilated small bowel and for a contrast study to confirm the site and degree of the obstruction. A small amount of water-soluble contrast medium was passed through the obstruction to the ascending colon, and thus the patient was suspected of having a partial obstruction on radiograph findings. At the time, laboratory tests showed only slight elevation of serum c-reactive protein (CRP) level (2.0 mg/dL). The WBC count was 7100/μL. However, more than 1,000 mL of intestinal fluid were drained via the long intestinal tube in 24 hours. Re-examination with sonography revealed an aperistaltic, dilated loop with slight mural thickening in the right lower abdomen, and increased amount of peritoneal fluid (Figure 9-37B). Slowly progressing strangulation obstruction was suspected on sonographic images contrary to his minimal clinical and radiograph findings. He was taken to the operating room for surgical intervention, which revealed a large amount of serobloody ascites and a congestive, hemorrhagic loop of bowel that was twisted and strangulated by an adhesive band. The strangulated loop was still viable and relieved by adhesiolysis.

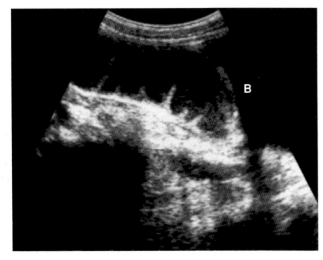

A

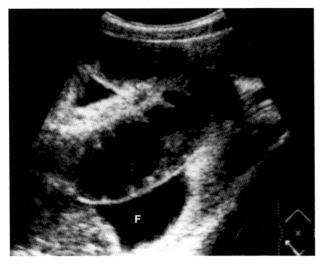

B

Figure 9-37. Sonograms of case 1. (A) An initial ultrasound examination revealed dilated loops of small bowel with peristaltic activity. B = bladder. (B) Reexamination with sonography revealed an akinetic, dilated loop with slight mural thickening and increased amount of peritoneal fluid (F) in the pelvis.

Commentary

Case 1 was an example of a patient who had a slowly progressing strangulation obstruction. The clinical picture of a strangulation obstruction varies by the severity of circulatory impairment, the length of strangulated loop, and the period after the onset. Diagnosis of strangulation small bowel obstruction is difficult preoperatively unless the patient presents with severe pain or peritoneal signs. In general, laboratory tests and plain radiographs are not diagnostic in the early stages of strangulation. Real-time sonography, however, can evaluate not only the morphological changes but also the physio-

logical changes observed in bowel obstruction. An aperistaltic, dilated loop distal to dilated loops with peristaltic activity is essential in the sonographic diagnosis of strangulation small bowel obstruction. The increase in the amount of peritoneal fluid, which is also diagnostic for strangulation, can be assessed by serial ultrasound examinations. In this particular case, the information provided by serial examinations was crucial in the decision process to proceed with an urgent laparotomy, and this prevented an enterectomy for hemorrhagic necrosis of the strangulated loop.

CASE 2

Patient Presentation

A 55-year-old man presented to the emergency department with a 5-day history of lower abdominal pain and watery diarrhea. He denied nausea and vomiting. He had a medical history of chronic hepatitis and cerebral infarction, and was a heavy smoker and heavy drinker.

On physical examination, his blood pressure was 145/84 mmHg; pulse, 110 beats per minute; and temperature, 38.4°C. His head, neck, pulmonary, and cardiovascular examinations were unremarkable. The abdominal examination was soft, diffusely tender, and without peritoneal signs.

Management Course

The patient remained hemodynamically stable in the emergency department. An upright chest radiograph and abdominal radiographs showed no evidence of bowel obstruction or gastrointestinal perforation. His urinalysis was normal. His laboratory tests showed an elevated serum CRP level (4.5 mg/dL) and leucocytosis (WBC 11,000/μL). An emergency ultrasound examination revealed no free intraperitoneal fluid but slightly thickened wall of the sigmoid colon (Figure 9-38A). Blood flow through the SMA was recognized on color Doppler. An abdominal CT scan was negative for intraperitoneal and retroperitoneal pathology. The patient was admitted for observation and treated conservatively with antibiotics and intravenous fluid therapy. Two days after the admission, he complained of having severe abdominal pain; a repeat bedside ultrasound examination revealed mural thickening of the sigmoid colon and turbulent peritoneal fluid, including gas echoes in the anterior pelvis (Figure 9-38B and C). He was taken to the operating room for an urgent laparotomy, which revealed feculent peritonitis due to perforative diverticulitis of the sigmoid colon.

Commentary

The patient in case 2 had an initial negative ultrasound examination and CT scan. Re-examination with bedside

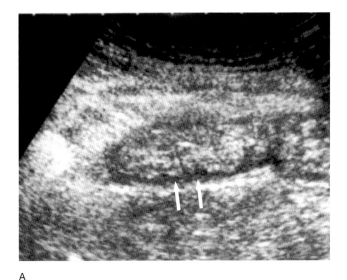

A

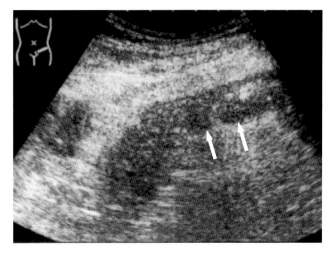

B

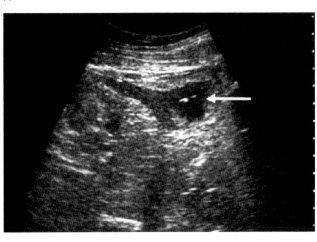

C

Figure 9-38. Sonograms of case 2. (A) No free peritoneal fluid but slightly thickened wall of the sigmoid colon (arrows) was revealed with an initial ultrasound examination. (B) Mural thickening of the sigmoid colon (arrows) was identified with reexamination. (C) Turbulent peritoneal fluid (arrow) including gas echoes was recognized in the anterior pelvis.

ultrasound revealed turbulent free peritoneal fluid and wall thickening of the sigmoid colon. These findings were suggestive of a sigmoid colon perforation due to acute diverticulitis, and thus, negated the need for a repeat CT scan while making a decision for surgical intervention. As abdominal sonography is available at the bedside, it should be repeated for a patient with an acute abdomen whose etiology is not yet defined.

CASE 3

Patient Presentation

A 26-year-old pregnant woman presented to the emergency department with complaints of right lower quadrant abdominal pain radiating to the right flank. She initially experienced epigastric pain accompanied by nausea and vomiting, which was followed by right lower quadrant pain. She denied urinary retention, dysuria, hematuria, diarrhea, and constipation. She was 18 weeks

pregnant and had no vaginal bleeding. She denied any significant medical history.

On physical examination, her blood pressure was 128/78 mmHg; pulse, 94 beats per minute; respirations, 18 per minute; and temperature, 37.0°C. She was anicteric. Her pulmonary and cardiovascular examinations were normal. The abdominal examination was soft but had significant peritoneal signs localized in the right lower quadrant laterally and superiorly deviated from McBurney's point. She also felt a severe pain on percussion in the costovertebral angle and right lumbar region. A gravid uterus, 3 cm below the umbilicus, was noted. The rectal examination revealed guaiac negative stool.

Management Course

The patient remained hemodynamically stable in the emergency department. No radiographs were taken because she was pregnant. Her urinalysis showed no red blood cells or bacteria. Her laboratory tests

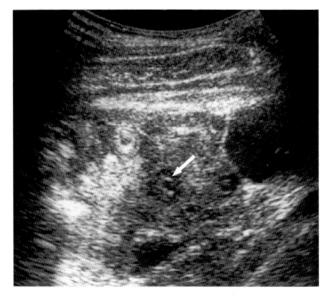

A

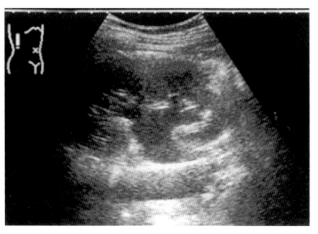

B

Figure 9-39. Sonograms of case 3. (A) An emergency ultrasound examination using a standard probe revealed a target figure of the appendix (arrow), which was draped over by omental tissues, in the right lower flank. (B) A coronal view in the right upper flank showed moderately dilated pyelocaliceal system within the right kidney.

demonstrated leukocytosis (WBC 12,000/μL) and elevated CRP level (10 mg/dL). An emergency ultrasound examination using a standard probe revealed a target figure of the appendix that was draped over by omental tissues (Figure 9-39A), dilated pyelocaliceal system in the right kidney (Figure 9-39B), and the fetus moving actively within the gravid uterus. There was no evidence of peritoneal fluid. The obstetrics and urologist consultants agreed with the attending surgeon's clinical and sonographic findings. The patient was suspected of having an acute appendicitis accompanied with acute

hydronephrosis on the basis of clinical and sonographic findings. Further diagnostic modalities to define the etiology of urinary system disorders were limited because she was pregnant. For the purpose of differential diagnosis and treatment, the urologist performed a retrograde ureteral catheterization under cystoscopic procedures. No evidence of pyuria or apparent obstructive lesions was confirmed, and subsequently, the patient was suspected of having a nonobstructive dilatation of the renal collecting system, which is occasionally recognized in pregnant women. The patient was taken to the operating room for an urgent laparotomy, which revealed an acute gangrenous appendix without abscess or apparent retroperitoneal infiltration. An appendectomy was performed and her postoperative course was uneventful. The right hydronephrosis was slightly reduced but lasted throughout pregnancy.

Commentary

Case 3 was an example of a pregnant patient who presented with an acute abdomen. She had acute appendicitis with puzzling symptoms and signs. The sonographic findings were compatible with her complicated clinical findings. The diagnosis of acute appendicitis in pregnant patients can be more challenging even when they present with a typical clinical picture for the disease. Abdominal sonography should be utilized for pregnant women and can assist physicians with their management strategy.

Nonobstructive dilatation of the collecting system occurs in normal pregnancy onward after 6–10 weeks, with both hormonal factors and pressure of the gravid uterus on the ureters considered to be likely causes. The dilatation is marked more on the right than on the left, and increases in severity throughout pregnancy. In this case, the retroperitoneal involvement of the inflammation from the appendicitis may have caused paresis of the ureter and, consequently, aggravated urinary retention.

▶ ACKNOWLEDGMENT

The author thanks the staff of the ultrasound section in the Kobe Nishi City Hospital and the Kobe City General Hospital for their assistance in obtaining the images used in this chapter.

REFERENCES

1. Gore RM, Gore MD: Ascites and peritoneal fluid collections. In: Gore RM, Levine MS, eds. *Textbook of Gastrointestinal Radiology*, 2nd ed. Philadelphia, PA: W.B. Saunders, 2000:1969.

2. Jeffrey RB, McGahan JP: Gastrointestinal tract and peritoneal cavity. In: McGahan JP, Goldberg BB, eds. *Diagnostic Ultrasound—A logical approach.* Philadelphia, PA: Lippincott-Raven, 1998:511.

3. Lim JH, Lee DH, Ko YT: Sonographic detection of duodenal ulcer. *J Ultrasound Med* 11:91, 1992.

4. Garcia SJM: Direct sonographic signs of acute duodenal ulcer. *Abdom Imaging* 24:226, 1999.

5. Winek TG, Mosely HS, Grout G, et al.: Pneumoperitoneum and its association with ruptured abdominal viscus. *Arch Surg* 123:709, 1988.

6. Williams N, Everson NW: Radiological confirmation of intraperitoneal free gas. *Ann R Coll Surg Engl* 79:8, 1997.

7. Jeffrey RB, Federle MP, Wall S: Value of computed tomography in detecting occult gastrointestinal perforation. *J Comput Assist Tomogr* 7:825, 1983.

8. Meiser G, Meissner K: Clinical relevance of sonography in acute diagnosis of perforated gastroduodenal ulcers. *Langenbecks Arch Chir* 368:197, 1986.

9. Chanda D, Kedar RP, Malde HM: Sonographic detection of pneumoperitoneum: an experimental and clinical study. *Australas Radiol* 37:182, 1993.

10. Kainberger P, Zukriegel M, Sattlegger P, et al.: Ultrasound detection of pneumoperitoneum based on typical ultrasound morphology. *Ultraschall Med* 15:122, 1994.

11. Braccini G, Lamacchia M, Boraschi P, et al.: Ultrasound versus plain film in the detection of pneumoperitoneum. *Abdom Imaging* 21:404, 1996.

12. Grechenig W, Peicha G, Clement HG, et al.: Detection of pneumoperitoneum by ultrasound examination: an experimental and clinical study. *Injury* 30:173, 1999.

13. Corn I: Intestinal Obstruction. In: Berk JE, ed. Bockus Gastroenterology, 4th ed., Vol. 3. Tokyo: W.B. Saunders, 1985:2056.

14. Ziter FMH Jr, Markowitz SK: Radiologic Diagnosis. In: Welch JP, ed. *Bowel Obstruction: Differential Diagnosis and Clinical Management.* Philadelphia, PA: W.B. Saunders, 1990:96.

15. Stephanie R, Wilson MD: Ultrasonography of the hollow viscera. In: Gore RM, Levine MS, eds. *Textbook of Gastrointestinal Radiology*, 2nd ed. Philadelphia, PA: W.B. Saunders, 2000:67.

16. Peck R: The small bowel. In: Meire H, Cosgrove D, Dewbury K, et al., eds. *Clinical Ultrasound* (Vol. 2, Abdominal and General Ultrasound), 2nd ed. New York: Churchill Livingstone, 1999:823.

17. O'Malley ME, Wilson SR: US of gastrointestinal tract abnormalities with CT correlation. *Radiographics* 23:59, 2003.

18. Fleischer AC, Dowling AD, Weinstein ML, et al.: Sonographic patterns of distended, fluid-filled bowel. *Radiology* 133:681, 1979.

19. Scheible W, Goldberger LE: Diagnosis of small bowel obstruction: The contribution of diagnostic ultrasound. *AJR* 133:685, 1979.

20. Meiser G, Meissner K: Ileus and intestinal obstruction: Ultrasonic findings as a guideline to therapy. *Hepatogastroenterology* 34:194, 1987.

21. Cho KC, Hoffman-Tretin JC, Alterman DD: Closed-loop obstruction of the small bowel: CT and sonographic appearance. *J Comput Assist Yomogr* 13:256, 1989.

22. Truong S, Arlt G, Pfingsten F, et al.: Importance of sonography in diagnosis of ileus. A retrospective study of 459 patients. *Chirurg* 63:634, 1992.

23. Schmutz GR, Benko A, Fournier L, et al.: Small bowel obstruction: Role and contribution of sonography. *Eur Radiol* 7:1054, 1997.

24. Ogata M, Imai S, Hosotani R, et al.: Abdominal ultrasonography for the diagnosis of strangulation in small bowel obstruction. *Br J Surg* 81:421, 1994.

25. Ogata M: Ultrasonographic findings in the intestinal wall with hemorrhagic necrosis caused by strangulation ileus. *Jpn J Med Ultrasonics* 17:19, 1990.

26. Czechowski J: Conventional radiography and ultrasonography in the diagnosis of small bowel obstruction and strangulation. *Acta Radiol* 37:186, 1996.

27. Ogata M, Imai S, Hosotani R, et al.: Abdominal sonography for the diagnosis of large bowel obstruction. *Jpn J Surg* 24:791, 1994.

28. Ogata M, Mateer JR, Condon RE: Prospective evaluation of abdominal sonography for the diagnosis of bowel obstruction. *Ann Surg* 223:237, 1996.

29. Russell JC, Welch JP: Pathophysiology of bowel obstruction. In: Welch JP, ed. *Bowel Obstruction: Differential Diagnosis and Clinical Management.* Philadelphia, PA: W.B. Saunders, 1990:28.

30. Suri S, Gupta S, Sudhakar PJ, et al.: Comparative evaluation of plain films, ultrasound and CT in the diagnosis of intestinal obstruction. *Acta Radiol* 40:422, 1999.

31. Weissberg DL, Scheible W, Leopld GR: Ultrasonographic appearance of adult intussusception. *Radiology* 124:791, 1977.

32. Holt S, Samuel E: Multiple concentric ring sign in the ultrasonographic diagnosis of intussusception. *Gastrointest Radiol* 3:307, 1978.

33. Puylaert JBCM: Acute appendicitis: US evaluation using graded compression. *Radiology* 158:335, 1986.

34. Jeffrey RB, Laing FC, Lewis FR: Acute appendicitis: High-resolution real-time US findings. *Radiology* 163:11, 1987.

35. Jeffrey RB, Laing FC, Townsend RR: Acute appendicitis: Sonographic criteria based on 250 cases. *Radiology* 167:327, 1988.

36. Schwerk WB, Wichtrup B, Rothmund M, et al.: Ultrasonography in the diagnosis of acute appendicitis: A prospective study. *Gastroenterology* 97:630, 1989.

37. Douglas DD, Macpherson NE, Davidson PM, et al.: Randomised controlled trial of ultrasonography in diagnosis of acute appendicitis, incorporating the Alvarado score. *BMJ* 321:919, 2000.

38. Terasawa T, Blackmore CC, Bent S, et al.: Systematic review: Computed tomography and ultrasonography to detect acute appendicitis in adults and adolescents. *Ann Intern Med* 141:537, 2004.

39. Skaane P, Schistad O, Amland PF, et al.: Routine ultrasonography in the diagnosis of acute appendicitis: A valuable tool in daily practice? *Am Surg* 63:937, 1997.

40. Pohl D, Golub R, Schwartz GE, et al.: Appendiceal ultrasonography performed by nonradiologists: Does it help in the diagnostic process? *J Ultrasound Med* 17:217, 1998.

41. Amgwerd M, Rothlin M, Candinas D, et al.: Ultrasound

diagnosis of appendicitis by surgeons—A matter of experience? A prospective study. *Lagenbecks Arch Chir* 379:335, 1994.

42. Williams RJ, Windsor AC, Rosin RD, et al.: Ultrasound scanning of the acute abdomen by surgeons in training. *Ann R Coll Surg Engl* 76:228, 1994.

43. Zielke A, Hasse C, Sitter H, et al.: Influence of ultrasound on clinical decision making in acute appendicitis: A prospective study. *Eur J Surg* 164:201, 1998.

44. Chen SC, Wan HP, Huang PM, et al.: Accuracy of ED sonography in the diagnosis of acute appendicitis. *Am J Emrg Med* 18:449, 2000.

45. Puylaert JBCM, Rioux M, Oostayen JA: The appendix and small bowel. In: Meire H, Cosgrove D, Dewbury K, et al., eds. *Abdominal and General Ultrasound*, 2nd ed. New York: Churchill Livingstone, 841, 1999.

46. Simonovsky V: Sonographic detection of normal and abnormal appendix. *Clin Radiol* 54:533, 1999.

47. Schwerk WB, Schwarz S, Rothmund M: Sonography in acute colonic diverticulitis. A prospective study. *Dis Colon Rectum* 35:1077, 1992.

48. Zielke A, Hasse C, Kisker O, et al.: Prospective evaluation of ultrasonography in acute colonic diverticulitis. *Br J Surg* 84:385, 1997.

49. Glazer G, Mann D: Acute pancreatitis. In: Monson J, Duthie G, O'Malley K, eds. *Surgical Emergencies*. Oxford, U.K.: Blackwell Science, 1999:134.

50. Balthazar EJ: Pancreatitis. In: Gore RM, Levine MS, eds. *Textbook of Gastrointestinal Radiology*, 2nd ed. Philadelphia, PA: W.B. Saunders, 2000:1767.

51. Jeffrey RB: The Pancreas. In: Jeffrey RB, ed. *CT and Sonography of the Acute Abdomen*. New York: Raven Press, 1989:111.

52. Cosgrove DO: The pancreas. In Meire H, Cosgrove D, Dewbury K, et al., eds. *Clinical Ultrasound* (Vol. 1, Abdominal and General Ultrasound), 2nd ed. New York: Churchill Livingstone, 1999:349.

53. Laing F: Ultrasonography of the acute abdomen. *Radiol Clin N Am* 30:389, 1992.

54. Ralls PW, Colletti PM, Lapin SA, et al.: Real-time sonography in suspected acute cholecystitis. *Radiology* 155:767, 1985.

55. Danse EM, Laterre PF, Van Beers BE, et al.: Early diagnosis of acute intestinal ischaemia: Contribution of colour Doppler sonography. *Acta Chir Belg* 97:173, 1997.

56. Teefey SA, Roarke MC, Brink JA, et al.: Bowel wall thickening: Differentiation of inflammation from ischemia with color Doppler and duplex US. *Radiology* 198:547, 1996.

CHAPTER 10

Renal

Stuart Swadron and Diku Mandavia

The kidney and bladder are two of the most sonographically accessible organs. Both are easily recognizable to those who are new to ultrasound and thus the urinary tract can be a simple starting point for learning-focused sonography in the acute care setting.

The primary focus of renal ultrasonography in the emergency setting has been to determine the presence or absence of hydronephrosis.[1-4] As with other areas of emergency ultrasound, physicians using the modality for this specific goal have begun to explore new indications for imaging the urinary tract. Ultrasound determination of bladder volume and evaluation of bladder filling before catheterization are two such examples.[5-14] Another important consideration that has arisen with the focused use of renal ultrasound is the management of unexpected or incidental findings, such as masses and cysts.[15-18]

▶ CLINICAL CONSIDERATIONS

For many years, the standard investigation in cases of suspected renal colic was the intravenous pyelogram (IVP). Although IVP is more specific than ultrasound for the detection and characterization of a ureteral stone,[19-23] it has several disadvantages in the emergency and acute care settings. Intravenous contrast dye, even in low ionic formulation, carries a small but real risk of allergy and nephrotoxicity.[24-27] For this reason, in patients with known allergy to contrast, diabetes mellitus, renal insufficiency, or pregnancy, renal ultrasound or computed tomography (CT) becomes the pre-ferred modality. Although routine determination of renal function tests in patients presenting with flank pain and hematuria is controversial, many radiology departments require these measurements before an IVP can be performed.

Ultrasound can be performed safely and quickly at the bedside with essentially no risks. Although it does not give information about renal function, the presence of unilateral hydronephrosis or hydroureter in the setting of hematuria and acute flank pain is very sensitive for the presence of a ureteral stone. Recent studies that combine the use of emergency renal ultrasound with a single plain abdominal film have found a sensitivity of 64–97% using IVP as a comparative standard.[19,20,22,23,28,29] Moreover, the degree of hydronephrosis, in combination with the patient's history, is helpful to determine the need for urgent consultation with a urologist. In this respect, bedside ultrasound often provides sufficient information to efficiently guide the treatment and disposition of the patient. Whereas a patient with mild to moderate hydronephrosis can, with few exceptions, be managed on an outpatient basis, the presence of severe hydronephrosis should prompt urgent consultation or close follow-up and further definition of the obstruction by CT.

Furthermore, ultrasound has the added value of providing anatomical information and identifying abnormalities that may be missed on IVP. In the course of utilizing ultrasound of the urinary tract to detect obstruction, practitioners are identifying other such abnormalities with increasing frequency. Some of these represent life- or kidney-threatening processes and may prompt timely definitive treatment. Ultrasound is especially sensitive for the presence of cysts and for distinguishing between solid and cystic masses.[30]

Because the differential diagnosis in patients with flank or abdominal pain involves other organs visualized well by bedside ultrasound, invaluable additional information may be available that cannot be obtained with IVP. Specifically, if no hydronephrosis is seen on ultrasound examination, the physician may proceed to visualize the gallbladder, common bile duct, and abdominal aorta.

One of the major advantages of bedside ultrasound is that it can be performed directly at the point of care without having to move the patient to the radiology suite. Sonography in this fashion is being performed by urologists evaluating patients in the emergency department and is also helpful in remote or austere locations where other imaging may not exist.[31,32]

Spiral CT has emerged as an important modality in the emergency and acute care settings for the evaluation of suspected renal colic.[33−35] Not only does CT provide excellent visualization of the urinary tract and of renal stones, it provides similar details for other abdominal structures and has a higher sensitivity for renal calculi.[36] Many physicians are now using CT in the place of both ultrasound and IVP, especially in older patients where the risk of abdominal aorta aneurysm (AAA) is greater. CT can reliably eliminate this life-threatening entity from the differential diagnosis. The sensitivity of CT scan in the detection of renal stone disease varies from 86–100%.[37−45] However, CT scanning remains less accessible, involves a considerable exposure to radiation, and probably is not necessary in younger patients with straightforward clinical presentations. The widespread use of CT has undergone scrutiny within the imaging community because of the large cumulative radiation dosage being delivered to patients. The successive and repetitive nature of renal colic virtually assures these patients (especially younger ones) a higher iatrogenic cancer risk and, thus, forms a logical argument for judicious use of CT in this population.[46,47]

▶ CLINICAL INDICATIONS

Possible indications for ultrasound examination of the urinary tract in the emergency and acute care setting are as follows:

- Acute flank pain/suspected renal colic
- Acute urinary retention and bladder size estimation
- Acute renal failure
- Acute pyelonephritis and renal abscess
- Possible renal mass
- Trauma

ACUTE FLANK PAIN/SUSPECTED RENAL COLIC

A focused emergency ultrasound examination of the kidneys is presently indicated for evaluation of the patient with suspected renal colic. Because of the prevalence of renal stone disease, this diagnosis is in the differential of all patients presenting with abdominal or flank pain. While ultrasonography is primarily utilized in patients presenting with flank pain and hematuria, its use also may be considered in the broader group of patients with undifferentiated abdominal pain and the absence of hematuria since renal stone disease may present in this fashion as well. While ultrasound most frequently does not detect an actual renal stone, its ability to detect hydronephrosis, an important consequence of obstructive uropathy, makes it an invaluable tool in the emergency setting.[48]

In the largest study comparing IVP with renal ultrasound, 288 patients admitted to hospital for intractable flank pain were studied.[28] Using IVP as the gold standard, the sensitivity of ultrasound alone for detecting renal stone disease was 93%, its specificity 83%, positive predictive value 93%, and negative predictive value 83%. When a kidney/ureter/bladder (KUB) radiograph was added to ultrasound, its specificity improved to 100%. In a study of 180 patients in the emergency department setting, Dalla Palma et al. found a sensitivity of 95% for the detection of renal stone disease using the combination of ultrasound and a KUB radiograph. The high negative predictive value of KUB radiograph and ultrasound in this study (95%) led these authors to conclude that IVP need not be performed when these are both negative.[20]

If microscopic hematuria is present and no hydronephrosis is seen, the consideration of other diagnoses should be made even though the diagnosis of renal stone is still possible. Those diagnoses that are immediately life threatening, such as a ruptured AAA, must be considered. Once the clinician is satisfied that more serious pathologies are not present, the patient may be discharged home for further workup as necessary on an outpatient basis, which may include an IVP, CT, or stone analysis if collected. The presence of a solitary kidney, renal failure, or urinary tract infection may be indications for admission or further investigation, despite the absence of significant hydronephrosis, when the diagnosis of renal stones is still under consideration. An algorithm for the evaluation of renal colic that incorporates the use of focused ultrasonography is outlined in Figure 10-1.

Patients who are dehydrated may fail to show the signs of hydronephrosis on ultrasound[49] and it is for this reason that oral or intravenous hydration is recommended before obstructive hydronephrosis can be excluded. Conversely, a patient with a full bladder

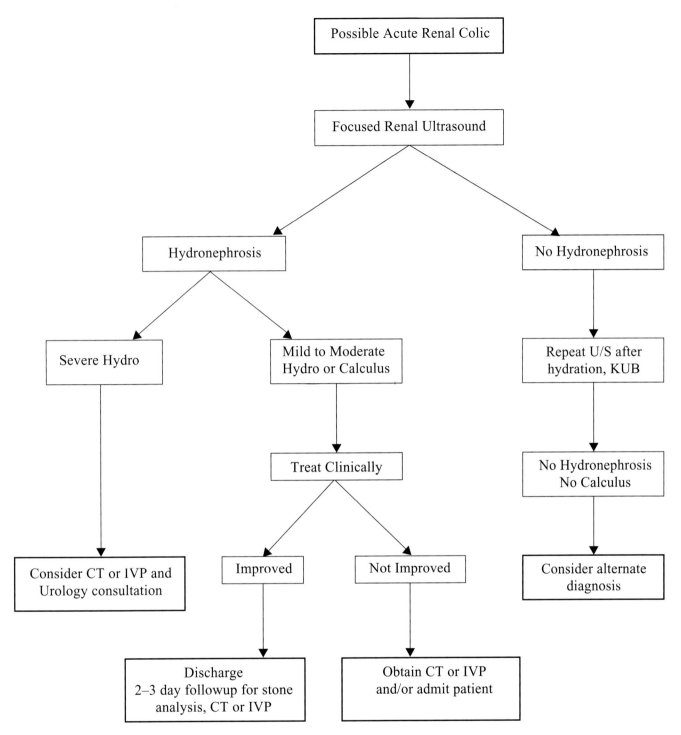

Figure 10-1. Algorithm for the evaluation of renal colic.

may have the appearance of bilateral hydronephrosis; if such a situation is encountered, the ultrasound examination should be repeated after the patient voids.[50] Because of these variations with state of hydration and bladder volume, it is extremely important to obtain images of both kidneys (for comparison) and the bladder, and to correlate the images with the clinical picture.

In a patient without hematuria, a negative KUB radiograph, and a negative bedside ultrasound examination for hydronephrosis, the diagnosis of renal colic becomes extremely unlikely; the negative predictive value of this combination is high, ranging from 75 to 95%.[19–21,28]

The persistence of bilateral hydronephrosis may indicate bladder outlet obstruction and further study is indicated. With long-standing hydronephrosis, a thinning of the medulla and cortex begin to occur.[30] The presence of right-sided hydronephrosis is a common finding in pregnancy and should not be confused for pathology.[50] Occasionally the finding of calyceal rupture will be noted by the presence of perinephric fluid with mild to moderate hydronephrosis. The finding of urinary extravasation is significant and should prompt urgent urological consultation.

An evolving technique in the evaluation of renal outflow obstruction involves the imaging of ureteral jets.[51,52] In the normal bladder, the intermittent ejection of urine into the bladder from the ureters can be visualized in real-time examination. In the presence of unilateral obstruction, ureteral jet flow to the ipsilateral side is impaired or not present. This can provide information on renal tract function and may be particularly useful when contrast dye administration is contraindicated.

ACUTE URINARY RETENTION AND BLADDER SIZE ESTIMATION

Bedside ultrasound can assist in the evaluation of patients with symptoms of acute urinary retention. At times it can be difficult to ascertain from history whether the patient has developed acute urinary retention. Although physical examination of the abdomen can demonstrate a distended bladder, this may not be accurate, especially in obese patients. Therefore, the placement of a urinary catheter for residual urine, as both a diagnostic and therapeutic procedure, has been the traditional approach when acute urinary retention is being considered. Although this approach does quantify the amount of urine retained, it is uncomfortable for patients and incurs a risk of infection. It is therefore preferable to avoid this procedure unless it is clear that urinary retention exists.

Ultrasound can immediately confirm and quantify the degree of obstruction and retention by imaging the urinary bladder and estimating its size. Many of the studies examining bladder volume have been performed by urologists in conjunction with urodynamic measurements.[5,7−12,53−59] In this setting, even small degrees of error may be unacceptable. By contrast, a qualitative estimate of bladder size may be very helpful in the emergency setting. Bedside pelvic ultrasound can easily classify the bladder volume as small, medium, or large, helping the clinician determine the need for emergent urinary catheterization. The presence of a large distended bladder mandates emergency urinary catheterization whereas an empty or small bladder on ultrasound suggests another cause for the patient's symptoms. An intermediate size may require bladder volume measurements to determine the need for catheterization. Whenever the bladder is imaged in this fashion, the kidneys should be examined for bilateral hydronephrosis, a concerning complication of long-standing bladder outlet obstruction.

Another potential indication for bedside ultrasound of the urinary tract is the assessment of bladder volume prior to urinary catheterization of children. Two recent studies have demonstrated that confirming the existence of urine in the bladder prior to catheterization can successfully reduce or even eliminate unsuccessful procedures, which are painful and often very traumatic. A minimum volume of 2 mL is necessary for accurate urinalysis. Because a calculated bladder index volume 2.4 cm^2, defined as the product of anteroposterior and transverse bladder diameters, corresponds to a bladder volume of 2 mL, catheterization should be deferred when the index is less than 2.4 cm^2.[13,14]

ACUTE RENAL FAILURE

Renal ultrasound can be a useful adjunct in the evaluation of acute renal failure. The clinical evaluation of acute renal failure begins with a determination of whether the cause is proximal to the kidneys (pre-renal failure), distal to the kidneys (post-renal failure), or intrinsic to the kidneys themselves ("renal" failure). Because post-renal causes such as obstruction of either ureteric or urethral outflow are readily reversible if identified in a timely fashion, these are most often considered first in the evaluation. Ultrasound is clearly an effective tool in the identification of post-renal obstruction, easily detecting bilateral hydronephrosis, and bladder distension. If only a solitary kidney is visualized and hydronephrosis is present, the need for acute decompression becomes particularly urgent. Moreover, prostatic enlargement, one of the most common causes of lower tract obstruction, can be identified on ultrasound.

After a post-renal cause has been excluded, renal ultrasound may provide still further diagnostic information. Whereas pre-renal causes of renal failure will not generally cause ultrasonographic abnormalities, several causes of acute and acute-on-chronic intrinsic renal failure will manifest themselves on ultrasound examination. Small, atrophic, and hyperechoic kidneys suggest chronic pathologic processes such as hypertensive nephropathy and chronic glomerulonephritis. The finding of enlarged kidneys with multiple cysts distorting the renal architecture suggests polycystic kidney disease as the cause of renal failure. Unfortunately, many causes of acute renal failure that are intrinsic, such as acute glomerulonephritis and acute tubular necrosis, may have nonspecific or minimal sonographic findings. Furthermore, different clinical entities may have different sonographic manifestations at different stages in their presentation. For this reason, other clinical methods, such as volume status determination, response to fluid therapy, microscopic urinalysis, and measurement of the fractional excretion of sodium must be utilized to distinguish between pre-renal and intrinsic causes of renal failure and guide therapy. Renal biopsy, often necessary to establish a definitive diagnosis, may be facilitated by ultrasound guidance.

ACUTE PYELONEPHRITIS AND RENAL ABSCESS

Acute pyelonephritis, an extremely common emergency diagnosis, does not necessarily require imaging. In fact, the sonographic appearance of the kidney in acute pyelonephritis is most commonly normal.[48] However, in complex cases or those not responding to medical management, ultrasound may be helpful in ruling out complications of pyelonephritis that require surgical management. For example, the formation of a renal abscess may complicate pyelonephritis. Renal abscesses are typically solitary, round hypoechoic masses, often with internal septations or mobile debris, and a degree of posterior acoustic enhancement.[48,50] Suspicious lesions identified in the course of the emergency ultrasound may prompt consultation with a urologist, a comprehensive sonographic study, and, in some cases, CT scanning to further characterize the lesion and formulate a treatment plan.[60] Perinephric abscesses extend beyond the kidney and may be visualized on ultrasound, but are better evaluated with CT. This modality should be sought when lesions are seen to extend beyond the kidney on ultrasound.[48]

One rare but life-threatening infection, emphysematous pyelonephritis, deserves special mention. Gas formation in the kidney by bacteria will cause echogenic areas that obscure the deeper structures. These echogenic areas could potentially be confused with renal stone disease; however, in the setting of pyelonephritis, this finding should prompt emergent surgical consultation. Patients with this infection are most frequently diabetic or immunocompromised for other reasons. Because patients with emphysematous pyelonephritis may have toxic and nonspecific presentations, suggestive findings on emergency ultrasound may prompt surgical intervention (either percutaneous drainage or open nephrectomy) that would have otherwise been overlooked or unduly delayed.[61−63]

RENAL MASSES

Renal masses are being seen with increasing frequency as a result of both emergency sonography and the incorporation of screening abdominal ultrasound into periodic health evaluations.[15,18,64−66] There is no question that the mortality and morbidity of malignancies detected in this incidental fashion are greatly reduced.[67−69] Although there is concern regarding the cost-effectiveness of routine use of ultrasound in the absence of specific symptomatology, a mechanism for the follow-up of abnormalities found in the emergency and acute care setting must be available. It cannot be overemphasized that the focused use of ultrasound to evaluate a patient for hydronephrosis is not a substitute for comprehensive sonography or other follow-up studies. Moreover, renal masses discovered on ultrasound almost always require further characterization with another modality, usually CT.[48] The majority of malignancies seen in the kidney are renal cell carcinoma (RCC).[16,66,70,71] These tumors are extremely heterogeneous in their sonographic appearance and may be isoechoic, hyperechoic, or hypoechoic to the adjacent parenchyma. It is also important to note that many of these tumors have a partially cystic presentation and may be mistaken for a simple benign cyst.[48]

Another common tumor seen in the kidney is the angiomyolipoma (AML).[48,70] These tumors are mostly benign and may be treated conservatively.[72] Whereas they are usually well-demarcated and brightly echogenic on ultrasound, there is a significant overlap in their sonographic appearance with that of echogenic renal cell carcinoma.[73] This serves to underscore the caution that is required in the interpretation of any mass found incidentally during ultrasound. Any such finding requires follow-up with a comprehensive ultrasound examination, a CT scan, or urological consultation.

Other tumors that are commonly seen on ultrasound are lymphomas and metastatic malignancies, which commonly appear as irregular nodules, either single or multiple. These may also be diffuse, grossly disturbing the renal architecture or infiltrative, extending into the perirenal and surrounding structures.[48] Transitional cell carcinoma (TCC), which is more commonly found in the bladder and ureter than in the renal pelvis, is frequently not visible on renal ultrasound. This is because it is frequently symptomatic (with gross hematuria) before sufficient tumor mass can be seen in the renal pelvis. Its sonographic appearance is one of a hypoechoic mass within the highly echogenic renal sinus.[48]

Renal cysts are an extremely common finding on ultrasound. Although simple cysts are benign, malignancies may present with a cystic appearance.[74] For this reason, caution needs to be exercised before dismissing a lesion seen on sonography as a simple cyst.

Polycystic kidney disease (PCKD) can be recognized as an abundance of cysts of varying sizes that both enlarge and distort the regular renal architecture.[48,50,74] Ultrasound is the modality of choice to evaluate this heritable disorder, which may present with hematuria, flank pain, hypertension, or renal failure. Cysts are frequently present in multiple organs in the body, and there is an association with cerebral aneurysms.[74] Urology or nephrology referral is indicated upon discovery of this disorder. Patients with chronic renal failure undergoing long-term dialysis also tend to develop multiple renal cysts. This disorder, known as acquired renal cystic disease (ARCD), is characterized by a huge increase in the incidence of renal malignancies, and for this reason regular surveillance of this condition is indicated.[48,74]

RENAL TRAUMA

On grey scale sonography, the primary indicator of major renal trauma is a subcapsular hematoma or perinephric hematoma. These findings may be recognized on the initial trauma ultrasound screening examination or on subsequent examinations. Patients with major trauma in whom injury of the renal pedicle is suspected are best evaluated with contrast CT, which provides information about renal function and is considered the modality of choice.[75] One study also showed standard B-mode sonography to have low sensitivity for patients with urological trauma.[76] If CT is not available, newer ultrasound techniques such as power color Doppler or contrast ultrasound may provide much more information than standard B-mode sonography.[77–80]

Ultrasound may also have a role in the follow-up and management of patients with identified parenchymal injury, such as hematomas and lacerations. These lesions are often well-visualized by ultrasonography and can be evaluated periodically to monitor their resolution.

▶ ANATOMICAL CONSIDERATIONS

COMPARTMENTS OF THE RETROPERITONEUM

Before describing the gross anatomy of the kidney, ureter, and bladder, it is first important to review where these structures lie within the abdominal cavity and their relation to their surroundings.

The retroperitoneal cavity is divided into three distinct compartments, with the kidneys occupying the middle or *perirenal* compartment. The anterior compartment contains the duodenum, pancreas, descending colon, celiac trunk, and superior mesenteric vessels, as well as associated fat. The posterior compartment, which lies anterior to the quadratus lumborum and psoas muscles, simply contains fat. The anterior and posterior compartments are also referred to as the *pararenal* compartments.

The perirenal compartment is bounded by *Gerota's fascia* both anteriorly and posteriorly, although many authors refer to the posterior component of the renal fascia as *Zuckerkandl's fascia*. This fascia, which invests the kidneys, adrenal glands, renal hila, proximal collecting system and perinephric fat, merges laterally to form the lateroconal fascia that extends to the parietal peritoneum of the lateral paracolic gutter. This completes the separation of the anterior and posterior retroperi-

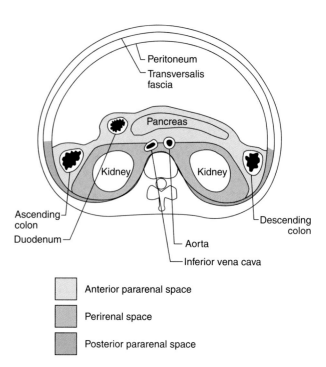

Figure 10-2. Anatomic compartments of the retroperitoneum.

toneal compartments. Thus, the kidneys are surrounded by two distinct layers of fat: the *perinephric fat*, which lies immediately outside the true fibrous capsule of the kidney, bounded by Gerota's fascia, and the *paranephric fat*, which lies in the pararenal compartments outside of Gerota's fascia.

This compartmentalization of the retroperitoneum is important clinically as it serves to localize various pathological processes. It also creates a barrier to the progression of various pathologic processes such as hemorrhage and infection. Collections of fluid in the anterior pararenal compartment, for example, are commonly related to pancreatitis or trauma, whereas collections of fluid in the posterior pararenal compartment are uncommon, usually representing spontaneous hemorrhage in patients with coagulopathy or related to trauma. Figure 10-2 demonstrates the compartments of the retroperitoneum.

ANATOMIC RELATIONSHIPS OF THE URINARY SYSTEM

There is significant asymmetry in the position of the two kidneys within the abdominal cavity. The right kidney is bounded anteriorly by the liver, which serves as an excellent acoustic window for sonography. It is usually slightly larger and slightly inferior to the left kidney. The left kidney is bounded anteriorly by several structures, including the pancreas, stomach, spleen, and large and small bowel, making it somewhat more difficult to image, as only the spleen serves as an acoustic window of equal quality to the liver. Superiorly and posteriorly, both kidneys have symmetrical relationships, with the diaphragms superiorly and the musculature of the retroperitoneum (psoas and quadratus) posteriorly. In the supine position, the superior pole of the left kidney is at the level of the 12th thoracic vertebrae and the inferior pole is at the level of the 3rd lumbar vertebrae. However, it is important to realize that the kidneys are mobile structures within the retroperitoneum, moving with changes in position and with the phases of respiration. Figure 10-3 demonstrates the anatomical relationships of the two kidneys.

The renal *hilum* is the specific area of the sinus where the renal artery enters and the renal vein and ureter exit the kidney on its medial concave surface. The ureters, which arise from the hila of each kidney, travel inferiorly toward the bladder in close relation to the psoas muscle, just anterior to the transverse process of the lumbar spine. As they enter the pelvis, they course medially to cross the iliac vessels and then laterally once again to parallel the margins of the bony pelvis before inserting posteriorly into the bladder.

The bladder, when empty, abuts the posterior aspect of the pubis. As it fills, it expands to fill more of the pelvis, displacing bowel loops into the abdomen. A distended bladder moves into the lower abdomen and gains relationships to the anterior abdominal wall.

RENAL ANATOMY

The kidneys are paired structures that lie obliquely with respect to every anatomic plane. They are situated so that their inferior poles are anterior and lateral to their superior poles. In addition, each hilum is directed obliquely as well in an anteromedially rather than simple medial orientation. The sonographic significance of this orientation is that the technique for imaging the kidneys must involve adjusting the probe obliquely in each plane to match the anatomy.[49,81]

Each kidney is between 9 and 13 cm in its maximum longitudinal measurement, and they decrease in size with advanced age and chronic renal failure. The approximate width and depth of the kidneys is 5 cm and 3 cm, respectively. Each kidney is surrounded by a true fibrous capsule and can be divided into two parts, the renal *parenchyma* and the renal *sinus*. The renal parenchyma, which surrounds the sinus on all sides except at the hilum, is composed of the outer *cortex*, consisting of the filtration components of the nephrons and the inner *medulla*, consisting of the reabsorptive components (loop of Henle). The cone-shaped medullary pyramids are oriented with their apices, or *papillae*, protruding inward toward the renal sinus. Thus, the functional unit of the kidney, or renal lobe, consists of a medullary pyramid and its surrounding cortex: urine being filtered by the cortex and then excreted through the papillae into the collecting system. There are between 8 and 18 such lobes in each kidney, bounded by

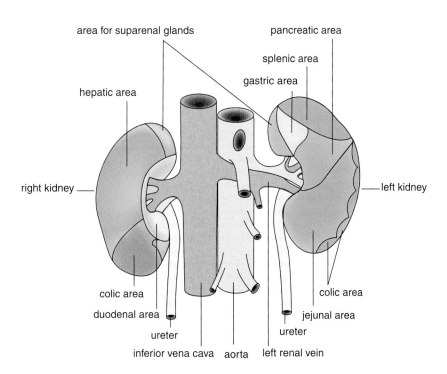

Figure 10-3. Anatomic relationship of the kidneys.

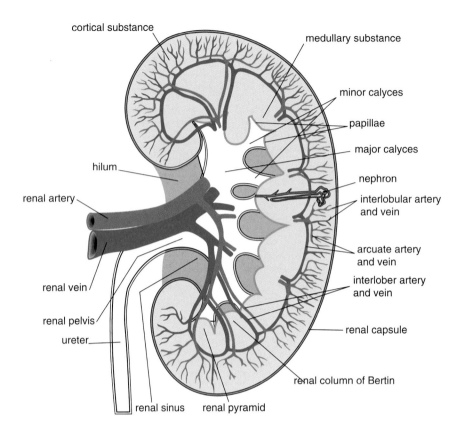

Figure 10-4. Gross anatomy of the kidney.

interlobar arteries and veins. The arcuate arteries, which branch from these interlobar arteries, are found at the base of the medullary pyramids and can serve as important landmarks in the interpretation of sonographic images.

The renal sinus, the central portion of the kidney, begins where the renal papillae empty their urine into the smallest subunit of the collecting system, the minor calyces. There are, therefore, between 8 and 18 minor calyces in each kidney corresponding to the pyramids. These minor calyces in turn coalesce into two to three major calyces. The major calyces merge with the renal *pelvis*, which is the dilated proximal end of the ureter as it joins the kidney. In addition to the collecting system, the renal sinus also contains the renal artery and vein, as well as fatty tissue, which is an extension of the perinephric fat bounded by Gerota's fascia. Figure 10-4 demonstrates the gross anatomy of the kidney.

▶ GETTING STARTED

Basic renal sonography can be performed with almost any machine suitable for bedside ultrasound. An ideal transducer would be a microconvex 3.5 MHz probe

which has a small footprint probe that allows easier navigation through the ribs. A larger curvilinear transducer can be used, but rib shadows may be problematic and could obscure critical areas. Images from a curvilinear probe will tend to be higher quality and resolution and show greater detail. A starting depth of 15 cm will suffice for most patients and can be adjusted as needed.

The right kidney is usually straightforward to visualize given its proximity to the liver, which provides an excellent acoustic window (Figure 10-5). The right kidney can usually be imaged well with the patient in a supine position (as in obtaining Morison's pouch in the FAST examination), but the left kidney may be difficult to image given the lack of a similar acoustic window on that side. For this reason, the left kidney is best imaged with the patient in the right lateral decubitus position (when clinically permissible), which allows the sonographer to easily access the far posterior aspects of the flank. Kidneys should first be imaged in the longitudinal plane, which is enhanced by orienting the beam of the probe in the same plane as the ribs. Once the longitudinal plane has been well visualized, the transducer should be rotated 90 degrees to obtain the transverse plane.

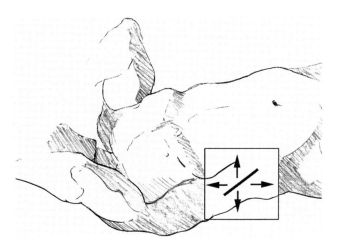

Figure 10-5. Transducer placement for imaging the right kidney. Central line represents the longitudinal axis of the kidney.

► TECHNIQUE AND NORMAL ULTRASOUND FINDINGS

While the kidneys are usually imaged using the 3.5 MHz transducer, a 5.0 MHz transducer may be used to yield greater anatomic detail in thin patients or in those patients with a transplanted kidney located in the pelvis. Images of both the affected and unaffected kidneys in both the longitudinal and transverse planes should be obtained, and, as with other structures, it is necessary to carefully scan through the kidneys in both of these planes to ensure that all of the parenchyma is imaged.[81] It is important to identify both kidneys for comparison to normal, and to rule out congenital or surgical absence. A focused ultrasound examination of the urinary tract should also include views of the bladder to access total filling and identify possible abnormalities.

RIGHT KIDNEY

The right kidney can usually be imaged with the patient supine, using the anterior subcostal approach (Figure 10-6). If clinically permissible, it may be necessary to have the patient turn toward their left side or prone. From a position inferior and lateral to the edge of the right costal margin, the transducer is moved incrementally medially and inferiorly until the kidney comes into view. Because of the kidney's oblique lie, it will be

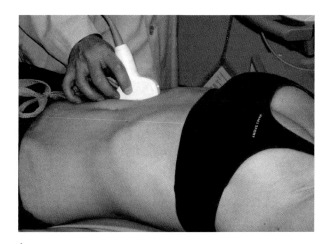

A

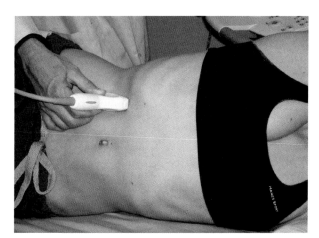

B

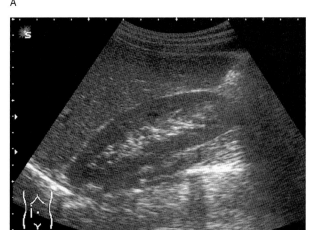

C

Figure 10-6. Longitudinal ultrasound view of the normal right kidney. Probe positon for supine patient (A), probe position for patient in lateral decubitus (B), and corresponding ultrasound image (C). Model is holding a deep breath for improved kidney imaging. (Courtesy of James Mateer, MD)

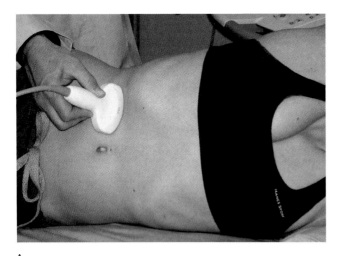

A

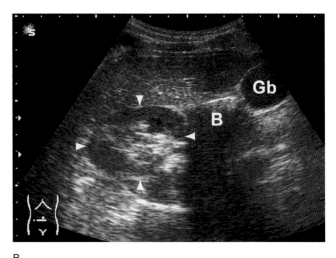

B

Figure 10-7. Transverse ultrasound view of the normal right kidney. Probe positon (A) and corresponding ultrasound image (B) with kidney border outlined (arrowheads). Gb = gallbladder, B = bowel with posterior shadowing. (Courtesy of James Mateer, MD)

necessary to rotate the transducer to obtain the image of the kidney in its maximal length. This is the longitudinal axis, and once the image is obtained, the transducer is swept medially and laterally to scan all of the parenchyma and sinus in this axis. In many patients it will not be possible to view the entire kidney longitudinally in one window, and separate images are often required of the superior and inferior poles. It also may be necessary to obtain some of the images using intercostal windows or by having the patient briefly hold their breath, moving the kidneys inferiorly to a subcostal window.

To obtain the transverse plane images, the transducer merely needs to be rotated 90 degrees from the longitudinal plane (Figure 10-7). Once in the transverse plane, the transducer can be moved either superiorly and medially or inferiorly and laterally to locate the renal hilum, with images superior representing the superior pole and images inferior representing the inferior pole. If intestinal gas is interfering with anterior views, coronal views of the right kidney should be used. This technique is described in detail in Chapter 5 (Trauma).

LEFT KIDNEY/BLADDER

Unlike the right kidney, with its generous acoustic window provided by the liver, the sonologist has to contend with interference from air in the stomach and intestine in order to obtain images of the left kidney. This may be circumvented by finding a more posterior window (usually through the spleen), with the patient turning toward the examiner in the right lateral decubitus position if possible.[49,81] To obtain the longitudinal images of the left kidney, the transducer is first placed in the midcoro-

nal plane, moving between the costal margin superiorly and the iliac crest inferiorly to find the kidney (Figure 10-8). As with the right kidney, it will be necessary to find the longest axis first before scanning the kidney throughout in this plane (Figure 10-9). With respect to imaging the entire kidney, using a combination of intercostal and subcostal views and subsequently obtaining transverse images by rotating the transducer, the same guidelines apply as for the right kidney. The coronal view is particularly helpful for imaging the inferior pole of the left kidney, which is often obscured by overlying gas within the descending colon. This technique is also described in detail in Chapter 5 (Trauma). The bladder is easily imaged with the transducer in the suprapubic position and

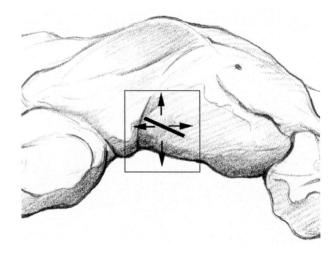

Figure 10-8. Transducer placement for imaging the left kidney. Central line represents the longitudinal axis of the kidney.

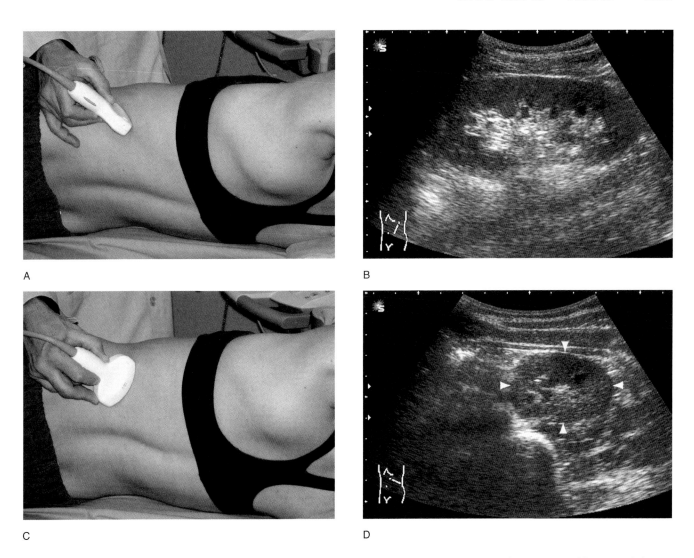

A

B

C

D

Figure 10-9. Normal left kidney. Longitudinal coronal probe position (A) and long-axis ultrasound image of the kidney (B). Transverse coronal probe position (C) and short-axis ultrasound image of the kidney (arrowheads) (D). (Courtesy of James Mateer, MD)

should be moderately filled for optimal imaging. Like the kidney it should be scanned thoroughly in both sagittal and transverse planes (Figure 10-10).

SONOGRAPHIC APPEARANCE OF THE KIDNEY, URETER, AND BLADDER

Each kidney is well demarcated by a brightly echogenic fibrous capsule surrounded by a variable amount of perinephric fat. The parenchyma typically has an echogenicity somewhat less than that of the liver. Within the parenchyma, the cortex can often be distinguished from the medullary pyramids, which because of their urine-filled tubules cut a less echogenic, saw toothed ribbon deep to the margin of the cortex. The sinus, which lies deep to the parenchyma, is highly echogenic because of its high fat content. In well-hydrated patients, anechoic

pockets of urine may be seen within the brightly reflective sinus. When scanned in real time, the continuity of these pockets within the renal pelvis can be demonstrated. Figures 10-6 and 10-7 show normal longitudinal and transverse ultrasound images of the right kidney. Although the normal ureter is not seen on ultrasound, a proximally distended ureter can often be visualized. The shape and relationships of the bladder on ultrasound examination depend on its degree of filling (Figure 10-10).

With urine in the bladder, its wall appears as a thin echogenic line surrounding an anechoic cavity. The normal prostate gland may be recognized as a hyperechoic ovular mass at the bladder neck (Figure 10-11). This is best seen on transverse views angled caudad, with a normal prostate size of up to 5 cm in width.

In patients with normal hydration and no ureteral obstruction, intermittent ureteral flow jets can be observed near the trigone area as urine flows into a filled

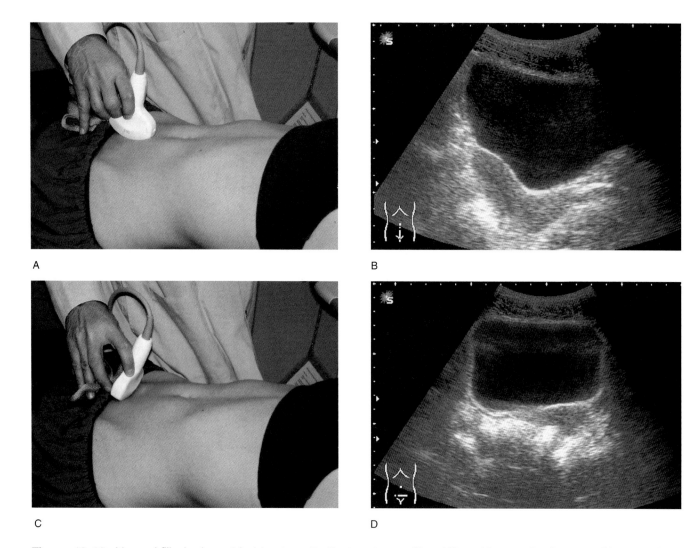

A

B

C

D

Figure 10-10. Normal filled urinary bladder. Longitudinal probe position (A) and long-axis ultrasound image of the bladder (B). Transverse probe position (C) and short axis ultrasound image of the bladder (D). (Courtesy of James Mateer, MD)

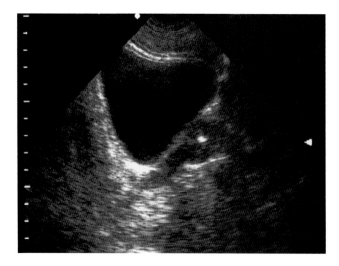

Figure 10-11. Longitudinal view of the male bladder reveals the prostate posteriorly that contains a small central calcification.

bladder. These can be visualized with gray scale sonography but are more obvious using color Doppler techniques (Figure 10-12).

► COMMON ABNORMALITIES

OBSTRUCTIVE UROPATHY

In hydronephrosis, large echo-free areas representing urine can be seen within the echogenic renal sinus. The degree of hydronephrosis seen is a continuum, although somewhat arbitrary designations of mild, moderate, and severe hydronephrosis are commonly used (Figures 10-13 and 10-14). The designation of severe hydronephrosis is generally reserved for kidneys that demonstrate some degree of cortical thinning. For those with chronic severe hydronephrosis, cortical atrophy will be more obvious (Figure 10-15). Acute ureteral obstruction may cause calyceal rupture. Occasionally high-grade obstruction with

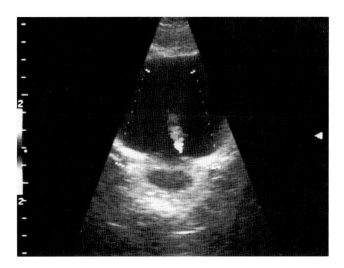

Figure 10-12. Transverse view of the male bladder reveals a normal ureteral flow jet on color Doppler (grayscale image) arising from the trigone area. A transverse view of the hypoechoic prostate gland is seen immediately below the bladder.

hydronephrosis can result in perinephric fluid signifying a ruptured calyx (Figure 10-16).

Stones can be seen within the kidney itself and, like gallstones, have a strongly echogenic appearance and cause acoustic shadowing (Figures 10-17 and 10-18). Stones are rarely visualized in the mid-ureter, but may occasionally be identified at the ureteropelvic junction (Figure 10-19) or uretovescicular junctions (Figure 10-20), two common locations of obstruction.

BLADDER VOLUME MEASUREMENT

This technique involves measuring the bladder in its maximal width, depth, and length, or by measuring the length and circumference and then inserting the value of these measurements into a mathematical formula. It has been used for more than 25 years and was first performed using B-mode imaging.[5,10] With real-time ultra-sound, most current machines contain automated calculators for volume measurement (Figure 10-21). As an alternate, the simple formula (L $\times$ W $\times$ H $\times$ 0.75) can be used as to estimate bladder volume.[11] Because of the inherent variability of bladder shape and the variation in this shape with differing degrees of filling, bladder volume measurements obtained in this fashion may have an error of between 15% and 35%.[5,9–12]

RENAL ABSCESS

Renal abscesses are typically solitary, round hypoechoic masses, often with internal septations or mobile debris and a degree of posterior acoustic enhancement. When these rupture or extend into the perinephric space, complex fluid may be appreciated surrounding a portion of the kidney (Figure 10-22).

RENAL MASSES

The majority of malignancies seen in the kidney are renal cell carcinoma.[16,66,70] These tumors are extremely heterogeneous in their sonographic appearance and may be isoechoic, hyperechoic, or hypoechoic to the adjacent parenchyma (Figure 10-23). It is also important to note that many of these tumors have a cystic presentation and may be mistaken for a simple benign cyst.[48]

Another common tumor seen in the kidney is the angiomyolipoma (AML).[72] Whereas they are usually well demarcated and brightly echogenic on ultrasound, there is a significant overlap in their sonographic appearance with that of echogenic renal cell carcinoma.[73]

RENAL CYSTS

Renal cysts are an extremely common finding on ultrasound. A benign cyst must meet all of the following criteria[48–50]:

1. smooth, round, or oval shaped;
2. no internal echoes or solid elements;

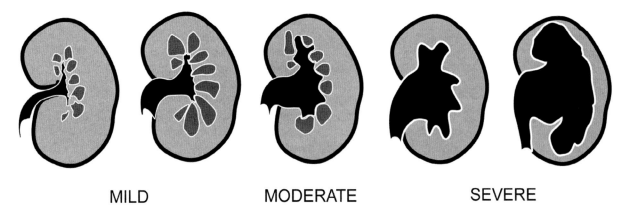

MILD   MODERATE   SEVERE

Figure 10-13. Grades of hydronephrosis.

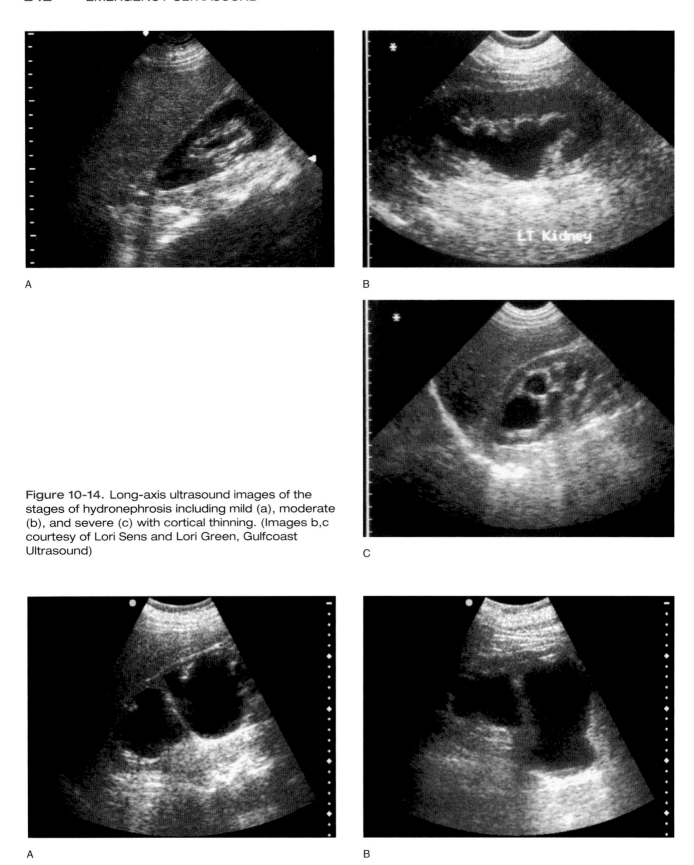

Figure 10-14. Long-axis ultrasound images of the stages of hydronephrosis including mild (a), moderate (b), and severe (c) with cortical thinning. (Images b,c courtesy of Lori Sens and Lori Green, Gulfcoast Ultrasound)

Figure 10-15. Chronic severe hydronephrosis. Coronal views of the kidney show severe hydronephrosis and cortical atrophy (a). Another view of the same kidney demonstrating severe urinary distention of the renal pelvis (b). (Courtesy of James Mateer, MD)

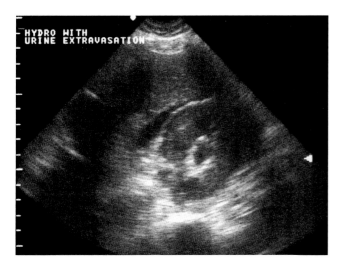

Figure 10-16. Hydronephrosis with acute calyceal rupture. Transverse view of right kidney (outlined by rib shadows) with hydronephrosis and urinary extravasation into the perirenal space.

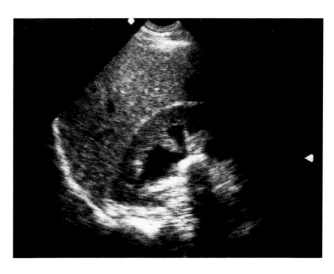

Figure 10-18. Longitudinal view of right kidney shows moderate hydronephrosis and a large stone within the renal pelvis.

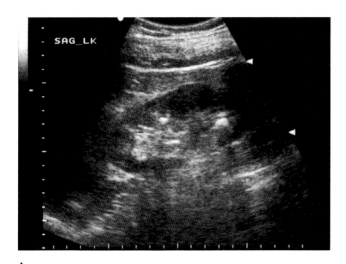

A

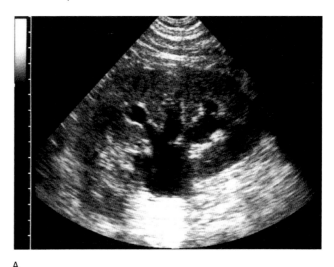

A

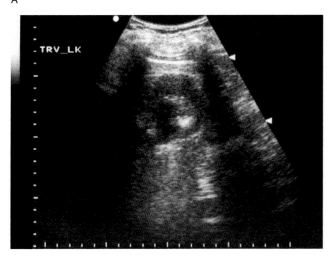

B

Figure 10-17. Longitudinal (a) and transverse (b) views of the left kidney show intrarenal stones (with posterior shadowing below the larger of the two stones). (Courtesy of Lori Sens, Gulfcoast Ultrasound)

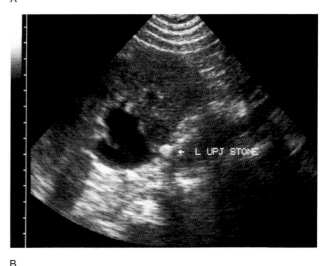

B

Figure 10-19. Ureteropelvic junction stone. Coronal view of the kidney (a) shows moderate hydronephrosis. A slightly different angle of the same kidney demonstrates a ureteropelvic junction stone (with posterior shadowing) as the cause of the urinary obstruction. (Courtesy of James Mateer, MD)

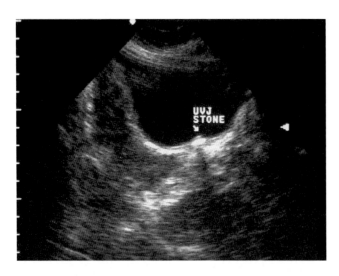

Figure 10-20. Ureterovescicular junction stone. Ureteral stone seen at the ureterovesical junction through a transverse view of the bladder.

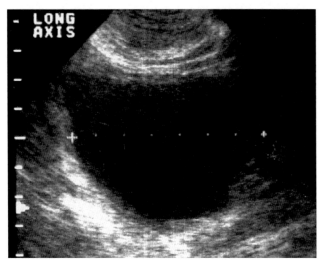

A

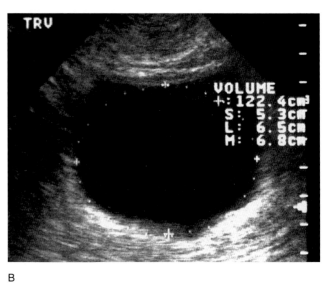

B

Figure 10-21. Longitudinal (a) and transverse (b) views of the bladder show the use of a software calculation program to determine bladder volume.

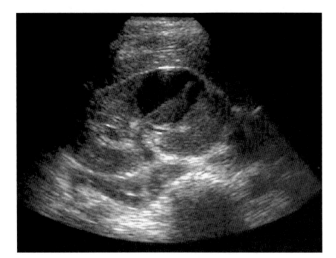

Figure 10-22. Longitudinal view of the kidney shows a large complex cyst in the mid portion of the cortex. The echogenic layer was persistent with probe angle and position (not an artifact) and was documented as inflammatory debris from a renal abcess (Reproduced with permission from Charles Lanzieri, MD, University Hospitals of Cleveland.)

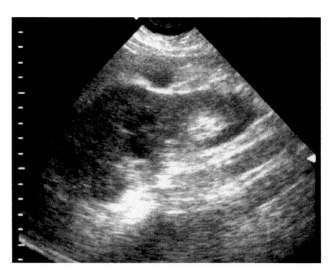

Figure 10-23. Renal cell carcinoma. Long-axis view through the right kidney showing renal cell carcinoma with enlargement of the upper pole including both solid and cystic elements.

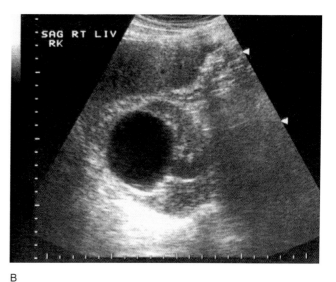

A

B

Figure 10-24. Renal cyst. Longitudinal (a) and transverse (b) views of the right kidney demonstrate the usual features of a simple cyst. (Courtesy of Lori Sens, Gulfcoast Ultrasound)

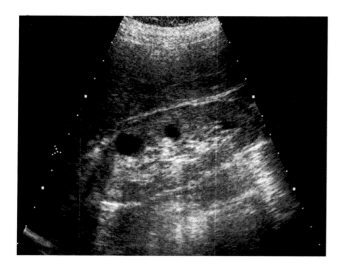

Figure 10-25. Longitudinal view of the right kidney with 2 small, simple appearing cysts within the middle and upper pole.

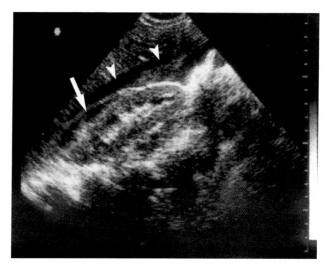

Figure 10-26. Renal trauma. Longitudinal view of the right upper quadrant shows fluid and clots in Morison's pouch (arrowheads) from hepatic injury and capsular elevation and a subcapsular hematoma of the kidney (arrow) related to blunt renal trauma. (Courtesy of James Mateer, MD)

3. well-defined interface between the cyst and the adjacent renal parenchyma in all planes and orientations; and

4. posterior echo enhancement beyond the cyst.

Figures 10-24 and 10-25 show the sonographic appearance of simple cysts.

RENAL TRAUMA

At present, sonography is not the definitive modality in the evaluation of renal trauma. The indicators of major renal trauma, subcapsular and perinephric hematomas

(Figure 10-26), must be differentiated from fluid in the hepatorenal space or in the posterior pararenal compartment of the retroperitoneum, which are not specific for renal trauma (Figure 10-27). Fluid in the anterior pararenal space is often difficult to visualize with ultrasound due to overlying bowel gas and lack of a distinct interface with solid organs.

A fracture of the kidney may be suspected when a hematoma of the kidney parenchyma is present. An organ hematoma will usually be isoechoic in the acute phase, making the ultrasound diagnosis difficult. Over

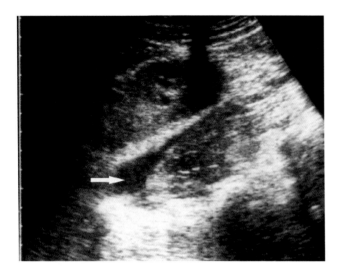

Figure 10-27. Coronal view of the kidney and psoas muscle demonstrates fluid in the posterior pararenal space (arrow). (Courtesy of James Mateer, MD)

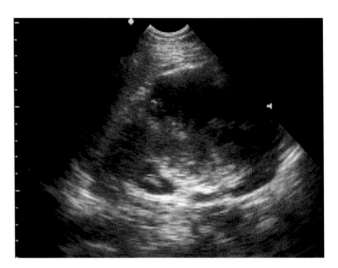

Figure 10-28. Longitudinal view of the kidney demonstrates a large complex subcapsular fluid collection and distorted cortical structure. This represents a subacute hematoma of the kidney.

time, a parenchymal hematoma will become hypoechoic compared to the surrounding tissue and more obvious on ultrasound (Figure 10-28). On color or power Doppler, an absence of flow will be seen in the portion of the kidney containing the hematoma.

► COMMON VARIANTS AND OTHER ABNORMALITIES

SONOLUCENT PYRAMIDS

In some patients, the medullary pyramids appear so sonolucent that they may be mistaken for the anechoic collections of urine seen with hydronephrosis.[49] They can be differentiated from distended calyces by the presence of cortex between them, by their triangular shape, and sometimes by the appearance of arcuate arteries, which appear as bright echogenic dots at the base of the pyramids (Figure 10-29).

HYPERTROPHIED COLUMNS OF BERTIN

Although identification of renal masses is not a goal of focused emergency ultrasound of the kidney, there is one common anomaly that deserves special mention because of its cause of potential to be mistaken for a renal mass. A "hypertrophied column of Bertin" refers to an invagination of renal cortical tissue into the renal sinus (Figure 10-30). This invagination can mimic a mass because it may cause an indentation and splaying of the sinus structures. It does, however, have the same echogenicity as the renal cortex and can be seen to be

continuous with the cortex in real time. In addition, these columns should not alter the outer contour of the kidney as commonly occurs with renal cell carcinoma.[48–50,74]

The dromedary (splenic) hump occurs on the left kidney as a normal variant in some patients and will appear as a symmetrical, rounded enlargement of the center portion of the cortex with homogenous echotexture. Since the contour of the kidney is altered, it is more difficult to confidently exclude renal cell carcinoma and a follow-up study is recommended (Figure 10-31).

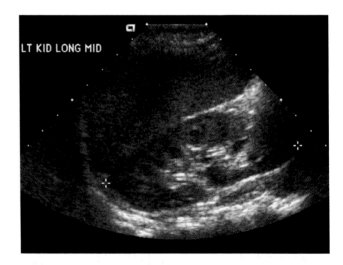

LT KID LONG MID

Figure 10-29. Right kidney in long axis with sonolucent renal pyramids. This corresponds with the medullary portions of the kidney. (Courtesy of James Mateer, MD, Waukesha Memorial Hospital)

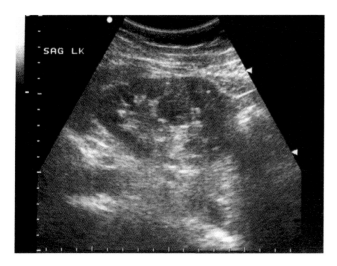

Figure 10-30. Long axis of the left kidney demonstrating a column of Bertin displacing the sinus structures. (Courtesy of Lori Sens, Gulfcoast Ultrasound)

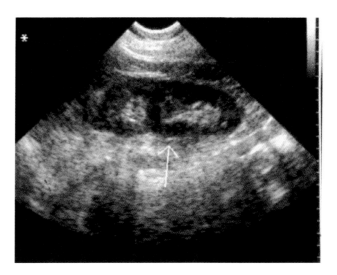

Figure 10-32. Partial duplex collecting system. Long-axis view of the kidney shows a distinct separation between the upper and lower portions of the collecting system within the kidney. (Courtesy of Lori Sens and Lori Green, Gulfcoast Ultrasound)

DUPLICATION OF THE COLLECTING SYSTEM

A duplex collecting system is one of the most common congenital renal anomalies and the degree of duplication can vary. A duplex collecting system may be sonographically detected as two central echogenic sinuses with normal bridging renal parenchyma between them (Figure 10-32). Hydronephrosis of the upper pole sinus and visualization of two distinct collecting systems and ureters is diagnostic of this condition.

ECTOPIC KIDNEY

If the kidney has an abnormal contour or is not found on the flank examinations as described above, then congenital abnormalities such as horseshoe kidney (Figure 10-33), pelvic kidney (Figure 10-34), or congenital absence of a kidney must be entertained. In any of these circumstances, consideration of comprehensive imaging and specialty consultation is indicated. All of these abnormalities place the patient with obstructive uropathy (and other renal pathologies) at increased risk for complications.

PROSTATE ENLARGEMENT

An enlarged prostate gland may be seen while imaging the bladder on transabdominal ultrasonography. It may be recognized as a hyperechoic ovular mass at the bladder neck with a transverse diameter greater than 5 cm (Figure 10-35).

POLYCYSTIC KIDNEYS

Polycystic kidney disease (PCKD) can be recognized as an abundance of cysts of varying sizes that both enlarge and distort the regular renal architecture (Figure 10-36).

CHRONIC RENAL DISEASE

The most common sonographic finding in chronic renal failure is that of bilaterally small and hyperechoic

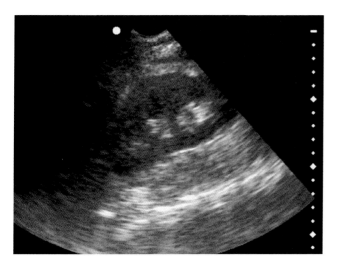

Figure 10-31. Long-axis view of the left kidney demonstrating the typical morphology of a dromedary hump. (Courtesy of James Mateer, MD)

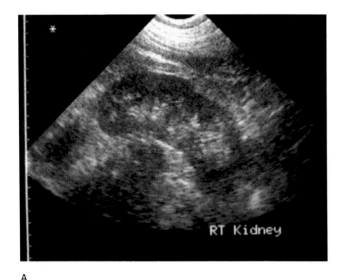

A

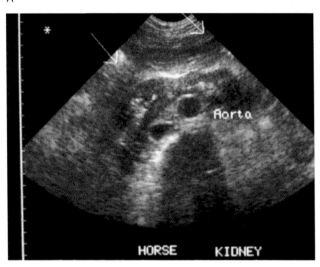

B

Figure 10-33. Horseshoe kidney. Longitudinal view of the right kidney shows a slightly unusual shape and an indistinct lower pole (a). The horseshoe kidney could have been missed if transverse views had not been done. Transverse views (b) clearly demonstrated a connection of the lower poles of both kidneys in the midline over the aorta (labeled). (Courtesy of Lori Sens and Lori Green, Gulfcoast Ultrasound)

kidneys. A variety of pathological processes ranging from diseases of the glomerulus (e.g., glomerulonephritis), infection (e.g., chronic pyelonephritis), and renal vascular disease may result in this sonographic finding. It is not specific to any particular etiology (Figure 10-37).

ADRENAL MASS

Although the normal adrenal glands may not be visualized during focused ultrasound of the urinary tract in the

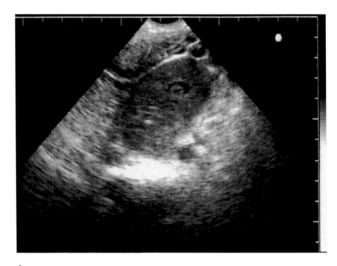

A

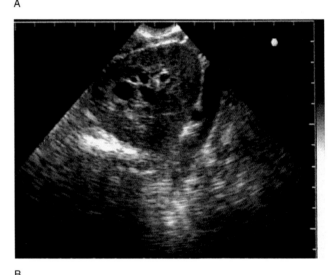

B

Figure 10-34. Pelvic kidney. Endovaginal image with a 7.5 MHz probe. Left adnexal mass is noted to be kidney shaped (a). Detail views demonstrated normal renal architecture and a position adjacent to the iliac vein (b). (Courtesy of James Mateer, MD)

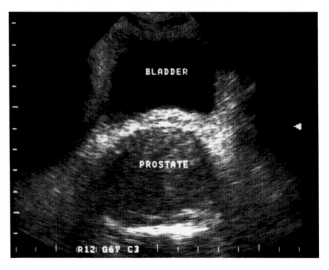

Figure 10-35. Transverse view of the bladder showing an enlarged prostate posteriorly.

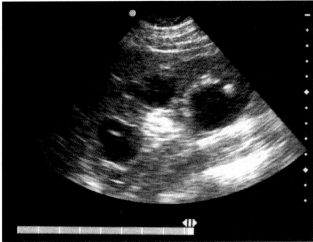

A

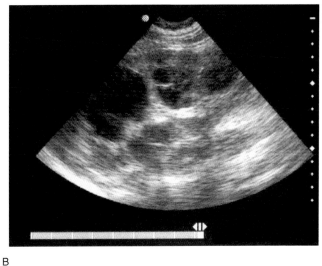

B

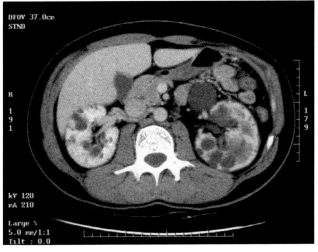

C

Figure 10-36. Polycystic kidneys. Coronal views of the right (a) and left (b) kidneys demonstrate adult polycystic kidney disease. CT scan of the same patient (c) for comparison. (Courtesy of James Mateer MD)

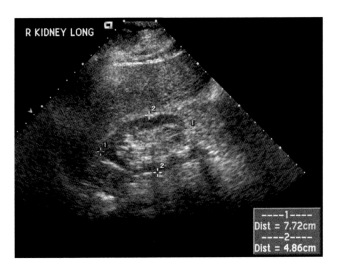

Figure 10-37. Chronic renal disease. This kidney demonstrates thinning of the cortex and a contracted size from chronic renal disease. (Courtesy of James Mateer, MD, Waukesha Memorial Hospital)

acute care setting, moderate and large adrenal masses may be seen anteromedially to the upper pole of the kidney. Because of the excellent acoustic window provided by the liver, right-sided masses are often better visualized. The appearance of adrenal masses is varied, as is the underlying pathology. Additional imaging with CT and biopsy may both be required to make a definitive pathological diagnosis (Figure 10-38).

BLADDER MASS

Bladder masses, both benign and malignant, may present as focal bladder wall thickening (Figure 10-39) or as an irregular echogenic mass projecting into the lumen (Figure 10-40). If such a mass is visualized, the possibility of upper tract obstruction should be addressed by visualizing the kidneys as well as examining for hydronephrosis. Further imaging and biopsy are required to make a definitive diagnosis.

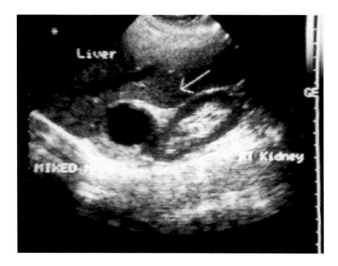

Figure 10-38. Adrenal mass. The right adrenal mass (arrow) has a thickened ring of tissue surrounding a cystic central portion. (Courtesy of Lori Sens and Lori Green, Gulfcoast Ultrasound)

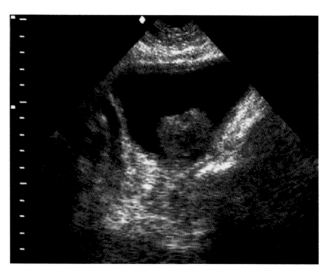

Figure 10-40. Large polypoid bladder mass noted in posterior bladder on an oblique view.

▶ PITFALLS

1. **Bedside ultrasound is limited in scope.** Any additional abnormalities that are recognized require a close follow-up.
2. **Hydronephrosis may be mimicked.** Several fairly common processes may mimic the presence of hydronephrosis, including prominent medullary pyramids, renal cortical cysts, an overdistended bladder, and pregnancy. Renal parapelvic cysts are less common but are eas-

ily confused with hydronephrosis due to their central location within the renal sinus. They can be differentiated from hydronephrosis due to their round shapes and their lack of communication with the fluid-filled renal pelvis. Extra-renal pelvis is a congenital variant in which the renal pelvis lies outside of the kidney. It can be confused with hydronephrosis. The visible anechoic area will be anatomically related to the sinus but will lie outside of the body of the kidney.[82] Both kidneys should always be scanned for comparison and the bladder should be evaluated for degree of filling.

3. **Presence of hydronephrosis may be masked by dehydration.** If ureterolithiasis is suspected, images should be obtained after the patient receives either an intravenous or an oral fluid bolus.
4. **The absence of hydronephrosis does not rule out a ureteral stone.** Small stones may not cause significant enough obstruction to produce hydronephrosis.
5. **Patients with an acute AAA often present with flank pain.** A ruptured AAA can present with a clinical picture suggesting acute renal colic. A large AAA can potentially compress the ureter and cause hydronephrosis. In patients older than 50 years with renal colic, one should always image the aorta in addition to the urinary tract (Figure 10-41).
6. **A bladder mass may be a hematoma.** In patients with gross hematuria, blood may accumulate in the bladder and appear as a mass on ultrasound. When suspected, this can be confirmed by resolution of the mass following bladder irrigation (Figure 10-42).

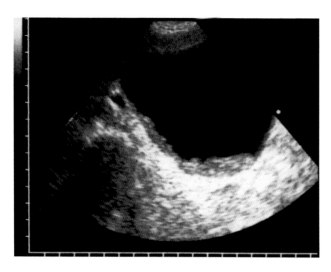

Figure 10-39. Bladder wall tumor. Transverse view of the bladder reveals a localized irregular thickening of the posterolateral bladder wall. (Courtesy of James Mateer, MD)

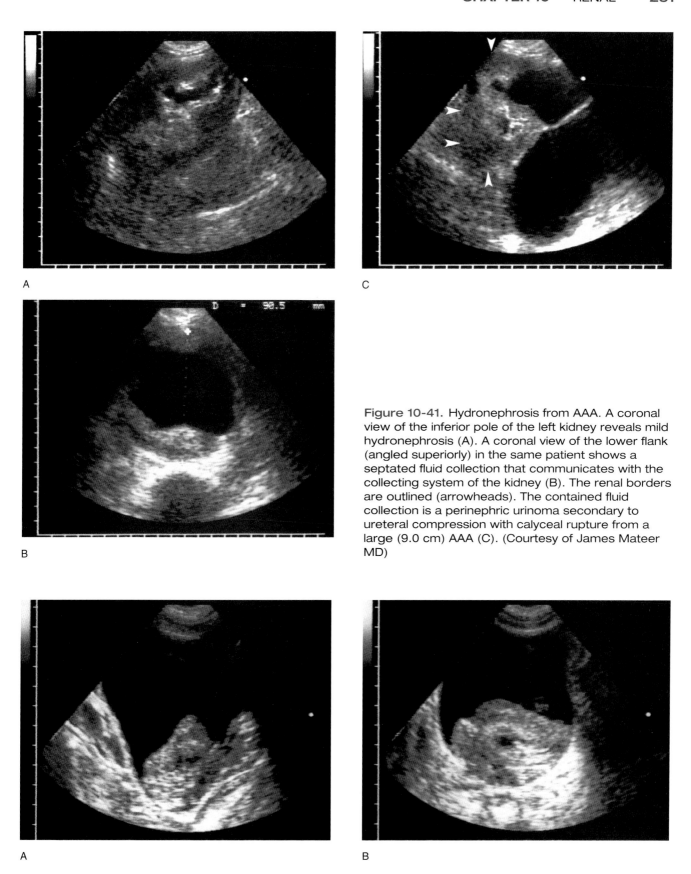

A

C

B

Figure 10-41. Hydronephrosis from AAA. A coronal view of the inferior pole of the left kidney reveals mild hydronephrosis (A). A coronal view of the lower flank (angled superiorly) in the same patient shows a septated fluid collection that communicates with the collecting system of the kidney (B). The renal borders are outlined (arrowheads). The contained fluid collection is a perinephric urinoma secondary to ureteral compression with calyceal rupture from a large (9.0 cm) AAA (C). (Courtesy of James Mateer MD)

A

B

Figure 10-42. Bladder hematoma. Longitudinal view of an enlarged bladder showing a posterior mass (a). Transverse views suggesting a laminar structure of the mass (b). This mass resolved following bladder irrigation. (Courtesy of James Mateer, MD)

▶ CASE STUDIES

CASE 1

Patient Presentation

A 38-year-old man presented to the emergency department at 3 AM after two hours of excruciating left flank pain and vomiting. He had similar pain the day prior but it was not as intense and subsided after a short period of time. He denied hematuria or dysuria. He had no previous history of renal colic.

On physical examination, he was noted to be in significant pain with difficulty getting comfortable. His blood pressure was 140/80 mmHg, heart rate 110 beats per minute, respirations 16 per minute, and his temperature 37.5°C. Head, neck, chest, and cardiovascular examinations were within normal limits. Examination of the abdomen revealed no significant anterior abdominal tenderness but he was noted to have tenderness at the left costovertebral angle. External genitourinary examination was normal.

Management Course

The patient was administered an intravenous narcotic for acute pain control and an antiemetic. Intravenous saline was initiated and basic laboratory tests were sent, including urinalysis. While awaiting laboratory tests, a bedside-focused ultrasound of the kidneys was performed by the treating physician. Ultrasound revealed moderate hydronephrosis of the left kidney confirming the clinical impression of acute renal colic (Figure 10-43). Two hours later, he was pain-free and urinalysis revealed 10–20 RBCs/hpf with no pyuria. He was given urology follow-up for the following day and oral analgesics on discharge.

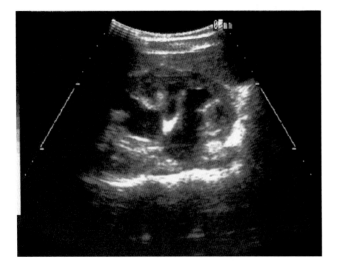

Figure 10-43. Case 1. Moderate hydronephrosis of the left kidney.

Commentary

Case 1 is a classic presentation of acute renal colic in a young adult. Many authors would recommend no testing except urinalysis in this scenario while others would argue for an imaging study for all cases. Even in classic presentations, a confirmatory test is desirable. Of the available modalities, ultrasound is the least expensive and fastest, and requires no ionizing radiation. This patient presented at 3 AM, which further complicates the case because of the limited imaging resources usually available at this hour in many practice settings. This patient may need further definitive imaging but bedside ultrasound provides enough information for acute diagnosis and disposition for emergency purposes.

CASE 2

Patient Presentation

A 26-year-old woman, gravida 2 para 1 at 11 weeks' gestation, presented to the emergency department with acute left flank and left lower quadrant pain. She had mild nausea but no vomiting. She denied any vaginal bleeding or any acute urinary symptoms and was previously healthy with no previous operations.

Physical examination revealed a young woman in moderate pain with a blood pressure of 100/60 mmHg, heart rate 100 beats per minute, respirations 14 per minute, and temperature 37.0°C. Head, neck, chest, and cardiovascular examinations were normal. Abdominal examination revealed left costovertebral angle tenderness and mild left lower quadrant tenderness without peritoneal signs. Pelvic examination revealed a nontender enlarged uterus with no cervical or adnexal tenderness.

Management Course

Intravenous saline was started and the patient received a small dose of intravenous narcotic for analgesia. Basic laboratory testing, including urinalysis, was obtained followed by a bedside ultrasound performed by the treating physician. The pelvis was quickly scanned through a transabdominal approach, revealing a live intrauterine pregnancy with no evidence of free pelvic fluid or abnormal mass. The left kidney revealed large hydronephrosis while mild hydronephrosis was seen in the right kidney (see, for example, Figures 10-14A,C). Urinalysis revealed 20–50 RBCs/hpf and 1–2 WBC/hpf with no bacteruria. Blood work was normal but she had persistent pain and admission to the antepartum ward was arranged along with urological consultation. Within 24 hours, she was feeling much better and repeat sonography at that time revealed resolving hydronephrosis. She was discharged home and had an uncomplicated delivery 6 months later.

Commentary

The above case illustrates the complex nature of evaluating abdominal pain in pregnancy. The physician has to consider an expanded differential diagnosis to include pregnancy-related conditions, while simultaneously being limited to fewer diagnostic adjuncts. In this case, the radiation and dye load associated with intravenous pyelography or CT is a relative contraindication to their use. Ultrasound provides ideal imaging for pregnant patients. The most important initial priority, the exclusion of an ectopic pregnancy, was done within minutes of arrival using a transabdominal scan. Hydronephrosis of the left kidney that was greater than the physiological hydronephrosis on the right side was significant in this case. Repeat sonography was also used to follow resolution of this patient's hydronephrosis.

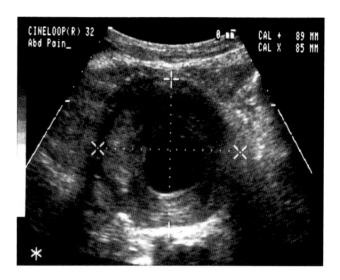

Figure 10-44. Case 3. Short-axis view of abdominal aortic aneurysm measuring 8.9 cm.

CASE 3

Patient Presentation

A 78-year-old man presented to the emergency department with left flank pain of 2 hours' duration. He denied nausea, vomiting, or any urinary symptoms. History was significant for chronic hypertension and nephrolithiasis requiring basket extraction 10 years prior.

Physical examination revealed an elderly man in moderate distress. Vitals signs revealed a blood pressure of 160/90 mmHg, heart rate 110 beats per minute, respirations 12 per minute, and temperature 37.7°C. Head, neck, chest, and cardiovascular examinations were within normal limits. Abdominal examination revealed an obese abdomen with diffuse tenderness without any definite discrete masses. The result from external genitourinary examination was normal, as was the rest of the physical examination.

Management Course

Intravenous access and blood work were immediately ordered. Cardiac monitor revealed sinus tachycardia and 12-lead electrocardiogram showed nonspecific ST changes. The emergency physician performed a focused abdominal ultrasound examining both the aorta and kidneys. The aorta was dilated with a maximum diameter of 8.9 cm and both kidneys appeared within normal limits (Figure 10-44). The diagnosis of AAA was made and he was taken immediately for surgery within 40 minutes of arrival. At laparotomy, the aneurysm was noted to have extensive retroperitoneal rupture but the patient had a successful repair and was discharged from the hospital 7 days later.

Commentary

Although uncomplicated renal colic itself does not present as an acute life-threatening emergency, the major differential in the elderly is a symptomatic abdominal aortic aneurysm. In the illustrated case, the patient had a history of previous renal colic complicating the clinical picture but bedside ultrasound was used to quickly evaluate both the kidneys and the aorta and thus clarified the emergent diagnosis. A "helical CT first" approach, which may delay the diagnosis and surgical consult, could have been catastrophic in this case.

REFERENCES

1. ACEP: *Emergency Ultrasound Imaging Criteria: Renal.* Statement Approved by ACEP Board, 2006.
2. Brown DF, Rosen CL, Wolfe RE: Renal ultrasonography. *Emerg Med Clin North Am* 15:877–893, 1997.
3. Use of ultrasound imaging by emergency physicians. *Ann Emerg Med* 38:469–470, 2001.
4. Noble VE, Brown D: Renal ultrasound. *Emerg Med Clin North Am* 22:641–659, 2004.
5. Kiely EA, Hartnell GG, Gibson RN, Williams G: Measurement of bladder volume by real-time ultrasound. *Br J Urol* 60:33–35, 1987.
6. Krupnick AS, Teitelbaum DH, Geiger JD, et al.: Use of abdominal ultrasonography to assess pediatric splenic trauma. Potential pitfalls in the diagnosis [see comments]. *Ann Surg* 225:408–414, 1997.
7. Mainprize TC, Drutz HP: Accuracy of total bladder volume and residual urine measurements: Comparison between real-time ultrasonography and catheterization. *Am J Obstet Gynecol* 160:1013–1016, 1989.
8. Topper AK, Holliday PJ, Fernie GR: Bladder volume estimation in the elderly using a portable ultrasound- based measurement device. *J Med Eng Technol* 17:99–103, 1993.

9. Poston GJ, Joseph AE, Riddle PR: The accuracy of ultrasound in the measurement of changes in bladder volume. *Br J Urol* 55:361–363, 1983.

10. Hartnell GG, Kiely EA, Williams G, Gibson RN: Real-time ultrasound measurement of bladder volume: A comparative study of three methods. *Br J Radiol* 60:1063–1065, 1987.

11. Chan H: Noninvasive bladder volume measurement. *J Neurosci Nurs* 25:309–312, 1993.

12. Ireton RC, Krieger JN, Cardenas DD, et al.: Bladder volume determination using a dedicated, portable ultrasound scanner. *J Urol* 143:909–911, 1990.

13. Chen L, Hsiao AL, Moore CL, Dziura JD, Santucci KA: Utility of bedside bladder ultrasound before urethral catheterization in young children. *Pediatrics* 115:108–111, 2005.

14. Milling TJ, Jr., Van Amerongen R, Melville L, et al.: Use of ultrasonography to identify infants for whom urinary catheterization will be unsuccessful because of insufficient urine volume: Validation of the urinary bladder index. *Ann Emerg Med* 45:510–513, 2005.

15. Spouge AR, Wilson SR, Wooley B: Abdominal sonography in asymptomatic executives: Prevalence of pathologic findings, potential benefits, and problems. *J Ultrasound Med* 15:763–767; quiz 769–770, 1996.

16. Ozen H, Colowick A, Freiha FS: Incidentally discovered solid renal masses: What are they? *Br J Urol* 72:274–276, 1993.

17. Zagoria RJ, Dyer RB: The small renal mass: Detection, characterization, and management. *Abdom Imaging* 23:256–265, 1998.

18. Mandavia DP, Pregerson B, Henderson SO: Ultrasonography of flank pain in the emergency department: Renal cell carcinoma as a diagnostic concern. *J Emerg Med* 18:83–86, 2000.

19. Henderson SO, Hoffner RJ, Aragona JL, Groth DE, Esekogwu VI, Chan D: Bedside emergency department ultrasonography plus radiography of the kidneys, ureters, and bladder vs intravenous pyelography in the evaluation of suspected ureteral colic [see comments]. *Acad Emerg Med* 5:666–671, 1998.

20. Dalla Palma L, Stacul F, Bazzocchi M, Pagnan L, Festini G, Marega D: Ultrasonography and plain film versus intravenous urography in ureteric colic. *Clin Radiol* 47:333–336, 1993.

21. Rosen CL, Brown DF, Sagarin MJ, Chang Y, McCabe CJ, Wolfe RE: Ultrasonography by emergency physicians in patients with suspected ureteral colic. *J Emerg Med* 16:865–870, 1998.

22. Haddad MC, Sharif HS, Shahed MS, et al.: Renal colic: Diagnosis and outcome. *Radiology* 184:83–88, 1992.

23. Ghali AM, Elmalik EM, Ibrahim AI, Abdulhameed E, el Tahir MI: Cost-effective emergency diagnosis plan for urinary stone patients presenting with ureteric colic. *Eur Urol* 33:529–537, 1998.

24. Gerlach AT, Pickworth KK: Contrast medium-induced nephrotoxicity: Pathophysiology and prevention. *Pharmacotherapy* 20:540–548, 2000.

25. Morcos SK: Contrast media-induced nephrotoxicity—questions and answers. *Br J Radiol* 71:357–365, 1998.

26. Waybill MM, Waybill PN: Contrast media-induced nephrotoxicity: Identification of patients at risk and algorithms for prevention. *J Vasc Interv Radiol* 12:3–9, 2001.

27. Berg KJ: Nephrotoxicity related to contrast media. *Scand J Urol Nephrol* 34:317–322, 2000.

28. Gorelik U, Ulish Y, Yagil Y: The use of standard imaging techniques and their diagnostic value in the workup of renal colic in the setting of intractable flank pain. *Urology* 47:637–642, 1996.

29. Sinclair D, Wilson S, Toi A, Greenspan L: The evaluation of suspected renal colic: Ultrasound scan versus excretory urography. *Ann Emerg Med* 18:556–559, 1989.

30. Zagoria R TG: *Genitourinary radiology: The Requisites.* St Louis, MO: Mosby-Yearbook, Inc, 1997:418.

31. Cramer JS, Forrest K: Renal lithiasis: Addressing the risks of austere desert deployments. *Aviat Space Environ Med* 77:649–653, 2006.

32. Surange RS, Jeygopal NS, Chowdhury SD, Sharma NK: Bedside ultrasound: A useful tool for the on-call urologist? *Int Urol Nephrol* 32:591–596, 2001.

33. Fielding JR, Silverman SG, Rubin GD: Helical CT of the urinary tract. *AJR Am J Roentgenol* 172:1199–1206, 1999.

34. Spencer BA, Wood BJ, Dretler SP: Helical CT and ureteral colic. *Urol Clin North Am* 27:231–241, 2000.

35. Rao PN: Imaging for kidney stones. *World J Urol* 22:323–327, 2004.

36. Fowler KA, Locken JA, Duchesne JH, Williamson MR: US for detecting renal calculi with nonenhanced CT as a reference standard. *Radiology* 222:109–113, 2002.

37. Boulay I, Holtz P, Foley WD, White B, Begun FP: Ureteral calculi: Diagnostic efficacy of helical CT and implications for treatment of patients. *AJR Am J Roentgenol* 172:1485–1490, 1999.

38. Chen MY, Zagoria RJ: Can noncontrast helical computed tomography replace intravenous urography for evaluation of patients with acute urinary tract colic? *J Emerg Med* 17:299–303, 1999.

39. Chen MY, Zagoria RJ, Saunders HS, Dyer RB: Trends in the use of unenhanced helical CT for acute urinary colic. *AJR Am J Roentgenol* 173:1447–1450, 1999.

40. Dalrymple NC, Verga M, Anderson KR, et al.: The value of unenhanced helical computerized tomography in the management of acute flank pain. *J Urol* 159:735–740, 1998.

41. Fielding JR, Steele G, Fox LA, Heller H, Loughlin KR: Spiral computerized tomography in the evaluation of acute flank pain: A replacement for excretory urography. *J Urol* 157:2071–2073, 1997.

42. Sheley RC, Semonsen KG, Quinn SF: Helical CT in the evaluation of renal colic. *Am J Emerg Med* 17:279–282, 1999.

43. Sheafor DH, Hertzberg BS, Freed KS, et al.: Nonenhanced helical CT and US in the emergency evaluation of patients with renal colic: Prospective comparison. *Radiology* 217:792–797, 2000.

44. Smith RC, Verga M, McCarthy S, Rosenfield AT: Diagnosis of acute flank pain: Value of unenhanced helical CT. *AJR Am J Roentgenol* 166:97–101, 1996.

45. Vieweg J, Teh C, Freed K, et al.: Unenhanced helical computerized tomography for the evaluation of patients with acute flank pain. *J Urol* 160:679–684, 1998.

46. Denton ER, Mackenzie A, Greenwell T, Popert R, Rankin SC: Unenhanced helical CT for renal colic—is the radiation dose justifiable? *Clin Radiol* 54:444–447, 1999.

47. Katz SI, Saluja S, Brink JA, Forman HP: Radiation dose associated with unenhanced CT for suspected renal colic:

Impact of repetitive studies. *AJR Am J Roentgenol* 186:1120–1124, 2006.

48. Thurston W, Wilson S: The urinary tract, In: Rumack C, Wilson S and Charboneau J, eds. *Diagnostic Ultrasound*. St. Louis, MO: Mosby, 1997.

49. Anderhub B: *General Sonography: A Clinical Guide,* St. Louis, MO: Mosby-Yearbook, Inc, 1995:414.

50. Williamson M: Renal ultrasound. In: Williamson M, ed. *Essentials of Ultrasound,* Philadelphia, PA: WB Saunders, 1996.

51. Burge HJ, Middleton WD, McClennan BL, Hildebolt CF. Ureteral jets in healthy subjects and in patients with unilateral ureteral calculi: Comparison with color Doppler US. *Radiology* 180:437–442, 1991.

52. Strehlau J, Winkler P, de la Roche J: The uretero-vesical jet as a functional diagnostic tool in childhood hydronephrosis. *Pediatr Nephrol* 11:460–467, 1997.

53. Alnaif B, Drutz HP: The accuracy of portable abdominal ultrasound equipment in measuring postvoid residual volume. *Int Urogynecol J Pelvic Floor Dysfunct* 10:215–218, 1999.

54. Riccabona M, Nelson TR, Pretorius DH, Davidson TE: In vivo three-dimensional sonographic measurement of organ volume: Validation in the urinary bladder. *J Ultrasound Med* 15:627–632, 1996.

55. Marks LS, Dorey FJ, Macairan ML, Park C, deKernion JB: Three-dimensional ultrasound device for rapid determination of bladder volume. *Urology* 50:341–348, 1997.

56. Ozawa H, Chancellor MB, Ding YY, Nasu Y, Yokoyama T, Kumon H: Noninvasive urodynamic evaluation of bladder outlet obstruction using Doppler ultrasonography. *Urology.* 56:408–412, 2000.

57. Rosseland LA, Bentsen G, Hopp E, Refsum S, Breivik H: Monitoring urinary bladder volume and detecting postoperative urinary retention in children with an ultrasound scanner. *Acta Anaesthesiol Scand* 49:1456–1459, 2005.

58. Rosseland LA, Stubhaug A, Breivik H: Detecting postoperative urinary retention with an ultrasound scanner. *Acta Anaesthesiol Scand* 46:279–282, 2002.

59. Van Os AF, Van der Linden PJ: Reliability of an automatic ultrasound system in the post partum period in measuring urinary retention. *Acta Obstet Gynecol Scand* 85:604–607, 2006.

60. Yen DH, Hu SC, Tsai J, et al.: Renal abscess: Early diagnosis and treatment. *Am J Emerg Med* 17:192–197, 1999.

61. Huang JJ, Tseng CC: Emphysematous pyelonephritis: Clinicoradiological classification, management, prognosis, and Pathogenesis. *Arch Intern Med* 160:797–805, 2000.

62. Wan YL, Lo SK, Bullard MJ, Chang PL, Lee TY: Predictors of outcome in emphysematous pyelonephritis. *J Urol* 159:369–373, 1998.

63. Stone SC, Mallon WK, Childs JM, Docherty SD: Emphysematous pyelonephritis: Clues to rapid diagnosis in the emergency department. *J Emerg Med* 28:315–319, 2005.

64. Siepel T, Clifford DS, James PA, Cowan TM: The ultrasound-assisted physical examination in the periodic health evaluation of the elderly. *J Fam Pract* 49:628–632, 2000.

65. Ueda T, Mihara Y: Incidental detection of renal carcinoma during radiological imaging. *Br J Urol* 59:513–515, 1987.

66. Tosaka A, Ohya K, Yamada K, et al.: Incidence and properties of renal masses and asymptomatic renal cell carcinoma detected by abdominal ultrasonography. *J Urol* 144:1097–1099, 1990.

67. Lanctin HP, Futter NG: Renal cell carcinoma: Incidental detection. *Can J Surg* 33:488–490, 1990.

68. Sweeney JP, Thornhill JA, Graiger R, McDermott TE, Butler MR: Incidentally detected renal cell carcinoma: Pathological features, survival trends and implications for treatment. *Br J Urol* 78:351–353, 1996.

69. Smith SJ, Bosniak MA, Megibow AJ, Hulnick DH, Horii SC, Raghavendra BN: Renal cell carcinoma: Earlier discovery and increased detection. *Radiology* 170:699–703, 1989.

70. Charboneau JW, Hattery RR, Ernst EC, III, James EM, Williamson B, Jr., Hartman GW: Spectrum of sonographic findings in 125 renal masses other than benign simple cyst. *AJR Am J Roentgenol* 140:87–94, 1983.

71. Helenon O, Correas JM, Balleyguier C, Ghouadni M, Cornud F: Ultrasound of renal tumors. *Eur Radiol* 11:1890–1901, 2001.

72. Belldegrun A deKernion J: Renal tumors, In: Campbell M and Walsh P, eds. *Campbell's Urology.* Philadelphia, PA: W.B. Saunders Company, 1998.

73. Forman HP, Middleton WD, Melson GL, McClennan BL: Hyperechoic renal cell carcinomas: Increase in detection at US. *Radiology* 188:431–434, 1993.

74. Drago J, Cunningham J: Ultrasonography of renal masses. In: Resnick M, Rifkin M, eds. *Ultrasonography of the Urinary Tract.* Baltimore, MD: Williams & Wilkins, 1991.

75. McGahan JP, Richards JR, Jones CD, Gerscovich EO: Use of ultrasonography in the patient with acute renal trauma. *J Ultrasound Med* 18:207–213; quiz 215–216, 1999.

76. McGahan PJ, Richards JR, Bair AE, Rose JS: Ultrasound detection of blunt urological trauma: A 6-year study. *Injury* 36:762–770, 2005.

77. Catalano O, Lobianco R, Sandomenico F, Mattace Raso M, Siani A: Real-time, contrast-enhanced sonographic imaging in emergency radiology. *Radiol Med (Torino)* 108:454–469, 2004.

78. Fang YC, Tiu CM, Chou YH, Chang T: A case of acute renal artery thrombosis caused by blunt trauma: Computed tomographic and Doppler ultrasonic findings. *J Formos Med Assoc* 92:356–358, 1993.

79. Poletti PA, Platon A, Becker CD, et al.: Blunt abdominal trauma: Does the use of a second-generation sonographic contrast agent help to detect solid organ injuries? *AJR Am J Roentgenol* 183:1293–1301, 2004.

80. Valentino M, Serra C, Zironi G, De Luca C, Pavlica P, Barozzi L: Blunt abdominal trauma: Emergency contrast-enhanced sonography for detection of solid organ injuries. *AJR Am J Roentgenol* 186:1361–1367, 2006.

81. Tempkin B: *Ultrasound Scanning: Priniciples & Protocols.* Philadelphia, PA: W.B. Saunders, 1993.

82. Hagen-Ansert S: Urinary system. In: Hagen-Ansert S, ed.: *Textbook of Diagnostic Ultrasound.* St. Louis, MO: Mosby, 1995.

CHAPTER 11

Testicular

Michael Blaivas

Acute testicular pain represents approximately 0.5% of the complaints presenting to an emergency department each year.[1] Causes of acute testicular pain include trauma, epididymitis, orchitis, torsion of the testicular appendage, and hemorrhage; however, testicular torsion is the diagnosis of the greatest concern in the emergency setting.

Previously, most young men who presented to an emergency or urgent care setting with a complaint of acute onset testicular pain were suspected of having testicular torsion.[2] Since the 1990s, this misconception has been dispelled and it is now known that the most common etiology of acute testicular pain is epididymitis.[2] The evaluation of acute testicular pain still presents a considerable challenge for emergency physicians since fully 50% of young men presenting to an emergency department with testicular torsion have already waited over 6 hours and are well on their way toward losing the torsed testicle.[3]

The issue of acute testicular pain is further complicated by the high potential for litigation associated with infertility after testicular loss due to torsion or disruption of the testicle from severe trauma. When the diagnosis of testicular torsion is missed, the majority of patients have been incorrectly classified as having epididymitis.[4] Despite the fact that the two disease processes would seem to be easily differentiated on the basis of history and physical examination, research and practice have demonstrated this not to be the case.[4]

► CLINICAL CONSIDERATIONS

The most important concern with testicular torsion is the potential for loss of the testicle or infertility. Other disease processes that may present with scrotal pain include torsion of the testicular appendage, epididymitis, orchitis, testicular trauma, hemorrhage into a testicular mass, and herniation of abdominal contents into the scrotum. High-resolution color Doppler ultrasonography has become widely accepted as the test of choice for evaluating acute scrotal pain, replacing scintigraphy in most institutions.[5] While scintigraphy requires less technical skill on the part of the radiologist consulted to evaluate the patient, there are major drawbacks to the technique. Scintigraphy is a time-consuming process that can add an hour or more to the evaluation of a patient who may already be several hours into the testicular torsion process.[5] Furthermore, the resultant hyperemia of the scrotal skin during testicular torsion can mask a lack of blood flow to the testicle itself and lead to a misdiagnosis in less experienced hands.[6] This nuclear medicine study also provides no information regarding testicular anatomy, a potentially critical issue if pathology other than torsion is present.

A careful history and physical examination are important and have been thought to enable an emergency physician to virtually exclude the diagnosis of testicular torsion without further testing in the majority of cases.[3] In practice, historical features of several disease processes can overlap. For example, duration of pain in testicular torsion, epididymitis, orchitis, and torsion of a testicular appendage frequently overlap.[7] In up to 20% of cases, testicular torsion is associated with trauma or physical exertion, such as heavy lifting.[8] Adding to the difficulty of making a diagnosis by history alone is the resistance of many young men to provide accurate histories regarding trauma.

Typical textbook clinical features of epididymitis, such as dysuria and urethral discharge, cannot be uniformly relied upon. Up to 50% of patients with acute epididymitis may not present with dysuria or urethral discharge.[4] Furthermore, many patients with epididymitis seem to complain of acute onset of pain. This is probably due to poor recall or the need for a threshold of discomfort to be crossed prior to the patient's recognition of pain. Another complicating factor is that if the body or tail of the epididymis is inflamed without affecting the head, the pain and swelling will be in a different location from what most physicians expect with epididymitis. Most physicians learn to feel for the head of the epididymis on their physical examination and do not realize that it may not be affected. Patients with testicular torsion who were initially misdiagnosed as epididymitis are most commonly misdiagnosed because of the presence of dysuria, pyuria, urethral discharge, or a history of prior vague testicular pain giving the impression of a less acute process.[1]

Ultrasonography of the acute scrotum is a relatively new application for bedside use in the emergency and acute care setting. Because of the time-sensitive nature of testicular torsion, ultrasonography is a tool to consider for the bedside diagnosis of possible torsion. Time is of the essence in diagnosing testicular torsion. Since inadequate funding and personnel limits have hurt the off-hours diagnostic imaging services provided by many hospitals, bedside ultrasonography for this indication should become a tool used by emergency physicians, urologists, and other interested clinicians.

▶ CLINICAL INDICATIONS

The clinical indications for emergency bedside ultrasound evaluation of the testicle include

- Acute testicular pain
- Acute scrotal mass
- Trauma

ACUTE TESTICULAR PAIN

An ultrasound examination of the testicle is indicated whenever testicular torsion is in the differential diagnosis after the history and the physical examination. The etiology of testicular torsion is related to laxity found in a redundant spermatic cord, typically known as the bell clapper deformity, which allows the testicle to twist about its own axis. The bell clapper deformity is most often found to be bilateral upon surgical exploration. Further increasing the likelihood of testicular torsion is a history of an undescended testicle.[9] Once blood flow is interrupted to the testicle, infarction and loss of the testicle can occur quickly. The urological literature demonstrates that salvage rates are approximately 100% at 3 hours, 83–90% at 5 hours, 75% at 8 hours, and 50–70% at 10 hours. When a testicle has been torsed for more than 10 hours, the rates of salvage decrease to 10–20%. After 24 hours, salvage of a testicle is rarely seen unless there has been intermittent detorsion.[10]

In general, urologists are reluctant to take patients to the operating room and explore a painful scrotum based solely on the clinical examination. Studies argue that such patients should not be routinely explored and that accurate diagnosis should be provided with power and pulse wave Doppler testing of the involved testicle.[11]

For the detection of testicular torsion, the sensitivity and specificity of ultrasonography approaches 100% for experienced sonologists. The literature regarding testicular ultrasound use by emergency physicians at the bedside is relatively limited.[12–17] This is in part because the technology needed to accurately diagnose or exclude testicular torsion includes both color or power and pulse wave Doppler. The price for this technology, although now found on basic machines for less than $30,000, was often out of reach for many emergency departments and clinics. Furthermore, the scrotal ultrasound examination carries a stigma of being a difficult and advanced level examination that will lead to dire consequences if misinterpreted.

The sonographic evaluation of acute testicular pain by emergency physicians has been studied. One group of authors evaluated 36 patients with acute testicular pain and demonstrated a sensitivity and specificity of 95% and 94%, respectively, for testicular torsion when surgical follow-up and radiology imaging were used as the criterion standard.[12] All three patients with testicular torsion were correctly identified. Other diagnoses found included epididymitis, orchitis, hemorrhage, and herniation. The authors demonstrated that emergency physicians could evaluate and diagnose a broad range of testicular pathology using ultrasonography. A larger retrospective study demonstrated good accuracy for a variety of pathology encountered in the emergency setting.[17]

A major limitation for any individual attempting to get enough experience with testicular ultrasonography may be the frequency of acute scrotal pain presentation at his or her facility. One study did show that testicular torsion could easily be simulated for training purposes by digital compression of the spermatic cord unilaterally, and this holds promise as an educational tool.[15]

The clinician benefiting most from scrotal ultrasonography would be the one without radiological or urological backup during a portion of the day. Determination that a testicle is intact or that normal testicular blood flow is present could allow avoiding, or at least delaying, costly or difficult transport to another facility.[18]

SCROTAL MASS

Painless scrotal masses are unlikely to represent an acute disease process. By history, patients often admit that the involved testicle had been slowly enlarging for some time and they had simply ignored it or grown accustomed to the difference until some factor finally made them seek medical assistance. Firm, nontender testicular masses commonly represent neoplasms that should be directed for expeditious follow-up with a urologist. When the patient presents complaining of pain from the testicular mass, it may be from hemorrhage into the neoplasm itself. The vast majority of soft, nontender testicular masses are hydroceles that may develop because of a number of disease processes or idiopathically. Many are congenital and result from a direct communication with the abdominal cavity. Hydroceles may result from trauma, infection, neoplasm, radiation therapy, and undiagnosed torsion.[19] Hernias can present with complaints of acute scrotal mass, and are generally painful. The presentation can be similar to that of torsion if the scrotum is erythematous.

TRAUMA

Blunt trauma to the scrotum can lead to damage of the testicle or associated structures. Assault, sports injury, bicycle crashes, and motor vehicle crashes are the most common causes of blunt testicular trauma. Injuries can be in the form of laceration, hemorrhage, or contusion of the testicle. Clinical features of testicular injury are a tender swollen testicle, often accompanied by ecchymosis. Accurate diagnosis by physical examination alone is often difficult secondary to marked swelling and pain in the traumatized scrotum, thus making ultrasound imaging a requisite. The goal of emergency ultrasound in patients presenting with acute trauma to the scrotum is to determine whether the testicle is damaged and requires operative intervention. Although a contusion or focal hemorrhage may simply require follow-up, fracture through the capsule of the testicle necessitates surgical intervention. Furthermore, since trauma can lead to testicular torsion, blood flow should be evaluated as well. High resolution ultrasound is sensitive for detecting major trauma to the testicle and, therefore, can be useful for screening patients. While the diagnostic accuracy of ultrasound in this trauma setting is heavily operator dependent, significant injury is relatively straightforward to diagnose.[20,21]

▶ ANATOMIC CONSIDERATIONS

The normal adult testes are located in the scrotum and are oval in shape. Average measurements obtained are 4 cm × 3 cm × 2.5 cm on ultrasound. Each adult testicle weighs between 10 and 19 grams. The testes are surrounded by the tunica vaginalis (Figure 11-1). Multiple septations arise from the tunica albuginea and run through the testicle. These septations result in the separation of the testicle into multiple lobules. The epididymis, an extratesticular structure, is made up of the head, body, and tail. The tail of the epididymis turns into the vas deferens as it travels superiorly out of the scrotum. The vas deferens, in turn, travels in the spermatic cord. The spermatic cord contains a number of important structures, including the testicular artery, cremasteric artery, deferential artery, lymphatic structures, and the genitofemoral nerve.

Sonographically, a testicle appears quite homogeneous in echotexture (Figure 11-2). The echogenicity of the testes is sometimes compared with that of the liver. Many structures such as the tunica albuginea are not seen under normal circumstances. The epididymis can be readily differentiated from the rest of the testicle in normal as well as pathological instances. It has similar echogenicity to the testicle but can appear slightly

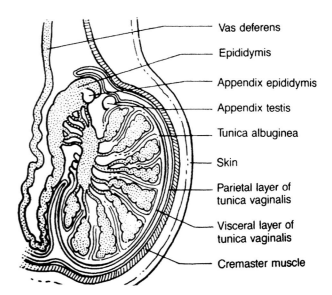

Figure 11-1. Normal testicular and scrotal anatomy. (From: Cohen HL. Hematocele, in Cohen HL, Civit CJ (eds): *Fetal and Pediatric Ultrasound: A Casebook Approach.* New York: McGraw-Hill, 2001, 541, Figure 105–6)

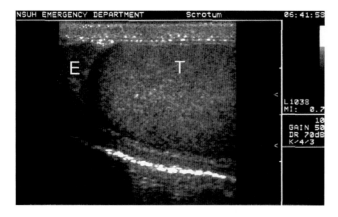

Figure 11-2. Longitudinal view of the normal testes. E: head of the epididymis, T: testicle.

brighter. While the head of the epididymis is readily seen, the body and tail may be harder to differentiate when no inflammation is present. The appendix testis is a small oval structure and is normally hidden by the epididymal head, thus making it nearly impossible to differentiate in normal examinations. If a hydrocele is present, the appendix testis often becomes outlined by the fluid and is seen as a defined structure (Figure 11-3). When torsed, it may cause not only local inflammation but also an epididymitis-like appearance due to diffuse inflammation of the epididymal head. The appendix testes may be located in different areas on the testicle. The epididymis can also have appendages as well.

Most of the arterial blood supply received by a testicle comes from the abdominal aorta by way of the testicular artery. A small portion of the arterial supply comes from the deferential and cremasteric arteries, which anastomose with the testicular artery. The deferential and cremasteric arteries supply the extratesticular structures of the scrotum, including the epididymis. Color and power Doppler can easily detect blood flow in

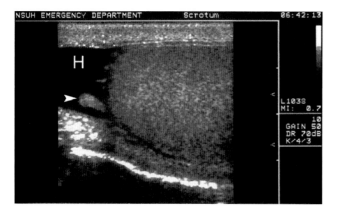

Figure 11-3. A small hydrocele outlines the appendix testis (arrowhead) in this patient presenting for chronic testicular pain. H: hydrocele.

these vascular structures in both normal and most pathological states. There is variability in normal anatomy and, in general, anything that appears abnormal should be compared to the contralateral side.

▶ GETTING STARTED

When approaching the testicular ultrasound examination, patient comfort is vital. A patient in severe pain can be problematical to scan. The main issue is having the patient lay still when performing power and pulse wave Doppler measurements. Both of these modalities are very sensitive to movement artifact. Thus, providing adequate analgesia is important. Once comfort is achieved, the patient will need to be disrobed from the waist down. A frog leg position allows good access to the scrotum and it may help prop pillows or blankets under each bent knee to allow relaxation of the legs. Typically, the ultrasound machine is parked on the patient's right. A linear, high-resolution transducer should be selected and, if available, a small parts or scrotal function should be chosen on the machine (Figure 11-4). A generous amount of ultrasound gel is required;

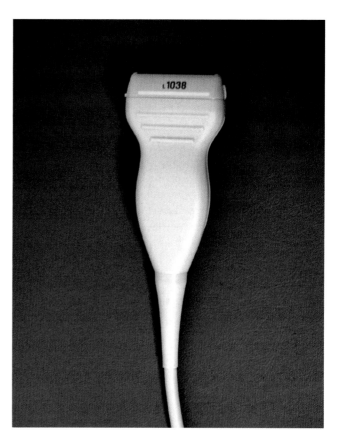

Figure 11-4. An example of a high-resolution linear array that can be used for testicular sonography.

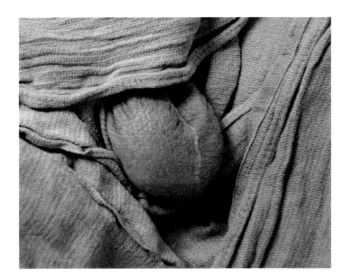

Figure 11-5. A properly exposed and draped patient with the scrotum supported in a sling of towels for improved patient comfort and visualization.

warmed gel is ideal. Cold gel may make the patient more uncomfortable by eliciting a cremasteric reflex. In cases of significant inflammation or torsion, activation of the cremasteric reflex may cause considerable pain. Placing a towel sling under the scrotum may also be beneficial (Figure 11-5). At this point, if not earlier, the sonologist should explain the examination details and its goals to the patient. This is very important in the adolescent who will likely feel more relaxed after an explanation.

The testes will not always lie vertically in the scrotum, but the ultrasound examination generally begins with that assumption. Although some would argue beginning the scan with a comparison view in transverse across both testes, this may not be ideal. In such a view, the transducer is held horizontally through the mid portion of both testes with the right one being on the left side of the ultrasound machine screen. For patient reassurance and comfort, starting with the unaffected side is important. Like any organ, the unaffected testicle is scanned in at least two planes, longitudinal (vertical) and transverse (horizontal), top to bottom, and side to side. It helps anchor the scanning hand whenever possible to something relatively immobile, like the patient's thigh or a bed rail. Essentially anything that will keep the scanning hand from moving or shaking unintentionally will help the examination significantly. Even a small amount of accidental movement will interfere to some degree.

Important tools to have on your ultrasound system for performing a testicular examination include power (or color) Doppler and pulse wave Doppler. Power Doppler activation will bring up a box-like window the size of which may or may not be changeable. This box can be moved around the screen to the portion of the tes-

ticle or scrotum of interest. If size of the power Doppler box or window is adjustable, it may or may not be helpful to enlarge so much that it covers the entire testicle. The drawback of covering such a large area can be a greatly decreased frame rate that most ultrasound machines will suffer as the territory covered by the power Doppler box becomes very large. Typically, a balance has to be achieved between too small a power Doppler window that requires frequent movement and does not capture the overall blood flow picture adequately and one that is too large and does not allow the machine to refresh the image frequently enough. Simply turning on the power Doppler box may not be enough if the presets on the machine are not set correctly. Adjusting the sensitivity settings to the lowest possible without having power Doppler signal swimming everywhere will allow for greater ease in detecting blood flow.

Once reliable power Doppler signals are being returned from the unaffected testicle, the pulse wave Doppler should be activated. A small gate, often two parallel lines, will appear on the screen (Figure 11-6). It is guided with a trackball or touch pad to the power Doppler signals inside the power Doppler box. Typically, some kind of update button will have to be pushed (the pulse wave button may have to be pushed a second time) when the parallel lines are placed over the power Doppler signal. Once activated, a running graph will appear showing the pulse wave Doppler signal (Figure 11-7). Turning up the pulse wave gain is acceptable to a point where the background around the graph baseline becomes brighter and shows some noise. This will allow the sonologist to be more sensitive to catching pulse wave venous and arterial flow. Venous flow is typically of one velocity with little variation in

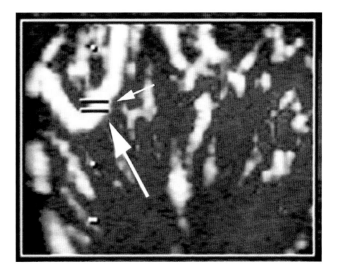

Figure 11-6. A close-up of the pulse wave Doppler gate is shown by arrows in this image.

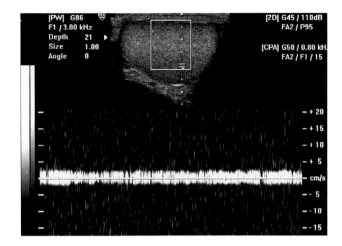

Figure 11-7. A pulse wave Doppler tracing is obtained from a testicle. A typical venous waveform is shown.

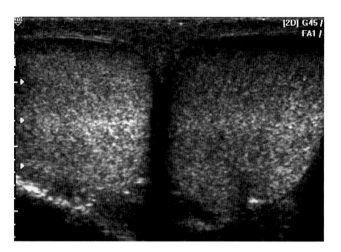

Figure 11-9. A side-by-side comparison image is shown. Both testicles are scanned at once with one linear transducer.

the testicle (Figure 11-7). Arterial flow has variation or pulsatility, although a triphasic pattern will rarely be seen in the testicle (Figure 11-8). Sampling should occur in multiple spots in the testicle. When producing a report for the medical record, it will be important to have pictures/printouts documenting the presence of normal (or abnormal) flow. Once the settings have been properly adjusted on the unaffected side, the transducer is moved to the painful testicle or hemiscrotum. If the machine's settings are left untouched when switching to the other side, the sonologist will quickly appreciate if blood flow in the affected testicle is similarly easy to obtain or not. In addition, grayscale comparison can quickly be made between the two sides. A side-by-side comparison of the two testes can be helpful and illustrates any difference in power Doppler detected blood flow or echogenicity very well in a single image (Figure 11-9).

▶ TECHNIQUE AND NORMAL ULTRASOUND FINDINGS

When evaluating the testes, a 7.5–10 MHz transducer is required in most situations, with a 5.0 MHz probe being utilized for large masses or very edematous scrotum (Figure 11-4). The increased resolution and magnification provided by these high-frequency linear probes is crucial for examining not only the parenchyma of the testicle but also the blood flow within it. Some imaging specialists will even utilize 12–15 MHz transducers to obtain the best details and Doppler resolution. This may not be possible if significant swelling exists and the testicle itself is several centimeters from the skin surface. High-resolution linear array transducers are used for a variety of applications in bedside ultrasound and are more common than ever before. Common applications have included detection of foreign bodies, central line placement, and for the evaluation of lower extremity deep venous thrombosis.[22–24]

In addition to a high-resolution probe, color and spectral Doppler are required when evaluating a patient for torsion. Power Doppler, a nondirectional version of color Doppler, is thought to be more sensitive for detecting blood flow, but omits the directional information.[5] It can, however, improve the sensitivity of the test, especially in the testicle, where blood flow tends to occur through relatively small diameter vessels and at lower speed. Knowing direction of blood flow is of little help in most cases of testicular ultrasound. Pulse wave Doppler is also an important component of the evaluation especially when incomplete torsion is present. It allows for documentation of both venous and arterial blood flow within the testicle. It is the venous component that is initially lost early in testicular torsion.

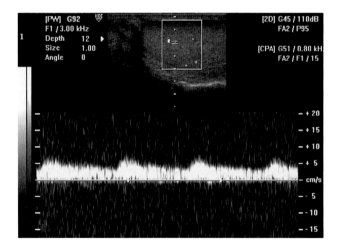

Figure 11-8. A pulse wave Doppler tracing is obtained from a testicle. A typical arterial waveform with a systolic and diastolic flow component is shown.

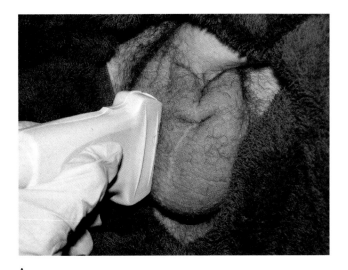

A

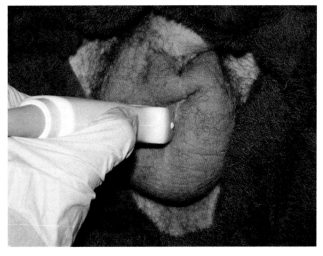

B

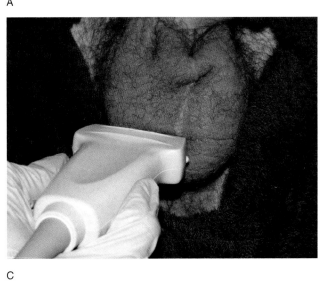

C

Figure 11-10. A longitudinal orientation to the transducer is shown on the right testicle (A). The transducer is held in transverse orientation of the right testicle and moved from upper pole (B) to lower pole (C).

The patient should be draped to preserve modesty and the scrotum placed in a sling designed from a towel to provide support and improve exposure (Figure 11-5). Although a frog leg position for the patient is preferred by most sonologists, some actually give up using a towel sling for better access.

Using only grayscale, the unaffected testicle is scanned in the longitudinal plane from side to side (Figure 11-10A). At this point the indicator on the transducer is typically pointed toward the patient's torso; however, if the testicle has an oblique lie, it is proper to orient the indicator toward the upper pole of the testicle. The sonologist may note any grayscale abnormalities such as edema, focal masses, or disruptions as well as measuring the length and thickness of the testes. The epididymis can also be evaluated in this view and measured. For the long-axis view, the image is usually adjusted so that the epididymal head is on the left side of the screen. Any epididymal abnormalities will often become evident on the longitudinal views. Turning transverse, still on the

unaffected side, the testicle should be scanned from top to bottom, again looking for any grayscale abnormalities (Figure 11-10B and 11-10C). Its width is measured in the central portion of the testicle. By now, the sonologist has had time to adjust the gain, depth, and resolution settings as appropriate for optimal grayscale image acquisition.

The transducer should now be oriented in the longitudinal plane of the testicle with the power Doppler feature turned on. Unless the machine presets happen to already be optimized for the testicular examination, some adjustments in gain, wall filter, and Pulse Repetition Frequency (PRF) will have to be made. The goal of these adjustments is to demonstrate as much blood flow as possible without introducing more than minimal artifact. Power Doppler is highly sensitive to any movement of the testicle or the sonologist's hand. Once areas of power Doppler signal are visualized, the sonologist should appreciate the overall level of blood flow in the testicle. With experience it will be obvious when there is too much blood flow, as in cases of inflammation, or too

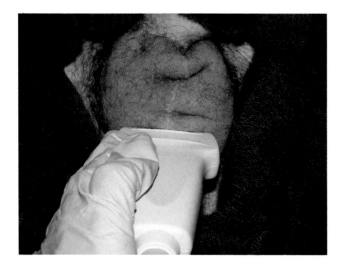

Figure 11-11. The transducer is held in transverse orientation across both testicles. This generates a comparison view of both testicles on the screen for gray scale and Doppler evaluation.

little blood flow, as in possible ischemia. Even in experienced hands, however, it is prudent to reserve judgment until the two sides can be compared, as long as the other testicle is present for comparison. At this point, the pulse wave Doppler is activated and its sample gate is placed over areas of power Doppler signal until both venous and arterial waveforms are obtained within the body of the testicle. Blood flow seen on the very edge of the testicle can be deceiving and should not be relied upon. Once this has been achieved, the sonologist can move on to the affected testicle.

This entire process should be repeated on the affected side; however, the examination is typically not finished at this point. In the majority of cases it is helpful to perform a transverse scan of the testes simultaneously (Figure 11-11). With the transducer turned horizontal and indicator toward the patient's right hip, the testes are scanned from upper to lower pole for comparison in grayscale. Representative images should be taken for the report, just as they were for blood flow demonstration with the pulse wave Doppler. Power Doppler should be turned on to evaluate the testes. This will often mean enlarging the power Doppler box, thus slowing the motion on the screen. Although a steady testicle and hand are required, this view is ideal for demonstrating any similarities or differences between testes in both grayscale and power Doppler. This is especially illustrative in cases of torsion, with one side showing ample blood flow and the affected side showing no blood flow in the same power Doppler box (Figure 11-12a,b). Similarly, when one testicle has significantly increased blood flow due to inflammation and the other has normal blood flow, the diagnosis is difficult to dispute when such an image appears in the written report (Figure 11-13). Despite which

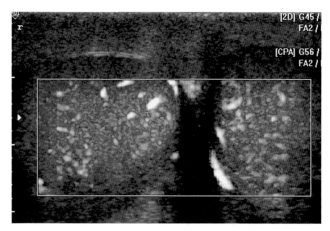

A

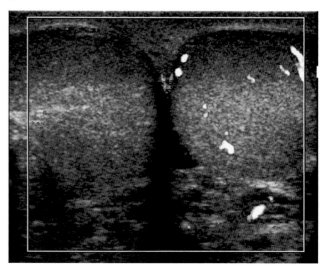

B

Figure 11-12. Power Doppler evaluation (grayscale copy). An equal amount of flow is shown in this comparison view of both testicles with power Doppler (A). In this side-by-side view, no flow is seen in the right testicle, which is displayed on the left side of the screen (B). Torsion was confirmed in the operating room.

order one chooses to perform the individual steps, the examination should be performed the same way each time for consistency.

▶ COMMON AND EMERGENT ABNORMALITIES

EPIDIDYMITIS

Infection of the epididymis or testicle usually results from retrograde spread of bacteria from the bladder or prostate via the vas deferens. Epididymitis is the most common type of scrotal inflammatory process.[3] Another inflammatory process that can present with signs and

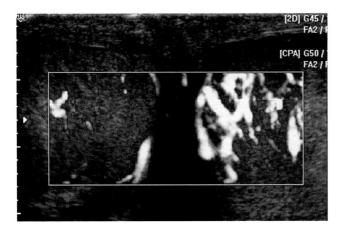

Figure 11-13. A side-by-side comparison view with power Doppler is shown. The left testicle, shown on the right side of the screen, has markedly increased flow in this example of orchitis.

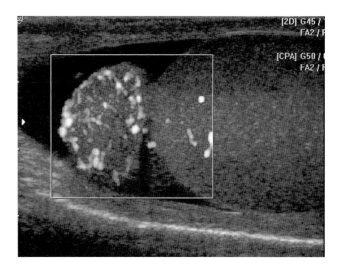

Figure 11-15. The enlarged epididymis is seen on the left side of the image with prominent blood flow shown by power Doppler (grayscale copy).

symptoms of epididymitis is torsion of the testicular appendage.

Sonographically, the affected epididymis appears enlarged, which is usually confirmed by measuring both the affected and unaffected sides (Figure 11-14). It will often have decreased echogenicity on standard B-mode examination. Occasionally, focal inflammation of a region of the epididymis is seen leading to an area of well-defined swelling or enlargement. This is usually either the head or the body of the epididymis. Epididymitis can cause accumulation of a reactive hydrocele similar to testicular torsion or torsion of the appendix testis. Thus, the presence of a small or moderate amount of fluid in the hemi-scrotum is not a reliable sign for differentiating between the disease processes.

Epididymal inflammation, either idiopathic or infectious, usually leads to increased blood flow that is easily noted on power Doppler when compared to the unaffected side (Figure 11-15). It is critical to realize that focusing on the head of the epididymis may cause novice sonologists to overlook the body and tail of the epididymis, which may be the site of isolated inflammation (Figure 11-16). The vas deferens may actually be inflamed first, before the epididymal tail, and would have markedly increased blood flow on power Doppler in its posterior location at the inferior pole of the testicle and epididymal tail. The tail of the epididymis can remain prominent after infection even with appropriate antibiotic therapy. Power Doppler should help

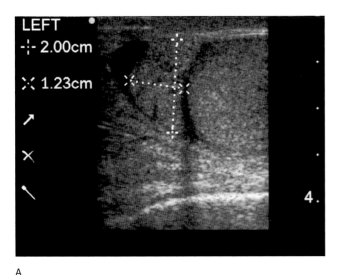

A

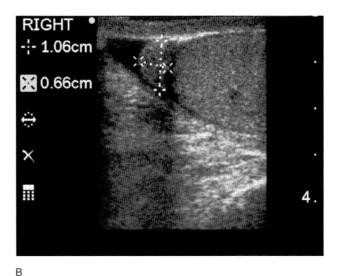

B

Figure 11-14. Epididymitis. The left epdidymal head is enlarged (A). Measurements for normal comparison on the right are included (B). (Courtesy of James Mateer, MD)

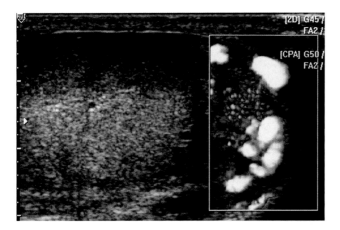

Figure 11-16. Prominent blood flow is shown in the power Doppler box located over the inflamed tail of the epididymis.

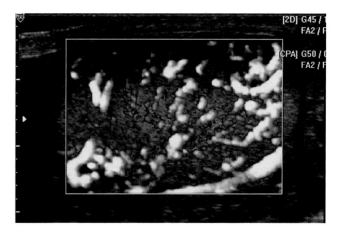

Figure 11-17. Marked increase in blood flow is seen with power Doppler throughout this testicle due to the presence of orchitis.

differentiate between an acutely inflamed epididymal tail and a prominent leftover from previous infection.

What clearly separates epididymitis from testicular torsion is the presence of increased blood flow in the testicle when compared to the contralateral side. Increased blood flow may be seen if the inflammation is spreading to the testicle. It is important to note that following detorsion the short-lived hyperemic response will also cause a transient increase in blood flow to the affected testicle, but should not last more than 15 minutes as long as the testicle has fully detorsed.

ORCHITIS

Orchitis is an acute infection of the testicle; most cases follow an initial episode of epididymitis.[3] The typical presentation includes a markedly tender and inflamed testicle. Standard B-mode ultrasound is not a reliable method to differentiate between orchitis and torsion unless the torsion is advanced and prominent changes are noted. For both orchitis and torsion, inflammation and edema can lead to decreased echogenicity of the testis. Activating power Doppler will quickly assist in differentiating between the two diagnoses since testicular blood flow will increase as a result of inflammation (Figure 11-17).

The inflammation and associated increase in blood flow seen on power Doppler may be regionalized, especially early in the process. Significant inflammation may be seen in one portion of the testicle (e.g., the inferior pole), but not in the rest of the testicle. The sonologist should take time to investigate the areas without markedly increased blood flow to make sure that all flow is not absent in them. Necrosis in one part of the testicle could lead to inflammation and increased flow in an adjacent portion and should this occur, urological consultation may be needed to evaluate for a possible

necrotic process. Furthermore, an area of absent blood flow can mean the presence of an abscess and would need to be followed carefully with urologic consultation (Figure 11-18). The increased blood flow of orchitis can mimic hyperemia seen after detorsion; if clinically suspicious, the sonologist may simply rescan the patient in 15 minutes. The hyperemia from a recent detorsion should have resolved and the pain should also have resolved. Increased blood flow from orchitis would still be present as would any discomfort that was there 15 minutes before, taking into account potential pain medication in the interim. Rarely, a chronic hyperemic state can be seen in chronic partial torsion as a result of subtle ischemia that leads to inflammation.

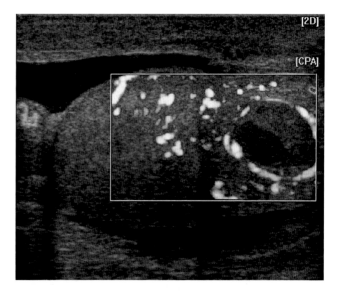

Figure 11-18. A complex hypoechoic area is seen in the testicle on the right side of the image. Power Doppler (grayscale copy) reveals flow in its periphery and elsewhere, but not inside this suspicious mass.

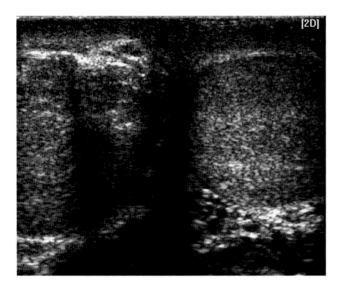

Figure 11-19. A side-by-side B-mode comparison view showing the right testicle (on the left side of the image) to be enlarged and less echogenic than the normal side (seen on the right side of the image).

TESTICULAR TORSION

A normal testicle has a diffusely homogenous sonographic appearance, with the exception of the mediastinum testis, which is an echogenic structure running through the center of the testicle. B-mode ultrasound allows for a good evaluation of the testicular parenchyma. This method, however, will detect torsion only when signs of edema or necrosis are already present (Figure 11-19). Power Doppler will reveal blood flow within the normal testicle (Figure 11-20). When blood flow is absent or severely compromised in the affected testicle, the diagnosis of testicular torsion is clear. When the degree of flow is similar between the affected and comparison testicle, pulse wave Doppler tracings should be obtained to confirm both arterial and venous flow. Power Doppler alone will not assure the sonologist that both venous and arterial flow is present. The absence of a venous pattern by pulse wave Doppler on the affected side suggests early torsion. This is better understood by reviewing the mechanism of torsion and loss of blood supply to the testicle.

During torsion, the testicle begins to twist around the axis of the spermatic cord. As the twisting progresses, venous flow is initially lost because of easily collapsible vessel walls and a lower pressure system. Venous obstruction is followed by a drop in arterial inflow that eventually progresses to complete obstruction of blood flow. Thrombosis occurs in the arteries and veins and results in necrosis of testicular tissue. Experimental studies have shown that complete arterial occlusion occurs at about 450–540 degrees of torsion.[27] Once the spermatic cord is fully torsed and no blood flow is present, the testicle begins to take on a diffusely edematous appearance on ultrasound (Figure 11-19). With the completion of testicular torsion, no power Doppler signal will be seen in the testicle (Figure 11-20).

In the presence of potential torsion, diagnostically, it is possible to take advantage of the most common mechanical cause for testicular torsion. The spermatic cord is in all likelihood twisting at some point in its course, and this twist may be visible on ultrasound. To check for the knot that is cutting off blood flow, the transducer can be advanced proximally from the superior pole of the testicle, following the incoming vessels up to the inguinal canal (Figure 11-21). The vessels frequently can

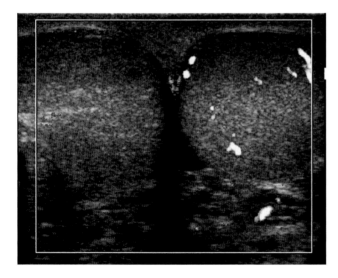

Figure 11-20. The same side-by-side comparison view as in Figure 10-19 but now with power Doppler (grayscale copy). The right testicle (seen on the left side of the image) is devoid of blood flow and was torsed at exploration.

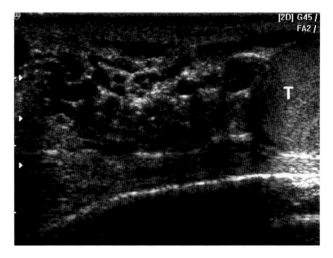

Figure 11-21. The transducer has been moved up proximal to the testicle (T) and cord vessels now fill the screen.

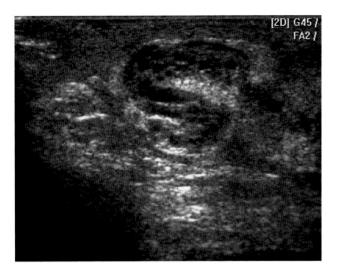

Figure 11-22. A longitudinal section above the testicle shows a complex area of knotting or twisting of the spermatic cord in a patient with torsion.

be followed for several centimeters until they disappear from view. A knot will appear to be an area of swirling of the spermatic cord on a longitudinal section when proceeding up the inguinal canal with the transducer oriented from the patient's feet to the head (Figure 11-22). Adding power Doppler may actually show flow in blood vessels approaching the knot from the pelvis but no flow leaving the knot and heading toward the testicle. Little else is needed to confirm the presence or torsion at that point. Conversely, being able to trace cord vessels proximally into the inguinal canal and showing blood flow throughout their course should be reassuring in excluding the diagnosis of testicular torsion.

If the diagnosis is in doubt due to continued pain or if torsion–detorsion is suspected, performing serial examinations at the bedside is helpful. Closely following the blood flow can allow the practitioner to detect worsening torsion or the presence of torsion and detorsion in a patient that may otherwise have been sent home. Repeated color/power Doppler imaging along with spectral Doppler examination in 45 minutes to an hour could catch subtle progression of torsion in a patient with continued suggestive pain but a normal initial examination. The presence of both venous and arterial blood flow in the testicle means it is not actively necrosing. Therefore, while continuing pain may be concerning, severe organ injury is not ongoing.

Torsion is not the only reason a patient may have testicular ischemia. Ischemia can result from spontaneous thrombosis of varicoceles or after corrective surgery. Severe edema following surgery or accidental vessel ligation during a vasectomy can also lead to vascular congestion and ischemia. The findings will be the same as in classic testicular torsion. A knot in the spermatic cord will not be identifiable in such cases.

SCROTAL TRAUMA

Scrotal trauma may result in damage to both the testes and the extratesticular structures. Visualization of a normal testicle on ultrasound examination virtually excludes any significant injury. Since surgical intervention is required for rupture of a testicle, the sonologist should have a heightened awareness for any abnormalities seen within the testicle on ultrasound. In these cases, further investigation or urology consultation is warranted. Ultrasound findings that suggest testicular rupture include focal areas of inhomogeneous echogenicity (Figure 11-23). These usually signal an area of hemorrhage or focal infarction. With larger hemorrhage, the testicle will lose its smooth contour (Figure 11-24). If the capsule of the testicle is intact, conservative treatment will often suffice. However, if a fracture line is seen crossing the capsule, then surgical intervention is required. While the sensitivity and specificity for ultrasound detection of testicular fracture vary in multiple studies, it remains an excellent diagnostic modality to begin evaluating the severity of injury.

Hemorrhage within the testicle can have an inconsistent appearance depending on the age of the bleed. Acute hemorrhage will appear inhomogeneously echogenic, but will later develop large anechoic regions within it. Although grayscale sonography can occasionally confuse hematomas and tumors, the use of color Doppler may differentiate the two processes. Tumors are often vascular structures while hematomas will not reveal blood flow internally. A mixture of findings can occur when a patient hemorrhages into a testicular mass.

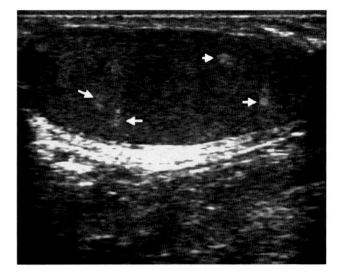

Figure 11-23. Arrows point to small focal hemorrhages after a blow to the groin. The patient was found to have no other testicular injury and recovered uneventfully.

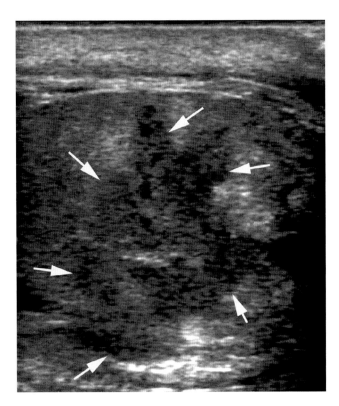

Figure 11-24. Testicular rupture has occurred after a sporting injury. Arrows outline an area of hemorrhage and testicular borders appear violated.

FOURNIER'S GANGRENE

Fournier's gangrene is another potential emergency that can present with acute scrotal pain and swelling. Fournier's gangrene is a polymicrobial infectious process that more commonly affects men with impaired immune function, including alcoholics.[25,26] Fournier's gangrene may be diagnosed solely on clinical grounds in advanced stages, where morbidity and mortality are highest. Since early detection and treatment are essential for decreasing morbidity and mortality, early imaging modalities may be required to differentiate Fournier's gangrene from scrotal cellulitis. Any delay in differentiating Fournier's gangrene from cellulitis or idiopathic scrotal edema may increase morbidity and mortality.

Ultrasound should be considered the imaging method of choice for the early evaluation of suspected Fournier's gangrene. Subcutaneous air on plain radiographs is not universally present, especially early in the disease process. Computed tomography does not visualize the scrotal structures as well as ultrasound, but more accurately detects small amounts of subcutaneous gas. Sonographic findings seen with early Fournier's gangrene include thickening of the scrotal skin and discrete focal regions of subcutaneous gas, which is pathognomonic for Fournier's gangrene (Figure 11-25).[16] The presence of gas in the scrotal wall should not be confused with gas sometimes seen in herniated bowel in the

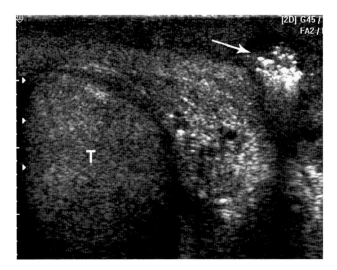

Figure 11-25. The testicle (T) is seen in the corner of the image, which shows thickened scrotal skin. A small area of subcutaneous gas is seen (arrow). This patient was found to have a scrotal abscess that was progressing to Fournier's gangrene.

scrotum. Since Fournier's gangrene may result from prostatitis or orchitis, signs of epididymo-orchitis may also be seen.

► COMMON VARIANTS AND SELECTED ABNORMALITIES

HYDROCELE

There is a potential space between the visceral and parietal layers of the tunica vaginalis that can collect fluid, resulting in a hydrocele. Hydroceles are usually visualized in the anterolateral aspect of the scrotum and may be bilateral or unilateral. Their location is due to the attachment of the tunica to the testicle and scrotum posteriorly. Many hydroceles are congenital and result from a direct communication with the abdominal cavity. Hydroceles can also result from trauma, infection, neoplasm, radiation therapy, and undiagnosed torsion.[19] Hydrocele can be seen as an isolated finding or in conjunction with acute or chronic pathology. They are occasionally seen as a lone finding in a patient who complains of acute scrotal pain.

On ultrasound examination, a hydrocele appears as an echo poor or dark area surrounding the testicle (Figure 11-26). Hydroceles can contain loculations, especially when an inflammatory process is present. Most acute hydroceles that form in reaction to infection are thin-walled. The collections of fluid seen as a result of trauma or torsion also tend to be small. Chronic hydroceles that have developed slowly from a secondary process are larger and may have irregular septations, which reflect previous hemorrhage or infection. As in most cases with ultrasonography, blood cannot be readily

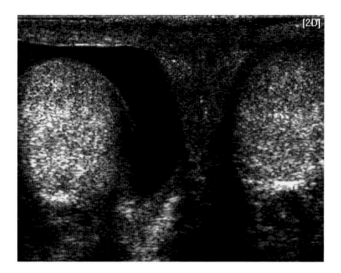

Figure 11-26. Side-by-side view showing the left and right testicle. The right testicle (seen on the left side of the image) is outlined by fluid of the hydrocele.

differentiated from serous fluid. A history of trauma, previously diagnosed neoplasm, or surgery would suggest a hematocele. A large number of echoes in the hydrocele may suggest the presence of pus in the proper clinical setting (Figure 11-27).

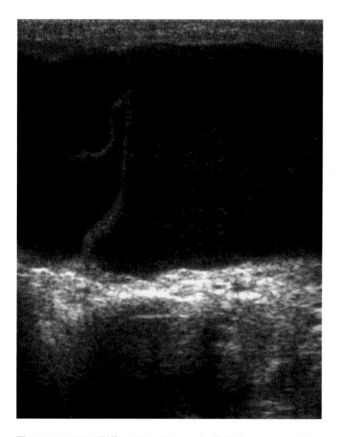

Figure 11-27. Diffusely echogenic fluid is seen in this image of a pyocele. On exploration, the scrotum was filled with pus that may have started with epididymitis.

VARICOCELE

Varicoceles occur in the presence of abnormal dilation and tortuosity of the veins in the pampiniform plexus located in the spermatic cord. Nearly 99% of all varicoceles are left-sided but they can present bilaterally.[16] This is due to the drainage of the spermatic vein on the right directly into the inferior vena cava. The left spermatic vein first drains into the left renal vein at nearly a 90 degree angle. This sharp angle prevents the spermatic vein from forming a valve.

Varicoceles are associated with decreased sperm motility and low sperm count. Acute thrombosis is a concern in young men and may lead to surgical intervention. On ultrasound examination, varicoceles appear as an extratesticular bundle of tubular structures (Figure 11-28). Occasionally, varicoceles may be confused with inflammation of the epididymal tail or bowel content in the scrotum. Having the patient perform a Valsalva maneuver should cause distention of the varices, and an obvious increase in blood flow through the venous structures. On rare occasions a varicocele may be seen extending into the testicle itself (Figure 11-29). It can be followed from its origin to differentiate it from other pathological processes. The addition of power Doppler, especially with a concomitant Valsalva maneuver, will demonstrate blood flow in the characteristic pattern (Figure 11-30).

Postoperative complications from repair of varicoceles can range from simple wound infection to scrotal abscess and, occasionally, testicular ischemia. Blood flow on the affected side should be confirmed whenever a postoperative patient presents with acute scrotal pain.

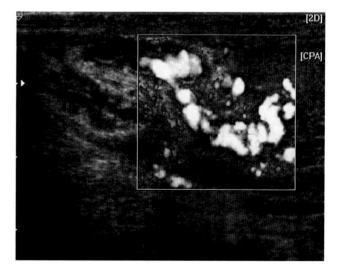

Figure 11-28. Tortuous vessels are seen on this image running from left to right (toward the testicle). A power Doppler window (grayscale copy) covering a portion of the varicocele shows prominent flow with a Valsalva maneuver.

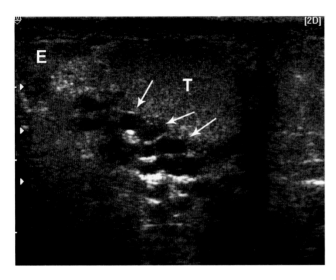

Figure 11-29. Extended varicocele. Tubular structures (arrows) are seen in the lower left corner of the testicle (T). The typical testicular architecture is disrupted. E-Epididymis.

It should not be assumed that surgical correction of a varicocele or a bell clapper deformity obviates the need for concern regarding testicular ischemia. While actual torsion by the spermatic cord may not be seen, thrombosis of the veins due to accidental or purposeful ligation may lead to testicular infarction and loss. Similarly, a large degree of postoperative edema can compromise blood flow.

HERNIATION

Herniation of abdominal content into the scrotum may lead to a patient presenting with acute testicular pain. In

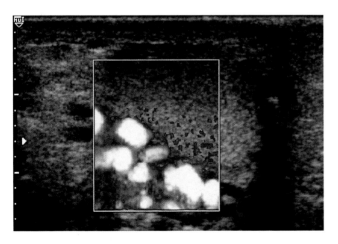

Figure 11-30. A power Doppler window now sits over the tubular structures seen in Figure 11-29. A significant amount of venous flow is seen with a Valsalva maneuver.

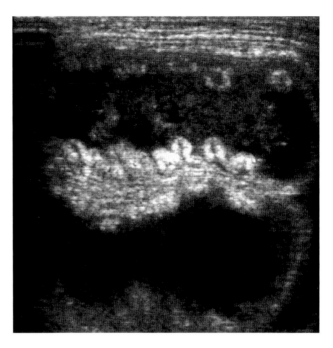

Figure 11-31. Scrotal hernia. Two loops of bowel are seen in the scrotum. Some fecal matter is seen in the nearfield loop.

some cases, the patient's history will be negative for previous hernias. The scrotum may be swollen and painful, thus simulating testicular torsion, epididymitis, or orchitis. Ultrasound evaluation can help identify the testes and often allows the examiner to visualize abdominal content, such as bowel loops or omentum (Figure 11-31). Occasionally, a loop of bowel can be clearly seen on ultrasound examination. In other cases, the sonologist will need to be guided by artifacts from gas within the loop of bowel. It is critical not to confuse gas gangrene with bowel gas seen in a hernia. The viability of a bowel segment identified can be grossly assessed with ultrasound. Obvious peristalsis typically means that the bowel has not yet infarcted. Complete absence of peristalsis with edematous bowel wall without any identifiable blood flow on power Doppler can mean that the bowel loop involved has already infarcted. Power Doppler identification of blood flow in the bowel wall is possible and suggests some viability. A surprising amount of blood flow picked up on Doppler can mean early ischemia with hyperemia that is preceding a further drop in perfusion and eventual necrosis. Omental fat can also be herniated into the scrotum and become strangulated just like bowel, leading to necrosis.

TESTICULAR MASSES

Testicular masses may present as either acute onset pain, especially if there is hemorrhage into a tumor, or chronic

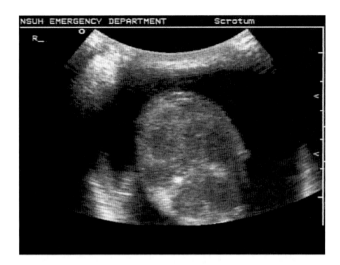

Figure 11-32. Testicular tumor. A long-axis view of the testicle reveals a surrounding hydrocele and multiple hypoechoic areas that replace the normal architecture. This tumor was discovered in a patient presenting complaining of acute testicular enlargement. On further questioning, the patient admitted that his testicle was slowly enlarging for over 2 years.

and painless testicular enlargement. In most cases, there is little for the clinician to do other than arrange rapid urological follow-up. If a large intratumor hemorrhage is detected, then immediate urological consultation may be needed. Patients who present with large painless testicular masses that may have been developing for years require careful consideration regarding discharge (Figure 11-32). Most testicular tumors are malignant germ-cell neoplasms, with only 5% being benign tumors.[28]

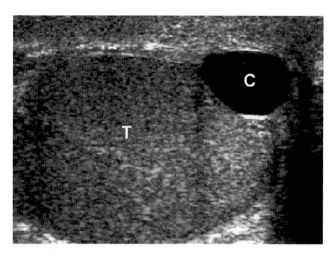

Figure 11-34. A cyst is seen in the tunica albuginea (C), in contact with the testicle (T).

Extratesticular masses can be encountered in emergency practice and those most often seen are benign cysts of the albuginea, epididymal cysts, or spermatoceles (Figure 11-33). Cysts of the albuginea typically present as small palpable masses and are echo-free on ultrasound (Figure 11-34). They are frequently located near the rete testis and epididymis. Epididymal cysts can be seen in up to one third of asymptomatic adults.[28] Spermatoceles are cystic collections of seminal fluid and are also fairly common. They are typically found within an efferent duct near the head of the epididymis and can result from trauma, inflammation, or vasectomy (Figure 11-35). Sonographic appearance is frequently that of multiple cystic fluid collections.

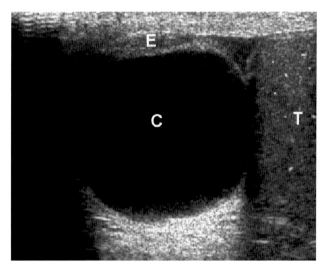

Figure 11-33. A large cyst (C) is seen in the epididymal head. A small wedge of compressed epididymal tissue (E) is seen just above the cyst. The testicle (T) is seen on the right side of the image.

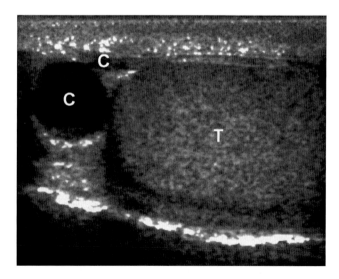

Figure 11-35. A medium-sized cyst is seen in the epididymal head (C) next to the testicle (T) as well as another smaller one just above and to the right of it.

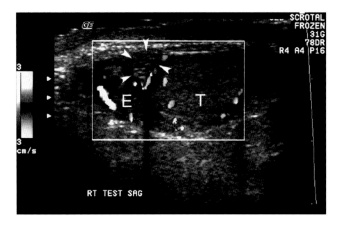

Figure 11-36. While increased flow was seen in the epididymis and testicle of this 8-year-old patient, no flow was noted within the suspected torsed appendix testis outlined by arrowheads. E: epididymis; T: testicle.

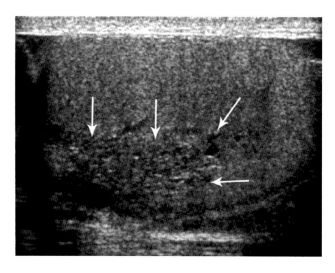

Figure 11-37. An area of dilated Rete testis is shown (arrows). This appearance is being seen more frequently with improved equipment and patient population changes.

TORSION OF THE APPENDIX TESTIS

Torsion of the appendix testis can present with similar symptoms to testicular torsion, but is often noted in a younger age group. Appendix testis torsion may result in inflammation of the epididymis and apparent epididymitis (Figure 11-36). The appendix occasionally will be seen next to and separate from the epididymal head and will have no blood flow noted inside it. The sonologist will need to carefully examine for the swollen appendix since the location of the appendix testis can be variable.

DILATED RETE TESTIS

Dilated rete testis is a common variant that may be more commonly found because of improved resolution on new ultrasound equipment. Dilated rete testis appears as a collection of small cysts or channels (Figure 11-37). They are an example of tubular ectasia secondary to obstruction in the epididymis of the efferent ductules. Rete testis is a nonpalpable lesion that is typically an incidental finding and found in patients who have undergone vasectomy. Power Doppler will reveal them to be avascular.

CALCIFICATIONS

Calcifications in the scrotal structures can involve the tunica albuginea, be intratesticular, or present in the form of scrotal pearls. Small testicular calcifications are known as microlithiasis (Figure 11-38).

UNDESCENDED TESTICLE

Patients may occasionally present with scrotal pain and are found to have only one testicle. While there can be congenital or surgically related absence of a testicle, it may be worthwhile to check for an undescended testicle, even in young adults. An undescended testicle may increase both the rate of infertility and testicular cancer. Some patients may not even be aware that one testicle

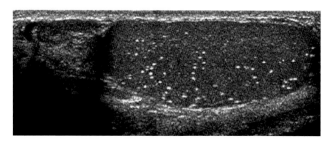

A

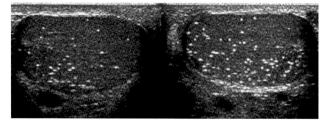

B

Figure 11-38. Longitudinal view of one testicle (A) and transverse views of both testicles (B) reveal multiple small symmetrical echogenic foci consistent with microlithiasis.

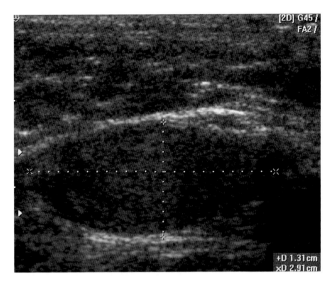

Figure 11-39. This small, prepubescent appearing testicle was located proximal to the scrotum in the patient's pelvis.

has not descended. Location of the testicle can be helpful and reassuring for the patient. Potential ischemia of the undescended testicle is present and blood flow should be checked (Figures 11-39 and Figure 11-40).

▶ PITFALLS

1. **Contraindication.** There are no absolute contraindications to evaluating the testicle with ultrasound. Examinations may be limited by severe pain, though, and analgesia will occasionally be required. Since minimal pressure is applied during the evaluation of the acute testicle, damage to a fractured testicle is not a concern.

2. **Prepubescent and infant boys.** Testicular blood flow in prepubescent boys and infants can be very difficult to detect. In cases of trauma, the testicular anatomy can still be accurately evaluated. It may require very sensitive equipment and considerable expertise to evaluate prepubescent testes. Some medical imaging departments even prefer to have nuclear medicine studies performed when experienced attending staff or sonographers are not available.

3. **Incomplete torsion.** Complete torsion occurs at approximately 450 degrees of twisting of the spermatic cord. Venous flow initially disappears followed by arterial blood flow. Careful comparison between the two sides is important to exclude incomplete torsion. Diagnosing torsion early in the disease process when it is still incomplete can be challenging with color Doppler alone; this method relies on subtle differences between the testes. Use of spectral Doppler to document both venous and arterial waveforms is optimal. Noting a venous waveform alone may be problematic. Figure 11-41 is from a patient who had no identifiable arterial waveforms in the affected testicle despite a careful search and even confirmation during a formal radiology ultrasound examination using an ultra-sensitive transducer. The patient was found to have incomplete torsion at surgical exploration that was prompted by these findings.

4. **Torsion–detorsion.** Some patients may exhibit torsion and detorsion. This usually presents as

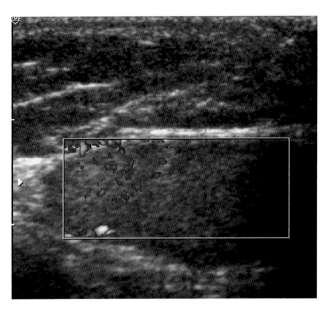

Figure 11-40. Power Doppler (grayscale copy) detected some flow in the undescended testicle with both venous and arterial flow patterns confirmed on pulse wave Doppler.

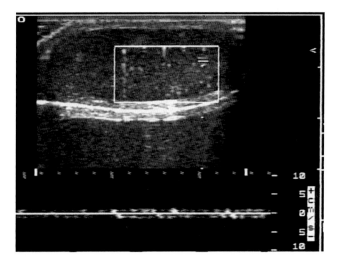

Figure 11-41. While an apparent venous flow pattern could be obtained in multiple parts of the testicle, no arterial flow was ever seen. The patient was found to have incomplete torsion at exploration.

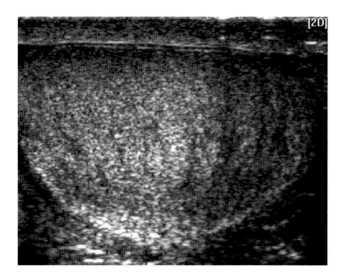

Figure 11-42. The testicle appears to have multiple vertical striations running through it. This was not a pathological state, rather the normal appearance of a testicle of this 55-year-old diabetic patient.

a waxing and waning pain that results from intermittent ischemia. This entity can make for a challenging diagnosis if the ultrasound examination is performed during a period of detorsion. Shortly after detorsion, hyperemia may be detected as increased blood flow in the affected testicle. This will usually not last much longer than 15 minutes and may be missed. Bedside ultrasonography may be helpful to evaluate this possibility as it allows for serial examinations. With the clinical acumen to observe the patient and perform serial ultrasound examinations, clinicians should be able to avoid this pitfall.

5. **Striated testis.** With the aid of modern high-resolution equipment, sonologists are more likely than ever to see details of testicular structure not previously noted on ultrasound. In fact, some structures may resemble abnormalities previously described in traditional texts. One such example is striated testes (Figure 11-42). This appearance can be confused with early changes seen with necrosis or other inflammatory process. Striated testes are most likely the result of testicular fibrosis or atrophy. It is most commonly seen in older patients and in diabetics.

► CASE STUDIES

CASE 1

Patient Presentation

A 21-year-old man presented to the emergency department with a complaint of right testicular pain. He stated that the pain started suddenly 5 hours prior to presentation. Since then, he also noted some swelling on the right. The patient denied being sexually active but did note being struck in the genitals the day before during a basketball game. He had an unremarkable medical history and did not smoke. The patient denied any history of sexually transmitted diseases and stated he was not having any urinary symptoms or urethral discharge.

Physical examination revealed a healthy young male in mild distress with normal vital signs. The abdominal examination was unremarkable, with no obvious hernias or costovertebral angle tenderness. Testicular examination revealed an erythematous right hemi-scrotum with moderate swelling. The testicle was enlarged and painful to the touch. The epididymis was tender and slightly enlarged on examination. The testicle had a horizontal lie and the cremasteric reflex could not be elicited. No cremasteric reflex was elicited on the contralateral side where the testicular and hemi-scrotum examinations were normal.

Management Course

The urine dip was negative. No urology service was available and the only radiology studies available at night were plain films, which were read by the emergency physician. A tertiary care hospital was approximately 90 minutes away by ambulance. Bedside emergency ultrasonography was available to the emergency physician. She performed an examination of the scrotum, noting enlargement and greatly increased blood flow to the right testicle and epididymis, with the epididymis being double the width compared to the contralateral side. A diagnosis of epididymitis with orchitis was made and the patient was discharged home with antibiotics, analgesics, and close follow-up and return instructions.

Commentary

Case 1 represents an example of the nonspecific signs, symptoms, and history that may be associated with the presentation of acute testicular pain. The patient acutely became aware of testicular discomfort and swelling although the disease process was probably slower in onset. The history of minor testicular trauma was a red herring but could not be ignored. The physical examination was often less helpful than described in many textbooks, especially when orchitis was present and the entire testicle was tender and swollen. Without the availability of bedside ultrasonography to evaluate the testicle, the emergency physician would have had to decide if transfer to an outside facility was mandated. If a lack of flow was seen in the testicle, arrangements could have been made for immediate transfer to a urology consultant and manual detorsion attempted. In this case, the diagnosis was made at the bedside with the aid of ultrasonography. An unnecessary transfer was avoided and the patient was discharged home with appropriate treatment and follow-up instructions.

CASE 2

Patient Presentation

An 18-year-old man presented to the emergency department 3 days after being kicked in the groin during a soccer match. The patient was seen at an outside facility shortly after the injury at which time an evaluation, including an ultrasound examination, revealed a small- to moderate-sized area of hemorrhage and no rupture through the testicular capsule. The patient was evaluated by a urologist and discharged home. He presents today because of increased swelling of the testicle. The scrotal skin is firm and erythematous, according to the mother, who is a pediatrician. The hydrocodone the patient was prescribed no longer relieves his pain. He denies any hematuria or other urinary symptoms.

Physical examination revealed an uncomfortable appearing man. The patient's vital signs were within normal limits. The cardiac, lung, and abdominal examinations were normal. Testicular examination revealed a swollen, enlarged, and erythematous left hemi-scrotum that was markedly tender to the touch. The testicle was clearly enlarged but difficult to differentiate within the scrotum. The contralateral testicle was nontender and appeared to be of normal size. A urinalysis shows no white or red blood cells and is within normal limits. The mother insists something has changed since his injury; however, when she contacted the urologist, he asked that she see him in 2 days and recommended increasing the patient's analgesic dose.

Management Course

An ultrasound examination in the medical imaging department is not available after hours. The nuclear medicine technician is in house performing a V/Q scan and could be ready for this patient in 60–90 minutes. The emergency physician performs a bedside ultrasound examination, and this reveals a large heterogeneous testicle with areas of acute and old hemorrhage. Normal color Doppler flow is present in the portion of the testicle that appeared normal. A fracture line could be defined through the parenchyma of the testicle and appeared to go through the capsule of the testicle. The urologist on call is contacted regarding the patient and comes in for evaluation. After a brief evaluation and review of the ultrasound examination on videotape, the patient is taken to the operating room for exploration. Surgical exploration reveals several areas of hemorrhage and a testicular rupture that is repaired. The patient is admit-

ted overnight. Follow-up shows slow resolution of the injury with 80% function of the testicle at 30 days. No further surgical intervention is required.

Commentary

Case 2 illustrates the utility of ultrasound in defining testicular anatomy. The patient had already been scanned almost 3 days ago and no severe pathology was noted. However, he bled more into the testicle and a fracture line going through the capsule was defined on re-examination. The patient harbored a finding that led directly to operative intervention. However, it would have been tempting to simply discharge him home for follow-up with his urologist once pain was better controlled. After all, the patient had already been imaged after the injury. The nuclear medicine scan may not have revealed any abnormalities as it is limited in defining anatomy.

CASE 3

Patient Presentation

A 34-year-old man presented to the emergency department, complaining of left scrotal pain. The patient noted awaking with severe pain approximately 6 hours prior to the admission. His medical history is remarkable for recent surgery to "fix" some varicoceles that had been causing him pain for years. He complained of scrotal pain, which was different from the incisional pain.

Physical examination revealed an afebrile patient in moderate distress. Examination of the abdomen was unremarkable. The genitourinary examination showed a slightly erythematous scrotum, more so on the left. There was moderate swelling of the left testicle and it was exquisitely tender. It had a normal lie and the epididymis could not be reliably palpated. The cremasteric reflex was elicited with difficulty bilaterally. There was no evidence of infection at the incision site.

Management Course

A urinalysis shows 3 red blood cell counts per high-powered field and 5 white blood cell counts per high-powered field. No bacteria are seen. An ultrasound examination performed by the emergency physician reveals the right testicle to have normal echotexture, size, and blood flow. The left testicle is found to be moderately enlarged and appears less echogenic than the unaffected testicle. No blood flow is seen within the testicle with either color or power Doppler. The urologist on call is notified and arrives to evaluate the patient, booking an operating room on her way into the hospital. The patient is taken for exploration and found to have an ischemic left testicle as a result of diffuse thrombosis of veins running in the cord and resultant vascular congestion.

Commentary

This case illustrates the difficulty in making a diagnosis without imaging in patients with postoperative scrotal pain. Sonologists who use bedside ultrasound are likely to make more accurate and confident diagnoses.

REFERENCES

1. Lewis AG, Bukowski TP, Jarvis PD: Evaluation of acute scrotum in the emergency department. *J Pediatric Surg* 30:277–280, 1995.
2. Fernandez MS, Dominguez C, Sanguesa C: The use of color Doppler sonography of the acute scrotum in children. *Cir Pediatr* 10:25–27, 1997.
3. Zoller G: Genitourinary trauma. In Rosen P, Barkin R, (eds): *Emergency Medicine Concepts and Clinical Practice*, 4th ed. St. Louis, MO: Mosby, 1997:2243–2245.
4. Knight PJ, Vassy LE: The diagnosis and treatment of the acute scrotum in children and adolescents. *Ann Surg* 200:664–666, 1984.
5. Albrecht T, Lotzof K, Hussain HK, Shedden D, Cosgove DO: Bruyn: Power Doppler US of the normal prepubertal testis: Does it live up to its promises? *Radiology* 203:227–231, 1997.
6. Fenner MN, Roszhart DA, Texter JH: Testicular scanning: Evaluating the acute scrotum in the clinical setting. *Urology* 10:25, 1991.
7. Jefferson RH, Perez LM, Joseph DB: Critical analysis of the clinical presentation of acute scrotum: A 9-year experience at a single institution. *J Urol* 158:1198–1201, 1997.
8. Cos LR, Rabinowitz R: Trauma-induced testicular torsion in children. *J Trauma* 22:223–225, 1982.
9. Prater JM, Overdorf BS: Testicular torsion: A surgical emergency. *Am Fam Emerg Physician* 44:834–840, 1991.
10. Lee TF, Winter DB, Madsen FA, et al.: Conventional color Doppler velocity sonography versus color Doppler energy sonography for the diagnosis of acute experimental torsion of the spermatic cord. *AJR* 167:785–790, 1996.
11. Kass EJ, Stone KT, Cacciarelli AA, Mithcell B: Do all children with an acute scrotum require exploration? *J Urol* 150:667–669, 1993.
12. Blaivas M, Sierzenski P, Lambert M: Emergency evaluation of patients presenting with acute scrotum using bedside ultrasonography. *Acad Emerg Med* 8:90–93, 2001.
13. Blaivas M, Sierzenski P: Emergency ultrasonography in the evaluation of the acute scrotum. *Acad Emerg Med* 8:85–89, 2001.
14. Blaivas M, Batts M, Lambert M: Ultrasonographic diagnosis of testicular torsion by emergency physicians. *Am J Emerg Med* 18:198–200, 2000.
15. Sierzenski P, Blaivas M, Belden M, Nielson T, Lambert M: Manual compression of the spermatic cord to simulate testicular torsion on ultrasound. A teaching model for emergency physicians. *Acad Emerg Med* 7:493, 2000.
16. Morrison D, Blaivas M, Lyon M: Emergency diagnosis of Fournier's gangrene with bedside ultrasound. *Am J Emerg Med* 23:544–547, 2005.
17. Blaivas M, Lyon M, Theodoro D: A two-year experience with bedside emergency ultrasound for acute scrotal pain in the emergency department. *Ann Emerg Med* 44:S82, 2004.
18. Lyon M, Blaivas M, Brannam L: Use of emergency ultrasound in a rural ED with limited radiology services. *Am J Emerg Med* 23:212–214, 2005.
19. Stewart R, Carroll B: The scrotum, In: Rumack CM, Wilson SR, Charboneau JW, eds. *Diagnostic Ultrasound*, vol 1. St. Louis, MO: Mosby, 1991:565–589.
20. Micallef M, Ahmad I, Ramesh N, Hurley M, McInerney D: Ultrasound features of blunt testicular injury. *Injury* 32:23–26, 2001.
21. Corrales JG, Corbel L, Cipolla B, et al.: Accuracy of ultrasound diagnosis after blunt testicular trauma. *J Urol* 150:1834–1836, 1993.
22. Blaivas M, Lambert JM, Harwood RA, Wood JP, Konicki J: Lower extremity doppler for deep venous thrombosis—Can emergency physicians be accurate and fast? *Acad Emerg Med* 7:120–126, 2000.
23. Hilty WM, Hudson PA, Levitt MA, Hall JB: Real-time ultrasound-guided femoral vein catheterization during cardiopulmonary resuscitation. *Ann Emerg Med* 29:331–337, 1997.
24. Hill R, Conron R, Greissinger P, Heller M: Ultrasound for the detection of foreign bodies in human tissue. *Ann Emerg Med* 29:353–356, 1997.
25. Benziri E, Fabiani P, Migliori G, et al.: Gangrene of the perineum. *Urology* 47:935–939, 1996.
26. Carroll PR, Cattolica EV, Turzan CW, et al.: Necrotizing soft-tissue infections of the perineum and genitalia: Etiology and early reconstruction. *West J Med* 144:174–178, 1996.
27. Netter F: *Scrotum: Reproductive System.* West Caldwell: CIBA, 73, 1989.
28. Hill MC, Sanders RC: Sonography of benign disease of the scrotum. In Sanders RC, Hill M, eds. *Ultrasound Annual.* New York: Raven Press, 1986:197–237.

CHAPTER 12

First Trimester Pregnancy

Robert F. Reardon and Scott A. Joing

Ultrasonography is the primary imaging modality used in pregnancy.[1-4] In first trimester pregnant patients who present with vaginal bleeding or abdominal pain, ultrasound can be used to distinguish ectopic pregnancy from threatened abortion or embryonic demise. The primary goal of emergency sonography of the pelvis in the first trimester is to identify an intrauterine pregnancy, which essentially excludes the diagnosis of ectopic pregnancy.[5] Secondary objectives are to detect extrauterine signs of an ectopic pregnancy, estimate the viability of an intrauterine pregnancy, and characterize other causes of pelvic pain and vaginal bleeding. In addition, sonographic detection of free fluid outside of the pelvis can help emergency physicians expedite the care of a patient with a ruptured ectopic pregnancy.[6] Emergency bedside sonography is not intended to define the entire spectrum of pelvic pathology in early pregnancy. A follow-up comprehensive pelvic ultrasound examination is indicated after the initial focused bedside examination, the timing of which is dictated by the clinical scenario.

► CLINICAL CONSIDERATIONS

Abdominal or pelvic pain and vaginal bleeding are common complaints during early pregnancy. Challenges to emergency or acute care physicians include making the diagnosis of pregnancy and then using available diagnostic tools to determine the etiology of the patient's complaint.

The development of sensitive pregnancy tests has made a missed diagnosis of early pregnancy unlikely. Modern qualitative urine tests for human chorionic gonadotropin (β-hCG) have a threshold of about 20 IU/L and allow detection of pregnancy as early as 1 week post-conception (3 weeks' gestational age). False-negative urine tests may occur when the urine is highly dilute (specific gravity <1.010), and obtaining a quantitative serum β-hCG should be considered in such cases.[7]

Once pregnancy is recognized in a symptomatic or high-risk patient, complications of early pregnancy, particularly ectopic pregnancy, must be considered. Those patients with pelvic or abdominal pain, vaginal bleeding, dizziness, syncope, or any risk factors for ectopic pregnancy need to have the status of their pregnancy evaluated. The location, viability, and gestational age of the pregnancy are important factors in establishing a diagnosis. Other findings such as free intraperitoneal fluid in the pelvis or a pelvic mass may also impact the patient's management.

Many diagnostic tests can be used to detect complications of early pregnancy. Serum β-hCG and progesterone levels, suction curettage, culdocentesis, and laparoscopy yield some information, but none can identify the entire spectrum of pathology like pelvic sonography. Furthermore, other imaging modalities, like CT and MRI, are not commonly used for detecting complications of early pregnancy.

The hormone β-hCG is produced by the trophoblasts during early pregnancy. Serum β-hCG levels rise exponentially in early pregnancy and can be used as a marker to date normal pregnancies. However, abnormal pregnancies have widely varying β-hCG levels, so a single level cannot differentiate a normal intrauterine pregnancy from an ectopic pregnancy or other abnormality.[8]

Progesterone is produced by the corpus luteum in early pregnancy and serum levels remain relatively high during a normal pregnancy. Serum levels are generally lower in abnormal pregnancies, including ectopic pregnancy, and fall with pregnancy failure. Clinicians who do not have bedside ultrasound immediately available have utilized progesterone levels to help differentiate between a normal pregnancy and a possible ectopic with some success.[9,10] These methods, however, have not proven to be as efficient or as accurate as protocols that incorporate initial transvaginal sonography. Preliminary reports suggest that progesterone may have a role in further categorizing patients who have an initial indeterminate transvaginal ultrasound. One study found that patients with a progesterone level $\geq$ 11 ng/mL are significantly more likely to have an early intrauterine pregnancy rather than an ectopic or an abortion (sensitivity 91%, specificity 84%).[11] Another study demonstrated a progesterone level less than 5 ng/mL to be 88% sensitive (although only 40% specific) in detecting ectopic pregnancy in the setting of an indeterminate (nonspecific free fluid or empty uterus) ultrasound.[12]

Suction curettage of the uterus can provide a definitive diagnosis of an intrauterine pregnancy if chorionic villi are identified. However, this test terminates an intrauterine pregnancy, making it applicable only when termination is desired or the pregnancy has obviously failed. Because it is invasive and other tests can provide similar information, suction curettage is rarely useful in the initial emergency evaluation during early pregnancy.

Culdocentesis is needle aspiration of the pelvic cul-de-sac through the posterior fornix of the vagina. Aspiration of blood is considered indicative of an ectopic pregnancy although blood in the cul-de-sac can be seen with an intrauterine pregnancy. However, culdocentesis is not very sensitive, especially for detecting nonruptured ectopic pregnancies.[5,13-15] It now has a very limited role and is recommended only when ultrasound is not available.[16]

Laparoscopy is an excellent test for visualizing extrauterine pelvic pathology, especially ectopic pregnancy.[17] However, it does not give any information about intrauterine contents or fetal viability. Recently laparoscopy has been utilized less frequently because sonography is noninvasive and can provide more information.[14] Laparoscopy can be used as a therapeutic tool and a diagnostic adjunct when sonography is nondiagnostic.

There are many advantages to using sonography in the first trimester of pregnancy. It is an ideal diagnostic tool in this setting since it can visualize both intrauterine contents and the extrauterine pelvic pathology. When used judiciously, ultrasound has no known adverse effects on the embryo and can be repeated as needed. Unlike curettage or culdocentesis, ultrasound is noninvasive and well tolerated by most patients.[18] Unlike curettage or laparoscopy, ultrasound can directly visualize the intrauterine or extrauterine location of a pregnancy.[19] Unlike serum markers, ultrasound can immediately identify an abnormal pregnancy or evaluate fetal viability. Also, ultrasound can accurately measure the gestational age of a pregnancy, whereas serum markers can only give a gross estimation. Finally, patients with an ectopic pregnancy can be risk-stratified using ultrasound by estimating the size of an extrauterine mass or the amount of free intraperitoneal blood.

A disadvantage of using ultrasound in early pregnancy is that a pregnancy may not be visible between 3 and 5 weeks' gestational age. During this time, sensitive urine pregnancy tests are positive but the gestation is usually too small to identify, even with transvaginal ultrasound. Another disadvantage of using ultrasound is that it is equipment and operator dependent. Clinicians who make important patient management decisions based on ultrasound results must know the limitations of each study based on who is performing the examination and what type of equipment is being used.

▶ CLINICAL INDICATIONS

Any patient who is at risk for complications of early pregnancy is a candidate for pelvic sonography. Symptoms and physical examination findings include pelvic or abdominal pain or tenderness, vaginal bleeding, dizziness, syncope, a pelvic mass, or uterine size that does not correlate with the gestational age. Risk factors for ectopic pregnancy include pelvic inflammatory disease, tubal ligation, tubal surgery, increased maternal age, intrauterine contraceptive devices, prior ectopic pregnancy, and a history of infertility.[20] Most patients with an ectopic pregnancy present with abdominal or pelvic pain, vaginal bleeding, or dizziness, but some are relatively asymptomatic. Since no specific sign or symptom is absolute, physicians must have a high index of suspicion so that subtle presentations are not overlooked. Also, any woman of childbearing age who presents with shock of unknown etiology should have an immediate abdominal and pelvic ultrasound examination, even before a pregnancy test is completed.[6]

The main indication for emergency pelvic sonography in the first trimester is to differentiate an intrauterine pregnancy from an ectopic pregnancy. Sonography can immediately establish one of these diagnoses in most patients with first trimester complaints.[19]

- Intrauterine pregnancy
- Ectopic pregnancy

Emergency pelvic sonography is also useful for the diagnosis of the following conditions in the first trimester of pregnancy:

- Pregnancy loss
- Multiple pregnancy
- Pelvic mass
- Ovarian torsion
- Gestational trophoblastic disease

▶ INTRAUTERINE PREGNANCY

A normal intrauterine pregnancy is the most common sonographic finding during the first trimester. Even novice sonologists can use pelvic ultrasound effectively because identifying an intrauterine pregnancy is straightforward and this finding virtually eliminates the possibility of an ectopic pregnancy.[21] About 70% of patients who present with abdominal pain or vaginal bleeding in the first trimester will have an intrauterine pregnancy visualized with bedside ultrasound and will not require further testing.[22] Care must be taken when using sonography between 3 and 5 weeks' gestational age because it is easy to confuse sonographic signs of an early intrauterine pregnancy with those of an ectopic pregnancy.

Identifying an intrauterine pregnancy with cardiac activity can give patients some reassurance about the outcome of their pregnancy. Those patients with a finding of embryonic cardiac activity have a much lower incidence of pregnancy loss than other patients with similar symptoms.[23,24] However, physicians should be careful not to give patients false hope about their pregnancy. Even when a normal intrauterine pregnancy is discovered, it is prudent to inform patients that emergency bedside sonography is a focused examination only and will not detect fetal anomalies. Also, patients with abdominal pain or vaginal bleeding still have a significant chance of pregnancy loss.

Dating an intrauterine pregnancy is not as important as excluding an ectopic pregnancy. However, when the uterine size does not correlate with the gestational age or when the last menstrual period is unknown, sonography is indicated to date the pregnancy. This is very common because about half of all pregnant women cannot remember their last menstrual period. Pregnancy dating is simple and rapid with modern ultrasound equipment. Sonographic dating during the first trimester is more accurate than dating later in pregnancy. A few minutes spent measuring an embryo will be much appreciated by the patient's obstetrician, especially in patients who have unclear menstrual dates or are noncompliant with prenatal care. This early measurement becomes more important near term when the obstetrician is considering induction of labor in a patient whose uterine size does not correlate with gestational age.

▶ ECTOPIC PREGNANCY

Ectopic pregnancy occurs in about 2% of all pregnancies in the United States.[13,14,25] However, symptomatic patients who present to an emergency setting have a much higher incidence, as high as 4.5–13% in some reports.[9,26–28] The incidence of ectopic pregnancy has quadrupled in the last 20 years.[13] During the same period of time, the case-fatality rate for ruptured ectopic pregnancies has decreased significantly. This decrease is due to earlier diagnosis and treatment secondary to increased awareness and improved diagnostic capabilities, such as transvaginal sonography.[14] Despite these improvements, a significant percentage of ectopic pregnancies is still missed.[29] Also, ectopic pregnancy remains the leading cause of maternal death during the first trimester of pregnancy.[30]

Heterotopic pregnancy, which is a concomitant intrauterine and extrauterine pregnancy, has also become more common in the last few decades. In 1948, the incidence of heterotopic pregnancy was estimated to be 1 per 30,000 pregnancies, based on a theoretical calculation and assuming an ectopic pregnancy rate of 0.37%.[31] Now that the ectopic pregnancy rate is about 2%, it is reasonable to expect that the rate of heterotopic pregnancy is higher than previously estimated. There is some suggestion that the incidence of heterotopic pregnancy may be as high as 1 in 8,000 pregnancies, but this may be practice specific.[31–36] The incidence is much higher in patients taking ovulation-inducing medications or undergoing in vitro fertilization (as high as 1 per 100 pregnancies).[37,38]

Emergency or acute care physicians have an important role in preventing morbidity and mortality from ectopic pregnancy.[39] Early diagnosis of ectopic pregnancy allows conservative treatment options, like methotrexate therapy.[14,40] Pelvic ultrasound is the main diagnostic modality that allows an early diagnosis to be made.

When emergency physicians perform bedside transvaginal sonography, pregnant patients have a shorter length of stay in the emergency department.[41–43] Also, bedside pelvic ultrasound screening by clinicians is more cost-effective than ordering comprehensive pelvic sonography on every patient with a possible ectopic pregnancy.[44] Most importantly, a protocol, which includes bedside transvaginal ultrasound by emergency physicians, has been shown to decrease the incidence of discharged patients returning with a subsequent ruptured ectopic pregnancy.[22,26,45]

ALGORITHM WITH TRANSVAGINAL SONOGRAPHY AND β-HCG DISCRIMINATORY ZONE

Prior to the development of ectopic pregnancy algorithms and the widespread use of transvaginal sonography, the diagnosis of about half of all ectopic pregnancies was missed, and about half of those ruptured prior to their next presentation.[26,46,47] In the 1980s, ectopic pregnancy was one of the leading causes of emergency physician malpractice suits.[48,49] Algorithms that incorporate transvaginal sonography and a β-hCG discriminatory zone have improved diagnostic accuracy and reduced the incidence of patients who are discharged and subsequently present with a ruptured ectopic pregnancy.[19,26]

One algorithm utilizes emergency bedside transvaginal sonography as the initial diagnostic step for all patients at risk for ectopic pregnancy, before a quantitative serum β-hCG is obtained (Figure 12-1).[4,26,45,47,50–59] Transvaginal sonography can establish a diagnosis of intrauterine pregnancy or ectopic pregnancy in 75% of patients at the time of their initial presentation.[19] If emergency bedside sonography demonstrates an intrauterine pregnancy or an ectopic pregnancy, then the work-up is complete. When no intrauterine pregnancy or ectopic pregnancy is identified, then the bedside ultrasound examination is indeterminate, and at this point a quantitative serum β-hCG level and a comprehensive pelvic ultrasound examination should be ordered. Again, if the comprehensive study shows an intrauterine pregnancy or an ectopic pregnancy, then the work-up is complete. If either the bedside or comprehensive ultrasound examination demonstrates nonspecific signs of an ectopic pregnancy, then the risk is very high. Therefore, this situation should be managed in the same manner as a clear ectopic pregnancy, and an obstetrics consult should be obtained. If both sonograms show no intrauterine pregnancy and no signs of an ectopic pregnancy, then the management depends on the serum β-hCG level. Patients with an indeterminate ultrasound examination and a β-hCG level above the discriminatory zone (β-hCG >1,000 mIU/mL) have a presumed ectopic pregnancy or embryonic demise and require an immediate obstetrics consultation. Those with an indeterminate ultrasound examination and a β-hCG level below the discriminatory zone (β-hCG < 1,000 mIU/mL) may have a small ectopic pregnancy, a very early intrauterine pregnancy, or embryonic demise. If hemodynamically stable and with an unremarkable physical examination, these patients can be discharged home without an obstetrics consult but they should be given

clear ectopic pregnancy discharge instructions and scheduled for close follow-up in 2–3 days for a repeat ultrasound examination and serum β-hCG level.[60]

Similar algorithms, incorporating emergency bedside transvaginal sonography, have been shown to improve the quality of patient care and to be more cost-effective than other approaches.[19,26,44,45]

QUANTITATIVE SERUM β-HCG AND DISCRIMINATORY ZONE

Serum β-hCG rises exponentially and predictably during the first 6–8 weeks of pregnancy and peaks at about 100,000 mIU/mL in a normal pregnancy. Serial β-hCG levels are useful for differentiating normal pregnancies from abnormal pregnancies. The serum level should increase by at least 66%, multiplying by 1.6, every 48 hours, and may even double between 36 and 48 hours. An abnormally slow rise in β-hCG indicates an abnormal pregnancy, either an ectopic pregnancy or embryonic demise. A normal or expected rise in β-hCG, however, does not necessarily exclude an ectopic.

Quantitative β-hCG measurements are currently standardized in relation to the International Reference Preparation (IRP). The reference standard for all β-hCG levels discussed in this chapter is the IRP. The standard method for reporting IRP β-hCG levels is in mIU/mL. Other reference standards are referred to in the literature, and it is important to distinguish between them since they are not equivalent. The Second International Standard is roughly equal to one half of the IRP and the Third International Standard is roughly equal to the IRP. In this chapter, β-hCG concentrations are reported in relation to the IRP, in mIU/mL.

A single serum β-hCG level is not as useful as serial levels because it does not differentiate a normal early intrauterine pregnancy from an ectopic pregnancy.[61] A common misconception is that a very low β-hCG level rules out ectopic pregnancy. Recent studies show that about 40% of ectopic pregnancies present with a β-hCG level less than 1,000 mIU/mL and about 20% present with a β-hCG level less than 500 mIU/mL.[19,62] In fact, patients who present with a β-hCG level less than 1,000 mIU/mL have a higher risk of ectopic pregnancy than other patients.[19,63,64] Furthermore, a low β-hCG level does not predict a benign course. Approximately 30–40% of ectopic pregnancies with a β-hCG level less than 1,000 mIU/mL will be ruptured at the time of diagnosis.[19,62,63]

The "discriminatory zone" is a concept that was developed to allow the complementary use of pelvic ultrasound and a single serum β-hCG level to help determine the likelihood of ectopic pregnancy. The discriminatory zone is the β-hCG level above which an intrauterine pregnancy should be consistently visualized by pelvic sonography. Patients with a β-hCG level above the discriminatory zone who do not have an intrauterine

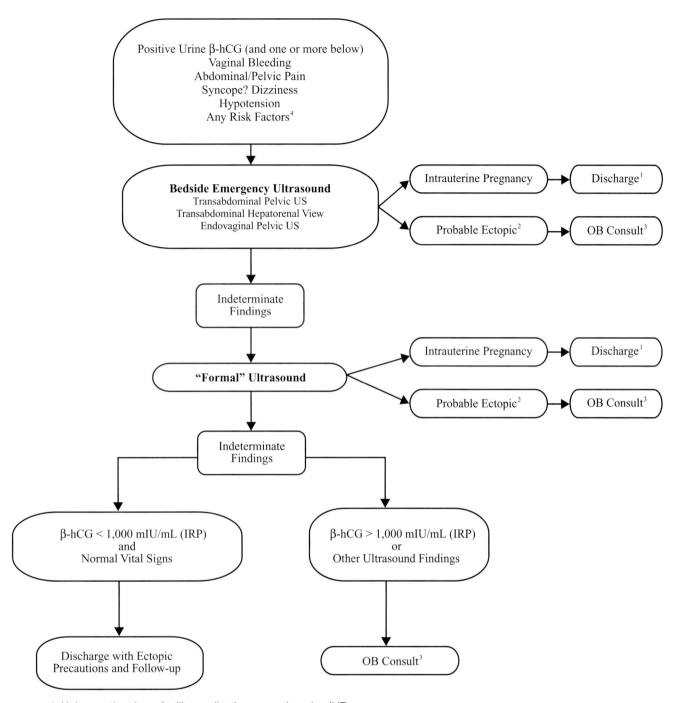

Figure 12-1. Ectopic pregnancy algorithm.

1. Unless patient is on fertility medications or undergoing IVF.
2. US criteria for probable ectopic pregnancy: extrauterine yolk sac or embryo, tubal ring, complex mass, or free fluid.
3. Surgery may be required if the patient has hypotension, a large ectopic sac (>4 cm), a large amount of pelvic free fluid, or hepatorenal free fluid.
4. Risk factors include: PID, tubal surgery or ligation, IUD's, prior ectopic, infertility, advanced age.

pregnancy on ultrasound examination are presumed to have an ectopic pregnancy until proven otherwise. This is the concept that led to the use of the discriminatory zone in previous ectopic pregnancy algorithms. Older algorithms used the β-hCG discriminatory zone to limit the use of pelvic sonography since it was thought that only patients with levels greater than 1,000 mIU/mL would benefit from an ultrasound examination.[47,52] When outdated algorithms are applied, however, a significant percentage of ectopic pregnancies will be missed.[47]

Recent studies clearly show the benefit of performing pelvic sonography on all patients with a possible ectopic pregnancy, regardless of their β-hCG level.[19,26,57,62,63,65] Although a normal pregnancy will not be visualized when the β-hCG level is low, many ectopic pregnancies are easily identified when the β-hCG level is less than 1,000 mIU/mL. In fact, transvaginal sonography can detect about half of ectopic pregnancies with β-hCG levels less than 1,000 mIU/mL.[19,60,62,63,66-68]

In this chapter's algorithm, the discriminatory zone serum β-hCG level is used to help guide the management of patients with indeterminate pelvic ultrasound examinations. The discriminatory zone β-hCG level of 1,000 mIU/mL was chosen because this is the level above which an intrauterine pregnancy can be consistently visualized by comprehensive transvaginal sonography.[30,53,62,69] Individual hospitals and clinics should choose their own discriminatory zone in collaboration with their obstetrics consultants and those who will perform their comprehensive ultrasound studies.

INDETERMINATE ULTRASOUND EXAMINATIONS

An "indeterminate" ultrasound examination in early pregnancy demonstrates no signs of intrauterine pregnancy or an ectopic pregnancy. One study attempted to subclassify patients with an indeterminate ultrasound examination based on their intrauterine findings.[70] Patients with a completely empty uterus and normal thin midline stripe had a 27% chance of an ectopic pregnancy and a 10% chance of an intrauterine pregnancy. Those with a nonspecific endometrial fluid collection had a 13% chance of an ectopic pregnancy and a 25% chance of an intrauterine pregnancy. Patients with intrauterine echogenic material had a 5% chance of ectopic pregnancy and none had an intrauterine pregnancy.

Approximately 15% of patients who are evaluated for a possible ectopic pregnancy have a β-hCG level greater than 1,000 mIU/mL and an indeterminate ultrasound.[19,70] Roughly 20% of these patients have an ectopic pregnancy.[58,59,70,71]

MANAGEMENT AND DISPOSITION

Patients diagnosed with an ectopic pregnancy have traditionally required surgery, which is usually a laparoscopic procedure. Although less successful compared to surgery,[72,73] medical therapy has become increasingly popular, with single-dose intramuscular methotrexate therapy being the most common regimen.[74] This regimen has a success rate ranging from 64 to 94%.[14,75-77] Clinical and sonographic criteria can help obstetricians decide which patients are candidates for medical ther-

apy instead of surgery. Higher serum β-hCG levels, especially above 10,000 mIU/mL, the presence of a yolk sac, and endometrial stripe thickness greater than 12 millimeters are associated with failure of methotrexate therapy.[40,75,77-81] Also, an adnexal mass greater than 4 cm in diameter, the presence of embryonic cardiac activity, a large amount of pelvic free fluid, and severe pain should be considered relative contraindications to medical management.[14,82] Clinical signs of shock along with free intraperitoneal fluid outside of the pelvis, such as in the hepatorenal space, are indications for surgery and contraindications to medical therapy.[6,14,30]

Patients with an unclear diagnosis of ectopic pregnancy need serial sonography and serial β-hCG levels. Obstetricians may be unwilling to initiate therapy in such patients for fear of interrupting an intrauterine pregnancy. Patients who have a β-hCG level greater than 1,000 mIU/mL and unclear or questionable sonographic findings should ideally be observed in the hospital. Repeat sonography and β-hCG level at 12–24 hours will make the diagnosis more clear. Those with no mass, free fluid, or other signs of ectopic pregnancy and a β-hCG level less than 1000 mIU/mL are safe to be discharged with early follow-up for repeat sonography and β-hCG level in 24–48 hours.[13,42,45,52]

The majority, up to 70% of all ectopic pregnancies, will spontaneously resolve without any treatment.[83,84] Therefore, expectant management may be reasonable in selected cases. Candidates for expectant management must have minimal symptoms, a small ectopic mass, and a low β-hCG level. Excellent clinical, sonographic, and laboratory follow-up must be ensured if expectant management is attempted.

▶ PREGNANCY LOSS

Diagnosing pregnancy loss is not as urgent as excluding an ectopic pregnancy. It is important, however, for emergency or acute care physicians to be aware of the sonographic features of pregnancy loss. It is helpful to know the risks of pregnancy loss related to specific ultrasound findings. This information will allow physicians to do a better job of counseling patients and making reasonable management plans for those with a threatened abortion.

Vaginal bleeding is a very common presentation and occurs in about 25% of all clinically apparent early pregnancies.[69,85,86] About 40–50% of these patients will eventually be diagnosed with pregnancy loss.[19,30,87-89] A threatened abortion is a significant source of anxiety for pregnant patients. Concern for the viability of the pregnancy is usually the primary reason for presentation. Pelvic sonography is very useful in patients with a threatened abortion because it provides an immediate diagnosis in about half of all patients with subsequent pregnancy loss.[87] Those without a definitive diagnosis require serial pelvic sonography and β-hCG levels.

Spontaneous abortion refers to expulsion of a nonviable pregnancy from the uterus before 20 weeks' gestational age. Microscopic identification of chorionic villi or obvious products of conception are required to make a definitive diagnosis. A completed spontaneous abortion can be diagnosed when all products of conception have been expelled. This usually occurs shortly after embryonic demise but may be delayed for days to weeks. Sonographically, an empty uterus should be seen after a completed spontaneous abortion. This finding indicates that the patient can be managed expectantly without curettage.[90–92]

Incomplete abortion is a nonspecific term used when a pregnancy has failed but all of the products of conception have not been expelled from the uterus. The terms embryonic demise, blighted ovum, and retained products of conception are all synonymous with incomplete abortion. Patients with an incomplete abortion may experience continued bleeding, infection, and anxiety, so it is important to make the diagnosis as soon as possible after embryonic demise has occurred. Patients with an incomplete abortion may require suction and curettage to remove retained products of conception.[92,93] Sonography is the only diagnostic modality that can directly assess intrauterine contents before a curettage is performed.

The term inevitable abortion implies that expulsion of uterine contents is in progress. Patients with an inevitable abortion have an open cervical os on physical examination. Pelvic sonography may show a separated gestational sac lying low within the uterus.[69] It is reasonable for physicians to use bedside pelvic sonography to help make initial management decisions in patients with a threatened abortion. However, it is prudent to confirm the diagnosis of embryonic demise with a comprehensive pelvic ultrasound prior to evacuation of intrauterine products. Also, it is important not to give patients false reassurance. Even when a completely normal intrauterine pregnancy is seen, they should be aware that there is still a chance of subsequent pregnancy loss.

Sonographic signs of a normal intrauterine pregnancy are reassuring and decrease the likelihood that a pregnancy will be lost.[23,87,94–96] In asymptomatic patients, those without threatened abortion, the rate of first trimester pregnancy loss decreases as the gestational age increases and as more normal structures can be identified with sonography. The rate of loss after only a gestational sac is identified is 11.5%. The rate decreases to 8.5% after a yolk sac is identified and to 7.2% after an embryo (2–5 mm) is identified. When a larger embryo is seen, the loss rate is even lower: 3.3% with a 6- to 10-mm embryo and 0.5% with an embryo greater than 10 mm. In addition, there is a 2% risk of pregnancy loss after the first trimester in pregnancies that previously appeared viable by ultrasound.[95]

As stated above, patients presenting with a first trimester threatened abortion have a 40–50% chance of pregnancy loss.[19,30,87–89] If embryonic cardiac activity can be seen, however, the rate of subsequent pregnancy loss is lower at 15–20%.[23,87] Also, as the gestational age and the size of the embryo increase, cardiac activity is more reassuring. Very early in the first trimester, when the embryo is less than 5 mm long, patients with a threatened abortion and cardiac activity have a loss rate of about 24%.[96] Those with a threatened abortion and cardiac activity near the end of the first trimester have a very low rate of pregnancy loss.[24]

▶ MULTIPLE PREGNANCY

Characterizing a multiple pregnancy (twins, triplets, etc.) is typically not in the realm of emergency medicine. However, timely pelvic sonography is indicated when menstrual dates do not correlate with the size of the patient's uterus. In such cases, sonographic pregnancy dating and evaluation for multiple pregnancy or molar pregnancy should be performed. Also, multiple pregnancies are often an incidental finding when sonography is performed for other indications, such as ruling out an ectopic pregnancy. Regardless of the indication for the sonogram, finding a multiple pregnancy is significant since the pregnancy will then be categorized as high risk and the patient will need close follow-up with an obstetrician.

Twin pregnancies are more likely to have fetal anomalies, premature delivery, and low birth weight. Early sonographic evaluation of a multiple pregnancy is important because differentiating dichorionic from monochorionic twins is much easier during the first trimester. Fraternal (dizygotic) twins are always dichorionic and diamnionic but identical (monozygotic) twins may be dichorionic, monochorionic, diamnionic, or monoamnionic, depending on when the zygote splits. Determining chorionicity is important since monochorionic twins have a mortality rate two to three times higher than dichorionic twins. Monochorionic twins share a single placenta, so they are at risk of twin transfusion syndrome, twin embolization syndrome, and acardiac parabiotic twin syndrome. In addition, determining amnionicity is important since monoamniotic twins are at risk for cord knots, wrapping of the cord around a cotwin, or locking of twins during delivery.

When imaging a multiple pregnancy, physicians should try to record quality images that clearly show the chorionicity and amnionicity. If chorionicity and amnionicity cannot be determined, then the patient should have a comprehensive ultrasound examination within several days. Also, it is important to inform patients that about 25% of twin pregnancies diagnosed during the first trimester will become singleton pregnancies by the second trimester.[97,98]

PELVIC MASSES

A pelvic mass may be noted in the first trimester of pregnancy during the physical examination or routine pelvic ultrasound examination. Physicians who perform bedside sonography need to have some basic knowledge of pelvic masses so they can make reasonable management plans. Most pelvic masses found in the first trimester are benign and require no treatment. They all, however, require close follow-up with serial sonography because some masses are at risk of hemorrhage, torsion, rupture, dystocia, and malignancy. Surgery will be required in about 1 per 1,300 pregnancies to exclude malignancy or to deal with one of the above complications. About 3% of all masses discovered during pregnancy have malignant potential.[99]

In general, patients with masses less than 5 cm in diameter in early pregnancy are treated conservatively and followed with serial sonography. Those presenting with peritoneal signs or severe pain may need immediate surgery because of rupture or torsion of a mass. Masses that are large, cause pain, or grow rapidly may require surgery. Those containing large solid areas, solid irregular areas, papillary excrescences, and irregular septae are at higher risk of malignancy. Also, the presence of ascites, in addition to a cystic pelvic mass, increases the chance of malignancy.[100] If surgery is required, then the optimal period is during the second trimester, when maternal and fetal risks are smallest.

The most common mass seen in early pregnancy is a corpus luteum cyst. The corpus luteum secretes progesterone to support the early pregnancy. A corpus luteum cyst is usually less than 5 cm in diameter and appears as a thin-walled unilocular structure surrounded by normal ovarian parenchyma. The appearance may vary substantially and the size may be greater than 10 cm. Hemorrhage into a corpus luteum cyst can cause the appearance of internal echogenic debris and septae.[30] Corpus luteum cysts usually regress spontaneously prior to 18 weeks of gestation.

A theca lutein cyst is an exaggerated corpus luteum and occurs in patients with very high β-hCG levels. Theca lutein cysts are commonly seen in patients with gestational trophoblastic disease and ovarian hyperstimulation from fertility medications. They appear as large multiseptated cystic masses. Theca lutein cysts usually resolve spontaneously once the abnormal stimulus is removed.

Uterine leiomyomas, or fibroids, are solid pelvic masses that are very common and may enlarge during pregnancy because of increased estrogen levels. They usually appear as relatively hypoechoic masses within the uterine wall and are sometimes confused with a simple muscular contraction of part of the uterine wall. Fibroids can have many different appearances, depending on the amount of smooth muscle and hyaline they contain and whether they have undergone hemorrhagic degeneration. They may contain calcifications or cystic areas of degeneration. Small fibroids tend to enlarge during the first and second trimesters but larger fibroids tend to enlarge only during the first trimester.[101] All fibroids tend to decrease in size during late pregnancy. Patients with multiple fibroids have a higher risk of bleeding, premature contractions, malpresentation, and retained products.[100] Large fibroids located in the lower part of the uterus during late pregnancy can obstruct labor and necessitate a cesarean section.

The most common complex mass seen in early pregnancy is a teratoma, or dermoid cyst.[99,100] These tumors arise from germ cells within the ovary and contain heterologous tissue like fat, skin, hair, and teeth. Sebaceous material within a dermoid can appear as a fluid–fluid level and teeth are very echogenic with distal shadowing. Dermoids are prone to torsion and rupture. Leaking of dermoid fluid can cause granulomatous peritonitis and sudden rupture can cause an acute abdomen.[100]

Mucinous and serous cystadenomas are ovarian epithelial neoplasms; they are the most common cystic tumors that enlarge during pregnancy.[102] Both of these tumors can appear as multicystic masses. Mucinous cystadenomas usually contain multiple thick internal septations and serous cystadenomas usually appear as unilocular structures. Again, pelvic masses that have internal septations and papillary excrescences are more likely to be malignant.[100]

Emergency sonologists typically do not attempt to characterize pelvic masses using sonography. However, these physicians will inevitably discover pelvic masses as incidental findings. When this occurs, most patients will need a comprehensive ultrasound examination and close follow-up with an obstetrician. Patients should be informed when a mass is found, and they should understand that bedside sonography is a screening tool and that further work-up is needed.

▶ ADNEXAL TORSION

Adnexal torsion is uncommon but about 20% of all cases occur during pregnancy.[103,104] Also, most cases occur during the first trimester.[99,105] Pregnant patients may be predisposed to torsion because of increased ovarian arterial flow and decreased ovarian venous flow, causing ovarian edema and enlargement. Torsion almost always occurs in the setting of an enlarged ovary or an ovarian mass; torsion rarely occurs in a normal size ovary.

Recently, ovarian hyperstimulation from fertility medications has been recognized as a risk factor for adnexal torsion because of ovarian enlargement.

Pain is the most common symptom of adnexal torsion. The diagnosis of torsion may be easily missed during pregnancy because pain may be attributed to the gravid uterus, the round ligament, or an adnexal mass. Further delay may occur because of the poor accuracy of Doppler ultrasound, which may miss up to 60% of cases of adnexal torsion.[106] Also, when a cystic ovarian mass is present, blood flow to the ovary may be difficult to visualize using pulse wave Doppler, even though torsion has not occurred.

Simple gray-scale pelvic sonography may be of some help in diagnosing adnexal torsion.[107,108] Finding a unilaterally enlarged ovary with multifollicular enlargement or any adnexal mass makes torsion more likely. Most patients with torsion have free fluid in the pelvic cul-de-sac, probably as a result of obstruction of venous and lymphatic drainage.[107,109] Finding normal-size ovaries and no pelvic free fluid makes the diagnosis of adnexal torsion highly unlikely.

Most diagnoses of adnexal torsion are delayed because of atypical clinical presentations and poor sensitivity of diagnostic modalities.[110] This may be especially detrimental in pregnancy causing maternal morbidity and fetal mortality. Therefore, it is prudent to have a high index of suspicion when there is no clear etiology for abdominal, pelvic, flank, or groin pain. Also, when the diagnosis is strongly suspected, negative diagnostic studies should not deter consultation and further evaluation.[111] Laparoscopy has been used during pregnancy as both a diagnostic and therapeutic modality.

▶ GESTATIONAL TROPHOBLASTIC DISEASE

Gestational trophoblastic disease (GTD) is a proliferative disease of the trophoblast. It occurs in about 1 per 1,700 pregnancies in the United States but is much more common in some other parts of the world.[112] GTD may occur with an intrauterine pregnancy or an ectopic pregnancy, or after a spontaneous abortion or full-term pregnancy. Most cases of GTD (80%) present as a benign hydatidiform mole. More malignant forms of GTD, invasive mole (12–15%), and choriocarcinoma (5–8%) may develop after a hydatidiform mole. Hydatidiform moles usually involve the entire placenta but a mole involving only part of the placenta can be associated with a live pregnancy.

Early in pregnancy, GTD may present with vaginal bleeding, uterine size that is too large for dates, persistent severe hyperemesis gravidarum, or early preeclampsia. Sometimes, the first clue to the diagnosis is a markedly elevated serum β-hCG level, usually greater than 100,000 mIU/mL. It has been shown that qualitative β-hCG urine assays may be falsely negative in the setting of GTD with markedly elevated serum β-hCG.[113] GTD is often discovered during routine pelvic sonography for pregnancy dating or other indications.

Ultrasound is the preferred modality for diagnosing GTD and both transabdominal and transvaginal sonography are usually diagnostic.[114] The classic finding, described as having a grape-like appearance, is an intrauterine echogenic mass containing diffuse small hypoechoic vesicles. In the first trimester, GTD may not be as obvious and can be confused with an incomplete abortion. In about half of cases of GTD, a theca lutein cyst is seen in the adnexa.

Early diagnosis and prompt treatment are the key to a favorable outcome. A hydatidiform mole usually resolves completely with evacuation of the uterus. Choriocarcinoma can metastasize to the lung, liver, and brain. It is very sensitive to chemotherapy but morbidity and mortality depend on the extent of metastases and early aggressive treatment.

▶ ANATOMIC CONSIDERATIONS

The uterus is located in the center of the true pelvis between the bladder anteriorly and the rectosigmoid colon posteriorly. The uterus is a thick-walled muscular structure that is about 6–7 cm long and about 3–4 cm in transverse and anterior–posterior diameters. It is shaped like an inverted pear and the uterine body is the widest portion. The cervix is the narrowest portion and is anchored to the posterior bladder by the parametrium. The cervix meets the vagina at the level of the bladder angle and protrudes into the anterior wall of the vagina. When the uterus is in the normal anteflexed position, the longitudinal axes of the uterus and vagina create an angle of about 90 degree. The fallopian tubes enter the body of the uterus laterally, in an area called the cornua. The fundus is the most superior portion of the uterine body above the cornua.

The uterine body and fundus lie inside the peritoneal cavity so intraperitoneal potential spaces exist both anterior and posterior to the uterus. The anterior cul-de-sac, between the bladder and uterus, is usually empty but can contain loops of bowel or free fluid. The posterior cul-de-sac, between the uterus and the rectosigmoid colon, is also known as the "pouch of Douglas" and it usually contains bowel loops. The posterior cul-de-sac is the most dependent intraperitoneal region when the patient is supine; therefore, it is the most common site for pooling of free pelvic fluid.

Lateral to the uterus, the peritoneal reflection forms the two layers of the broad ligament. The broad ligament extends from the uterus to the lateral pelvic sidewalls. The fallopian tubes extend laterally from the body of the uterus in the upper free margin of the broad ligament. The ovaries are attached to the posterior surface of the broad ligament. They are also attached to the body of the uterus by the ovarian ligaments and to the lateral pelvic sidewalls by the suspensory ligaments of the ovary. Normal ovaries are about 2 cm wide and 3 cm long. The ovaries are usually located in a depression on the lateral pelvic walls called the ovarian fossa. However, since the ligaments are not rigid structures, the ovaries may be seen in a number of other locations, especially in women who have previously been pregnant.

▶ GETTING STARTED

While working with a stable patient in need of early first trimester pregnancy evaluation in the emergency department, ultrasonography of the pelvis is most efficiently accomplished immediately following the pelvic examination. This allows for uninterrupted presence of a chaperone that may have assisted with the pelvic examination. Sonographic findings of very early pregnancy and nonpregnant patients can be difficult to distinguish. Therefore, it is often advisable to wait to perform the pelvic examination and subsequent ultrasound evaluation after pregnancy status has been confirmed, usually by urine qualitative β-hCG. Occasionally patients will communicate that they are pregnant when in reality they are not. Waiting for laboratory confirmation of pregnancy status helps avoid the misuse of time and resources looking for a pregnancy that does not exist. On the other hand, if the patient's last menstrual period suggests a sufficiently advanced gestational age, immediate transabdominal ultrasonography can confirm pregnancy and eliminate the need for urine or serum β-hCG.

During transabdominal pelvic ultrasound, the bladder should be full. A longitudinal image of the uterine midline should initially be obtained to determine the location of the body of the uterus, the cervix, and the pouch of Douglas. Significant axial pressure should be applied to produce the best images if this can be tolerated by the patient. After imaging the long axis of the uterus, the probe should be rotated transversely 90 degrees in its long axis to find the ovaries and scan the adnexa. The ovaries are located lateral to the widest portion of the uterus in the transverse plane next to the internal iliac artery and vein. The broad ligament should be followed laterally from the cornual region of the uterus to the ovary on each side.

During transvaginal ultrasonography, the bladder should be empty. The uterus and cervix should serve as anatomic landmarks and initially be visualized longitudinally. Because of anatomic variability, the midline of the uterus may not be in the same plane and consistent with the midline of the patient's body. Ovaries are most easily visualized in the transverse plane after following the broad ligament laterally from the cornual region of the uterus. Evaluation of specific structures such as the uterus, ovaries, or adnexal masses may be enhanced by placement of the probe tip directly over the area of interest. Just as the examiner's hand is used to palpate structures during a routine physical examination, gentle application of axial force on the probe may elicit tenderness and provide important diagnostic information.

▶ TECHNIQUE AND NORMAL ULTRASOUND FINDINGS

Transabdominal and transvaginal sonography are complementary imaging techniques and should be used together. In general, transvaginal imaging should not be performed without also performing a transabdominal scan, but this may not be practical in a busy clinical setting. Transvaginal imaging allows the probe tip to be placed very close to the organ of interest so that high-frequency probes can be used to generate high-resolution images. However, transvaginal probes have a limited field of view and objects more than a few centimeters away from the probe tip may not be seen. Transabdominal sonography uses lower frequency probes so the field of view is much larger and a better overview of pelvic structures can be obtained. The main drawback of transabdominal scanning is that the resolution is lower, so details of small pelvic structures are not as discernible, particularly ovaries and early pregnancies.

NORMAL NONPREGNANT PELVIS

Transabdominal Scanning

Transabdominal scanning is usually accomplished using a 3.5 5 MHz ultrasound probe. The bladder is used as a window in transabdominal scanning, so it should be full to obtain optimal images. In the emergency setting, transabdominal scanning may be performed without a full bladder because it is not practical to have patients drink fluid and wait for an hour while their bladders fill. Intravenous fluid administration will typically lead to rapid bladder filling. Quality images are usually obtained without bladder filling in thin women and those with an anteflexed uterus. Gentle pressure on the probe can also be used to produce good-quality transabdominal images without filling the bladder.

The best transabdominal view for evaluating the uterus and its contents is the standard midline sagittal view (Figure 12-2). To obtain this view, the probe is placed on the abdominal wall in the midline just above the pubic bone, with the probe indicator pointing

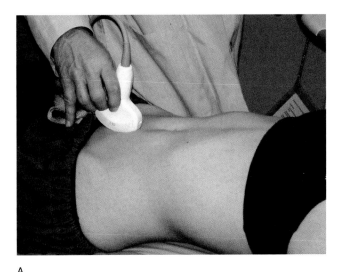

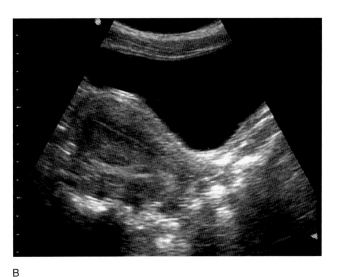

A   B

Figure 12-2. Transabdominal midline sagittal view of the normal pelvis. Probe position (A) and corresponding ultrasound image (B). (A, Courtesy of James Mateer, MD)

cephalad (Figure 12-3). By convention, the indicator on the probe should correlate with the left side of the monitor so that in sagittal images cephalad structures are on the left side. This view provides a longitudinal image of the uterus and the entire midline stripe should be visible. The cervix is seen just posterior to the bladder angle with the body of the uterus to the left of the angle and the vaginal stripe to the right. The ovaries can be seen by sliding the probe laterally, with the

probe indicator still pointing cephalad, and aiming the beam toward the contralateral adnexa, using the bladder as a window. Sometimes when the bladder is very full or a large pelvic mass is present, better images can be obtained by placing the probe directly over the adnexa.

In some cases it may be easier to visualize the ovaries and other adnexal structures with the standard transabdominal transverse view (Figure 12-4). This view

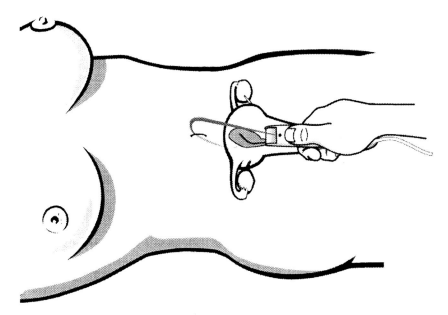

Figure 12-3. Scan plane for the transabdominal midline sagittal view. The marker dot is pointed cephalad.

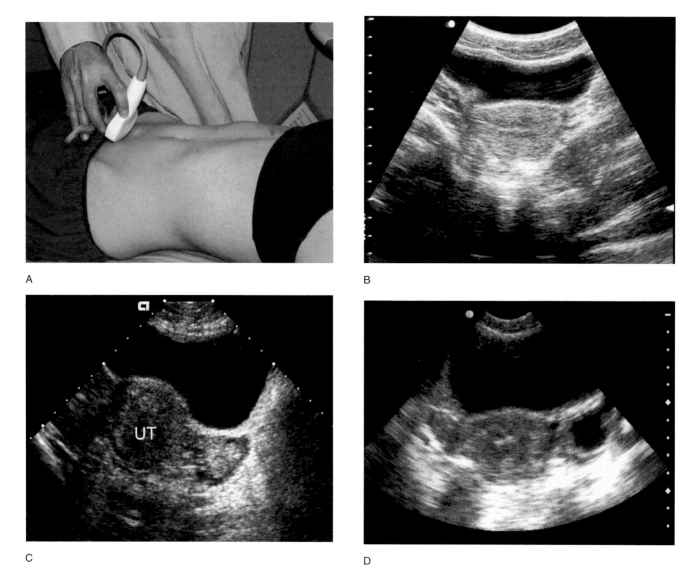

A

B

C

D

Figure 12-4. Transabdominal transverse ultrasound views of the normal pelvis. Probe position (A) and corresponding transverse midline ultrasound view (B). Transverse view of left adnexa and left ovary (C), (UT = Uterus) (courtesy of Waukesha Memorial Hospital), Transverse ultrasound view of the uterus and both ovaries (D). The right ovary is small and of similar echogenicity as the uterus, the left ovary is more prominent because of a contained cyst. (A, D, Courtesy of James Mateer, MD)

is obtained by placing the probe in the midline of the abdominal wall just above the pubic bone, with the probe indicator pointing to the patient's right side. This view provides a transverse image of the uterus and allows the midline of the uterus and the adjacent adnexa to be seen in the same image if the anatomy cooperates. In transverse images, anatomic structures have the same orientation as on a CT scan: right-sided structures are on the left side of the monitor and left-sided structures are on the right. To examine the entire pelvis in transverse planes, the probe should be kept in the midline suprapubic region with the probe indicator pointed to the patient's right and the beam should be aimed cau-

dad and cephalad (Figure 12-5). This motion will allow the uterus to be viewed in transverse sections from the cervix to the fundus respectively.

The ovaries are most commonly found between the body of the uterus and the pelvic sidewall. In their normal location, the ovaries are bound posteriorly by the internal iliac artery and superiorly by the external iliac vein. These structures can be identified and used to help locate the ovaries. Normal ovaries appear as small discrete hypoechoic structures. Individual ovarian follicles are usually not visible with transabdominal imaging. Normal ovaries are not always seen with transabdominal sonography because they are relatively small and may be

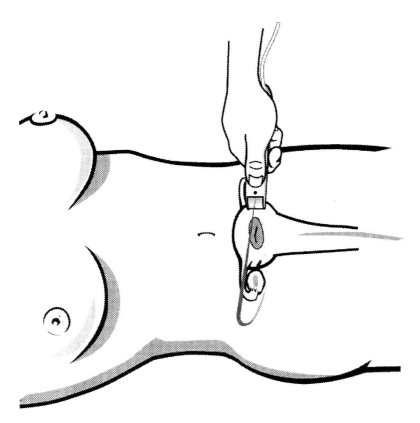

Figure 12-5. Scan plane for the transabdominal transverse view. The marker dot is pointed toward the patient's right side.

camouflaged by bowel or other surrounding structures with similar echogenicity. However, adnexal masses are frequently larger and very easy to identify with transabdominal imaging (Figure 12-4D).

Transvaginal Sonography

Transvaginal scanning is different from other ultrasound techniques because the ultrasound probe is placed inside the vagina and very close to the organs of interest. Transvaginal sonography is accomplished using a specialized probe with a 5–7.5 MHz transducer. The probe has an indicator, similar to other ultrasound probes, which should correlate to the left side of the monitor screen. The sound beams may emanate straight out from the tip of the probe (end-fire) or at an angle from the tip of the probe (offset). End-fire probes are more versatile and make imaging planes easier to understand. This discussion of scanning planes will assume that an end-fire probe is being used.

Before the transvaginal probe is used, it must be thoroughly cleansed and covered by a rubber or vinyl sheath. Conducting gel should be placed inside the sheath before the probe is covered for appropriate sound transmission. Most sonologists use specially made latex condoms as probe covers while some prefer to use vinyl gloves as probe covers.[115] Water-based lubricant, not

conducting gel, should be used to lubricate the outside of the sheath before insertion into the vagina. Ultrasound conducting gel may be irritating to the vaginal mucosa. Patients should empty their bladder before transvaginal scanning is performed. A full bladder will straighten the angle between the uterus and vagina and move the body of the uterus away from the probe. Patient positioning is important in obtaining good transvaginal scans. The operator must be able to aim the probe anterior enough to see the fundus of an anteverted uterus. Scanning is best accomplished while the patient is in lithotomy stirrups or by elevating her pelvis on a pillow while she is in a frog-leg position. Many clinicians prefer to use lithotomy stirrups and perform transvaginal sonography as part of their pelvic examination, after the speculum and bimanual examinations.

Before inserting the transvaginal probe, the procedure should be explained to the patient. It is usually best to explain that transvaginal sonography is similar to the bimanual pelvic examination but visual rather than tactile information is obtained. Transvaginal sonography should not be painful and is usually very well tolerated by patients. Anxious patients may be given the option of inserting the probe into the vagina themselves.

The probe is initially inserted with the probe indicator pointed toward the ceiling (Figures 12-6 and 12-7). The uterus is easily recognized upon insertion of the

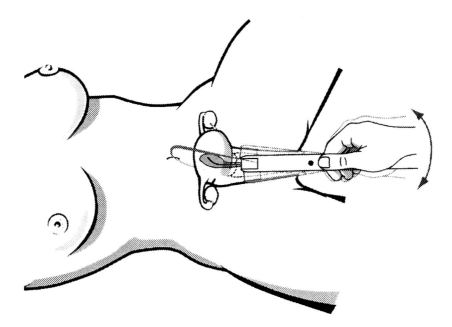

Figure 12-6. Scan plane for the transvaginal sagital view (frontal perspective). The marker dot is pointed toward the ceiling.

probe. This is the standard transvaginal sagittal view; it produces a longitudinal image of the uterus similar to the transabdominal sagittal view but rotated 90 degree counterclockwise (Figure 12-8). The entire uterine midline stripe should be seen in this view. If the uterus is not seen immediately, then it may be extremely anteverted and the probe should be aimed upward toward the anterior abdominal wall, keeping the indicator pointed toward the ceiling. Lateral movement of the probe can be used to scan from side to side through the entire pelvis (Figure 12-6). The uterus appears as a relatively hypoechoic structure with thick walls and a well-defined border. The endometrial midline stripe is thin during the proliferative phase and thick during the secretory phase of the menstrual cycle (Figures 12-9 and 12-10). The cervix can be seen by pulling the probe back a few centimeters and aiming the probe tip downward toward the patient's back (Figure 12-11). In this view, the posterior cul-de-sac should be inspected for any evidence of free fluid.

After the uterus is identified, the ovaries can be found by their position relative to the uterus. They are usually found just lateral and posterior to the body of the uterus, between the uterus and the lateral pelvic wall. The sonographic appearance of the ovaries is distinct. They are relatively hypoechoic structures containing multiple anechoic follicles (Figures 12-12, 12-13, and 12-14). To find the ovaries in sagittal oblique planes, the

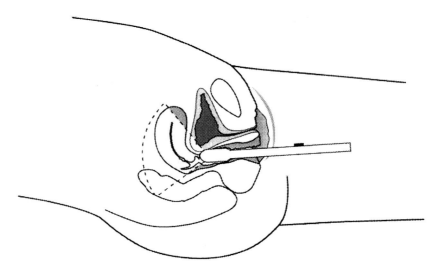

Figure 12-7. Scan plane for the transvaginal sagital view (saggital perspective). The marker dot is pointed toward the ceiling.

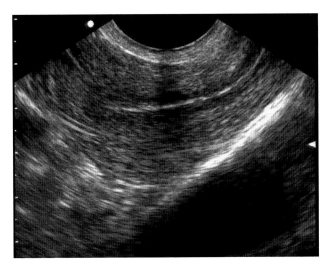

Figure 12-8. Transvaginal midline sagittal ultrasound view of the normal pelvis. The thin endometrial stripe represents the early proliferative phase.

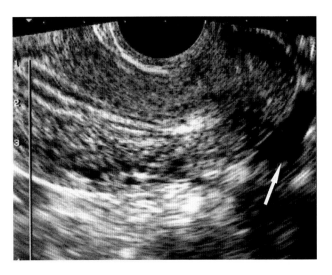

Figure 12-11. Transvaginal sagittal view of the uterine body and cervix. A small (physiologic) fluid collection is present in the posterior cul-de-sac (arrow).

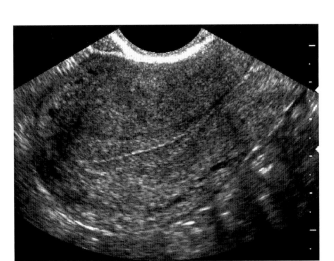

Figure 12-9. Transvaginal midline sagittal ultrasound of the uterus during the late proliferative menstrual phase. The endometrial stripe is slightly thickened, but not very echogenic.

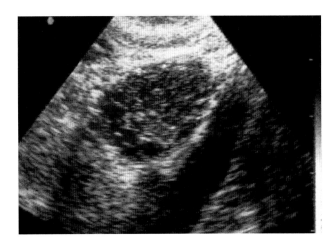

Figure 12-12. Transvaginal view of a normal left ovary. The ovary is recognized by the oval shape, peripheral follicles and echogenicity similar to the myometrium of the uterus. This ovary is adjacent to the iliac vein. (contributed by James Mateer, MD)

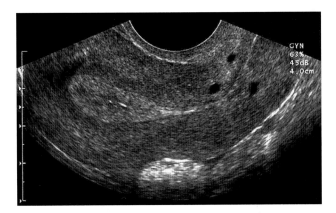

Figure 12-10. Transvaginal midline sagittal ultrasound of the uterus during the secretory menstrual phase. The endometrium is thickened and echogenic. Three nabothian cysts are seen in the cervix.

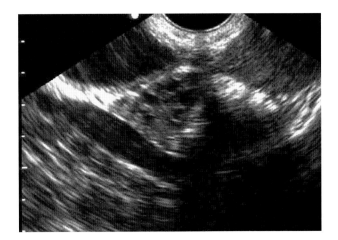

Figure 12-13. Transvaginal view of a normal ovary. This ovary (center of the image) is surrounded by the bladder (above-left), iliac vein (below), intestine with gas and shadows (below-right), and the uterus (above-right).

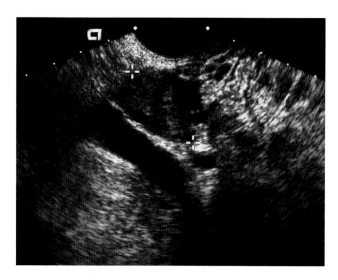

Figure 12-14. Transvaginal ultrasound of the normal right ovary in long axis. The external iliac vein is below and to the left of the ovary on the image while a cross section of the internal iliac artery (or vein) is directly below and to the right. (Contributed by James Mateer, MD, Waukesha Memorial Hospital)

probe is aimed laterally, with the probe indicator still toward the ceiling (Figure 12-6). The internal iliac artery and vein can often be identified and used as a guide because the normal position of the ovary is adjacent to these structures. Sometimes the ovaries cannot be identified with transvaginal sonography.[116]

The standard transvaginal coronal view may be better for surveying the entire pelvis. This view is obtained by turning the probe indicator toward the patient's right side (Figures 12-15 and 12-16). The coronal view gives a transverse image of the uterus and allows the uterus and ovaries to be seen in the same plane. The entire pelvis can be explored with oblique coronal planes by aiming the probe up toward the anterior abdominal wall and down toward the patient's back, keeping the probe indicator pointing toward the patient's right side (Figure 12-17).

Transvaginal sonography is a dynamic imaging technique. To visualize structures, they need to be very close to the tip of the probe. When structures are not readily visualized, operators should use their free hand to palpate the patient's anterior abdominal wall, similar to performing a bimanual pelvic examination.[30,69,115] Pressure on the anterior abdominal wall will often bring an ovary or a mass into the field of view. Also, the abdominal hand and the transvaginal probe can be used together to manipulate pelvic contents and observe how the organs move in relation to one another. An ovary may be easier to identify if it is seen as a discrete structure moving independently from adjacent loops of bowel. Also, structures that appear as complex masses may be composed of multiple smaller structures that move independently of each other. Holding the transvaginal probe very still and observing for bowel peristalsis is a good method for differentiating bowel from other pelvic structures. Finally, the tip of the transvaginal probe can be used to try to localize pelvic pain. This may help the physician narrow the differential diagnosis when a mass or other abnormality is visualized.

Although several standard imaging planes have been described, the pelvis can often be scanned without

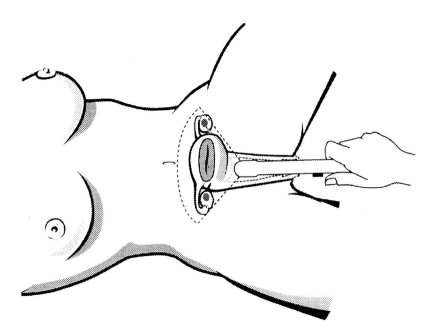

Figure 12-15. Scan plane for the transvaginal coronal view (frontal perspective). The marker dot is pointed toward the patient's right side.

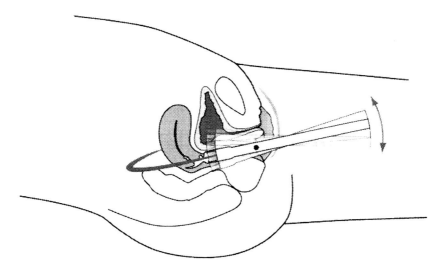

Figure 12-16. Scan plane for the transvaginal coronal view (saggital perspective). The marker dot is pointed toward the patient's right side.

concern for specific planes. Once an organ or a mass is identified, the probe can be turned in any direction that helps the operator obtain better images. Also, as long as the entire pelvis is imaged in a systematic organized manner, the use of specific planes is probably not crucial.[117]

NORMAL EARLY PREGNANCY

Both transvaginal and transabdominal sonography can be used to detect an early intrauterine pregnancy. Transvaginal ultrasound can identify an intrauterine pregnancy at about 5 weeks' gestational age (3 weeks postconception), about 7–10 days earlier than transabdominal ultrasound. The convention when referring to

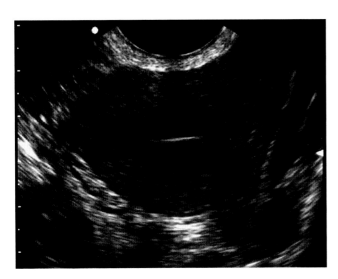

Figure 12-17. Transvaginal coronal ultrasound view of the normal pelvis.

the age of a pregnancy is gestational age, which is the date from conception plus 2 weeks. An approximate correlation can be made between gestational age, β-hCG level, and pelvic ultrasound findings (Table 12-1).[4,30,53,69,118–124]

Transvaginal sonography is now the standard modality for evaluating early pregnancy. The following descriptions pertain to transvaginal sonography, except where specifically noted. The transvaginal technique is referred to as "endovaginal" sonography by some authors. The first sonographic sign of early pregnancy, the intradecidual sign, can be seen at 4–5 weeks (Figure 12-18). The intradecidual sign is a small sac, only a few millimeters in diameter, which is completely embedded within the endometrium on one side of the uterine midline, not deforming the midline stripe.[30,124,125] There is a focal echogenic thickening of endometrium surrounding the sac. The intradecidual sign can be seen only by using a high-resolution technique (5 MHz or higher) and is not an accurate indicator of intrauterine pregnancy.[125]

A gestational sac can be clearly identified at about 5 weeks. With transvaginal sonography, a gestational sac can be seen in most patients with β-hCG levels of 1,000–2,000 mIU/mL and in all patients with levels above 2,000 mIU/mL.[123] A gestational sac is characterized by a sonolucent center (chorionic sac) surrounded by a thick symmetric echogenic ring, known as the chorionic rim. This finding is seen in most intrauterine pregnancies but can also be seen surrounding a pseudogestational sac associated with an ectopic pregnancy.[69] Doppler ultrasound can be used to measure peritrophoblastic flow in order to distinguish a true gestational sac from a pseudogestational sac.[126] However, since this is outside the realm of bedside emergency sonography, identification of a simple gestational sac should not be used as definitive evidence of an intrauterine pregnancy.

► TABLE 12-1. **CORRELATION OF GESTATIONAL AGE, β-HCG LEVEL, AND PELVIC ULTRASOUND FINDINGS**

Gestational Age	β-hCG[*,†,‡] (mIU/mL)	Transvaginal U.S. Findings	Transabdominal U.S. Findings
4–5 weeks	<1000	Intradecidual sac	N/A
5 weeks	1,000–2,000	Gestational sac (±DDS)	N/A
5–6 weeks	>2,000	Yolk sac (±embryo)	Gestational sac (±DDS)
6 weeks	10,000–20,000	Embryo with cardiac activity	Yolk sac (±embryo)
7 weeks	>20,000	Embryonic torso/head	Embryo with cardiac activity

*Significant individual variation in β-hCG levels at a given gestational age may occur.
†In multiple pregnancy (twins, triplets, etc.), β-hCG levels will be much higher at a given gestational age.
‡β-hCG reference standard is the International Reference Preparation (IRP).

Many authors consider a clear double decidual sign as the first definitive evidence of an intrauterine pregnancy.[30,69,127] The double decidual sign is two concentric echogenic rings surrounding a gestational sac (Figure 12-19). The inner ring is the same structure as the chorionic ring and is called the decidua capsularis.

The outer ring is called the decidua vera, derived from the stimulated endometrium of the uterus, while the thin hypoechoic layer between them is the endometrial canal.[30,127,128] A gestational sac with a vague or an absent double decidual sign is not diagnostic of an intrauterine pregnancy and may be a pseudogestational sac. If two

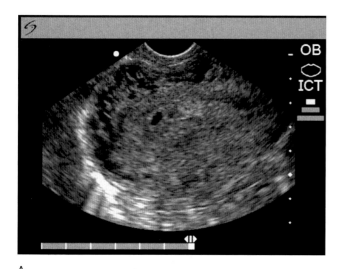

A

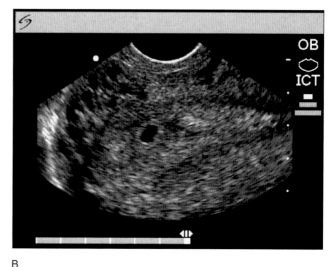

B

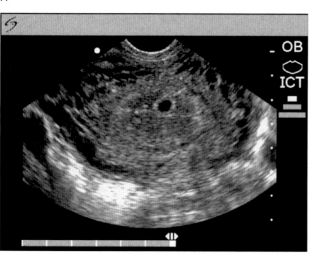

C

Figure 12-18. Intradecidual sign. Longitudinal transvaginal view of the uterus at 7.5 MHz (a). Magnified long-axis view of the endometrium shows a 5-mm gestational sac within a slightly thickened endometrium (b). Transverse view of the same patient demonstrates the location within the upper portion of the endometrium and the lack of deformation of the midline stripe (c). All views show a prominent arcuate venous plexus (a variant of normal) within the myometrium of the uterus for this patient. (Courtesy of James Mateer, MD)

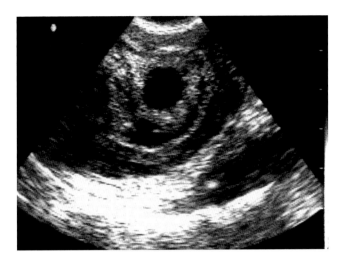

Figure 12-19. Double decidual sign surrounding an intrauterine gestational sac. Normal early pregnancy. Transvaginal image. This sign is often subtle and usually only noticeable along one side of the gestational sac but is very distinct in this example. (Courtesy of James Mateer, MD)

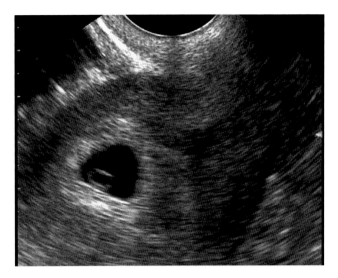

Figure 12-20. Yolk sac within an intrauterine gestational sac. Normal early pregnancy. Transvaginal image.

clear rings are seen, an intrauterine pregnancy is very likely. Unfortunately, the double decidual sign is present in only about half of all intrauterine pregnancies and is not 100% accurate.[129]

The yolk sac is the first structure that can be seen inside the gestational sac (Figure 12-20). Some authors consider the yolk sac the first definitive evidence of intrauterine pregnancy.[53,124] It is probably prudent for inexperienced sonologists to visualize the yolk sac before

making a diagnosis of an intrauterine pregnancy, avoiding misinterpretation of more subtle findings like the double decidual sign. The yolk sac is a symmetric circular echogenic structure at the edge of the gestational sac. The yolk sac has a role in the transfer of nutrients to the embryo during the first trimester and early hematopoiesis takes place there. The yolk sac can first be seen by transvaginal sonography at about 5–6 weeks and then shrinks and disappears by about 12 weeks.[130]

The embryo appears as a thickening or small mass that is seen at the margin of the yolk sac between 5 and 6 weeks Figure 12-21A). The normal embryo will grow

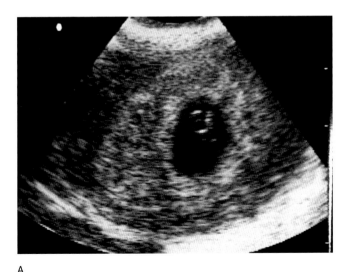

A

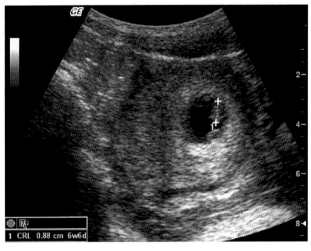

B

Figure 12-21. Small embryo and yolk sac within an intrauterine gestational sac (A). The 5-mm embryo is positioned along the right side of the yolk sac in this image and cardiac pulsations were visible during real-time sonography. Transvaginal image at 7.5 MHz (courtesy of James Mateer, MD). Embryonic pole is separated from the yolk sac and measures 6 weeks + 6 days via crown rump length (B). Transabdominal longitudinal view with empty bladder. (Courtesy of Hennepin County Medical Center)

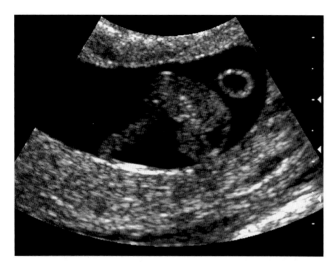

Figure 12-22. Intrauterine embryo and yolk sac. Normal pregnancy at 8 weeks. Transvaginal image.

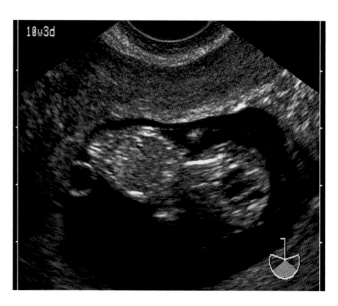

Figure 12-23. Intrauterine fetus and yolk sac with amnion surrounding the embryo. Normal pregnancy at 10 weeks. Transvaginal image.

rapidly, about 1 mm per day. The embryo can first be seen when it is only 2–3 mm and cardiac activity may not be detectable initially. By 6 weeks, the embryo is a distinct structure separate from the yolk sac (Figure 12-21B). Also, the tiny vitelline duct, which connects the yolk sac to the base of the cord, can sometimes be seen between the yolk sac and the embryo.

Cardiac activity should be detected within the embryo at about 6 weeks. Any embryo measuring greater than 5 mm should have cardiac activity when transvaginal sonography is used. At 7 weeks, the embryo will be about 12 mm and the head of the embryo will be clearly distinguished. At this age, the embryo's head contains a single large cerebral ventricle and has an appearance similar to the yolk sac.[69] At 8 weeks, the head of the embryo is about the same size as the yolk sac and limb buds begin to appear (Figure 12-22). Also, the physiologic midgut herniation can be visualized as an echogenic mass anterior to the trunk of the embryo. The bowel becomes intra-abdominal and the hernia disappears by 12 weeks. At 8 weeks and beyond, a thin echogenic line, the amnionic sac, may be seen surrounding the embryo.

At 10 weeks, organogenesis is complete and the embryo is now referred to as a fetus (Figure 12-23). Between 10 weeks and the end of the first trimester, the contours of the fetus become much more obvious. The fingers and toes can be identified and counted. Limb movements can be observed and bones and joints can be recognized. In the head, the falx cerebri becomes very distinct and the prominent choroid plexus can be seen in each of the lateral ventricles. The kidneys and bladder can be evaluated at 12 weeks. The heart and the stomach can also be identified inside the trunk and

a four-chamber heart can be recognized by the end of the first trimester. Finally, the face and palate can be easily recognized late in the first trimester.

Routine screening for fetal abnormalities is not typically performed during the first trimester; the optimal time for this is at 18–20 weeks. However, some obvious abnormalities may be identified and it is important to know which structures are usually seen during the first trimester. There is some utility to evaluating nuchal thickness with transvaginal sonography, between 11 and 14 weeks, as a screening test for exomphalos and trisomies 18 and 13, but this is outside the realm of emergency bedside sonography.

PREGNANCY DATING

Measurements of both the gestational sac and the embryo are accurate in the first trimester. Tables and formulas are available for calculating the gestational age using these measurements.[4,131] However, modern ultrasound software automatically calculates gestational age when calipers are placed on the structures of interest and appropriate presets are used.

The earliest measurement that can be used for pregnancy dating is mean sac diameter (MSD) of the gestational sac. MSD is the average of three orthogonal measurements of the gestational sac: (length + width + depth)/3. Pregnancy dating using MSD is only useful at 5–6 weeks, when the gestational sac is present but an embryo is not yet seen.

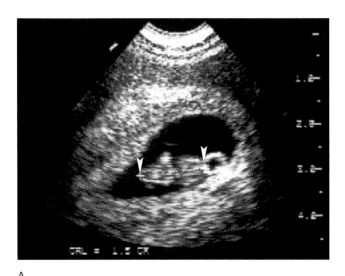

A

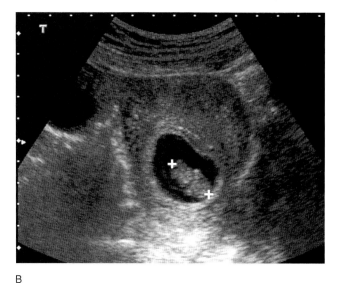

B

Figure 12-24. Crown rump length. Transvaginal ultrasound that shows proper placement of cursors for CRL measurement (A). Measure the maximal embryo length, excluding the yolk sac (Courtesy of James Mateer, MD). Transabdominal transverse ultrasound of a 9-week IUP (B). (Courtesy of Hennepin County Medical Center)

When an embryo is visible, at about 6 weeks, measurement of the crown-rump length (CRL) of the embryo should be used to date the pregnancy.[53] When measuring CRL, it is important to measure the maximal embryo length, excluding the yolk sac (Figure 12-24). Errors can occur when the calipers are not carefully placed at the margins of the embryo. Also, the embryo can flex and extend slightly, changing the measurement. Nevertheless, gestational age determination by CRL is accurate to within 5–7 days.[30]

Measurement of the biparietal diameter (BPD) of the fetal skull is used for pregnancy dating at the end of the first trimester and during the second trimester. The BPD is a transverse measurement of the diameter of the skull at the level of the thalamus. The calipers should be positioned from the leading edge of the skull (outer table) on the near side to the leading edge of the skull (inner table) on the far side (Figure 12-25). Errors can be made by measuring the wrong part of the skull or if the image plane is not a true transaxial section through the fetal head. Pregnancy dating by BPD is also very accurate, especially prior to 20 weeks.[69]

MULTIPLE PREGNANCY

Documentation of the chorionicity and amnionicity of a multiple pregnancy is important early in the pregnancy because it may be hard to determine later in pregnancy. There are several sonographic criteria that can be used

to determine chorionicity and amnionicity in the first trimester. Two clear gestational (chorionic) sacs may be seen as early as 6 weeks; this is good evidence of dichorionic twins (Figure 12-26). Later in the first trimester, dichorionicity can be established by finding a thick septum separating the two chorionic sacs (Figure 12-27). If the septum separating the two pregnancies is thin, then it may be difficult to determine whether it is the wall of a chorionic sac or an amnionic membrane. When the

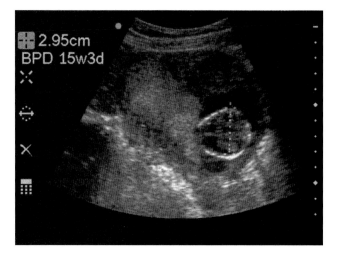

Figure 12-25. Biparietal diameter. Endovaginal ultrasound shows correct imaging plane of the head and cursor placement for accuracy. (Courtesy of James Mateer, MD)

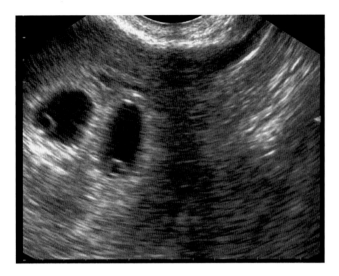

Figure 12-26. Dichorionic twins. Two chorionic sacs and two yolk sacs are clearly seen. Transvaginal image.

septum is thin, identification of a chorionic peak can confirm a dichorionic twin pregnancy. A chorionic peak is a triangular projection of tissue, of the same echogenicity as the placenta, emanating from the placenta and tapering to a point in the intertwin membrane.[30]

The amnionicity of a monochorionic pregnancy can also be determined by first trimester sonography. Counting the number of yolk sacs is the easiest way to determine amnionicity; if there are two yolk sacs, then there must be two amnions.[69] After about 8 weeks, amnionic membranes should be visible and diamnionic pregnancies should have a separate amnion surrounding each twin.

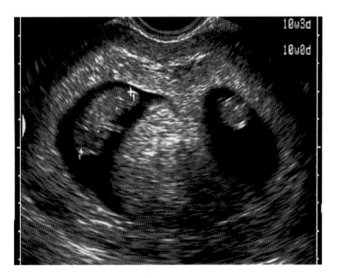

Figure 12-27. Dichorionic twins. Calipers mark the crown-rump length of one of the embryos. Gestational age is 10 weeks 0 days. Transvaginal image.

► COMMON AND EMERGENT ABNORMALITIES

ECTOPIC PREGNANCY

Definite Ectopic Pregnancy

A live extrauterine embryo with cardiac activity can be seen with transvaginal sonography in up to 15–20% of ectopic pregnancies (Figure 12-28).[54,58] An extrauterine gestational sac containing an embryo or yolk sac is also diagnostic and is seen in a significant percentage of ectopic pregnancies (Figure 12-29).[58]

Nonspecific Signs of Ectopic Pregnancy: Free Fluid, Tubal Ring, and Complex Mass

There are several nonspecific sonographic findings that are not diagnostic but are highly suggestive of an ectopic pregnancy in pregnant patients with an empty uterus (Table 12-2).[26,54,56–59,132–134] Some of these findings are subtle and may be easily missed, especially if transvaginal sonography is not available or an inexperienced sonologist performs the scan. Therefore, emergency physicians should obtain a comprehensive ultrasound examination if no intrauterine pregnancy or ectopic pregnancy is identified with emergency bedside sonography.

Free Pelvic or Intraperitoneal Fluid

Free fluid in the posterior pelvic cul-de-sac or in other intraperitoneal sites is suggestive of ectopic pregnancy (Figure 12-30).[56,59,134,135] Transvaginal sonography is very sensitive for detecting free fluid in the posterior

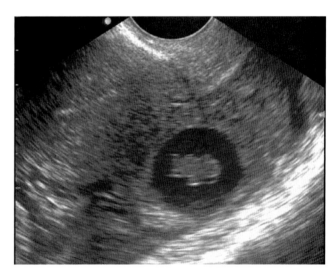

Figure 12-28. Ectopic pregnancy. Living embryo in the adnexa and empty uterus (endometrial echo is visible in the left upper portion of the image). Embryonic cardiac activity was present on real-time imaging. Transvaginal image.

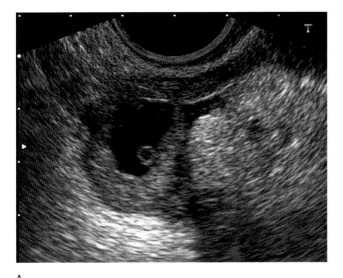
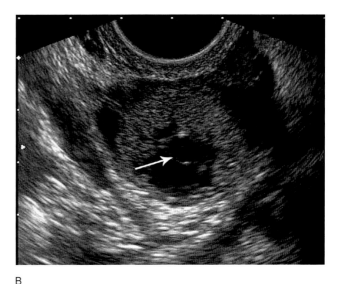

A   B

Figure 12-29. Ectopic pregnancy. Extrauterine gestational sac with a thick echogenic ring and a yolk sac within (A). A small stripe of free fluid is present as well as bowel gas artifact surrounding the structure. Transvaginal image. A thick concentric echogenic ring in the adnexa is surrounded by free fluid (B). A subtle yolk sac is contained within the structure (arrow). (Courtesy of Hennepin County Medical Center)

cul-de-sac.[30] Only about one third of ectopic pregnancies have no free fluid in the cul-de-sac.[136] Also, free fluid is the only abnormal sonographic finding in about 15% of ectopic pregnancies.[134] The greater the volume of free intraperitoneal fluid, the greater the likelihood of ectopic pregnancy (Figures 12-31 and 12-32).[69,135] In fact, patients with a moderate to large amount of free pelvic fluid have about an 86% chance and those with hepatorenal free fluid have a nearly 100% chance of having an ectopic pregnancy.[59] Although a large amount of fluid predicts ectopic pregnancy, it is not a reliable indicator of tubal rupture. Only about 60% of those with a large amount of free fluid have a ruptured tube.[56,137] Free fluid may be due to leaking of blood from the end of the fallopian tube, which can occur slowly.

Echogenic fluid is more likely to represent blood, and this also increases the chances of an ectopic pregnancy (Figure 12-30). If bleeding is brisk, clots may be seen in the pelvic cul-de-sac instead of fluid. Although

a small amount of hypoechoic free pelvic fluid may be normal, it must be considered suspicious in the setting of a pregnant patient with an empty uterus.[56,57,59,134] The definition of "small amount" is fluid that is confined to the cul-de-sac and covering less than one third of the inferior posterior uterus. As stated, anything more than a small amount is almost always associated with an ectopic pregnancy.[56,58,59]

Abdominal sonography of the hepatorenal space (Morison's pouch) should be performed on every patient

▶ **TABLE 12-2. NONSPECIFIC SONOGRAPHIC SIGNS OF ECTOPIC PREGNANCY**

Sonographic Findings	Likelihood of Ectopic Pregnancy (%)
Any free pelvic fluid	52
Complex pelvic mass	75
Moderate or large free pelvic fluid	86
Tubal ring	>95
Mass and free fluid	97
Hepatorenal free fluid	~100

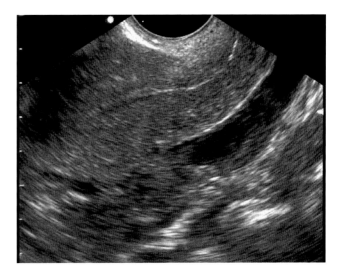

Figure 12-30. Ectopic pregnancy. Empty uterus and free fluid in the posterior cul-de-sac. Transvaginal sagittal image.

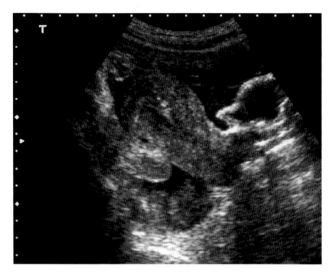

Figure 12-31. Ectopic pregnancy. Transabdominal longitudinal view shows an empty uterus. Complex fluid from liquid and clotted blood is present in both the anterior and posterior cul-de-sac areas. The bladder is collapsed around a Foley catheter balloon. (Courtesy of Hennepin County Medical Center)

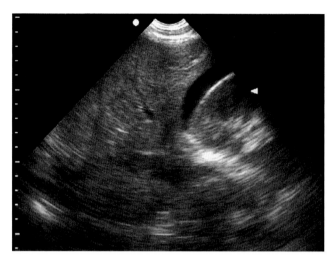

Figure 12-33. Ectopic pregnancy. Free fluid in the hepatorenal space. Transabdominal image.

Tubal Ring

A tubal ring is nearly diagnostic of ectopic pregnancy.[54,58,132,134] A tubal ring is a concentric hyperechoic structure found in the adnexa (Figures 12-34, 12-35, and 12-36). It is created by the trophoblast of the ectopic pregnancy surrounding the chorionic sac and is the equivalent of a gestational sac.[30] A tubal ring, in general, has a different sonographic appearance than a corpus luteum or other ovarian cysts because it has a relatively thick and brightly echogenic, round, symmetric wall. Ovarian cysts have walls of varying thickness and are surrounded by normal ovarian follicles. With transvaginal sonography, it may be possible to identify a tubal ring in more than 60% of ectopic pregnancies.[54,58]

with a possible ectopic pregnancy.[30,69] Free fluid in the hepatorenal space (Figure 12-33), or elsewhere outside the pelvis, is evidence of a large amount of intraperitoneal fluid.[138] In a pregnant woman with an empty uterus, this must be considered bleeding secondary to an ectopic pregnancy. Finding free fluid in the hepatorenal space with emergency bedside sonography reduces the time to diagnosis and treatment of ectopic pregnancy.[6] A finding of hepatorenal free fluid "should give the surgeon a greater sense of urgency."[30]

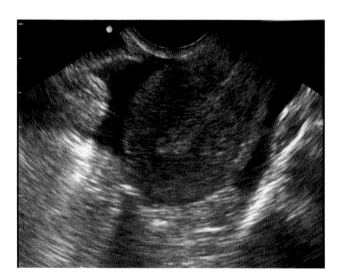

Figure 12-32. Ectopic pregnancy. Free fluid surrounding an empty uterus. Transvaginal image.

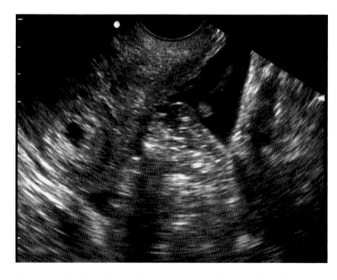

Figure 12-34. Ectopic pregnancy. Tubal ring (2 cm). Free pelvic fluid with floating bowel. Transvaginal image.

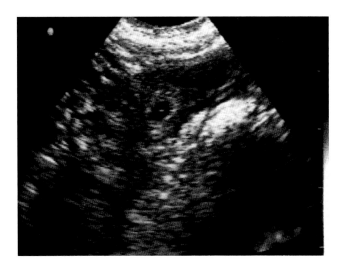

Figure 12-35. Tubal ring. Transvaginal view of the right adnexa shows a tiny (7 mm) brightly echogenic ring-like structure. This was determined to be a very early ectopic pregnancy. (Courtesy of James Mateer, MD)

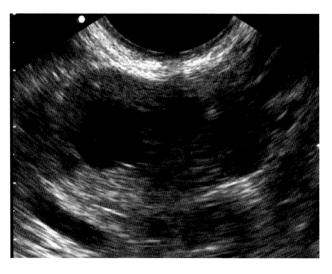

Figure 12-37. Ectopic pregnancy. Complex right adnexal mass located above the iliac vein on the image. Transvaginal technique.

When a tubal ring is seen, the likelihood of ectopic pregnancy is greater than 95%.[58]

Complex Mass

The most common sonographic finding in ectopic pregnancy is a complex adnexal mass (Figures 12-37 and 12-38).[52] A complex adnexal mass may represent a tubal hematoma, ectopic trophoblastic tissue, or distorted contents of an ectopic gestational sac.[54,58,59,69,133,134] A complex mass contains a mixture of cystic and solid components. This is a sensitive sonographic sign of ectopic

pregnancy. When an experienced sonologist performs a transvaginal scan, it may be seen in up to 85% of cases.[58] However, a complex mass may be subtle and easily missed.[69] The mass may blend into adjacent structures with similar echogenicity and may have an appearance similar to the bowel or ovaries.

Several sonographic signs may help differentiate a complex mass from the surrounding pelvic structures. Identifying the ovaries and then searching between the ovaries and the uterus is the best technique for locating an adnexal mass. To differentiate a mass from other pelvic structures, sonologists should press down on the

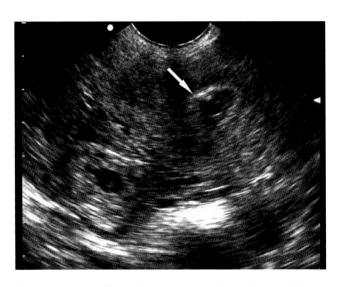

Figure 12-36. Ectopic pregnancy. Pseudogestational sac in the uterus (arrow) and 2.5 cm brightly echogenic tubal ring in the adnexa. Transvaginal image.

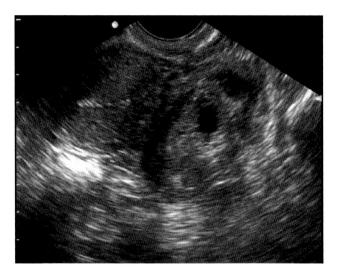

Figure 12-38. Ectopic pregnancy. An empty uterus is seen in transverse transvaginal view and is identified by the endometrial stripe. The complex mass is in the left adnexa and adjacent to the uterus.

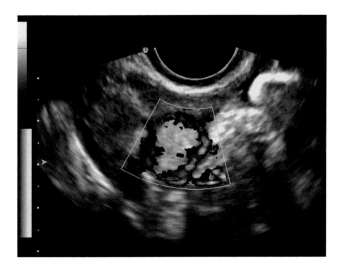

Figure 12-39. Ring of fire. Transvaginal ultrasound of the adnexa demonstrates ectopic mass with surrounding power Doppler signal. (Courtesy of J. Christian Fox, MD)

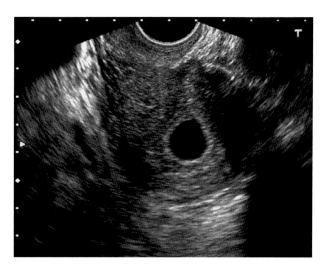

Figure 12-40. Early embryonic demise. Empty intrauterine sac consistent with 6.5-week gestational sac size, contains no yolk sac or embryo. Transvaginal image. (Courtesy of Hennepin County Medical Center)

patient's lower abdomen with their free hand during transvaginal scanning, in a manner similar to performing a bimanual pelvic examination. This will cause pelvic structures to move in relation to one another and examiners can recognize a mass as a separate structure, moving independently from the ovary and bowel. Also, if the transvaginal probe is held very still, peristalsis of the bowel can be seen, differentiating it from other pelvic structures.

Color Doppler has been used in an attempt to differentiate surrounding structures from an adnexal mass. High velocity, low impedance trophoblastic flow can sometimes be seen surrounding an ectopic sac; this is referred to as the "ring of fire"[139] (Figure 12-39). Although some authors suggest that color Doppler provides little additional information and is not more accurate than grey-scale sonography for determining whether an adnexal mass is an ectopic pregnancy.[30,104,140] More recent studies and case reports suggest asymmetric adnexal color Doppler flow is a useful clue.[141,142]

PREGNANCY LOSS

Embryonic Demise

There are several sonographic signs that can reliably predict embryonic demise. The earliest sign is a gestational sac without a yolk sac or embryo (Figure 12-40). With high-resolution transvaginal sonography ($\geq$ 6.5 MHz), a yolk sac is usually seen within the gestational sac when MSD is $\geq$ 10 mm and an embryo is usually seen when MSD is $\geq$ 16 mm.[30,121,143,144] However, with a 5 MHz transvaginal probe or with transabdominal scan-

ning, a yolk sac may not be seen until the MSD is $\geq$ 20 mm.[69,145,146] For the purposes of emergency bedside transvaginal sonography, an empty gestational sac $\geq$ 20 mm is a good predictor of embryonic demise; this is referred to as a blighted ovum. The nonobstetrics clinician should refrain from proclaiming this to the patient and simply note that normal structures are not seen and it may be too early to make a firm diagnosis.

Another good indicator of embryonic demise is lack of embryonic cardiac activity (Figure 12-41). With transvaginal sonography, cardiac activity should be seen in all embryos greater than 5 mm long by crown-rump length.[30,69,96,147] With transabdominal sonography, cardiac activity should be seen in all embryos greater than 10 mm long.[69] When searching for embryonic cardiac activity, it is important to be sure that the embryo is clearly seen. This is easier at 7–8 weeks when the embryonic head and torso can be identified. Also, it is essential to use a high frame rate and turn off the frame-averaging mode when looking for cardiac activity.[30]

Several more subtle signs are also suggestive of embryonic demise or poor fetal outcome. Embryonic bradycardia predicts a poor prognosis[148,149] The normal heart rate for an embryo longer than 5 mm by crown-rump length (6.3 weeks' gestational age) is greater than 120 beats per minute (bpm). The lower the heart rate is below 120 bpm, the lower the survival rate of the embryo. Embryos longer than 5 mm with heart rates below 100 bpm have a survival rate of only 6%.[149] Very early pregnancies, with embryos less than 5 mm in length, normally have slower heart rates, but a rate less than 90 bpm is nearly always associated with embryonic demise.[148,149]

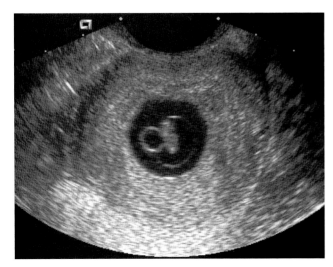

A

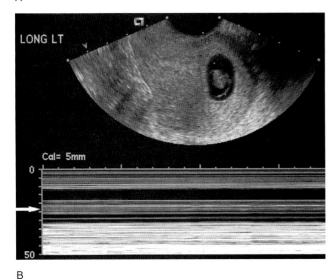

B

Figure 12-41. Embryonic demise. Transvaginal image of the fetal pole which measured 7 weeks via CRL (a). The yolk sac appears slightly enlarged and the amnion is clearly visible. There was no cardiac activity on real-time sonography and this was documented by the M-Mode examination (b). Note the lack of any motion in the fetal band (arrow). (Courtesy of James Mateer, MD, Waukesha Memorial Hospital)

An abnormal yolk sac is another subtle sign of demise or abnormal pregnancy. A very small yolk sac (less than 2 mm diameter) between 8 and 12 weeks is usually associated with an abnormal pregnancy.[150] A very large yolk sac (>6 mm diameter) between 5 and 12 weeks is predictive of embryonic demise or a significant chromosomal abnormality.[30,151] Also, prior to 12 weeks, inability to visualize the yolk sac when an embryo is clearly present is strong evidence of impending embryonic demise.[151] Yolk sac shape is not associated with adverse pregnancy outcome. Pregnancies with a normal

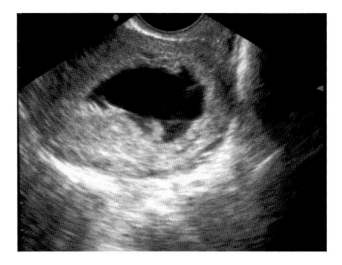

Figure 12-42. Embryonic demise. Distorted gestational sac. Transvaginal image

size but irregularly shaped yolk sac have a normal outcome in nearly all cases.[30]

An odd-shaped or grossly distorted gestational sac is reportedly a good indicator of pregnancy failure, but this finding is subjective (Figure 12-42).[145] A gestational sac low in the uterus, with or without a yolk sac or embryo, is generally considered a sign of inevitable abortion (Figures 12-43 and 12-44). Also, a weakly echogenic or thin (<2 mm wide) trophoblastic reaction surrounding a gestational sac may indicate imminent demise. Finally, a gestational sac, which is not more than 5 mm MSD larger than the crown-rump length of the embryo, is probably abnormal.[146,152]

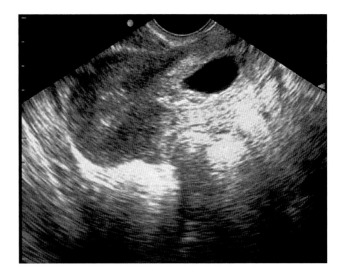

Figure 12-43. Inevitable abortion. The fundus is on the left of the image and the gestational sac is approaching the cervical portion of the uterus. Transvaginal image.

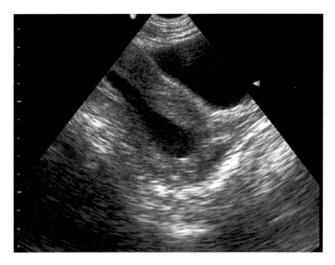

Figure 12-44. Embryonic demise with inevitable abortion. Large empty distorted intrauterine sac that is bulging toward the cervical canal. Transabdominal longitudinal view with the bladder and vaginal stripe along the right side of the image.

Subchorionic hemorrhage is bleeding between the endometrium and chorionic membrane. This is a common finding late in the first trimester. Sonographically, part of the chorionic membrane and placenta are separated from the decidua vera (the endometrium) (Figure 12-45).[30] Acutely, the hemorrhage may appear hyperechoic or isoechoic relative to the placenta, with only slight elevation noted. Over the next week or two, the blood becomes hypoechoic. Patients who present with threatened abortion and have a subchorionic hemorrhage probably have a higher incidence of embryonic

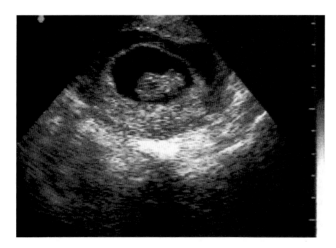

Figure 12-45. Subchorionic hemorrhage. An echolucent crescent-shaped stripe is located between the decidua capsularis and the decidual vera (endometrium) from implantation hemorrhage. Transvaginal images. (Courtesy of James Mateer, MD)

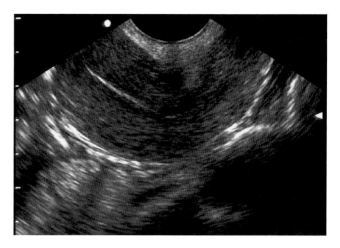

Figure 12-46. Empty uterus after a completed spontaneous abortion. Transvaginal image.

demise.[153,154] Those with large subchorionic hemorrhages may have a much higher rate of pregnancy loss.[153]

Physicians should be conservative when interpreting findings of embryonic demise and give the pregnancy the benefit of the doubt in all cases. Ordering a comprehensive ultrasound and obtaining an obstetrics consult is prudent when the diagnosis is unclear.

Completed Spontaneous Abortion

The uterus should be empty after a completed spontaneous abortion (Figure 12-46). A small amount of blood or clot may also be present.

Retained Products of Conception

Patients with intrauterine echogenic material or a thickened midline stripe ($\geq$10 mm wide) after a spontaneous abortion probably have retained products of conception (Figure 12-47).[90,92,155] When curettage is performed in such cases, chorionic villi are identified in about 70%.[92] Many patients with retained products will do well with expectant management but they may require curettage and should be followed closely for bleeding and infection.[156]

► COMMON VARIANTS AND SELECTED ABNORMALITIES

Several normal anatomic variants may make transabdominal and transvaginal pelvic sonography more difficult. Retroversion of the uterus occurs in about 10% of women. It has little clinical significance but it makes transabdominal imaging difficult. Retroversion means that the body of the uterus bends posterior toward the rectosigmoid colon instead of toward the anterior

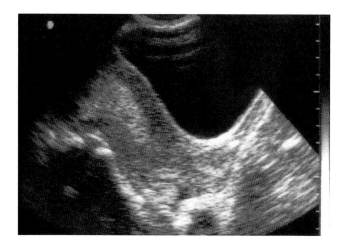

Figure 12-47. Intrauterine echogenic material (2–3 cm thick), consistent with retained products of conception. Transabdominal longitudinal image. (Courtesy of James Mateer, MD)

abdominal wall. The body of the uterus is then too far away from the transabdominal probe and resolution is poor (Figure 12-48A). Transvaginal sonography is much better for imaging a retroverted uterus because the probe can still be placed close to the body of the uterus (Figure 12-48B). When the uterus is retroverted, the ovaries usually lie anterior and lateral to the body of the uterus.

Lateral deviation of the uterus is another normal variant that makes pelvic ultrasound difficult. When transabdominal or transvaginal scanning is performed and the uterus is not seen in the midline, then the probe should be aimed laterally, and sagittal oblique images

obtained. It is not uncommon to find the body of the uterus bending toward the lateral pelvis. If this is the case, then the midline stripe may be difficult to see in just one plane. Lateral and coronal images may be helpful in this situation. When the uterus is deviated laterally, it may displace the ovary out of its usual location. The ovary may then be found superior to the uterus or in the posterior cul-de-sac.

Variation in the location of the ovaries can also make pelvic ultrasound difficult. Transvaginal sonography is required to visualize most normal ovaries. Even with transvaginal scanning, however, they may be difficult to find. In women who have previously been pregnant, the ovaries may be found lateral, posterior, or superior to the uterus. In patients with an enlarged uterus, those who are pregnant or have uterine fibroids, the ovaries are often displaced superior to the uterus. When the ovaries are superior to the uterus, they are difficult to see with transvaginal sonography.

The fallopian tubes are not normally seen on transabdominal ultrasound ultrasound. If the tubes are filled with fluid secondary to scarring or pelvic inflammatory disease, then they may be easily recognized. They will be found in the adnexa lateral to the uterine body. When imaged longitudinally, the fallopian tubes will appear as anechoic tubal structures; when imaged transversely, they will appear as cystic structures. If multiple redundant loops of the tube are adjacent to one another, then this may be misinterpreted as a large multicystic mass. Using the endovaginal approach, healthy fallopian tubes are frequently imaged at their uterine origin and may be traced near each ovary if there is no bowel gas interference.

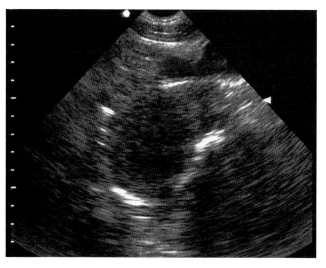

A

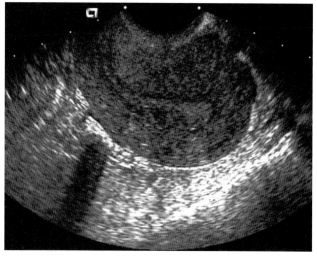

B

Figure 12-48. Transabdominal sagittal view of a retroverted uterus (A). The uterine body and fundus are not well visualized because of the uterine position and empty bladder. A transvaginal longitudinal view of the uterus (B) provides improved resolution. Note that with a retroverted uterus, the fundus is projected to the right side of the image and the cervix to the left. (B, Courtesy of James Mateer, MD, Waukesha Memorial Hospital)

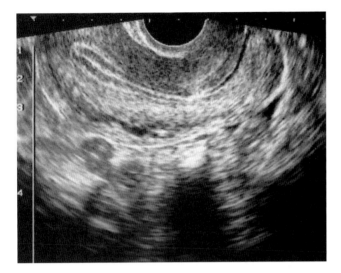

Figure 12-49. Transvaginal sagittal view of the normal anteflexed uterus. Note that the fundus is displayed on the left side of the monitor. Minimal (physiologic) free fluid can be seen in the posterior cul-de-sac below the cervix. The patient has a moderately prominent arcuate venous plexus which does not represent free fluid.

A small amount of fluid in the posterior cul-de-sac can be normal. This fluid may not be seen with transabdominal sonography but is easily visualized with transvaginal imaging (Figure 12-49).

PELVIC MASSES

Corpus Luteum Cyst

Corpus luteum cysts are the most common pelvic masses found in early pregnancy. They are usually unilocular and have thin walls (Figure 12-50). Internal hemorrhage may result in internal septations and echogenic material

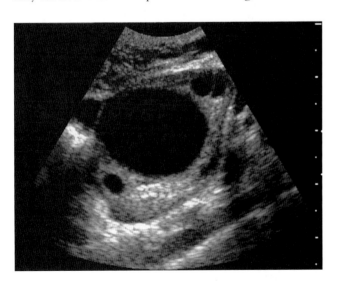

Figure 12-50. Corpus luteum cyst. Transvaginal image.

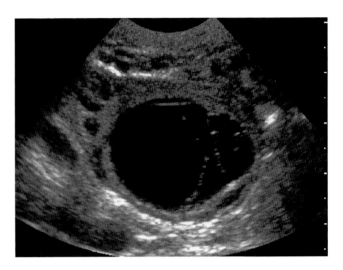

Figure 12-51. Corpus luteum cyst with fine septations from internal hemorrhage. Transvaginal image.

(Figure 12-51). The corpus is solid in appearance in up to 50% of cases.

Leiomyomas

Uterine fibroids are very common and may grow during pregnancy. They are located in the uterine wall and have a variable sonographic appearance. They often cause dispersion of ultrasound and distortion of pelvic images (Figure 12-52).

Malignant Pelvic Masses

The most common tumors that enlarge during pregnancy are ovarian cystadenomas. Internal septations and

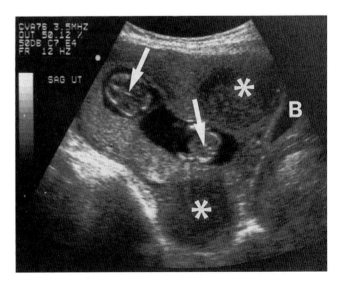

Figure 12-52. Uterine fibroids (*) with pregnancy (arrows). (From *Williams Obstetrics*, 21st ed. New York, McGraw-Hill, 2001; Figure 35–13, p. 929)

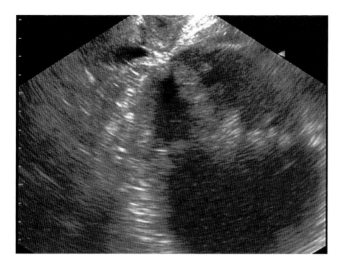

Figure 12-53. Large complex pelvic mass with papillary excrescences and septations. Possible malignancy. Transvaginal image.

papillary excrescences are suggestive of malignancy (Figure 12-53).

ADNEXAL TORSION

Most cases of adnexal torsion occur in the presence of an enlarged ovary or an ovarian mass (see Chapter 14). Finding a normal ovary makes the diagnosis much less likely.

GESTATIONAL TROPHOBLASTIC DISEASE

Most cases of GTD present as a benign molar pregnancy. Those with an invasive mole or choriocarcinoma usually have a history of a molar pregnancy. The classic finding is the appearance of a cluster of "grapes," an intrauterine mass with diffuse hypoechoic vesicles (Figure 12-54). The appearance is not always classic in the first trimester, and the diagnosis may be missed (Figure 12-55).

▶ PITFALLS

ECTOPIC PREGNANCY

1. **Not performing pelvic sonography because of a recent last menstrual period or a low β-hCG**. Patients with a positive pregnancy test who present with abdominal pain or vaginal bleeding should undergo a pelvic ultrasound examination regardless of their reported last menstrual period or β-hCG level. Patients may misinterpret vaginal spotting during pregnancy for a menstrual

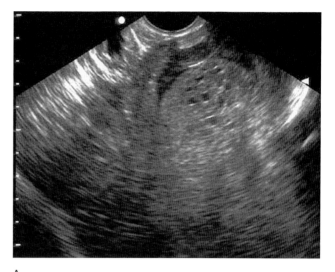

A

B

Figure 12-54. Molar pregnancy. Transvaginal images.

period; thus, obtaining a menstrual history is not an accurate method for excluding ectopic pregnancy. Also, it is not uncommon for patients to have a low β-hCG level and a ruptured ectopic pregnancy.

2. **Attributing an empty uterus to a very early intrauterine pregnancy or a completed spontaneous abortion**. More than 40% of ectopic pregnancies have a β-hCG level less than 1,000 mIU/mL; therefore, an empty uterus with a low β-hCG level should not be considered normal and the entire pelvis should be scanned for signs of an ectopic pregnancy.[62] Also, the only definitive evidence of a completed spontaneous abortion is passage of obvious products of conception or chorionic villi. Without definitive evidence of a completed abortion, the diagnosis of ectopic pregnancy must be ruled out.[46]

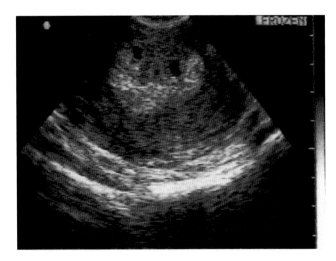

Figure 12-55. Early molar pregnancy. Transverse transvaginal image reveals a thick, echogenic endometrial echo with a few scattered irregular cystic areas in a patient with a high hCG level. (Courtesy of James Mateer, MD)

3. **Mistaking a pseudogestational sac for a gestational sac.** Visualizing an intrauterine pregnancy essentially excludes the diagnosis of ectopic pregnancy in most patients. The intradecidual sign and gestational sac are early signs of an intrauterine pregnancy, but neither is 100% reliable.[121,124,125] Sonologists should be careful not to mistake a pseudogestational sac associated with an ectopic pregnancy for a gestational sac.[30,69,126] A pseudogestational sac, also known as a decidual cast, is an intrauterine fluid collection surrounded by a single decidual layer (Figures 12-36). A pseudogestational sac occurs in 5%–10% of ectopic pregnancies and appears as an elongated and odd-shaped sac in the center of the endometrial cavity with inconsistent thickening of the endometrium.[69] A pseudogestational sac can usually be differentiated from a gestational sac using transvaginal sonography.[100] Also, Doppler ultrasound may help by finding high-velocity low impedance peritrophoblastic flow surrounding a true gestational sac, but the reliability of this is not 100%.[126,139]

4. **Misidentifying an early intrauterine pregnancy.** Clinicians should avoid making the diagnosis of an intrauterine pregnancy when only a small gestational sac is visible. A clear double decidual sign is the first reliable evidence of an intrauterine pregnancy.[30,127] A yolk sac and embryo are obvious signs of an intrauterine pregnancy and should be seen when an inexperienced sonologist makes the diagnosis of an intrauterine pregnancy.[121] Cardiac activity should be seen in all embryos greater than 5 mm long, and this is regarded as the best evidence of an intrauterine pregnancy. It may be prudent for novice sonologists to see cardiac activity before diagnosing an intrauterine pregnancy.

5. **Overestimating the ability to identify subtle signs of ectopic pregnancy.** Although an empty uterus, free intraperitoneal fluid in the hepatorenal space, and free fluid in the pelvis are easy to identify, complex adnexal masses and tubal rings may be subtle. An experienced sonologist should repeat indeterminate bedside scans to look for these subtle signs.

6. **Performing a transvaginal ultrasound without a transabdominal scan.** The transabdominal pelvic view allows a broader view of the pelvis and may detect masses that are outside the field of view of the transvaginal probe and may be a helpful starting point in some patients. Also, the hepatorenal space should always be scanned to look for free intraperitoneal fluid.[69] Some patients may have minimal symptoms and normal vital signs despite a ruptured ectopic pregnancy with a large amount of intraperitoneal blood.

7. **Identifying a normal appearing pregnancy but not recognizing its location in relation to the uterus.** An ectopic pregnancy may appear to be an intrauterine pregnancy if its extrauterine location is not carefully noted (Figure 12-56). Also, an interstitial ectopic pregnancy may appear to be intrauterine but careful imaging will reveal that it lies on the margin of the uterine wall

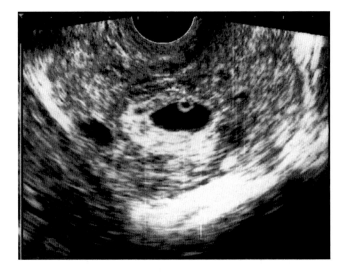

Figure 12-56. Ectopic pregnancy. Extrauterine gestational sac with a bright thick echogenic ring and a yolk sac within. A cursory examination could mistake the surrounding mid-level echoes as uterine tissue, but note the absence of any endometrial echo. Transvaginal image.

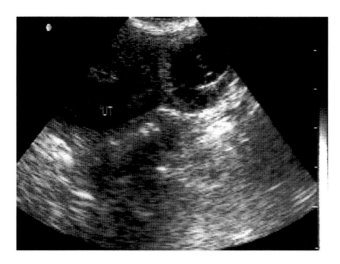

Figure 12-57. Interstitial ectopic. Transverse transvaginal ultrasound reveals a small fluid collection within the endometrium of the uterus (UT). The round echogenic ectopic ring was partially imbedded within the uterine myometrium. (Courtesy of James Mateer, MD)

and not in the intrauterine cavity. Transabdominal sonography will help clarify the big picture in cases of possible ectopic pregnancy.

8. **Mistaking an interstitial pregnancy for an intrauterine pregnancy**. An interstitial pregnancy may be mistaken for an intrauterine pregnancy.[157] Interstitial pregnancies comprise about 2–5% of all ectopic pregnancies.[69] Most ectopic pregnancies occur in the ampullary segment of the fallopian tube but interstitial ectopic pregnancies occur in the cornual region (Figure 12-57). They are partially enveloped by the myometrium. Because of the rich myometrial blood supply, an interstitial pregnancy can grow larger and rupture later than most ectopic pregnancies. When rupture occurs, intraperitoneal bleeding (potentially arterial) and vaginal bleeding may be brisk and profuse. Many of these patients exsanguinate and die before reaching the hospital. It may be difficult to identify an interstitial pregnancy because the gestational sac may be completely surrounded by the uterus. However, an interstitial pregnancy usually appears to be at the margin of the uterine wall rather than inside the uterine cavity.[158] The eccentrically located gestational sac is surrounded by an asymmetric myometrial mantle with a free wall thickness usually less than 5–8 mm. The "interstitial line sign" is a fine echogenic line extending from the endometrial stripe to the interstitial gestational sac. This finding is diagnostic of an interstitial ectopic pregnancy. If the diagnosis is not made early, prior to rupture, up to 50% of patients may require a hysterectomy.[69]

9. **Failure to identify heterotopic pregnancy**. Failure to obtain a history of fertility medications or in vitro fertilization may lead to this pitfall. The risk of heterotopic pregnancy in such patients is as high as 1%, so finding an intrauterine pregnancy does not exclude the diagnosis of ectopic pregnancy. Also, patients without these risk factors may have a heterotopic pregnancy.[33,159] Therefore, it is prudent to scan the entire pelvis looking for free pelvic fluid or an adnexal mass, even after an intrauterine pregnancy has been identified.

OTHER PITFALLS

1. **Fetal anomalies**. Failure to diagnose fetal anomalies by ultrasound has recently become a significant source of malpractice litigation. To avoid this problem, patients should be informed that emergency bedside sonography is a focused examination only and is not designed to detect embryonic abnormalities.

2. **Embryonic demise**. Many potential pitfalls are associated with the diagnosis of embryonic demise. When poor resolution or poor quality scans are obtained, normal structures may not be visualized, leading to the errant diagnosis of a blighted ovum. Also, inability to identify embryonic cardiac activity can occur secondary to mistaking another structure for the embryo or using a frame-averaging ultrasound mode. These pitfalls can be avoided by positively identifying the embryo and by using a high frame rate setting when searching for embryonic cardiac activity. Before the diagnosis of embryonic demise is made, the pregnancy should be given the benefit of the doubt. Sonography by an experienced operator and consultation with obstetrics is prudent before the patient is informed of the definitive diagnosis.

3. **Multiple Pregnancy**. When twins are identified by bedside ultrasound, it is important to inform the patient that about 25% of twin pregnancies diagnosed in the first trimester will become singleton pregnancies by the second trimester.

4. **Pelvic Masses**. The most common pitfall when identifying a pelvic mass is neglecting to arrange close follow-up and informing the patient of the finding. Pelvic masses may enlarge during pregnancy and are usually incidental findings on pelvic sonography. Ovarian malignancy may rarely present during pregnancy.

5. **Pelvic pain**. Pelvic pain is a common complaint in early pregnancy. A common pitfall of using pelvic ultrasound in these patients is that the

finding of an intrauterine pregnancy often ends the work-up for the etiology of the patient's symptoms. Once ectopic pregnancy is excluded, the patient's pelvic pain may be attributed to the pregnancy and diagnoses such as appendicitis or adnexal torsion may not be considered. Physicians should remember that appendicitis is relatively common in pregnancy and 20% of adnexal torsion occurs during pregnancy.

6. **Gestational Trophoblastic Disease**. Molar pregnancy is usually obvious on pelvic ultrasound. However, early in pregnancy, the findings may be subtle. Serum β-hCG will always be very high in GTD. A potential pitfall is assuming that this diagnosis is excluded because it is not seen on bedside ultrasound. Such patients need close follow-up and repeat ultrasound examinations.

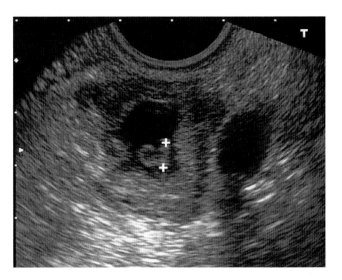

Figure 12-58. Case 1. Bedside transvaginal ultrasound showed an empty uterus and a 3 × 3 × 4 cm right adnexal mass adjacent to the right ovary, containing a gestational sac, yolk sac, and embryo. (Courtesy of Hennepin County Medical Center)

► CASE STUDIES

CASE 1

Patient Presentation

A 20-year-old woman, gravida 3, para 0, at about 3–6 weeks' gestation, because she was unsure of her last menstrual period, complained of several hours of heavy vaginal bleeding and low, central abdominal cramping. She denied any history of sexually transmitted disease, intrauterine device, ectopic pregnancy, or pelvic surgery. Previous pregnancies ended in early spontaneous abortions. She denied vomiting, fever, and urinary symptoms.

On physical examination, her blood pressure was 105/71 mmHg, heart rate, 87 beats per minute; respirations, 14 per minute; and temperature, as 36.8°C. She was in no distress. Her head, neck, pulmonary, cardiovascular, and back examinations were unremarkable. Abdominal examination revealed a soft abdomen with mild suprapubic tenderness. Speculum examination revealed a closed cervical os with a small amount of blood in the vaginal vault. Bimanual pelvic examination revealed no tenderness or mass.

Management Course

Urinalysis was unremarkable, but the urine pregnancy test was positive. Bedside transvaginal ultrasound performed immediately after the pelvic examination showed an empty uterus and a 3 × 3 × 4 cm right adnexal mass adjacent to the right ovary, containing a gestational sac, yolk sac, and embryo (Figure 12-58). Estimated gestational age by crown rump length was 6 weeks and 2 days. Trace free fluid was noted in the right adnexa, but the pouch of Douglas and Morison's pouch were negative for free fluid. Intravenous access was obtained, and the obstetrics service was consulted. The serum β-hCG level was 14,358 mIU/mL and the blood type was B positive. A repeat ultrasound examination in the radiology department confirmed the above bedside findings. The patient was taken to the operating room where a laparoscopic right salpingectomy was performed without complications. The patient recovered well and subsequently was discharged home.

Commentary

Case 1 was an example of a patient with an unruptured ovarian ectopic pregnancy. This diagnosis was made rapidly by the emergency physician using bedside transvaginal ultrasound immediately after the routine pelvic examination. This case demonstrated that the bimanual pelvic examination is unreliable for detecting significant pelvic pathology. Given the patient's serum β-hCG level greater than 10,000 mIU/mL and adnexal mass diameter of 4 cm, medical therapy with methotrexate would likely fail.

CASE 2

Patient Presentation

A 36-year-old woman, gravida 2, para 1 at 11 weeks stated gestational age, presented to the emergency department via ambulance 15 minutes after the acute onset of painless vaginal bleeding. She reported that she had been dealing with multiple episodes of vomiting over the previous 5 days, which was unlike her previous pregnancy. She denied any other significant symptoms or medical history.

On physical examination, her blood pressure was 110/68 mmHg, heart rate, 110 beats per minute; respirations, 20 per minute; and temperature, 36.7°C. She appeared older than her stated age. Her head, neck, pulmonary, cardiovascular, and back examinations were unremarkable. Abdominal examination revealed a prominently gravid abdomen, noted to appear larger than expected for the patient's stated gestational age. Mild epigastric tenderness was present. Emergency department pelvic examination was deferred in consideration of vaginal bleeding and advanced gestational age.

Management Course

A urine pregnancy test was positive. The patient received intravenous fluids and an antiemetic. Bedside transabdominal pelvic ultrasound in the emergency department showed a "snowstorm" appearance with cystic structures within the uterus, concerning for gestational trophoblastic disease (Figure 12-59). Serum β-hCG measured 2,354,000 mIU/mL. The patient's blood type was A positive. The obstetrics service was consulted and a comprehensive ultrasound examination detailed an enlarged uterus filled with tissue and cysts consistent with complete molar pregnancy. The patient underwent a suction dilation and curettage. Her nausea and vomiting improved and she was discharged home on postoperative day 1 with plans for serial β-hCG measurements and clinic follow-up.

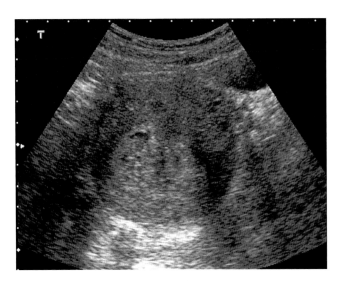

Figure 12-59. Case 2. Bedside transabdominal pelvic ultrasound showed a "snowstorm" appearance of the uterus and cystic structures within the endometrium consistent with gestational trophoblastic disease. (Courtesy of Hennepin County Medical Center)

Commentary

Case 2 exemplified the utility of bedside ultrasound in the rapid diagnosis of pathologic conditions not routinely encountered in the emergency department. Recognition of normal and abnormal findings on bedside ultrasound helped focus the differential diagnosis. Although hyperemesis, a prominently gravid abdomen, and a markedly elevated serum β-hCG level were clues to this patient's final diagnosis, definitive diagnosis and management would not have taken place without ultrasound imaging.

CASE 3

Patient Presentation

A 28-year-old woman arrived in the emergency department late in the evening, complaining of nausea, weakness, and episodic loss of consciousness over the past few hours. She did not know when her last menstrual period was. She felt confused, but denied any significant pain. She was unwilling to provide any further history, citing nausea and weakness.

Upon physical examination, her blood pressure was 82/40 mmHg, heart rate, 86 beats per minute; respirations were 22 per minute; and temperature was 36.9°C. The patient was diaphoretic and appeared uncomfortable. Her head, neck, pulmonary, and back examinations were unremarkable. Cardiac examination revealed a grade I/VI systolic murmur. Abdominal examination was significant for mild bilateral lower quadrant tenderness with no rebound or guarding. Genitourinary examination revealed a closed cervical os and no bleeding. She had mild cervical motion and bilateral adnexal tenderness.

Management Course

A urine pregnancy test was ordered as the emergency physician performed a transabdominal ultrasound examination. This revealed a hypoechoic sac in the uterus, a tubal ring in the left adnexa, and a small amount of free pelvic fluid (Figure 12-60). A scan of the upper abdomen revealed free fluid in the hepatorenal space. A urine pregnancy test was positive. After 2 L of intravenous normal saline, the patient's blood pressure was 94/52 mmHg with a heart rate of 84 beats per minute; infusion of O-negative packed red blood cells was initiated. The on-call obstetrician was immediately contacted and the operating room was prepared. While the obstetrician was en route, an emergency bedside transvaginal ultrasound examination confirmed a definite ectopic pregnancy with a yolk sac in the left adnexa. The patient was taken directly to the operating room when the obstetrician arrived. A ruptured ectopic pregnancy and

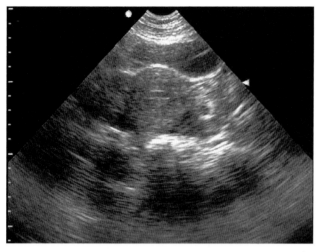

A

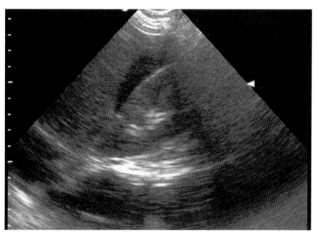

B

Figure 12-60. Case 3. Pseudogestational sac within the uterus and tubal ring in the left adnexa. Transabdominal transverse image (A). Free fluid in the hepatorenal space. Transabdominal right upper quadrant image (B).

2–3 L of free intraperitoneal blood were found at surgery. The patient required a left salpingectomy. Her serum β-hCG level was 917 mIU/mL.

Commentary

Case 3 illustrated a patient with a ruptured ectopic pregnancy. She was in shock and required immediate resuscitation. She could not provide a reliable history and was not aware that she was pregnant. She had relatively mild abdominal symptoms and was not tachycardic, which is not uncommon with acute intraperitoneal blood loss. Transabdominal sonography revealed hepatorenal free fluid and a tubal ring. Hepatorenal free fluid alone, in a young pregnant woman with nontraumatic hypotension, is nearly diagnostic of a ruptured ectopic pregnancy and was enough evidence to proceed to surgery. In addi-

tion, this patient had a tubal ring, which is also nearly diagnostic of an ectopic pregnancy. Immediate bedside transvaginal scanning by the emergency physician allowed a more detailed view of the mass and revealed a definite ectopic pregnancy.

REFERENCES

1. American College of Emergency Physicians: Clinical policy for the initial approach to patients presenting with a chief complaint of vaginal bleeding. American College of Emergency Physicians. *Ann Emerg Med* 29:435–458, 1997.
2. American College of Emergency Physicians: American College of Emergency Physicians: ACEP emergency ultrasound guidelines-2001. *Ann Emerg Med* 38:470–481, 2001.
3. American College of Emergency Physicians. Use of ultrasound imaging by emergency physicians. *Ann Emerg Med* 38:469–470, 2001.
4. Reardon & Jehle In *Emergency Medicine: A Comprehensive Study Guide*. New York: McGraw-Hill, 2000:737–748.
5. Brennan DF: Ectopic pregnancy–Part II. Diagnostic procedures and imaging. *Acad Emerg Med* 2:1090–1097, 1995.
6. Rodgerson JD, Heegaard WG, Plummer D, et al.: Emergency department right upper quadrant ultrasound is associated with a reduced time to diagnosis and treatment of ruptured ectopic pregnancies. *Acad Emerg Med* 8:331–336, 2001.
7. Cartwright PS, Victory DF, Moore RA, et al.: Performance of a new enzyme-linked immunoassay urine pregnancy test for the detection of ectopic gestation. *Ann Emerg Med* 15:1198–1199, 1986.
8. Marill KA, Ingmire TE, Nelson BK: Utility of a single beta HCG measurement to evaluate for absence of ectopic pregnancy. *J Emerg Med* 17:419–426, 1999.
9. Stovall TG, Kellerman AL, Ling FW, Buster JE: Emergency department diagnosis of ectopic pregnancy. *Ann Emerg Med* 19:1098–1103, 1990.
10. Stovall TG, Ling FW, Andersen RN, Buster JE: Improved sensitivity and specificity of a single measurement of serum progesterone over serial quantitative beta-human chorionic gonadotrophin in screening for ectopic pregnancy. *Hum Reprod* 7:723–725, 1992.
11. Valley VT, Mateer JR, Aiman EJ, et al.: Serum progesterone and endovaginal sonography by emergency physicians in the evaluation of ectopic pregnancy. *Acad Emerg Med* 5:309–313, 1998.
12. Dart R, Ramanujam P, Dart L: Progesterone as a predictor of ectopic pregnancy when the ultrasound is indeterminate. *Am J Emerg Med* 20:575–579, 2002.
13. Krause Janicke In *Emergency Medicine: A Comprehensive Study Guide* (eds Tintinalli). New York: McGraw-Hill, 2000, 686.
14. Lipscomb GH, Stovall TG, Ling FW: Nonsurgical treatment of ectopic pregnancy. *N Engl J Med* 343:1325–1329, 2000.
15. Vermesh M, Graczykowski JW, Sauer MV: Reevaluation of the role of culdocentesis in the management of ectopic pregnancy. *Am J Obstet Gynecol* 162:411–413, 1990.

16. Vande Krol L, Abbott JT: The current role of culdocentesis. *Am J Emerg Med* 10:354–358, 1992.

17. Brennan DF: Diagnosis of ectopic pregnancy. *J Fla Med Assoc* 84:549–556, 1997.

18. Pelsang RE: Diagnostic imaging modalities during pregnancy. *Obstet Gynecol Clin North Am* 25:287–300, 1998.

19. Kaplan BC, Dart RG, Moskos M, et al.: Ectopic pregnancy: prospective study with improved diagnostic accuracy. *Ann Emerg Med* 28:10–17, 1996.

20. Peterson HB, Xia Z, Hughes JM, et al.: The risk of ectopic pregnancy after tubal sterilization. U.S. Collaborative Review of Sterilization Working Group. *N Engl J Med* 336:762–767, 1997.

21. Loffredo AJ, Dyne PL: Emergency Medicine Residents can perform bedside ultrasound with a high degree of sensitivity and specificity to detect intrauterine pregnancy with cardiac activity. *Acad Emerg Med* 8:547–547, 2001.

22. Durham B, Lane B, Burbridge L, Balasubramaniam S: Pelvic ultrasound performed by emergency physicians for the detection of ectopic pregnancy in complicated first trimester pregnancies. *Ann Emerg Med* 29:338–347, 1997.

23. Cashner KA, Christopher CR, Dysert GA: Spontaneous fetal loss after demonstration of a live fetus in the first trimester. *Obstet Gynecol* 70:827–830, 1987.

24. Wilson RD, Kendrick V, Wittmann BK, McGillivray B: Spontaneous abortion and pregnancy outcome after normal first trimester ultrasound examination. *Obstet Gynecol* 67:352–355, 1986.

25. Van Den Eeden SK, Shan J, Bruce C, Glasser M: Ectopic pregnancy rate and treatment utilization in a large managed care organization. *Obstet Gynecol* 105:1052–1057, 2005.

26. Mateer JR, Valley VT, Aiman EJ, et al.: Outcome analysis of a protocol including bedside endovaginal sonography in patients at risk for ectopic pregnancy. *Ann Emerg Med* 27:283–289, 1996.

27. Tayal VS, Cohen H, Norton HJ: Outcome of patients with an indeterminate emergency department first trimester pelvic ultrasound to rule out ectopic pregnancy. *Acad Emerg Med* 11:912–917, 2004.

28. Condous G, Okaro E, Khalid A, et al.: A prospective evaluation of a single-visit strategy to manage pregnancies of unknown location. *Hum Reprod* 20:1398–1403, 2005.

29. Braen Krause, Wolfson AB: In: *Harwood-Nuss' Clinical Practice of Emergency Medicine* Harwood-Nuss, A. ed. Philadelphia, PA: Lippincott Williams & Wilkins, 2005: 500.

30. Lyons, Levi Dashefsky In: Diagnostic ultrasound eds. Rumack, CM, Wilson, SR & Charboneau, JW. Mosby, 1999: 975–1011.

31. DeVoe, Pratt: Simultaneous intrauterine and extrauterine pregnancy. *Am J Obstet Gynecol* 56:1119–1126, 1948.

32. Bright DA, Gaupp FB: Heterotopic pregnancy: A reevaluation. *J Am Board Fam Pract* 3:125–128, 1990.

33. Jerrard D, Tso E, Salik R, Barish RA: Unsuspected heterotopic pregnancy in a woman without risk factors. *Am J Emerg Med* 10:58–60, 1992.

34. Reece EA, Petrie RH, Sirmans MF, et al.: Combined intrauterine and extrauterine gestations: A review. *Am J Obstet Gynecol* 146:323–330, 1983.

35. Richards SR, Stempel LE, Carlton BD: Heterotopic pregnancy: Reappraisal of incidence. *Am J Obstet Gynecol* 142:928–930, 1982.

36. Richards SR, Stempel LE, Carlton BD: Heterotopic pregnancy. *Am J Obstet Gynecol* 148:227–228, 1984.

37. Berger MJ, Taymor ML: Simultaneous intrauterine and tubal pregnancies following ovulation induction. *Am J Obstet Gynecol* 113:812–813, 1972.

38. Gamberdella FR, Marrs RP: Heterotopic pregnancy associated with assisted reproductive technology. *Am J Obstet Gynecol* 160:1520–1522; discussion 1522–1524, 1989.

39. Nederlof KP, Lawson HW, Saftlas AF, et al.: Ectopic pregnancy surveillance, United States, 1970–1987. *MMWR CDC Surveill Summ* 39:9–17, 1990.

40. Lipscomb GH, McCord ML, Stovall TG, et al.: Predictors of success of methotrexate treatment in women with tubal ectopic pregnancies. *N Engl J Med* 341:1974–1978, 1999.

41. Burgher SW, Tandy TK, Dawdy MR: Transvaginal ultrasonography by emergency physicians decreases patient time in the emergency department. *Acad Emerg Med* 5:802–807, 1998.

42. Schlager D, Whitten D, Tolan K: Emergency department ultrasound: Impact on ED stay times. *Am J Emerg Med* 15:216–217, 1997.

43. Shih CH: Effect of emergency physician–performed pelvic sonography on length of stay in the emergency department. *Ann Emerg Med* 29:348–351; discussion 352, 1997.

44. Durston WE, Carl ML, Guerra W, et al.: Ultrasound availability in the evaluation of ectopic pregnancy in the ED: Comparison of quality and cost-effectiveness with different approaches. *Am J Emerg Med* 18:408–417, 2000.

45. Mateer JR, Aiman EJ, Brown MH, Olson DW: Ultrasonographic examination by emergency physicians of patients at risk for ectopic pregnancy. *Acad Emerg Med* 2:867–873, 1995.

46. Abbott J, Emmans LS, Lowenstein SR: Ectopic pregnancy: Ten common pitfalls in diagnosis. *Am J Emerg Med* 8:515–522, 1990.

47. Barnhart K, Mennuti MT, Benjamin I, et al.: Prompt diagnosis of ectopic pregnancy in an emergency department setting. *Obstet Gynecol* 84:1010–1015, 1994.

48. Holbrook J: A computerized audit of 15,009 emergency department records. *Ann Emerg Med* 19:139–144, 1990.

49. Trautlein JJ, Lambert RL, Miller J: Malpractice in the emergency department—Review of 200 cases. *Ann Emerg Med* 13:709–711, 1984.

50. Barnhart K, Coutifaris C: Diagnosis of ectopic pregnancy. *Ann Emerg Med* 29:295–296, 1997.

51. Barnhart KT, Simhan H, Kamelle SA: Diagnostic accuracy of ultrasound above and below the beta-hCG discriminatory zone. *Obstet Gynecol* 94:583–587, 1999.

52. Braffman BH, Coleman BG, Ramchandani P, et al.: Emergency department screening for ectopic pregnancy: A prospective US study. *Radiology* 190:797–802, 1994.

53. Timor-Tritsch In: *Transvaginal Sonography of the Normal and Abnormal Fetus* (eds Bronshtein & Zimmer). New York: Parthenon Publishing, 2001:7–34.

54. Cacciatore B: Can the status of tubal pregnancy be predicted with transvaginal sonography? A prospective comparison of sonographic, surgical, and serum hCG findings. *Radiology* 177:481–484, 1990.

55. Nyberg DA, Filly RA, Laing FC, et al.: Ectopic pregnancy. Diagnosis by sonography correlated with quantitative HCG levels. *J Ultrasound Med* 6:145–150, 1987.

56. Sadek AL, Schiøtz HA: Transvaginal sonography in the management of ectopic pregnancy. *Acta Obstet Gynecol Scand* 74:293–296, 1995.

57. Shalev E, Yarom I, Bustan M, et al.: Transvaginal sonography as the ultimate diagnostic tool for the management of ectopic pregnancy: Experience with 840 cases. *Fertil Steril* 69:62–65, 1998.

58. Brown DL, Doubilet PM: Transvaginal sonography for diagnosing ectopic pregnancy: Positivity criteria and performance characteristics. *J Ultrasound Med* 13:259–266, 1994.

59. Mahony BS, Filly RA, Nyberg DA, Callen PW: Sonographic evaluation of ectopic pregnancy. *J Ultrasound Med* 4:221–228, 1985.

60. ACEP Clinical Policies Committee and Clinical Policies Subcommittee on Early Pregnancy. American College of Emergency Physicians: Clinical policy: critical issues in the initial evaluation and management of patients presenting to the emergency department in early pregnancy. *Ann Emerg Med* 41:123–133, 2003.

61. Stovall TG, Ling FW: Ectopic pregnancy. Diagnostic and therapeutic algorithms minimizing surgical intervention. *J Reprod Med* 38:807–812, 1993.

62. Dart RG, Kaplan B, Cox C: Transvaginal ultrasound in patients with low beta-human chorionic gonadotropin values: how often is the study diagnostic? *Ann Emerg Med* 30:135–140, 1997.

63. Counselman FL, Shaar GS, Heller RA, King DK: Quantitative B-hCG levels less than 1000 mIU/mL in patients with ectopic pregnancy: Pelvic ultrasound still useful. *J Emerg Med* 16:699–703, 1998.

64. Kohn MA, Kerr K, Malkevich D, et al.: Beta-human chorionic gonadotropin levels and the likelihood of ectopic pregnancy in emergency department patients with abdominal pain or vaginal bleeding. *Acad Emerg Med* 10:119–126, 2003.

65. Condous G, Kirk E, Lu C, et al.: Diagnostic accuracy of varying discriminatory zones for the prediction of ectopic pregnancy in women with a pregnancy of unknown location. *Ultrasound Obstet Gynecol* 26:770–775, 2005.

66. Bernaschek G, Rudelstorfer R, Csaicsich P: Vaginal sonography versus serum human chorionic gonadotropin in early detection of pregnancy. *Am J Obstet Gynecol* 158:608–612, 1988.

67. Kadar N, Bohrer M, Kemmann E, Shelden R: The discriminatory human chorionic gonadotropin zone for endovaginal sonography: A prospective, randomized study. *Fertil Steril* 61:1016–1020, 1994.

68. Nyberg DA, Mack LA, Laing FC, Jeffrey RB: Early pregnancy complications: endovaginal sonographic findings correlated with human chorionic gonadotropin levels. *Radiology* 167:619–622, 1988.

69. Weston In: *Clinical Ultrasound: A Comprehensive Text* (eds Dewbury, Meire and Cosgrove) London: Churchill Livingstone, 2001:151–187.

70. Dart R, Howard K. Subclassification of indeterminate pelvic ultrasonograms: Stratifying the risk of ectopic pregnancy. *Acad Emerg Med* 5:313–319, 1998.

71. Parvey HR, Maklad N: Pitfalls in the transvaginal sonographic diagnosis of ectopic pregnancy. *J Ultrasound Med* 12:139–144, 1993.

72. Lewis-Bliehall C, Rogers RG, Kammerer-Doak DN, et al.: Medical vs. surgical treatment of ectopic pregnancy. The University of New Mexico's six-year experience. *J Reprod Med* 46:983–988, 2001.

73. Sowter MC, Farquhar CM: Ectopic pregnancy: An update. *Curr Opin Obstet Gynecol* 16:289–293, 2004.

74. American College of Obstetricians and Gynecologists: ACOG practice bulletin. Medical management of tubal pregnancy. Number 3, December 1998. Clinical management guidelines for obstetrician-gynecologists. *Int J Gynaecol Obstet* 65:97–103, 1999.

75. Stika CS, Anderson L, Frederiksen MC: Single-dose methotrexate for the treatment of ectopic pregnancy: Northwestern Memorial Hospital three-year experience. *Am J Obstet Gynecol* 174:1840–1846; discussion 1846–1848, 1996.

76. Stovall TG, Ling FW: Single-dose methotrexate: An expanded clinical trial. *Am J Obstet Gynecol* 168:1759–1762; discussion 1762–1765, 1993.

77. Potter MB, Lepine LA, Jamieson DJ: Predictors of success with methotrexate treatment of tubal ectopic pregnancy at Grady Memorial Hospital. *Am J Obstet Gynecol* 188:1192–1194, 2003.

78. Hung TH, Shau WY, Hsieh TT, et al.: Prognostic factors for an unsatisfactory primary methotrexate treatment of cervical pregnancy: a quantitative review. *Hum Reprod* 13:2636–2642, 1998.

79. Takacs P, Chakhtoura N, De Santis T, Verma U: Evaluation of the relationship between endometrial thickness and failure of single-dose methotrexate in ectopic pregnancy. *Arch Gynecol Obstet* 272:269–272, 2005.

80. Nazac A, Gervaise A, Bouyer J, et al.: Predictors of success in methotrexate treatment of women with unruptured tubal pregnancies. *Ultrasound Obstet Gynecol* 21:181–185, 2003.

81. Bixby S, Tello R, Kuligowska E: Presence of a yolk sac on transvaginal sonography is the most reliable predictor of single-dose methotrexate treatment failure in ectopic pregnancy. *J Ultrasound Med* 24:591–598, 2005.

82. Hammer & Milad In: *Gynecology and Obstetrics* Sciarra ed. Philadelphia, PA: Lippincott Williams & Wilkins, 2000: 1–14.

83. Shalev E, Peleg D, Tsabari A, et al.: Spontaneous resolution of ectopic tubal pregnancy: Natural history. *Fertil Steril* 63:15–19, 1995.

84. Elson J, Tailor A, Banerjee S, Salim R, Hillaby K, Jurkovic D: Expectant management of tubal ectopic pregnancy: prediction of successful outcome using decision tree analysis. *Ultrasound Obstet Gynecol.* 23:552–556, 2004.

85. Everett C: Incidence and outcome of bleeding before the 20th week of pregnancy: Prospective study from general practice. *BMJ* 315:32–34, 1997.

86. Wilcox AJ, Weinberg CR, O'Connor JF, et al.: Incidence of early loss of pregnancy. *N Engl J Med* 319:189–194, 1988.

87. Falco P, Milano V, Pilu G, et al.: Sonography of pregnancies with first trimester bleeding and a viable embryo: A study of prognostic indicators by logistic regression analysis. *Ultrasound Obstet Gynecol* 7:165–169, 1996.

88. Filly In: *Ultrasonography in Obstetrics and Gynecology* Callen ed, Philadelphia, PA: WB Saunders, 1994:63–85.

89. Scott In: *Danforth's Obstetrics and Gynecology.* Scott, DiSaia & Hammond eds. Philadelphia, PA: Lippincott, 1994:175.

90. Cetin A, Cetin M: Diagnostic and therapeutic decision-making with transvaginal sonography for first trimester spontaneous abortion, clinically thought to be incomplete or complete. *Contraception* 57:393–397, 1998.

91. Mansur MM: Ultrasound diagnosis of complete abortion can reduce need for curettage. *Eur J Obstet Gynecol Reprod Biol* 44:65–69, 1992.

92. Rulin MC, Bornstein SG, Campbell JD: The reliability of ultrasonography in the management of spontaneous abortion, clinically thought to be complete: A prospective study. *Am J Obstet Gynecol* 168:12–15, 1993.

93. Jurkovic D, Ross JA, Nicolaides KH: Expectant management of missed miscarriage. *Br J Obstet Gynaecol* 105:670–671, 1998.

94. Goldstein SR: Early detection of pathologic pregnancy by transvaginal sonography. *J Clin Ultrasound* 18:262–273, 1990.

95. Goldstein SR: Embryonic death in early pregnancy: A new look at the first trimester. *Obstet Gynecol* 84:294–297, 1994.

96. Levi CS, Lyons EA, Zheng XH, et al.: Endovaginal US: Demonstration of cardiac activity in embryos of less than 5.0 mm in crown-rump length. *Radiology* 176:71–74, 1990.

97. Landy HJ, Weiner S, Corson SL, et al.: The "vanishing twin": Ultrasonographic assessment of fetal disappearance in the first trimester. *Am J Obstet Gynecol* 155:14–19, 1986.

98. Sampson A, de Crespigny LC: Vanishing twins: The frequency of spontaneous fetal reduction of a twin pregnancy. *Ultrasound Obstet Gynecol* 2:107–109, 1992.

99. Whitecar MP, Turner S, Higby MK: Adnexal masses in pregnancy: A review of 130 cases undergoing surgical management. *Am J Obstet Gynecol* 181:19–24, 1999.

100. Fleischer AC, Shah DM, Entman SS: Sonographic evaluation of maternal disorders during pregnancy. *Radiol Clin North Am* 28:51–58, 1990.

101. Lev-Toaff AS, Coleman BG, Arger PH, et al.: Leiomyomas in pregnancy: Sonographic study. *Radiology* 164:375–380, 1987.

102. Beischer NA, Buttery BW, Fortune DW, Macafee CA: Growth and malignancy of ovarian tumours in pregnancy. *Aust N Z J Obstet Gynaecol* 11:208–220, 1971.

103. Bider D, Mashiach S, Dulitzky M, et al.: Clinical, surgical and pathologic findings of adnexal torsion in pregnant and nonpregnant women. *Surg Gynecol Obstet* 173:363–366, 1991.

104. Fleischer In: *Ultrasound: A Practical Approach to Clinical Problems* Bluth, Arger, Benson, Ralls, Siegel eds. New York: Thieme, 2000:273–280.

105. Grendys EC, Barnes WA: Ovarian cancer in pregnancy. *Surg Clin North Am* 75:1–14, 1995.

106. Peñ JE, Ufberg D, Cooney N, Denis AL: Usefulness of Doppler sonography in the diagnosis of ovarian torsion. *Fertil Steril* 73:1047–1050, 2000.

107. Albayram F, Hamper UM: Ovarian and adnexal torsion: Spectrum of sonographic findings with pathologic correlation. *J Ultrasound Med* 20:1083–1089, 2001.

108. Lambert MJ, Villa M: Gynecologic ultrasound in emergency medicine. *Emerg Med Clin North Am* 22:683–696, 2004.

109. Warner MA, Fleischer AC, Edell SL, et al.: Uterine adnexal torsion: Sonographic findings. *Radiology* 154:773–775, 1985.

110. Houry D, Abbott JT: Ovarian torsion: A fifteen-year review. *Ann Emerg Med* 38:156–159, 2001.

111. Abbott & Thickman In: *Diagnostic Radiology in Emergency Medicine* Rosen St. Louis, eds. MO: Mosby-YearBook, 1992:581–589.

112. Freedman RS, Tortolero-Luna G, Pandey DK, et al.: Gestational trophoblastic disease. *Obstet Gynecol Clin North Am* 23:545–571, 1996.

113. Davison CM, Kaplan RM, Wenig LN, Burmeister D: Qualitative beta-hCG urine assays may be misleading in the presence of molar pregnancy: A case report. *J Emerg Med* 27:43–47, 2004.

114. Teng FY, Magarelli PC, Montz FJ: Transvaginal probe ultrasonography. Diagnostic or outcome advantages in women with molar pregnancies. *J Reprod Med* 40:427–430, 1995.

115. Zimmer & Bronshtein In: *Transvaginal Sonography of the Normal and Abnormal Fetus* Bronshtein & Zimmer eds. New York: Parthenon Publishing, 2001:48–50.

116. DiSantis DJ, Scatarige JC, Kemp G, et al.: A prospective evaluation of transvaginal sonography for detection of ovarian disease. *Am J Roentgenol* 161:91–94, 1993.

117. Rottem S, Thaler I, Goldstein SR, et al.: Transvaginal sonographic technique: Targeted organ scanning without resorting to "planes." *J Clin Ultrasound* 18:243–247, 1990.

118. Filly In: *Ultrasonography in Obstetrics and Gynecology* (eds Callen) Philadelphia, PA: WB Saunders, 1988:19–46.

119. Fossum GT, Davajan V, Kletzky OA. Early detection of pregnancy with transvaginal ultrasound. *Fertil Steril* 49:788–791, 1988.

120. Keith SC, London SN, Weitzman GA, et al.: Serial transvaginal ultrasound scans and beta-human chorionic gonadotropin levels in early singleton and multiple pregnancies. *Fertil Steril* 59:1007–1010, 1993.

121. Nyberg DA, Mack LA, Harvey D, Wang K: Value of the yolk sac in evaluating early pregnancies. *J Ultrasound Med* 7:129–135, 1988.

122. Pellicer A, Calatayud C, Miró F, et al.: Comparison of implantation and early development of human embryos fertilized in vitro versus in vivo using transvaginal ultrasound. *J Ultrasound Med* 10:31–35, 1991.

123. Sengoku K, Tamate K, Ishikawa M, et al.: [Transvaginal ultrasonographic findings and hCG levels in early intrauterine pregnancies]. *Nippon Sanka Fujinka Gakkai Zasshi* 43:535–540, 1991.

124. Yeh HC, Goodman JD, Carr L, Rabinowitz JG: Intradecidual sign: A US criterion of early intrauterine pregnancy. *Radiology* 161:463–467, 1986.

125. Laing FC, Brown DL, Price JF, et al.: Intradecidual sign: Is it effective in diagnosis of an early intrauterine pregnancy? *Radiology* 204:655–660, 1997.

126. Dillon EH, Feyock AL, Taylor KJ: Pseudogestational sacs: Doppler US differentiation from normal or abnormal intrauterine pregnancies. *Radiology* 176:359–364, 1990.

127. Nyberg DA, Laing FC, Filly RA, et al.: Ultrasonographic differentiation of the gestational sac of early intrauterine pregnancy from the pseudogestational sac of ectopic pregnancy. *Radiology* 146:755–759, 1983.

128. Bradley WG, Fiske CE, Filly RA: The double sac sign of early intrauterine pregnancy: Use in exclusion of ectopic pregnancy. *Radiology* 143:223–226, 1982.

129. Parvey HR, Dubinsky TJ, Johnston DA, Maklad NF: The chorionic rim and low-impedance intrauterine arterial flow in the diagnosis of early intrauterine pregnancy: Evaluation of efficacy. *Am J Roentgenol* 167:1479–1485, 1996.

130. Stampone C, Nicotra M, Muttinelli C, Cosmi EV: Transvaginal sonography of the yolk sac in normal and abnormal pregnancy. *J Clin Ultrasound* 24:3–9, 1996.

131. Kurtz In: *Ultrasonography in Obstetrics and Gynecology: A Practical Approach* Benson, Arger & Bluth eds. New York: Thieme, 2000:112–121.

132. Fleischer AC, Pennell RG, McKee MS, et al.: Ectopic pregnancy: Features at transvaginal sonography. *Radiology* 174:375–378, 1990.

133. Nyberg DA, Mack LA, Jeffrey RB, Laing FC: Endovaginal sonographic evaluation of ectopic pregnancy: A prospective study. *Am J Roentgenol* 149:1181–1186, 1987.

134. Nyberg DA, Hughes MP, Mack LA, Wang KY: Extrauterine findings of ectopic pregnancy of transvaginal US: Importance of echogenic fluid. *Radiology* 178:823–826, 1991.

135. Dart R, McLean SA, Dart L: Isolated fluid in the cul-de-sac: How well does it predict ectopic pregnancy? *Am J Emerg Med* 20:1–4, 2002.

136. Russell SA, Filly RA, Damato N: Sonographic diagnosis of ectopic pregnancy with endovaginal probes: What really has changed? *J Ultrasound Med* 12:145–151, 1993.

137. Frates MC, Brown DL, Doubilet PM, Hornstein MD: Tubal rupture in patients with ectopic pregnancy: Diagnosis with transvaginal US. *Radiology* 191:769–772, 1994.

138. Abrams BJ, Sukumvanich P, Seibel R, et al.: Ultrasound for the detection of intraperitoneal fluid: The role of Trendelenburg positioning. *Am J Emerg Med* 17:117–120, 1999.

139. Taylor KJ, Ramos IM, Feyock AL, et al.: Ectopic pregnancy: Duplex Doppler evaluation. *Radiology* 173:93–97, 1989.

140. Achiron R, Goldenberg M, Lipitz S, et al.: Transvaginal Doppler sonography for detecting ectopic pregnancy: Is it really necessary. *Isr J Med Sci* 30:820–825, 1994.

141. Blaivas M: Color doppler in the diagnosis of ectopic pregnancy in the emergency department: Is there anything beyond a mass and fluid? *J Emerg Med* 22:379–384, 2002.

142. Ramanan RV, Gajaraj J: Ectopic pregnancy—The leash sign. A new sign on transvaginal Doppler ultrasound. *Acta Radiol* 47:529–535, 2006.

143. Kobayashi F, Sagawa N, Konishi I, et al.: Spontaneous conception and intrauterine pregnancy in a symptomatic missed abortion of ectopic pregnancy conceived in the previous cycle. *Hum Reprod* 11:1347–1349, 1996.

144. Levi CS, Lyons EA, Lindsay DJ: Early diagnosis of nonviable pregnancy with endovaginal US. *Radiology* 167:383–385, 1988.

145. Nyberg DA, Laing FC, Filly RA: Threatened abortion: Sonographic distinction of normal and abnormal gestation sacs. *Radiology* 158:397–400, 1986.

146. Rowling SE, Coleman BG, Langer JE, et al.: First-trimester US parameters of failed pregnancy. *Radiology* 203:211–217, 1997.

147. Pennell RG, Needleman L, Pajak T, et al.: Prospective comparison of vaginal and abdominal sonography in normal early pregnancy. *J Ultrasound Med* 10:63–67, 1991.

148. Doubilet PM, Benson CB: Embryonic heart rate in the early first trimester: What rate is normal? *J Ultrasound Med* 14:431–434, 1995.

149. Doubilet PM, Benson CB, Chow JS: Long-term prognosis of pregnancies complicated by slow embryonic heart rates in the early first trimester. *J Ultrasound Med* 18:537–541, 1999.

150. Green JJ, Hobbins JC: Abdominal ultrasound examination of the first trimester fetus. *Am J Obstet Gynecol* 159:165–175, 1988.

151. Lindsay DJ, Lovett IS, Lyons EA, et al.: Yolk sac diameter and shape at endovaginal US: Predictors of pregnancy outcome in the first trimester. *Radiology* 183:115–118, 1992.

152. Bromley B, Harlow BL, Laboda LA, Benacerraf BR: Small sac size in the first trimester: A predictor of poor fetal outcome. *Radiology* 178:375–377, 1991.

153. Bennett GL, Bromley B, Lieberman E, Benacerraf BR: Subchorionic hemorrhage in first trimester pregnancies: Prediction of pregnancy outcome with sonography. *Radiology* 200:803–806, 1996.

154. Nyberg DA, Cyr DR, Mack LA, et al.: Sonographic spectrum of placental abruption. *Am J Roentgenol* 148:161–164, 1987.

155. Kurtz AB, Shlansky-Goldberg RD, Choi HY, et al.: Detection of retained products of conception following spontaneous abortion in the first trimester. *J Ultrasound Med* 10:387–395, 1991.

156. Nielsen S, Hahlin M, Platz-Christensen J: Randomised trial comparing expectant with medical management for first trimester miscarriages. *Br J Obstet Gynaecol* 106:804–807, 1999.

157. DeWitt C, Abbott J: Interstitial pregnancy: A potential for misdiagnosis of ectopic pregnancy with emergency department ultrasonography. *Ann Emerg Med* 40:106–109, 2002.

158. Jafri SZ, Loginsky SJ, Bouffard JA, Selis JE: Sonographic detection of interstitial pregnancy. *J Clin Ultrasound* 15:253–257, 1987.

159. Somers MP, Spears M, Maynard AS, Syverud SA: Ruptured heterotopic pregnancy presenting with relative bradycardia in a woman not receiving reproductive assistance. *Ann Emerg Med* 43:382–385, 2004.

CHAPTER 13

Second and Third Trimester Pregnancy

Bradley W. Frazee and Chandra Aubin

Over the last 30 years, ultrasound has played an essential role in the care of the obstetric patient. The body of knowledge and expertise in obstetric sonography is now enormous. Ultrasound is the primary imaging modality for evaluation of uterine, cervical, and amniotic fluid abnormalities; placental and umbilical cord problems; and determination of gestational age, fetal congenital abnormalities, multiple gestation, and fetal presentation.[1] While some of these applications are of limited relevance in the emergency setting, certain information can be rapidly obtained with bedside ultrasound that is potentially critical to the emergency care of an obstetric patient.

This chapter discusses the use of emergency ultrasound to evaluate pregnant patients in the second and third trimesters. During this time period, the major indications for its use are the initial assessment of the pregnant trauma patient, evaluation of vaginal bleeding and preterm labor, and evaluation of abdominal pain. Emphasis will be placed on a focused or goal-directed ultrasound examination to rapidly measure fetal cardiac activity, estimate gestational age, and exclude placenta previa. Additional applications include assessment of amniotic fluid volume, cervical length and fetal position, and the evaluation of nonobstetrical causes of abdominal pain.

▶ CLINICAL CONSIDERATIONS

Confirming the presence of an intrauterine pregnancy when symptoms arise in the first trimester is now considered a standard application of emergency ultrasound. The clinical indications for performing the examination, the limited information sought, and the recommended technique are all widely agreed upon and well described. In contrast, the role of emergency ultrasound in the second and third trimesters of pregnancy is not well established. Yet, emergency physicians are frequently faced with evaluating women in the latter part of pregnancy. Pregnant women may present to the emergency department because of trauma, profuse vaginal bleeding, or severe abdominal pain. Depending on the practice setting, obstetrical consultation may not be rapidly available and patients may have had no prior prenatal care. Increasingly, ultrasound is immediately available in the emergency setting and clinicians are adept at its use. Clearly, there are a number of clinical situations during the second and third trimesters of pregnancy where a rapid, goal-directed ultrasound examination can both expedite diagnosis and improve the overall care of mother and fetus.

A discussion of the use of emergency ultrasound in the second and third trimesters of pregnancy must begin by addressing the following questions:

1. What are the standard clinical indications for emergency ultrasound in the second and third trimesters of pregnancy? In what clinical situations should emergency ultrasound be routinely employed?
2. What focused ultrasound applications are reasonable uses for the clinician?
3. For the major clinical indications, what are the goals of the ultrasound examination?
4. Are there alternative imaging modalities to ultrasound that should be considered?

What are the standard clinical indications for emergency ultrasound in the second and third trimesters of pregnancy? The concept that emergency ultrasound should remain focused, or goal-directed, helps define its appropriate use in the latter part of pregnancy. In this setting, the focused concept takes on particular importance for the following reasons. First of all, because the scope and quantity of information potentially available through ultrasound in late pregnancy is enormous, the physician performing ultrasound in the emergency setting must have a distinct, clinically relevant scanning goal in mind before placing the probe on the abdomen. It would be inappropriate, for example, to assess fetal cardiac morphology in the emergency department. Similarly, the idea of performing a screening ultrasound examination on a clinically stable patient with established pregnancy, simply to confirm gestational age or fetal well-being, may not be an appropriate indication for emergency ultrasound. Even in the hands of obstetric ultrasound specialists, the impact of screening ultrasound on perinatal outcome remains debatable.[2] Second, the medicolegal ramifications of basing clinical decisions on emergency ultrasound in the obstetric patient mandate caution. In one analysis of malpractice claims involving diagnostic ultrasound, obstetric ultrasound constituted 75% of the cases.[3] Not only should the information sought with each application be carefully limited, but ultrasound should be used only for emergency indications where the immediate benefit of the information outweighs the possibility of a missed diagnosis.

Major clinical indications for the use of emergency ultrasound that seem to satisfy these constraints include the initial evaluation of a pregnant trauma patient, mid- and late-trimester vaginal bleeding, preterm labor, and abdominal pain of unclear etiology in a pregnant patient.

What focused ultrasound applications are reasonable uses for the clinician? Several standard emergency ultrasound applications are indicated in late pregnancy and are considered safe and accurate in this setting. These include the focused assessment with sonography for trauma (FAST) examination to exclude hemoperitoneum, a right upper quadrant ultrasound ex-

amination to assess for gallstones and signs of cholecystitis, and a renal ultrasound examination to evaluate for severe hydronephrosis. In addition, the following focused applications are unique to the obstetric setting. Ultrasound may be used to rapidly visualize fetal cardiac activity. The fetal heart rate can be measured using M-mode scanning. In the second and third trimesters, gestational age may be estimated by measuring biparietal diameter or femur length. Transabdominal scanning can be used to evaluate for possible placental abruption, to exclude placenta previa, to assess amniotic fluid volume, and to ascertain the position of the fetus. Transvaginal or translabial scanning may be used to clarify the relationship of the placenta to the internal os and to measure cervical length.

For the major clinical indications, what are the goals of the ultrasound examination? In other words, given the patient's clinical problem, what clinically important question(s) can be answered rapidly with a focused ultrasound examination? For example, in a trauma patient who is comatose and appears to be possibly pregnant, the following questions could be answered with emergency ultrasound: Is the patient pregnant? Is there evidence of free intraperitoneal fluid (from hemoperitoneum or uterine rupture)? Is the fetus alive? What is the gestational age of the fetus (and might it survive in the extrauterine environment)? Is there obvious retroplacental hematoma? Figure 13-1 presents a goal-directed approach to emergency ultrasound in the second or third trimester of pregnancy based on the patient's clinical problem.

Are there alternative imaging modalities to ultrasound that should be considered? The emergence of ultrasound as the main imaging modality in pregnancy is based in part on its being considered extremely safe for the fetus. Human organogenesis largely takes place before the 10th week of gestation, when diagnostic ultrasound is often used. The absence of an association between ultrasound and fetal structural anomalies supports its safety in early pregnancy.[4] The critical period of brain development is during the 14th to 22nd week of gestation. The theoretical adverse affect of ultrasound on the fetal brain, due to production of thermal energy and cavitation, has been the topic of several important epidemiologic studies, all of which have found no deleterious effects on cognitive development.[1,5,6] By contrast, the risk to the fetus associated with exposure to ionizing radiation, particularly from abdominal computed tomography (CT), is considered significant.

For assessment of fetal well-being, alternatives to sonography include the handheld Doppler stethoscope for measurement of fetal heart tones and cardiotocography to continuously monitor fetal heart rate and uterine activity. Cardiotocography is a form of fetal assessment that simultaneously records fetal heart rate, fetal movements, and uterine contractions to investigate hypoxia.

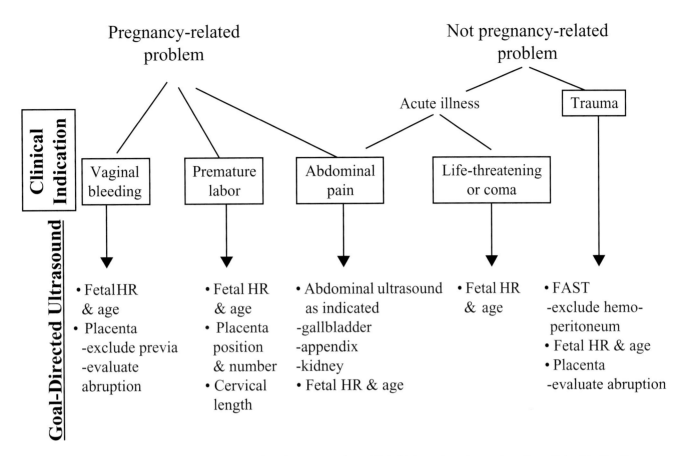

Figure 13-1. Goal-directed ultrasound in the second and third trimesters based on the clinical indication.

Cardiotocography is a sensitive, although indirect, test for the diagnosis of placental abruption after trauma, and remains the cornerstone of that evaluation. In the absence of a reliable menstrual history, a very rough estimate of gestational age can be obtained by measuring fundal height. This crude test represents the only alternative to sonography for estimating the age of the fetus if the history is not available.

For the evaluation of vaginal bleeding in late pregnancy, sonography has supplanted the traditional double setup examination as a means of excluding placenta previa. Placental abruption is usually diagnosed on clinical grounds, with the assistance of cardiotocography. Use of magnetic resonance imaging has been described in the work-up of relatively stable patients with unexplained vaginal bleeding, but it has not been widely adopted.[7]

Ultrasound frequently plays a complimentary role to the physical examination and cardiotocography in the evaluation and management of preterm or precipitous labor. Ultrasound is the only imaging modality used in this setting to assess cervical length, amniotic fluid volume, and fetal position.

Abdominal pain of unclear etiology is the single major clinical indication for use of emergency ultrasound in late pregnancy where alternative imaging modalities— such as plain radiography, CT, and pyelography—are commonly employed in the nonpregnant patient.

▶ CLINICAL INDICATIONS

The clinical indications for performing emergency ultrasound in the second and third trimesters of pregnancy are

- trauma,
- vaginal bleeding,
- premature labor, and
- abdominal pain.

▶ TRAUMA

Trauma occurs in 6% of pregnant patients[8] and is a leading cause of nonobstetrical mortality.[9] Furthermore, fetal loss as a result of trauma far exceeds maternal mortality.[10] Emergency ultrasound has the potential to play a critical role in the initial evaluation of obstetrical trauma. Use of the FAST examination to evaluate maternal intra-abdominal hemorrhage has been shown to be beneficial.[11] Because fetal well-being is dependent on adequate maternal circulation, a tenant of trauma care is that resuscitation of the mother and assessment of maternal injuries is the initial priority. Besides maternal shock, processes that contribute to fetal loss include direct fetal injury, uterine rupture, placental abruption, ruptured membranes, and premature labor. Of these, placental abruption is the most common and may occur after relatively minor trauma and in the absence of other injuries.[12] While cardiotocography and observation for the occurrence of frequent contractions remain the cornerstone of the evaluation,[8] ultrasound may rapidly confirm the presence of significant abruption, usually in the setting of a high clinical suspicion.[12] In addition, and perhaps more importantly, emergency ultrasound may be used to rapidly demonstrate fetal cardiac activity and determine gestational age.[11]

FETAL CARDIAC ACTIVITY IN TRAUMA

Fetal assessment begins with measurement of fetal cardiac activity to establish fetal viability. This step is recommended early, not only in evaluation of the pregnant trauma patient,[12] but in patients with vaginal bleeding[13] and preterm labor as well.[14] The normal fetal heart rate following the first trimester is 120–160 beats per minute. Sustained bradycardia is associated with fetal hypoxia and acidemia. Historically, in emergency medicine, fetal cardiac activity was established by measuring fetal heart tones with a handheld Doppler stethoscope.

Bedside ultrasound is an attractive alternative to the handheld Doppler stethoscope for initial detection of fetal cardiac activity. Using B-mode scanning of the gravid uterus, locating the fetal heart and assessing the presence of cardiac motion is relatively straightforward. Using M-mode scanning, the waveform produced by cardiac motion can be recorded. Fetal heart rate is then determined rapidly and accurately with the aid of obstetrics software, contained in most ultrasound machines. In the setting of significant trauma, assessment of fetal cardiac activity can be done as an adjunct to the FAST examination. Furthermore, sonography should be used to confirm fetal cardiac activity whenever cardiotocography is not immediately available, or if a fetal heart rate signal cannot be detected by the Doppler probe on this device.[8]

ESTIMATION OF GESTATIONAL AGE IN TRAUMA

Knowledge of gestational age is critical in this setting since decisions need to be made for emergency cesarean section, such as in the setting of maternal cardiac arrest.[15] In a stable trauma patient, gestational age may influence the decision to proceed to exploratory laparotomy.[11] In addition, the gestational age and fetal maturity influence the management of placenta previa, preterm labor, rup-

ture of membranes, eclampsia, and other severe medical illnesses in late pregnancy. In the setting of trauma, sonographic assessment of gestational age, along with fetal heart rate, can be performed as an adjunct to the initial FAST examination.

When assessing gestational age, the following general points should be borne in mind. By current convention, obstetric dating begins with the first day of the last normal menstrual period, referred to as gestational age or menstrual age, and is equal to the fetal or conceptual age plus 14 days. Fetal viability should be assumed when the gestational age is greater than 24 weeks. The pregnancy is considered term at 38 weeks. Sonographic estimates of gestational age are progressively less accurate (less predictive validity) the later in pregnancy they are obtained, due to increasing variation in biological size of the fetus (Table 13-1). A simple rule that reinforces this principle is that the variability (2 SD from the mean) of a gestational age estimate is equal to approximately 8% of the predicted age.[16] An ultrasound measurement of biparietal diameter that yields a gestational age of 32 weeks has a variability of ±19 days. Nevertheless, estimates based on biparietal diameter, obtained as late as 20 weeks, still outperform menstrual history for predicting onset of labor.[17] If possible, gestational age should be based on results of a formal ultrasound examination performed prior to 20 weeks, or on a reliable menstrual history. Beyond 20 weeks, use of emergency ultrasound to estimate gestational age may be necessary if there has been no prenatal care, menstrual dates seem unreliable, or when the mother has an altered mental status.

In the first trimester, crown-rump length is the preferred biometric measurement for establishing gestational age. In the second and third trimesters, measurements that are commonly used and well validated to estimate gestational age include biparietal diameter (BPD), head circumference (HC), and femur length (FL). Modern ultrasound machines generally come equipped with software that will automatically calculate gestational age based on any one of these parameters. In choosing which biometric parameter to measure, the established

▶ **TABLE 13-1. VARIABILITY OF GESTATIONAL AGE ESTIMATES***

Parameter Measured	Gestational Age Interval (weeks)			
	14–20	20–26	26–38	32–42
BPD	1.4	2.1	3.8	4.1
HC	1.2	1.9	3.4	3.8
FL	1.4	2.5	3.1	3.5

*Two standard deviations, in weeks.
BPD = biparietal diameter; FL = femur length; HC = head circumference.
Source: Adopted with permission from Benson CB, Doubilet PM. Sonographic prediction of gestational age: accuracy of 2nd and 3rd trimester measurements. Am J Radiol 157:1275–1277, 1991.

predictive validity of the parameter (Table 13-1) should be considered, and the ease and speed with which it can be obtained. A parameter that has excellent predictive validity according to the obstetric literature, but is difficult to measure and therefore prone to error, may not be well suited to the emergency setting.

In the second trimester, BPD and HC are the most widely used measurements.[16,18] Although in expert hands, HC has a somewhat better predictive validity than BPD, measurement of BPD is preferable in the emergency setting because of the relative ease and, therefore, accuracy with which it is obtained. While HC must be calculated in a particular plane, BPD can be measured in any plane, provided the line of measurement intersects the thalamus and third ventricle.[16,19] Of particular relevance to the emergency setting is a study that directly correlated neonatal survival in premature infants with various biometric measurements obtained by ultrasound shortly before birth. Based on analysis of receiver operator curves, a BPD of greater than 54 mm was the single best predictor of survival.[20]

In the third trimester, FL is a frequently used alternative to BPD for estimating gestational age.[16,21] In late pregnancy, measurement of BPD may be difficult because the fetal skull is frequently located within the maternal pelvis and obscured by acoustic shadowing. The predictive validity of FL is slightly better than BPD at this stage.[18] Femur length is relatively easy to measure because the transducer need only be parallel to the femoral long axis.[16,22]

In late third trimester, identification of ossified epiphyses around the knee represents a potentially very rapid means of estimating gestational age, and is therefore attractive in the emergency setting. Appearance of the distal femoral epiphyseal ossification center indicates a gestational age of 29 weeks or greater, whereas its absence means that the gestational age is less than 34 weeks.[23] Similarly, appearance of an ossified proximal tibial epiphysis suggests a gestational age of at least 35 weeks and that the fetus is at or very near term.[16]

ABRUPTION FROM TRAUMA

The term placental abruption refers to the separation of a normally implanted placenta from the uterus prior to the birth of the fetus. Any significant trauma occurring beyond the first trimester may potentially result in placental abruption, but particular attention must be given to victims of motor vehicle crashes, falls from height, and domestic violence.[8,24,25] When trauma results in major maternal injuries, the reported incidence of abruption is as high as 35%.

Abruption requiring emergent delivery is possible even when the maternal physical examination is normal.[12] A heightened index of suspicion is made even more critical, given the variable and sometimes subtle presentation of abruption. While the classic presentation is the triad of vaginal bleeding, uterine tenderness, and labor, patients may manifest few, if any, signs or symptoms early in their course. The evaluation may be further complicated by the presence of distracting injuries, drawing attention away from early clues to the diagnosis. Finally, abruption is a dynamic process demanding close observation and ongoing monitoring for fetal–maternal effects. A trauma-induced abruption may be self-limited or continue to evolve up to 24 hours after the inciting event.[8]

The diagnosis of abruption following trauma remains largely clinical, beginning with a meticulous search for evidence of vaginal bleeding, uterine tenderness, labor or fetal distress, the latter being the key to diagnosis. Uterine contractions are present in nearly all cases of abruption although they may be difficult to appreciate by either the physician or patient. Contractions are characteristics of high frequency but low amplitude. Pearlman et al. demonstrated that 6 hours of cardiotocographic monitoring after trauma was 100% sensitive for predicting all subsequent complications.[12] A similar study confirmed that even rare cases of late-onset abruption or fetal distress after trauma were heralded in each instance by early abnormalities on cardiotocography.[25] Hence, an absence of signs of uterine irritability or fetal distress remains an excellent indicator of maternal–placental well-being, suggesting that abruption is either absent or clinically insignificant. Cardiotocography should be a routine part of the initial evaluation of every pregnant trauma patient, even those who are asymptomatic. The stable patient without evidence of uterine irritability for 6 hours may be discharged home with appropriate follow-up and instructions. If the patient demonstrates any degree of uterine irritability during the 6-hour observation period, it is recommend that monitoring be continued for 24 hours.

As stated above, the role of ultrasound in the pregnant trauma patient remains first and foremost the assessment of free intraperitoneal fluid, fetal viability, and gestational age. Ultrasound has a limited role in the diagnosis and management of placental abruption. Fewer than 50% of sonographic studies are positive in the setting of known abruption.[26] While it is reasonable to include a rapid assessment of the placenta as part of the FAST examination, one must interpret the findings in the context of other supporting evidence for abruption. Given the poor sensitivity and specificity of sonography for abruption, any result that contradicts other clinical or cardiotocographic evidence for or against abruption must be viewed with skepticism. One scenario where the diagnostic utility of ultrasound is enhanced is that of the pregnant trauma patient with vaginal bleeding originating from the cervix, where the main considerations are placenta previa or abruption. In this setting, ultrasound can effectively diagnose abruption by excluding previa as the cause of the bleeding.[27]

Several laboratory markers are available to assist in the evaluation of potential abruption. Coagulation tests indirectly implicate abruption by showing evidence of fibrinolysis and disseminated intravascular coagulation. These markers, however, are neither specific nor sensitive for the diagnosis of abruption. The Kleihauer–Betke test, which assesses the presence of fetal hemoglobin in the maternal circulation, has been suggested as another screening test for abruption because, on average, abruption causes 15 mL of fetal blood to be mixed into the maternal circulation. Drawbacks of this test include the long processing time and general lack of prognostic value.[28] Multiple studies have shown the Kleihauer–Betke test to be of little clinical value in the overall management of placental abruption.[8,28]

UTERINE RUPTURE

Uterine rupture is a rare complication of blunt trauma in pregnancy, occurring in only about 0.6% of cases,[8] and is much more common as a complication of labor. Traumatic uterine rupture usually results from a high-energy mechanism. Uterine rupture invariably results in fetal demise; accompanying maternal mortality is approximately 10%.[8] Traumatic uterine rupture is likely to be diagnosed by emergency ultrasound during the initial FAST examination or while attempting to establish fetal viability.[11]

During labor, uterine rupture and uterine dehiscence usually occur at the site of a previous uterine incision, such as for cesarean section or myomectomy. Uterine rupture is defined as complete disruption of the fetal membranes, causing communication between the uterine and peritoneal cavities, and usually involves extensive tearing of the uterine scar and severe hemorrhage.[29] The clinical presentation of uterine rupture is variable, but often dramatic. It may include pain described as "tearing," vaginal hemorrhage, maternal shock, and loss of station of the fetus. Uterine dehiscence, by definition, leaves the uterine serosa and fetal membranes intact. It often involves only a small rent in an old myometrial scar and may cause only minor additional symptoms during labor. The overall incidence of uterine rupture and dehiscence is approximately 0.05% of pregnancies, rising to 0.8% of those involving labor after prior cesarean section.[29]

▶ VAGINAL BLEEDING

Vaginal bleeding beyond 20 weeks' gestation complicates 5% of pregnancies. It is caused by placental abruption 13% of the time and by placenta previa 7% of the time.[30,31] Placenta previa and abruption account for the vast majority of cases requiring transfusion or cesarean section, as opposed to the approximately 80% of vaginal bleeding cases that are due to early labor, lower genital lesions or remain undiagnosed. Overall, vaginal bleeding in the second and third trimesters is associated with fetal mortality or adverse outcome in nearly one third of all cases.[32–34]

PLACENTA PREVIA

In placenta previa, the placenta is implanted in the lower pole of the uterus instead of high up in the fundus; it is located either over or very near the internal os. Placenta previa has traditionally been subdivided into complete, meaning that the entire os is covered by placenta, and partial, meaning that, when dilated, the os is partially covered. This distinction, however, is usually irrelevant to the sonographic evaluation prior to the onset of labor.

Placenta previa is present at term in only approximately 0.5% of pregnancies. Yet, routine ultrasound in early second trimester has found low-lying placenta in up to 45% of patients and an apparent placenta previa in 5%.[35–37] This paradox is widely referred to as placental migration. In fact, it is due not to reimplantation of the placenta at a more superior location on the uterus, but rather to the relatively rapid elongation of the lower uterine segment, effectively drawing the placenta away from the os.[24]

Maternal risk factors for placenta previa include advanced age, multiparity, non-Caucasian race, previous cesarean section, and prior history of placenta previa.[24] Placenta previa usually presents as painless vaginal bleeding. However, pain from contractions sometimes accompanies the hemorrhage. The first episode of bleeding typically occurs in the third trimester, but may not occur until after the 36th week in up to one third of cases.[24]

The evaluation of possible placenta previa begins with transabdominal scanning since it is rapid, noninvasive, and reliable in locating a non–low-lying placenta. Also, a digital vaginal examination can precipitate severe hemorrhage in the presence of placenta previa. Ultrasound can be used to locate the placenta and exclude placenta previa prior to vaginal examination, obviating the traditional "double set-up" examination. Because its sensitivity for diagnosing placenta previa is 92%–98%,[38,39] a placenta seen to be located at or near the fundus by transabdominal ultrasound effectively excludes previa. After excluding the diagnosis of placenta previa, the clinician can then proceed to evaluate the patient for placental abruption. On the other hand, if the placenta is clearly seen to cover the entire os, particularly in the third trimester, the diagnosis of placenta previa is generally confirmed. However, when the placenta appears on transabdominal ultrasound to be low lying or partially covering the os, or if an adequate view cannot be obtained, further evaluation with transvaginal or translabial scanning is generally indicated. With the transabdominal approach, the relationship of the inferior edge of the cervix to the internal os is frequently obscured by patient obesity, an overdistended bladder, myometrial contractions, a posterior placenta, or the ossified fetal skull.[40,41] In one study of patients with suspected previa, assessment of the placenta–os relationship was impossible in 31% of transabdominal scans.[42] Diagnosis of placenta previa by transabdominal scanning has a high false-positive rate, up to 17% in one large study.[43] Nevertheless, in the case of severe hemorrhage, if findings on transabdominal ultrasound appear consistent with previa, the patient should proceed directly to the operating room. A double setup examination may then be performed in the operating room at the obstetrician's discretion.

Transvaginal sonography is a widely accepted modality for further evaluation of possible placenta previa when transabdominal scanning reveals a low-lying placenta or is nondiagnostic.[24,30] Since the late 1980s, numerous studies have documented that it is safe and more accurate than transabdominal scanning.[38,43–46] Optimal imaging is usually obtained with the endovaginal probe no closer than 3 cm to the cervix,[42] and there have been no reported cases of the procedure precipitating or worsening hemorrhage. In all but one study, sensitivity for the diagnosis of placenta previa has been 100%, where an internal os–placenta distance of less than 2 cm is taken as positive. Transvaginal scanning is able to image the internal os–placenta relationship and eliminates the majority of false-positive transabdominal scans.[43] In a study that is particularly relevant to the emergency setting, Oppenheimer et al. demonstrated that when the distance from the placenta edge to the internal os was greater than 2 cm, vaginal delivery was possible in every case. Cesarean section for vaginal bleeding was required in 7 of 8 cases in which the distance was less than or equal to 2 cm.[44] Transvaginal scanning also has the technical advantage over transabdominal scanning that the bladder need not be fully distended.

Translabial, or transperineal, sonography is an increasingly accepted alternative to transvaginal scanning.[24,47] As with transvaginal scanning, the os-placenta relationship is almost always well visualized, thereby clarifying the findings of transabdominal scanning[40,48] and a full bladder is not required. The advantages of translabial scanning over transvaginal scanning are that it is noninvasive, theoretically safer, and does not require an endovaginal probe. Translabial scanning can be performed immediately after an apparently positive or nondiagnostic transabdominal scan without changing probes. It therefore may be particularly well suited to the emergency setting

The approach to management of placenta previa depends largely on the sonographic assessment of fetal well-being and gestational age. Although cesarean section is the definitive treatment, vaginal bleeding due to confirmed placenta previa is frequently managed in an expectant fashion. The rationale for expectant management are (1) bleeding prior to the third trimester is often self-limited and can be treated by transfusion, if necessary; (2) vaginal bleeding represents little direct risk to the fetus in the absence of significant abruption or maternal shock; and (3) delaying delivery, to maximize fetal maturity, improves perinatal outcome.[24] Obviously, confirmation of fetal well-being is a prerequisite to expectant management. A rapid initial measurement of fetal cardiac activity can be performed in the emergency setting with transabdominal ultrasound, although cardiotocography is then required for ongoing fetal monitoring. Other measures of fetal well-being, such as amniotic fluid volume and biophysical profile, also may have an impact on management.

A determination of gestational age also is required to guide treatment decisions.[13] The following general guidelines have been proposed with regard to management of previa based on gestational age. When gestational age is less than 24 weeks, delivery is indicated only for hemorrhage that is life threatening to the mother. Between 24 and 34 weeks, fetal distress and life-threatening hemorrhage are indications for delivery. Beyond 34–37 weeks, delivery is indicated for significant bleeding or labor.[24]

PLACENTAL ABRUPTION

Any abnormal separation of the placenta occurring after 20 weeks' gestation is defined as a placental abruption. Prior to this date, placental separation is considered part of the overall process of spontaneous abortion. While it affects less than 1% of all pregnancies, abruption accounts for more than a quarter of all perinatal mortality.[13,24] The epidemiology of placental abruption suggests a variety of risk factors contribute to its development, many of which relate to more general microvascular disease. One of the strongest associations is with maternal hypertension, both chronic and pregnancy-induced.[49] Cigarette smoking and cocaine abuse have also been linked to higher rates of abruption.[50,51] Trauma is an uncommon but important cause of abruption.

Hemorrhage begins at the point of separation between the placenta and the uterus, or the placenta and the amnion. The timing and degree of subsequent bleeding from the cervix is dependent on the size of the hemorrhage and its location relative to the placenta. The amount of vaginal bleeding is not a reliable guide to the degree of placental abruption or the severity of hemorrhage. In 20% of cases, patients may experience no vaginal bleeding despite significant placental separation. The amount of vaginal bleeding must never be taken as a guide to degree of internal hemorrhage. Similarly, the presence of abdominal pain, considered a hallmark symptom for abruption, will be absent in nearly half of all cases.[13,24] It follows, therefore, that any evaluation of painless vaginal bleeding in pregnancy must consider the possibility of abruption.[12,24,29] The most consistent finding in abruption will be the presence of uterine irritability and contractions.[12] These may be unappreciated by both patient and physician without the aid of cardiotocography.

Because neither the character of the bleeding nor the presence of pain can be relied upon to differentiate placental abruption from previa, it is recommended that the evaluation of vaginal bleeding in the second and third trimesters always begin with an ultrasound examination to exclude placenta previa. Once previa is excluded sonographically, abruption becomes the major diagnostic consideration. The diagnosis of abruption is usually made clinically, rather than with imaging, and rests on cardiotocographic findings of uterine irritability and fetal distress. While ultrasound will show evidence of placental hemorrhage in up to 50% of cases, it lacks sufficient sensitivity and specificity to serve as a reliable diagnostic standard. Use of magnetic resonance imaging has been described in the work-up of relatively stable patients with unexplained vaginal bleeding, but it has not been widely adopted.[7]

Once diagnosed, immediate Cesarean section remains the definitive treatment for placental abruption. Decisions regarding the manner and timing of any intervention will necessarily reflect an overall assessment of maternal–fetal well-being. If the fetus is immature and the abruption is judged to be mild, an expectant approach may be attempted. Signs of preterm labor may be difficult to distinguish from mild abruption.[24] If there is no evidence of fetal distress, a cautious trial of tocolytic or magnesium therapy may be considered. Evidence suggests that such pregnancies can be successfully prolonged without serious consequence to the fetus. A term fetus or evidence of uterine irritability refractory to tocolytic therapy should prompt expedited delivery. Similarly, fetal distress or maternal signs of abruption indicate a need for immediate cesarean section.[24,30]

▶ PREMATURE LABOR

Approximately 7% of newborns are premature at birth, resulting in both mental and physical impairment.[52] Preterm labor is defined as regular uterine contractions accompanied by characteristic changes in the cervix, occurring prior to 37 weeks' gestation. The main goal of the emergency evaluation of preterm labor is assessment of the potential for premature delivery. Ultrasound plays a pivotal role in this setting, as it is a safe, rapid, and accurate method of imaging the cervix for signs of labor. In addition, ultrasound may be used to estimate gestational age and confirm the presence of a fetal heart rate. Fetal well-being may be further assessed sonographically through the biophysical profile and measurement of amniotic fluid volume. Amniotic fluid volume and biophysical profile are of potential utility in the setting of any severe maternal illness, when expectant management versus active management depends on fetal well-being. Finally, when the clinician is faced with a patient in active labor, ultrasound can be invaluable in rapidly identifying fetal lie, or the presence of multiple gestations.

CERVICAL EFFACEMENT

The primary indication for assessing the cervix in late pregnancy is to confirm the onset of labor in the setting of regular contractions prior to 37 weeks. As labor begins, the cervix undergoes effacement followed by dilation. While the digital examination has traditionally been used to evaluate such cervical change, ultrasound has emerged as a safer, more accurate means to do so.[53] Sonographic measurement of cervical length represents an objective way to quantify effacement.

There are several justifications for using an ultrasound examination rather than the digital examination in this setting. First, a direct contraindication to digital examination may exist, such as placenta previa or ruptured membranes. Digital examination in these settings can produce life-threatening bleeding or chorioamnionitis, respectively. A transabdominal or translabial ultrasound examination obviates the need for an invasive examination. Second, an ultrasound examination has been shown in numerous studies to be more accurate than digital examination in estimating cervical length and predicting preterm labor, in part because the anterior–superior portion of the cervix is located beneath the bladder, inaccessible to the examining finger.[53] Funneling (dilatation of the internal os) occurs when amniotic contents begin to protrude into the cervical canal and is one of the earliest signs of labor. Because the internal os cannot be palpated manually, this sign is assessed strictly by sonography.[53–57]

There are three methods for imaging the cervix with ultrasound: transabdominal, transvaginal, and translabial (transperineal). The transabdominal and the translabial approaches have the advantage of being noninvasive. The transabdominal approach is the least reliable, successfully imaging the cervix in only 46% of patients without, and 86% with, a full bladder.[58] Presenting fetal parts and a large maternal habitus may obscure the cervix. The transvaginal technique produces the most consistent findings, touted to result in visualization of the cervix in up to 100% of patients.[54] The limitation of this technique lies in its invasive nature and need for an endocavitary probe. It carries a theoretical risk of chorioamnionitis if rupture of membranes has occurred. Translabial (or transperineal) ultrasound is considered the most technically difficult method. In the hands of a skilled sonographer, however, this approach provides an adequate view of the cervix in up to 95% of patients.[54,59] In the emergency setting, a reasonable approach is to begin with transabdominal scanning and proceed to translabial scanning with the same probe if the cervix is poorly visualized.

From studies involving all three techniques, it has become clear that cervical measurements can predict the risk of preterm delivery. In a seminal study of nearly 3,000 women at 24–28 weeks' gestation, Iams et al. demonstrated a positive correlation between short cervical length (<30 mm) and risk for preterm birth before 35 weeks[55] (Figure 13-2). Another study of patients between 16 and 28 weeks' gestation found a 79% rate of preterm delivery in those with cervical funneling of greater than 50%.[60] Subsequent studies have confirmed the predictive value of both short cervical length and the presence of funneling, and have extended the findings to twin pregnancies.[54,57,61] For the most part, subjects in these studies were asymptomatic outpatient patients, limiting applicability to the emergency setting. Moreover, the impact of such findings on clinical management, such as the need for cervical cerclage, remains uncertain.

Using ultrasound to determine the presence or absence of cervical changes can help the emergency physician risk stratify patients with symptoms suggestive of labor. The critical cervical length appears to be 30 mm; preterm delivery becomes likely when less than 30 mm.

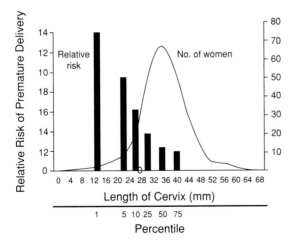

Figure 13-2. Relative risk of premature delivery (solid bars) versus cervical length, measured by transvaginal ultrasound at 24 weeks. Cervical length is expressed both in millimeters and percentiles of the normal distribution. The number of subjects versus cervical length is also shown (solid curve). (Reprinted, with permission, from Iams JE, Goldenberg RL, Meis PJ, et al. The length of the cervix and the risk of spontaneous premature delivery. *N Engl J Med* 334:567, 1996.)

Cervical sonography should be used in conjunction with clinical variables—such as results of the biophysical profile, gestational age, and history of preterm births—to influence management decisions. The goal of such an evaluation is to identify patients who would benefit from admission and tocolysis versus candidates for outpatient follow-up. The utility of cervical sonography in preterm labor was retrospectively evaluated at one facility. Women were hospitalized only if they had a cervical length less than 30 mm. This protocol produced a decrease in hospital days of 48% without affecting the rate of preterm births.[62]

FETAL POSITION AND NUMBER

Lie refers to the relationship of the fetus to the long axis of the uterus while presentation describes what fetal part is nearest the cervix. In normal deliveries the fetal lie is longitudinal and the presentation is cephalic. Transverse lie and breech presentation—where the fetal sacrum or feet, respectively, are engaged in the pelvis—are referred to as malpresentations. The classification of breech presentations is presented in Figure 13-3.

In the emergency setting, it is absolutely essential to know the presenting fetal part. Even with good prenatal care, fetal presentation is often unknown because prior to 25 weeks the fetus frequently changes position. Breech presentations, which account for some 3%–4% of all deliveries, are fraught with complications such as asphyxia, cord prolapse, and spinal cord injuries to the fetus.[63] Knowledge of the presentation allows the emergency physician to mobilize the appropriate equipment and support staff needed for delivery. In an emergency vaginal delivery, the presenting part is discovered easily by physical examination of the vagina or perineum. Prior to this point, determining fetal position by palpation may be difficult, particularly for a nonobstetrician. Moreover, when preterm labor is accompanied by vaginal bleeding or premature rupture of membranes, vaginal examination is contraindicated. In such cases, an ultrasound examination can be used to establish fetal position.

As important as the fetal position is determination of the number of fetuses. Ultrasound is invaluable in identifying the "surprise twin" prior to labor and delivery.[64,65] Perinatal death occurs seven times more frequently in twin deliveries as compared to singletons.[66] Like breech presentations, delivery of twins requires additional expertise, support, and equipment.

AMNIOTIC FLUID VOLUME

Besides providing a perfect acoustic window for the sonographer, amniotic fluid serves multiple functions for the developing fetus. It cushions, regulates temperature,

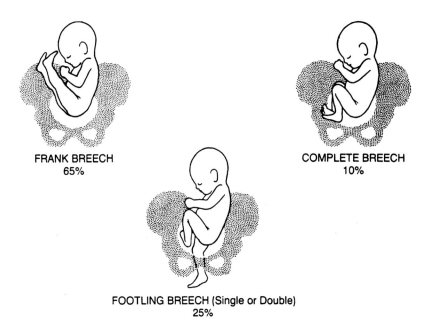

FRANK BREECH
65%

COMPLETE BREECH
10%

FOOTLING BREECH (Single or Double)
25%

Figure 13-3. Types of breech presentation. In a frank breech presentation (the most common), the thighs are flexed at the hips with the legs and knees extended. In complete breech (the least common), the thighs are flexed at the hips, and there is flexion of the knees as well. One or both hips and knees are extended in the footling breech. The risk of cord prolapse is greatest with footling breech and least with a frank breeh. *(Reprinted with permission from Callen PW. The obstetric ultrasound examination. In: Callen PW, ed. Ultrasonography in obstetrics and gynecology, 4th ed. Philadelphia: WB Saunders, 13, 2000.)*

helps prevent infection, and provides fluid and nutrients to the developing embryo. Late in pregnancy, the main source of amniotic fluid is the kidney. Thus, a normal amount of amniotic fluid is considered a sign of at least one functioning kidney. Fetal swallowing and intramembranous absorption are the main sources of elimination.[67,68]

In addition to being an important, measurable component of the biophysical profile, amniotic fluid volume is often used by itself to monitor maternal–fetal well-being. Alterations in amniotic fluid volume have been found to correlate with numerous maternal and fetal problems. Hence, some familiarity with amniotic fluid volume measurement is essential for the emergency sonographer. Like the full biophysical profile, measurement of amniotic fluid volume is most likely to be done in the emergency setting when sonographic indicators of maternal–fetal health might influence the course of management.

A number of semi-quantitative methods for assessing amniotic fluid volume by ultrasound have been proposed. Amniotic fluid index is considered by many investigators to be the most accurate measurement technique, but also the most time-consuming. It is also the most widely used by many obstetricians. For a more

rapid assessment, either the largest vertical pocket or the two-diameter pocket techniques can be used. Compared to the largest vertical pocket, the two-diameter pocket technique is more sensitive in detecting oligohydramnios. In the case of multiple gestations, the largest vertical pocket may be superior in quantifying amniotic fluid volume associated with each fetus.[68,69] In the emergency setting, any one of these techniques is reasonable and the choice will depend on the clinician's experience.

Although its significance is controversial, oligohydramnios is defined as less than 300 mL of amniotic fluid volume and can be divided into acute and chronic presentations. Acute oligohydramnios is usually due to premature rupture of membranes. The emergency provider should be aware that in these patients, a low amniotic fluid volume is associated with a shorter latency time from rupture to delivery.[68] Chronic oligohydramnios is commonly associated with postdate pregnancies, as the fetus outgrows the placenta. Uteroplacental insufficiency, often from maternal hypertension or autoimmune disorders, causes shunting of blood away from the kidneys toward more vital organs such as the brain. This results in oligohydramnios. Common fetal anomalies, pulmonary hypoplasia, low Apgar scores, and need for cesarean section have all been associated with

▶ **TABLE 13-2. CRITERIA FOR FIVE COMPONENTS OF THE FETAL BIOPHYSICAL PROFILE***

Biophysical Variable	Normal (score = 2)	Abnormal (score = 0)
Fetal breathing movements	One or more episode of ≥20 s duration in 30 min	Absent or no episode of ≥20 s in 30 min
Gross body movements	Two or more discrete body/limb movements in 30 min (episodes of active continuous movement considered as single movement)	Less than two episodes of body/limb movements in 30 min
Fetal tone	One or more episode of active extension with return to flexion of fetal limb(s) or trunk (opening and closing of hand considered normal tone)	Slow extension with return to partial flexion, movement of limb in full extension, absent fetal movement, or partially open fetal hand
Reactive fetal heart rate	Two or more episodes of acceleration of ≥15 bpm and of >15 s associated with fetal movement in 20 min	One or no episode of acceleration of fetal heart rate or acceleration of <15 bpm in 20 min
Qualitative amniotic fluid volume	One or more pockets of fluid measuring ≤2 cm in vertical axis	Either no pockets or largest pocket <2 cm in vertical axis

*A score of 8 or more is considered normal.
Source: Manning FA. Fetal biophysical profile. *Obstet Gynecol Clin North Am* 26(4):557, 1999.

oligohydramnios. Despite these associations, many investigators have found no correlation with fetal morbidity or mortality.[67,68] Present in up to 1.7% of pregnancies, polyhydramnios (>2,000 mL) is usually found at prenatal evaluation of a "large-for-dates" pregnancy. Polyhydramnios can also be divided into acute and chronic presentations. The acute form usually occurs in the second trimester and is found when the mother or fetus is very ill. Chronic presentations outnumber acute presentations 50 to 1, and can be divided into maternal (15%), fetal (13%), and unknown (67%) causes. The most common maternal cause is glucose intolerance, which leads to fetal macrosomia. Other causes are infection (syphilis, rubella, cytomegalovirus, toxoplasmosis, and parvovirus) and fetal central nervous system and gastrointestinal malformations. For the obstetrician, polyhydramnios prompts a more thorough work-up, including amniocentesis for chromosome analysis, antibody screening, glucose screening, and the drawing of TORCH [Toxoplasmosis, Other (Syphilis), Rubella, Cytomegalovirus, Herpes Simplex] titers.[68] In the emergency setting, chronic polyhydramnios is of little significance in an otherwise well-appearing patient.[68]

BIOPHYSICAL PROFILE

There are multiple noninvasive measures by which to evaluate the health of the unborn child. Traditionally, non-stress testing and amniotic fluid volume measurement have been used. The biophysical profile is a more sophisticated instrument that combines non-stress testing and amniotic fluid volume with three additional sonographic parameters—fetal tone, movement, and breathing—to derive an objective score that reflects overall fetal well-being (Table 13-2).[69,71,72] The idea behind the biophysical profile is that the central nervous system, which is very sensitive to hypoxia, controls all of the measured parameters. Thus, a low biophysical profile score may indicate either acute or chronic fetal hypoxia.[73,74] Results of the biophysical profile are always considered together with gestational age and maternal and fetal comorbidities, but in general, lower scores have increased risk of fetal hypoxia, and scores above 8 are considered normal.[72–79]

▶ ABDOMINAL PAIN

Abdominal pain arising in the second and third trimesters of pregnancy represents a significant challenge for the clinician. Besides the usual complement of etiologies, obstetrical causes of pain must be added to the list. The impact of any diagnostic or management decisions on both mother and fetus must also be weighed. The anatomic and physiologic changes of pregnancy may alter the traditional presentation of many disorders. The symptomatology of pregnancy itself may overlap with that of early abdominal pathology. Concerns over ionizing radiation or medication teratogenicity may limit choices of diagnostic imaging or therapy. All of these elements conspire to confuse the clinical picture, delay definitive diagnosis, and alter therapy, which risk higher morbidity for both mother and fetus. Ultrasound offers the safest and most effective means of deciphering these complex anatomic and pathophysiologic relationships.

Nonobstetrical causes of abdominal pain in pregnancy occur at rates similar to that of the nonpregnant

▶ **TABLE 13-3. DEFFERENTIAL DIAGNOSIS OF ABDOMINAL PAIN IN THE SECOND AND THIRD TRIMESTER**

Obstetric causes
   Labor
   Placental abruption
   Placental previa
   Chorioamnionitis
   Pre-eclampsia/HELLP
Nonobstetric causes
   Appendicitis
   Cholecystitis
   Peylonephritis
   Nephrolithiasis
   Hepatitis
   Peptic ulcer disease and reflux

▶ **TABLE 13-4. QUALITATIVE RADIATION RISK CATEGORIES AND ESTIMATED FETAL DOSE BY TYPE OF RADIOGRAPH**

Qualitative radiation risk categories	
Risk category	Dose range (mGy)*
Low	<10
Intermediate	10–250
High	>250
Fetal dose estimation by type of radiograph	
Diagnostic procedure	Estimated dose (mGy)*
Conventional radiograph	2 mGy/exposure
CT (abdomen or pelvis)	5 mGy/slice
Fluoroscopy (pelvis or abdomen)	10 mGy/min

*10 mGy = 1 rad.
Source: Mann F, Nathens A, Langer S, et al. Communicating with the family the risks of medical radiation to conceptuses in victims of major blunt-force truama. *J Trauma* 48(2):354, 2000.

population. Similarly, the need for urgent abdominal surgery appears to parallel that of the general population, once ectopic pregnancy and cesarian section are excluded.[80,81] However, the morbidity associated with virtually every abdominal emergency remains higher in the pregnant patient due in large part to the challenge of early diagnosis.[82]

The evaluation of abdominal pain in the second and third trimesters demands maintaining a broad differential and an awareness of the altered presentation of various abdominal disorders common to the emergency setting. Table 13-3 lists the more common obstetrical and nonobstetrical causes of abdominal pain, including several extrauterine etiologies specific to pregnancy. Every work-up begins with a careful history and physical examination that should significantly narrow the differential. Laboratory tests must be interpreted in the context of pregnancy-induced changes (e.g., leukocytosis and relative anemia) and are frequently of limited diagnostic value.

Sonography is the next diagnostic step in most cases and stands to substantially narrow the differential diagnosis, if not confirm the diagnosis. As an example, right upper quadrant pain in the third trimester engenders a broad differential that should include biliary disease, pyelonephritis, nephrolithiasis, appendicitis, and liver disorders. Normal laboratory tests and urinalysis would quickly reduce the list of likely possibilities to gallstone-related and appendicitis (although up to 15% of patients with renal colic may present without hematuria). Ultrasound would then be used to confirm or exclude both of these disorders while providing additional information on the pregnancy itself.

Ultrasound is the traditional first-line imaging modality for abdominal pain in pregnancy because it offers excellent anatomic and functional information about the mother and fetus without exposing either to the ef-

fects of ionizing radiation. Intrauterine exposure to radiation may have both oncogenic and teratogenic effects. Case-controlled studies of childhood cancer show a slight but significant increase in relative risk among the children of female radiologists exposed to 1,000 mrems of radiation.[81] Potential for teratogenicity and carcinogenesis appear to be greatest in the period of 2–15 weeks and decreases proportionally as the fetus nears term. In the first trimester, *in utero* radiation exposure is graded as low, moderate, and high as a function of total dose, with the clearest evidence for harm above a threshold level of 150 mGy (Table 13-4).[83] Significant variability exists, however, depending on gestational age, body habitus, and type of study. Exposure in the second and third trimesters is less critical with an estimated relative increase in cancer risk of 64% per rad (10 mGy), which corresponds to a 0.05% relative increase in rate of childhood malignancies. Fortunately, the majority of abdominal radiographic tests fall well below these threshold levels and plain radiography and CT remain viable diagnostic tools in the gravid patient with abdominal pain.[83] That said, the decision to use radiography in the pregnant patient must take into account a number of competing elements: the risk of radiation to the developing fetus, the risk of delayed diagnosis if available imaging techniques are not used, and the relative suitability of alternative imaging or management strategies. There are also the intangible concerns of mother and physician about radiation exposure that, while not supported by data, nevertheless push toward alternative imaging. The use of diagnostic radiography in the pregnant patient is often appropriate provided the risks and benefits are weighed in a manner that ensures the best outcome for the mother and fetus. Nevertheless, ultrasound assumes a position of primacy in the evaluation of the pregnant

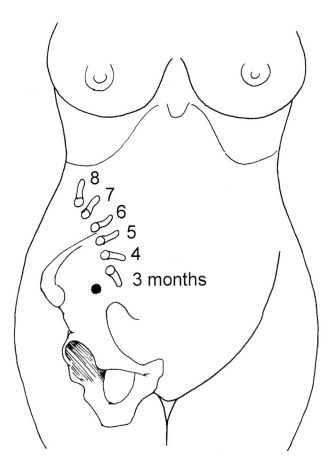

Figure 13-4. Location of the appendix during succeeding months of pregananry.

patient with abdominal pain, given its safety and unique ability to assess fetal well-being.

As pregnancy advances into the second and third trimesters, a number of anatomic and physiologic changes occur. These changes in turn alter the way a variety of common disease processes may present. The primary sonographic approach to these disorders must change accordingly. As the uterus develops, the intestinal tract is displaced upward, backward, and to the sides. Correspondingly, the appendix moves to the right upper quadrant and away from the omentum (Figure 13-4). Increased intra-abdominal pressure leads to increased esophageal reflux while the gravid uterus compresses the ureters, vena cava, and bladder.[80,81] The pregnant woman commonly experiences varying degrees of anorexia, nausea, vomiting, and back and flank pain, which are all related to the compressive and postural effects of the gravid uterus. These same symptoms, likely to be dismissed as "normal," may in fact herald a serious intra-abdominal process. Alternative presentations, masked signs and symptoms, and distorted anatomy all serve to prevent timely diagnosis and treatment in the pregnant patient.

OBSTETRICAL CAUSES OF ABDOMINAL PAIN

The primary obstetrical causes of abdominal pain in the second and third trimesters are preterm labor, placental abruption, and chorioamnionitis.[80-85] Preterm labor can often be diagnosed by history alone with its characteristic periodicity and crescendo–decrescendo pain. It is important to remember that while preterm labor is usually idiopathic, it may be in response to any general abdominal or systemic disorder. The diagnosis is confirmed with tocodynamometry. Ultrasound may play an important role in determining gestational age, fetal position, state of the cervix, and fetal well-being, all of which will help define patient management. Similar to preterm labor, mild placental abruption may present only with signs of early labor. Contractions are typically high frequency but low amplitude. Vaginal bleeding is common but may be absent in 20% of cases. Pain and tenderness range from mild to severe, crampy to constant, but also will be absent in over half of all patients. Ultrasound lacks sufficient sensitivity to confirm or exclude the diagnosis of abruption. Diagnosis and management decisions are based largely on clinical information in conjunction with cardiotocography. Chorioamnionitis refers to an infection of the amniotic fluid, typically following a rupture of membranes, or rarely as a complication of diagnostic amniocentesis. In rare cases, infection may occur without membrane rupture causing pain, preterm labor, and systemic signs of infection. Diagnosis can be made by ultrasound-guided amniocentesis.[80-85]

There are several disorders unique to pregnancy that may cause abdominal pain in rare situations. Severe pregnancy-induced hypertension is complicated by the HELLP syndrome in 5–10% of cases, which is characterized by hemolysis, low platelets, and elevations in liver function tests. Midepigastric or right upper quadrant pain may be present in 25% of cases. Spontaneous liver or spleen subcapsular hematomas can also develop, usually, but not always, in association with pregnancy-induced hypertension. Patients may experience right or left upper quadrant pain, mild coagulopathy but normal liver function tests. Hematoma rupture results in diffuse peritonitis and hemorrhagic shock. The diagnosis is often difficult since early this condition may resemble uterine rupture or abruption. Ultrasound can be useful in differentiating these conditions.[81,86]

APPENDICITIS

Appendicitis is the most common surgical emergency in pregnancy, accounting for two thirds of all laparotomies.[86,87] In the first half of pregnancy, the clinical presentation of appendicitis remains similar to that of nonpregnant patients. Thereafter, the clinical picture becomes more atypical.[87] As mentioned above, early constitutional symptoms are often subtle or dismissed as pregnancy-related. The abdominal pain is predominantly right-sided and corresponds to the right upper quadrant location of the appendix. Leukocytosis is a common but inconsistent finding and 20% of patients demonstrate a sterile pyuria. The differential diagnosis includes ovarian torsion, ovarian mass or cyst, and other sources of right upper quadrant pain, specifically cholecystitis, pyelonephritis, or hepatitis.[80,81,88]

Once suspected on clinical grounds, the diagnosis may be confirmed by graded compression ultrasound, reported to be highly accurate for the diagnosis of appendicitis during pregnancy. In one study of 45 pregnant women, graded compression ultrasound demonstrated a sensitivity of 100% and specificity of 96% for the diagnosis of appendicitis.[89] However, earlier studies found a considerably lower sensitivity of 75–89%, although with similar specificities.[90,91] These results, along with its well-established diagnostic performance in nonpregnant patients, would suggest that ultrasound for appendicitis in pregnancy should be regarded as a diagnostic test that is specific, but of limited sensitivity. A negative ultrasound examination in the setting of an intermediate or high pretest probability would demand further testing.

The sonographic evaluation of appendicitis is challenging and highly operator dependent. During pregnancy, this assessment is further complicated by the upward and outward displacement of the appendix by the growing uterus. A graded compression test is performed with additional attention paid to overall appendiceal diameter, wall thickening or the presence of surrounding fluid and debris. The specific sonographic findings of appendicitis are discussed in Chapter 8. In the third trimester, the sheer size of the uterus may preclude adequate visualization, despite a proper high-lateral approach.[89] Placing the patient in the left lateral decubitus position may resolve this obstacle.

As an alternative, abdominal CT may be considered. Although increasingly common in the evaluation of nonpregnant patients with suspected appendicitis, there are no studies describing its reliability during pregnancy. Concerns over fetal radiation exposure make any large comparison studies unlikely. Finally, laparoscopy or laparotomy may be indicated. It has been recommended that surgeons maintain a lower threshold for surgical exploration in the setting of pregnancy and possible appendicitis, given the variability of clinical signs and the increased morbidity associated with diagnostic delay. Negative exploration rates as high as 40% in the third trimester are commonplace and considered acceptable.[91] The functional absence of the omentum in pregnancy means that a ruptured appendix is less likely to be walled off, resulting in earlier peritonitis. Perinatal

mortality rises from 4.8% in unperforated appendicitis to 27.8% when the appendix ruptures.[87]

CHOLELITHIASIS AND CHOLECYSTITIS

Acute gallbladder disease appears to be slightly more common in pregnancy than in the nongravid population, which is a fact that reflects a higher prevalence of gallstones in fertile women (3.5–11%).[92,93] Signs and symptoms are essentially the same as the general population: abrupt onset of stabbing or colicky right upper quadrant abdominal pain accompanied by nausea and vomiting. While the presence of fever and a Murphy's sign suggest acute cholecystitis, mild elevations in the white blood cell count, amylase, and alkaline phosphatase can be normal during pregnancy. The differential diagnosis includes appendicitis, pyelonephritis, nephrolithiasis, and rare entities such as the HELLP syndrome or subcapsular hematoma. The pregnant patient with right upper quadrant pain should invariably undergo imaging tests to secure the diagnosis.

As in the nonpregnant population, sonography is the imaging modality of choice; its technique and diagnostic performance are essentially unaltered by pregnancy. Oral cholecystograms and HIDA scans are effective but less attractive options in the pregnant patient due to the attendant risks of radiation exposure. Ultrasound will identify virtually all gallstones.[93] The presence of gallbladder wall thickening or pericholecystic fluid is a strong sonographic indicator of gallbladder inflammation. Most patients with acute cholecystitis can be managed conservatively with IV hydration, analgesia, and antibiotics. The risk of fetal loss with cholecystectomy approaches 5% but appears to be lowest when performed in the second trimester. However, surgery must not be delayed if the patient becomes toxic or develops pancreatitis since the fetal loss rate may reach 50% in such cases.[93]

URINARY TRACT DISORDERS

The anatomy and physiology of the urinary tract are altered in pregnancy, affecting both the incidence of urinary tract infections and the sonographic appearance of the collecting system. The unifying theory appears to be increased urinary stasis due to mechanical pressure on the bladder and ureters, incomplete emptying of the bladder, and progesterone-induced relaxation of ureteral peristalsis.[94] Because of the compressive effects of the gravid uterus, asymptomatic dilatation of one or more of the collecting systems may be seen in 41%–93% of patients.[95] The right ureter is often slightly more dilated than the left. This obstructive effect may occur at as early as 15–20 weeks' gestation and persist throughout pregnancy. By 6 weeks postpartum, the collecting systems have reverted to normaly.[95]

Because of increased stasis, the incidence of urinary tract infection rises during pregnancy. This affects between 1% and 2% of all pregnant women. Pregnant women with cystitis complain of urinary urgency and frequency and suprapubic discomfort, all symptoms common to pregnancy without infection. Dysuria is less often encountered in normal pregnancy and is perhaps a more specific indicator of lower tract infections. If undiscovered, a third of cases of cystitis may progress to pyelonephritis, which present with typical symptoms of fever, chills, nausea, vomiting, and flank pain. Diagnosis is based on the clinical picture together with urine demonstrating an infection. Pyuria is present in 20% of appendicitis cases, but bacteriuria will be absent.[85,94]

Despite the higher incidence of urinary stasis and infection, there is no apparent increased risk of nephrolithiasis during pregnancy. Patients present with the usual abrupt onset of unilateral flank pain, nausea, and hematuria. It is estimated that up to 15% of nephrolithiasis will not exhibit hematuria, making this a challenging diagnosis.

Traditional imaging modalities such as intravenous pyelogram (IVP) and spiral CT do not lend themselves well to the pregnant patient due to concerns over ionizing radiation. Hydronephrosis revealed on sonography, normally taken as strong indirect evidence of a ureteral stone, must be interpreted cautiously. Similarly, a urinary tract infection in the setting of hydroureter should not necessarily imply infection with obstruction. On the other hand, pregnancy alone rarely causes marked ureteral distention (over 1 cm) and such a finding on the same side as the pain would strongly suggest the presence of an obstructing stone.[80,84,95] Ultrasound may occasionally allow direct visualization of a calyceal or uretovesicular junction stone. Patient management should be directed at relief of symptoms and a meticulous search for infection and alternative causes of pain. Most patients with nephrolithiasis can be managed successfully with IV fluids and analgesia with the eventual spontaneous passage of the stone. Rarely, ureteral stenting or basket retrieval will be needed.

ACID PEPTIC DISEASE

Reflux esophagitis is a common complication of pregnancy and may mimic a number of the more serious abdominal disorders. The increased intra-abdominal pressure and compressive effects of the gravid uterus on gastric emptying make reflux symptoms pervasive during the latter stages of pregnancy. Women will complain of episodic pain in the epigastrium, nausea, vomiting, and early satiety. Changing dietary patterns, patient positioning, and adding antacid therapy may mitigate these symptoms. In contrast, peptic ulcer disease is an infrequent occurrence in pregnancy. A reduction in gastric acid secretion and intestinal motility combined with increased mucus production during pregnancy explain this phenomena.[80,84]

▶ ANATOMIC CONSIDERATIONS

By the 13th week, or the beginning of the second trimester, the fundus of the gravid uterus is easily palpable above the pelvic brim and, by 20 weeks, it normally reaches the level of the umbilicus. Beyond 20 weeks, the distance in centimeters from the pubic symphysis to the fundus approximates gestational age in weeks (Figure 13-5). As the uterus and developing fetus grow, the intestines are displaced posteriorly, superiorly, and toward the flanks. As a result, by the third trimester, the appendix is normally found in the right upper quadrant (Figure 13-4). The growing uterus also compresses the ureters, frequently resulting in asymptomatic hydroureter, which occurs more often on the right side.

A thorough familiarity with the anatomy of the lower uterine segment, the cervix, and surrounding

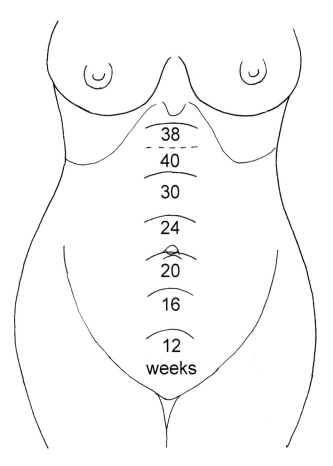

Figure 13-5. Estimation of gestational age of a singleton pregnancy by height of the fundus.

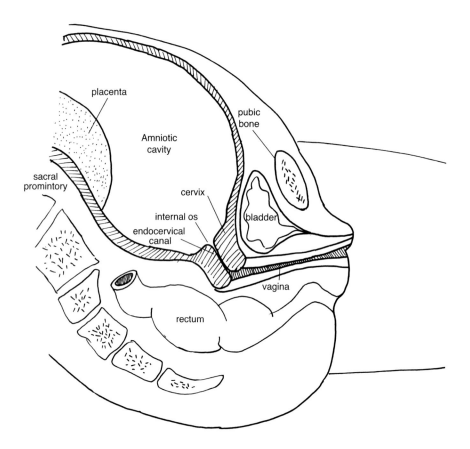

Figure 13-6. Diagram of cervix and surrounding structures, sagittal view.

pelvic structures is essential for sonographic evaluation of placenta previa and cervical length (Figure 13-6). The normal cervix is a 3–5 cm long, mouth-like structure at the uterine opening. In late pregnancy, the inner one third of the cervix, or isthmus, elongates to form the lower uterine segment. The long axis of the cervix is defined by the endocervical canal and normally it lies at a right angle to the vagina. An area of glandular tissue, which may be hypoechoic or hyperechoic, surrounds the endocervical canal. This glandular zone disappears after 31 weeks of gestation, indicative of cervical ripening, making the canal difficult to locate sonographically.[54,64] The bladder, with its echogenic wall and anechoic urine, lies anterior to the vagina and cervix. As the bladder distends, it impinges on the anterior wall of the lower uterine segment. The rectum and sacral promontory lie posterior to the cervix and lower uterus.

Understanding the sonographic appearance of placental abruption in its various forms requires familiarity with the underlying uterine and placental anatomy. The placenta is primarily a fetal organ, with its size, thickness, and texture reflecting the health and gestational age of the developing fetus. By the early phase of the second trimester, the placenta is easily visible sonographically as a homogeneous, hyperechoic rim of tis-

sue around the gestational sac.[96] The thickness of the placenta in millimeters will approximate the gestational age in weeks and rarely exceeds 4 cm.[97] By the latter part of the second trimester, the relevant anatomic segments of the placenta become more established. These include (from outside in) the myometrium, decidua basalis (endometrial–placental interface), intervillous space (area of maternal–fetal exchange), chorion (membrane that envelopes the fetal vessels), and amnion (membrane that overlies the placenta, separating it from amniotic fluid) (Figure 13-7). Fetal (umbilical) vessels course within the chorion whereas maternal (endometrial) vessels are located within the decidua.

The sonographic appearance of these layers is variable. Prominent endometrial arteries and veins within the decidua may appear as hypoechoic bands of tissue separating the myometrium from the fetal placenta, which is termed the retroplacental hypoechoic complex.[96] In the intervillous space, sonolucent pools of maternal blood, called villous lakes, can lend a heterogeneous appearance to this middle layer. The addition of Doppler in both of these cases may help determine the vascular nature of a sonolucent area. Lastly, the subchorionic segment may undergo cystic changes associated with fibrin deposition in up to 20% of patients. These echogenic, cyst-like lesions can grow to

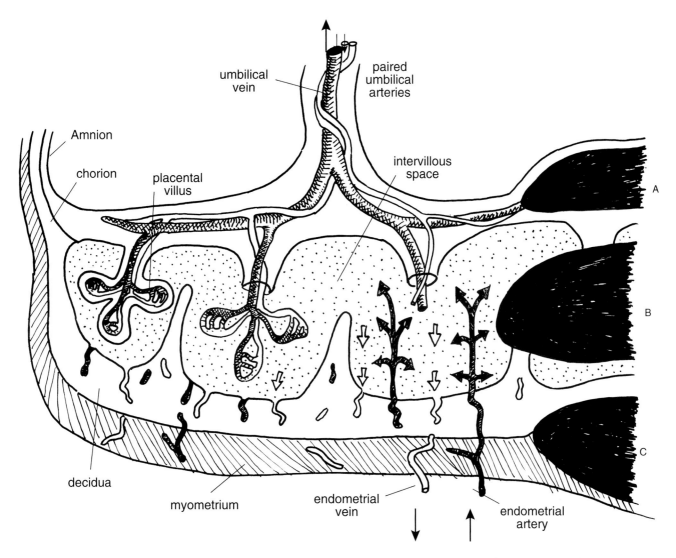

Figure 13-7. Diagram of the anatomy of the third trimester placenta. The location of three types of placental abruption is also shown: A, preplacental, B, subchoionic, C, retroplacental. (Adapted from Moore KL, Persaud TVN. *The Developing Human,* 6th ed. Philadelphia, PA: WB Saunders, 1999)

1 cm in size but are of no clinical significance.[96,97] The normal occurrence of these lesions conspire to limit the specificity of the ultrasound in the evaluation of possible abruption.

A discussion of fetal anatomy and development is beyond the scope of this chapter and has limited relevance to emergency ultrasound. Fetal anatomic landmarks that must be recognized for the biparietal diameter and femur length measurements are described in the Technique and Normal Ultrasound Findings section.

▶ TECHNIQUE AND NORMAL ULTRASOUND FINDINGS

FETAL HEART RATE DETERMINATION

Fetal heart rate should be determined by transabdominal scanning using a 3.5 MHz probe. The ultrasound machine should be set for simultaneously B-mode and M-mode recording and obstetrical measurements. Scan plane is unimportant, although fanning the probe in a plane transverse to the fetal spine is one method of rapidly locating the heart. The cursor on the B-mode image should be positioned over a clearly oscillating portion of the heart, such as the mitral valve, for several cycles. Once a continuous waveform is evident on the M-mode tracing at a depth corresponding to the heart, the image should be frozen. Finally, with the ultrasound machine set for fetal heart rate determination, the distance of one or two cycle lengths should be measured (depending on the ultrasound machines software) and fetal heart rate should be automatically displayed (Figure 13-8). Sonologists should avoid using pulse wave, continuous wave, or color Doppler, particularly on a first-trimester gestation, as these modalities transmit higher energy.

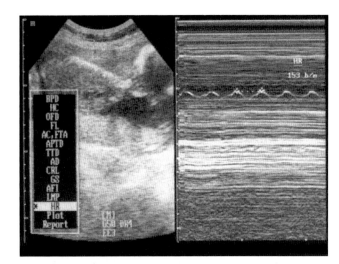

Figure 13-8. Fetal heart rate determination. B-mode image and M-mode tracing are simultaneously displayed. Doppler cursor passes through fetal heart. Cardiac oscillations are evident on M-mode tracing. With image frozen, a cardiac cycle length is automatically calculated and displayed with obstetrics measurement software.

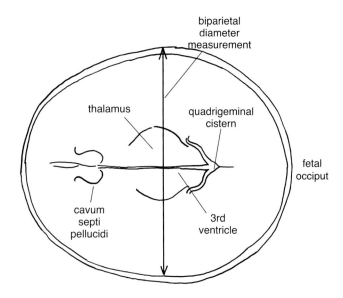

Figure 13-9. Schematic diagram of fetal anatomic landmarks used to loacate the correct plane for biparietal diameter measurement. The "arrow sign" arises from the junction of third ventricle (shaft of the "arrow") and quadrigeminal cistern (forms the "arrowhead") which points toward the fetal occiput.

SONOGRAPHIC DETERMINATION OF GESTATIONAL AGE

Biparietal Diameter

Because of its good predictive validity and relative ease of measurement, BPD is the biometric measurement of choice for estimating gestational age after 14 weeks, when it supplants crown-rump length. Determinations of gestational age during the second and third trimesters should be performed by transabdominal scanning using a 3.5–5 MHz transducer. By widely accepted convention, the BPD should be measured at the level of the third ventricle, paired thalami, quadrigeminal cistern, and cavum septi pelucidi.[18,21] Although counterintuitive, the fetal ventricles and subarachnoid space are echogenic compared to brain due to the relative prominence of the choroid plexus and pia-arachnoid matter. The junction of the hyperechoic third ventricle and quadrigeminal cistern forms an easily recognizable sonographic landmark, referred sometimes to as the arrow sign (Figure 13-9). It has been proposed that BPD be measured in any plane as long as the line of measurement crosses the thalami and the third ventricle.[19] The endpoints of measurement should be either from outer edge of the near calvarial wall to the inner edge of the far wall or from the middle of the near calvarial wall to the middle of the far wall. The near and far calvarial walls should appear symmetric. Care should be taken not to include overlying soft tissue and scalp in the measurement (Figure 13-10).[19]

Femur Length

Beyond 26–32 weeks' gestation, FL is an alternative to BPD, and may be easier to measure. Femur length is actually a measurement of the ossified portion of the diaphysis and metaphysis only, and does not include the cartilaginous portions of the bone. The endpoints of measurement are the junction of the ossified metaphysis

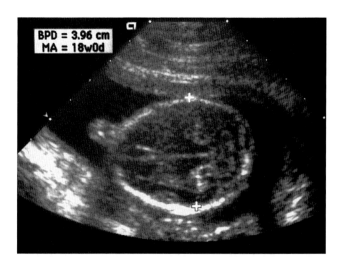

Figure 13-10. Biparietal diameter to estimate gestational age. Measurement is taken from outer wall of calvarium to inner wall (see marker cursors), in a line that crosses the paired thalami and third ventricle. In the plane shown, the cavum septi pellucidi is seen.

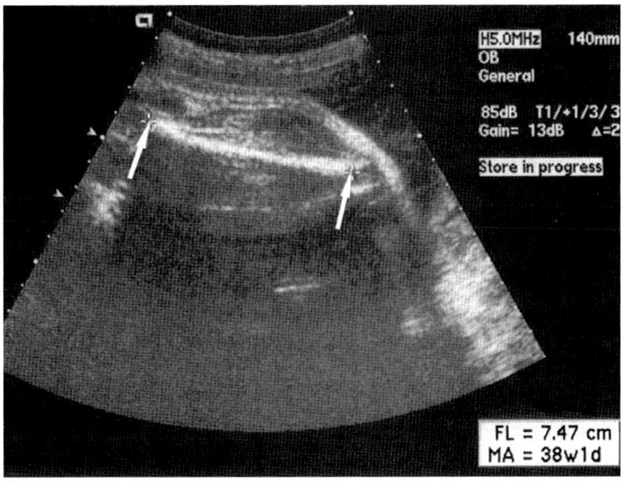

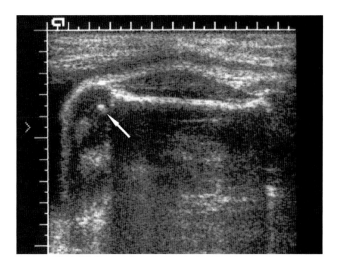

Figure 13-11. Femur length to estimate gestational age. Inclusion of cartilaginous greater trochanter and lateral condyle in the image assures proper long axis plane. However, measurement includes only the ossified (Brightly hyperechoic) portion of bone (arrows).

Figure 13-12. Distal femoral epiphesis. Longitudinal view of the femoral shaft with bent knee on the left. Appearance of a distal femoral epiphesis (arrow) indicates that the gestational age is at least 29 weeks.

and the cartilaginous diaphysis at either end. The distal femoral epiphysis, a secondary ossification center, is not included. Femur length can be measured in any plane as long as it is parallel to the long axis of the bone and includes the accepted endpoints. To avoid an oblique, falsely short measurement, the plane of section should include the femoral head or greater trochanter and the distal femoral condyle, all of which are cartilaginous (Figure 13-11).[22] Although not included in the FL measurement, the distal femoral and proximal tibial epiphyses should be sought, whether or not they are ossified (Figure 13-12).

voided. A full bladder may create a false impression of placenta previa by pushing the anterior wall of the lower uterus against the posterior wall, thereby shortening the distance between the artificially long cervix and the placenta (Figure 13-14). Myometrial contractions, which in the second trimester may not be felt by the mother, also may result in a false-positive diagnosis of previa. A myometrial thickness of greater than 2 cm is suggestive of a contraction.[96] Repeat scanning in 20–30 minutes has been suggested to avoid a false-positive diagnosis of previa due to contractions; however, this option may be unrealistic in the emergency setting. In cases where the

LOCATION OF THE PLACENTA

Transabdominal Approach

To exclude placenta previa, the sonographic evaluation of vaginal bleeding should begin with transabdominal scanning using a 3.5–5.0 MHz transducer. The placenta should be located and scanned in a sagittal plane to determine whether it extends into the lower uterine segment (Figure 13-13). If so, transverse and oblique scans should be performed to determine whether it is centrally or laterally located. When the placenta is low lying, measurement of the os placenta distance by transabdominal ultrasound is often difficult because the endocervical and inferior placental edge are not in the same sagittal plane.[98]

The bladder should be full to best visualize the lower uterine segment and internal os. However, if the placenta appears to approach the os with the bladder full, scanning should be repeated after the patient has

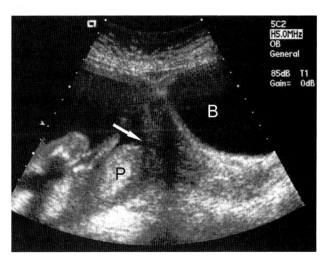

Figure 13-13. Posterior marginal placenta previa (P). Transabdominal approach, sagittal plane. The endocervical canal (arrow) is obscured by edge artifact emanating from the bladder (B).

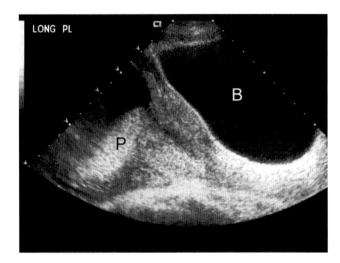

Figure 13-14. Posterior marginal placenta previa (P). Transabdominal approach, sagittal plane. In this case, an overdistended bladder (B) may be compressing the lower uterine segment, causing a false positive impression of previa.

fetal presenting part obscures the region of the internal os, an attempt can be made to manually elevate the fetus by placing the patient in the Trendelenburg position and applying sustained pressure on the lower abdominal segment on either side of the midline.

Transvaginal Approach

Transvaginal or translabial sonography should be employed to clarify the internal os–placenta relationship when transabdominal scanning is nondiagnostic. The main contraindication to these techniques is ruptured or bulging membranes.[96] Transvaginal ultrasound is considered safe in the setting of second and third trimester bleeding because optimal images usually are obtained with the probe inserted only about 2.5 cm beyond the introitus and no closer than 3 cm to the cervix.[44,45] Also, the angle between the probe and the cervix is usually sufficient to prevent the probe from inadvertently slipping into the cervix. The technique should be performed using a 5.0–7.5 MHz endovaginal probe covered by scanning medium and a sterile condom. The examination should begin with sagittal scanning and the probe subsequently can be rotated and its angle changed to gain a longitudinal view of the placenta and fully image its inferior edge. Care should be taken to thoroughly investigate the lateral walls of the uterus. If the inferior placental edge appears near the internal os, the os–placental distance should be measured. To do so, the endocervical canal, which appears sonographically as a faint, hyperechoic or hypoechoic line, must first be located. The internal os is assumed to be located at the junction of endocervical canal and the anterior cervical wall.

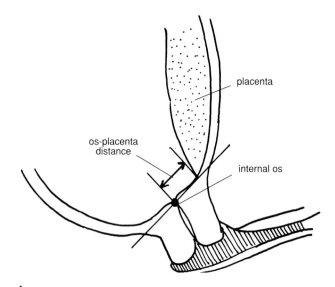

A

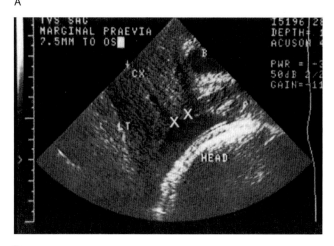

B

Figure 13-15. (A) Diagram of measurement of os-placental distance. (B) Transvaginal ultrasound of os-placental distance. *(Reprinted with permission from Cunningham et al. Williams Obstetrics, 21st ed. New York: McGraw-Hill, 2001.)*

The probe should be angled and rotated until the imaging plane contains both the os and the lowest part of the placenta, at which point the image should be frozen and a measurement taken (Figure 13-15).

Translabial Approach

A translabial (or transperineal) ultrasound examination is performed using a 3.5–5.0 MHz transducer to which scanning medium is applied, then a sterile cover, and finally a thin layer of sterile jelly over the cover. If available, a phased array transducer with a small footprint is preferable. The bladder should be empty. The probe should be placed over or between the labia majora, posterior to the urethra and anterior to the vaginal introitus.

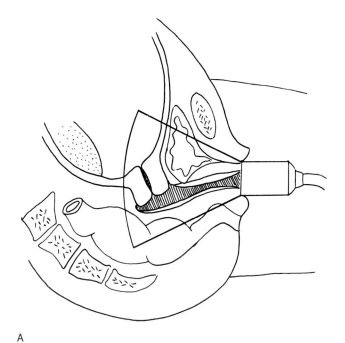

A

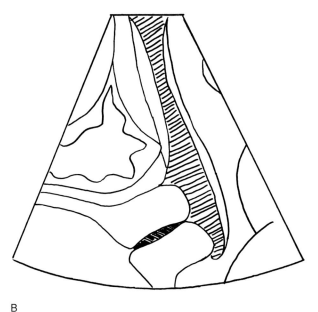

B

Figure 13-16. Diagram of translabial ultrasound of the cervix and **low lying placenta** (A). Image acquistion in the sagittal plane and standard image projection are shown (B).

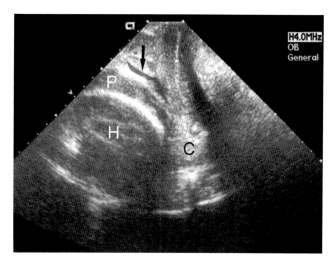

Figure 13-17. Translabial ultrsound showing the fetal head (H) overlying internal os and a low lying placenta (P). The bladder is collapsed (arrow) and the vaginal stripe is seen beetween the transducer and cervix (black C).

measured. In addition, it has been proposed that previa can be excluded by translabial scanning when a fetal part is visualized directly adjacent to the cervix or when the cervix is separated from a fetal part only by amniotic fluid without intervening placental tissue.[43]

CERVICAL LENGTH ASSESSMENT

The three scanning approaches available for measuring cervical length—transabdominal, transvaginal, and translabial—are essentially identical to those described above for assessing placenta previa. The transabdominal approach tends to suffer from various impediments to visualizing the entire cervix, such as large maternal habitus, intervening presenting part, or a shadow from the bony pubis. A distended bladder provides an advantageous acoustic window, but may create an artificially lengthened cervix by pushing the anterior wall of the lower uterine segment against the posterior wall (Figure 13-18). If transabdominal scanning fails to provide an adequate view of the cervix, transvaginal or translabial scanning is required.

The translabial approach to measuring cervical length generally requires more experience to perform because proper image acquisition and interpretation are somewhat difficult. With the presenting part toward the left on the monitor, the imaging plane should be adjusted so that the vagina courses directly away from the transducer between the bladder and the rectum. The cervical canal is normally at a right angle to the vagina (Figure 13-19).[59] In translabial scanning, rectal gas can obscure the distal cervix and the pubic symphysis may obscure

Scanning should be performed in a sagittal plane, with the bladder to the left on the monitor (Figures 13-16 and 13-17). Once the cervical os and placenta are visualized, the transducer should be angled laterally to image the entire surface of the cervix and lateral walls of the lower uterine segment.

When a low-lying placenta is encountered by translabial scanning, the os–placenta distance should be

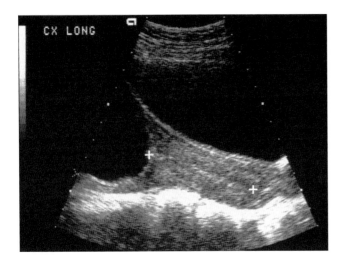

Figure 13-18. Normal cervical length measurement, taken from external os to interal os (see cursors). Transabdominal approach, sagittal plane.

the proximal cervix.[54,64] A left-side down decubitus position and partially full bladder may facilitate imaging. Translabial scanning of the cervix is particularly difficult prior to 20 weeks or with a posteriorly directed cervix.[54]

Regardless of the approach employed, cervical measurements are made in a sagittal plane, from internal os to external os. The first task should be to locate the endocervical canal, which may appear hypo- or hyperechoic. The internal os is located at the junction of the endocervical canal and the anterior cervical wall. To locate the external os, the anterior and posterior lips of the cervix should be visualized (Figure 13-18). The cervix is a dynamic organ, and thus should be observed for

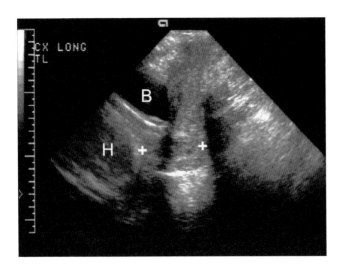

Figure 13-19. Normal cervical length measurement (5 cm by cursors), translabial approach, sagittal plane. The vaginal canal is visualized in the near field and the cervix lies at right angle to the vaginal canal. B = bladder; H = fetal head.

3–5 minutes before any measurements are made.[54,64] In general, the shortest cervical length should be recorded. This measurement will provide a conservative estimate of risk of preterm delivery. The normal cervix measures between 2.9 and 5 cm in length.[99] At the same time as cervical length is measured, an assessment of any cervical funneling should be made.

FETAL POSITION AND NUMBER

While usually straightforward, assessment of fetal number and position by bedside sonography should be performed systematically and carefully. Not only does the recognition of breech presentation or twins have important management ramifications, but also correctly interpreting sonographic images of a moving, near term fetus can be difficult. Position should be documented using the maternal bladder as the reference point.[64] The presenting part should be scrutinized in multiple imaging planes to confirm cephalic or breech presentation versus transverse lie. It may be helpful to deliberately scan the fetal spine in both a long axis and transverse plane (Figure 13-20). In the case of an established breech presentation, an attempt should be made to characterize it as frank, complete, or footling breech (Figure 13-3). To avoid missing a multiple gestation, the clinician should systematically interrogate the entire uterine cavity, making sure to image the attachment of the fetal head to the fetal body in view.[65]

ASSESSMENT OF AMNIOTIC FLUID VOLUME

There are three techniques for measuring amniotic fluid volume. A 3.5–5.0 MHz sector, convex or linear transducer is recommended for making these measurements.[100]

To obtain an amniotic fluid index, the uterus is divided into four quadrants using the umbilicus and the linea nigra as external landmarks (Figure 13-21). Fluid should be measured vertically in each quadrant, with the transducer parallel to the maternal sagittal plane. The sum of the largest pocket measured in each quadrant should be between 5 and 20 cm. A sum value below or above this range is considered oligohydramnios or polyhydramnios, respectively. If the amniotic fluid index measures less than 8 cm, the examination should be repeated three times and the results averaged. Of note, fetal movements should not affect amniotic fluid index.[96] In twin pregnancies, a separate amniotic fluid index can be calculated for each amniotic sac and the normal range is the same as for singleton gestations.[101]

For the largest vertical pocket technique, the single deepest pocket should be measured in the vertical

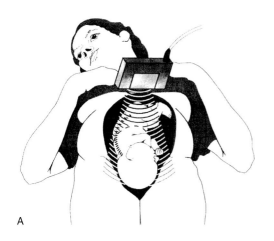

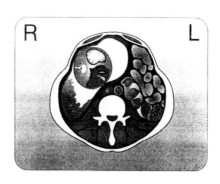

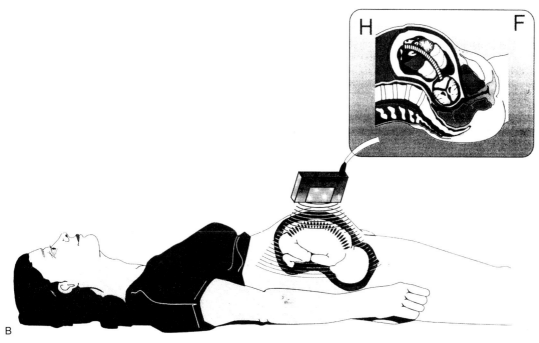

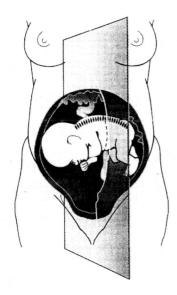

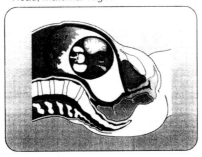

Transverse Lie
Head, Maternal Right

Figure 13-20. Sonographic technique for dtermining fetal position: (A) Transverse scan of longitudinal lie, vertex presentation; (B) Sagittal scan of longitudinal lie, vertex presentation. (C) Sagittal scan of transverse lie. (Reprinted with permission from Callen PW. The obstetric ultrasound examination. In: Callen PW, ed. *Ultrasonography in Obstetrics and Gynecology,* 4th ed. Philadelphia, PA: WB Saunders, 10, 2000)

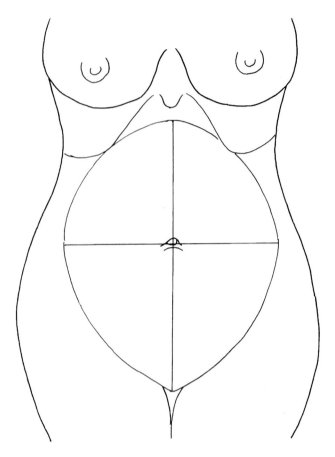

Figure 13-21. Amniotic fluid index measurement. The uterus is divided into four quadrants, using the linea nigra and umbilicus as landmarks. Measure the deepest pocket in each quadrant, scanning in the sagittal plane. Add these four values to obtain the amniotic fluid index.

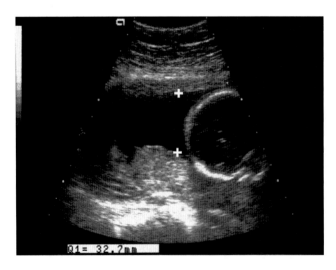

Figure 13-22. Largest vertical pocket measurement to estimate amniotic fluid volume. The pocket shown is 3.27 cm deep; 2 to 8 cm is considered normal.

plane (Figure 13-22). A value between 2 and 8 cm is considered to be normal. Both largest vertical pocket and amniotic fluid index are prone to overestimate amniotic fluid volume if the pocket measured is long but narrow (Figure 13-23).[69] In the two-diameter pocket method, the single deepest pocket of fluid should be sought, but should be measured both vertically and horizontally. The product of these measurements should be between 15 and 50 cm^2. Compared to the largest vertical pocket technique, this method is felt to be more sensitive and have a lower false-negative rate in detecting oligohydramnios.[102]

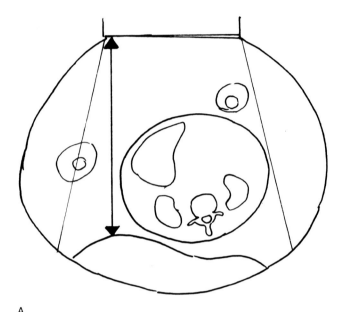

A

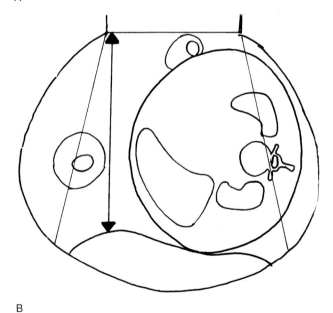

B

Figure 13-23. Diagram illustrating how vertical measurements of amniotic fluid pockets, as done in the amniotic fluid index and largest vertical pocket, can lead to overestimation of amniotic fluid volume if the pocket is long but thin.

BIOPHYSICAL PROFILE

As mentioned above, the biophysical profile involves assessment of the following five parameters, four of which are purely sonographic: amniotic fluid volume, fetal breathing, fetal movement, fetal tone, and a nonstress test. The assessment of each sonographic component is detailed in Table 13-2. In scoring the biophysical profile, each variable is assigned a maximum value of 2, giving a maximum overall score of 10. A score of 8/10 or greater is considered normal, provided the amniotic fluid volume component is normal.[70,103] Taking advantage of this scoring system, many obstetricians will eliminate the nonstress test portion because it is the most time consuming part of the assessment, requiring 30 minutes to conduct, and longer if the fetus is asleep. Eliminating the nonstress test makes the biophysical profile a fairly rapid, purely sonographic test. The nonstress test is included only if another parameter is abnormal (i.e., without it the score would be less than 8). Further modifications of biophysical profile scoring have been proposed based on the amniotic fluid volume component. For each type of amniotic fluid volume measurement, two normal criteria have been proposed: a two-diameter pocket at least 2×2 cm versus a two-diameter pocket 1×1 cm, and largest vertical pocket of at least 1 cm versus largest vertical pocket of at least 2 cm.[64,103,104]

► COMMON AND EMERGENT ABNORMALITIES

PLACENTA PREVIA

The term placenta previa refers to a placenta that completely covers the internal cervical os. When the placental edge is located within 3 cm of the internal os, it is termed marginal placenta previa. The term low-lying placenta is useful for describing the case of a placenta located in the lower portion of the uterus in which the exact os–placenta relationship cannot be defined, or for describing an apparent placenta previa when seen in the second trimester (Figures 13-13 and 13-24).

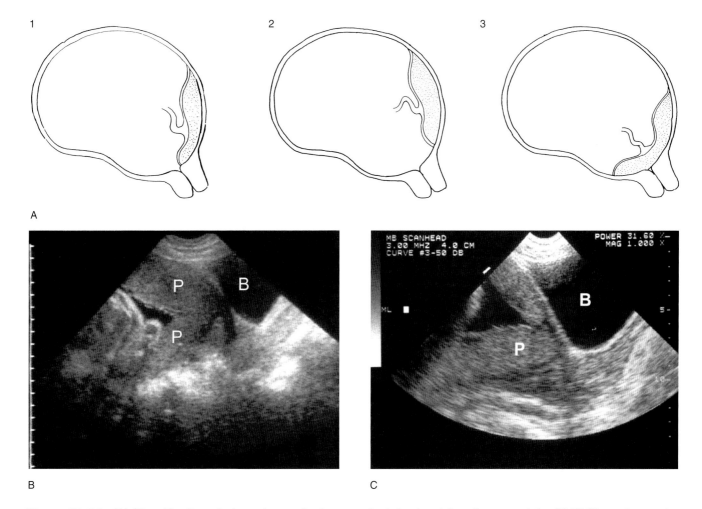

Figure 13-24. (A) Classification of placenta previa: 1 = marginal; 2 = low lying; 3 = complete. (B,C) Placenta previa. Transabdominal longitudinal ultrasound demonstrates complete previa (B) and partial previa (C). B = bladder; P = placenta. (Sonograms courtesy of L. Sens and L. Green, Gulfcoast Ultrasound)

Transabdominal scanning can exclude placenta previa when the placenta is clearly visualized in the fundus. If the placenta appears low lying by transabdominal scanning, then translabial or transvaginal scanning is often required to clarify the os–placenta relationship (see Figures 13-15 and 13-17).

PLACENTAL ABRUPTION

During placental abruption, a hemorrhage occurs within a layer of the placenta causing separation from the adjacent uterine wall.[105] This separation and hemorrhage may remain partial and self-limited or progress on to complete abruption. The clinical manifestations of abruption and its prognosis are directly determined by the extent to which placental circulation is compromised, which in turn depends on both its size and location. Hemorrhage confined to the edge of the placenta is referred to as marginal. The degree or size of placental-uterine separation is graded as mild (grade 1), partial (grade 2), or complete (grade 3) (Figure 13-25).[27,32] These categories correlate reasonably well with the clinical presentation and prognosis. Grade 1 separations are usually marginal, involve less than a few centimeters of the placental border, and are usually not clinically significant. In contrast, grade 3 abruption can be fatal to both the fetus and the mother. Abruption is further categorized by the anatomic location of the hematoma relative to the placenta: retroplacental (in the decidua basalis, between placenta and uterine wall), subchorionic (between decidua and the membranes), and preplacental (between placenta and amniotic fluid, immediately beneath the amnionic membrane) (Figure 13-7).[106] These distinctions also have significant prognostic implications, but primarily for fetal outcome. While retroplacental hemorrhage of 60 mL or more carry a 50% fetal mortality rate, similar-sized subchorionic hemorrhage translate to only a 10% rate of fetal demise. Preplacental hemorrhage is often self-limited and clinically silent, with 30% detected only after delivery.[32,106] They appear sonographically as an irregular bulge along the inner border of the placenta. Rupture of these hematomas results in the classic "port-wine" staining of the amniotic fluid.

While vaginal bleeding is considered a hallmark for abruption, its overall reliability as a diagnostic indicator is poor since it depends on the anatomic location of the hemorrhage and its proximity to the edge of the placenta (Figure 13-25). Abruption in which the hemorrhage does not communicate with the external os is referred to as concealed.

The most consistent sonographic finding in abruption is hemorrhage and hematoma, the appearance of which will depend not only on its quantity and location but also on the timing of the ultrasound in relation

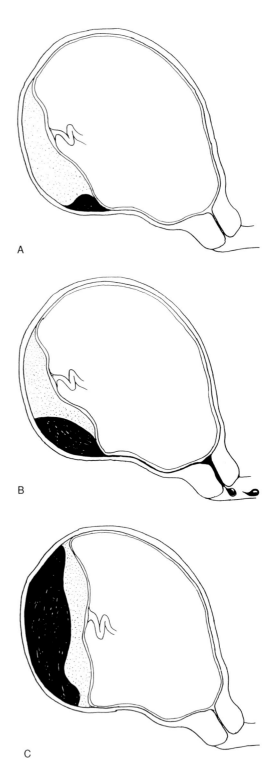

Figure 13-25. Classification of placental abruption. (A) Grade 1, mild abruption—as in this diagram, usually marginal in location. Presentation may be subtle or subclinical, affords best prognosis. (B) Grade 2, partial abruption—presentation and prognosis determined by location of separation and degree of compromise of maternal-fetal circulation. (C) Grade 3, complete abruption—worst prognosis. In this diagram, the hemorrhage is concealed by the tamponading effect of the placental margins.

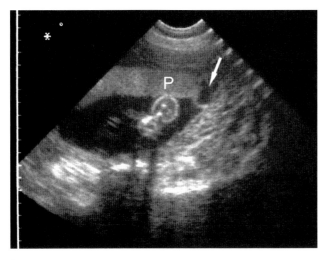

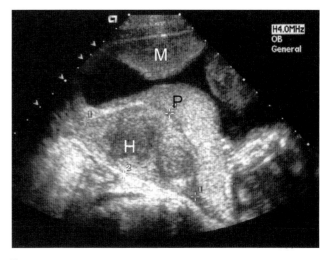

A

B

Figure 13-26. (A) Placental abruption. Transabdominal long-axis scan shows an anterior placenta with a contained marginal abruption (arrow). *(Courtesy of L. Sens and L. Green, Gulfcoast Ultrasound.)* (B) Placental abruption. Transabdominal scan, sagittal plane, demonstrating retroplacental hematoma (H) in an 18-week pregnancy. The placenta (P) is located on the posterior wall. A myometrial contraction (M) of the anterior wall is evident.

to the onset of hemorrhage. Acute hemorrhage appears isoechoic to slightly hyperechoic relative to the highly vascular normal placenta (Figure 13-26).[107,108] This is analogous to the situation of splenic hematomas where subcapsular and intraparenchymal hemorrhage may be indistinguishable from the adjacent normal spleen. Gradually over 1–2 weeks, the hematoma becomes sonolucent and more easily distinguished from the adjacent placenta. Hence, sonograms obtained 1–2 weeks after the onset of abruption may identify sonolucent hematoma not apparent on an initial study. Isoechoic hematomas may be suspected if a portion of the placenta appears unusually thick or heterogeneous in texture. For this same reason, hematomas of abruption are occasionally mistaken for uterine leiomyomas. Another obstacle to sonographic diagnosis is that acute hemorrhage may spontaneously decompress to an adjacent area or out through the vagina, such that the amount of retroplacental blood remaining is inadequate for visualization by ultrasound examination.[16,30,32]

CERVICAL CHANGES IN LABOR

Labor is heralded by regular contractions associated with cervical change. Cervical change consists of effacement of the cervix followed by dilation of the external os. The degree of effacement can be quantified sonographically by assessment of cervical length and the presence or absence of funneling. As a general guideline, a cervical length of 1.5 cm and 1 cm represents 50% and 75% effacement, respectively. Funneling is a phenomena that occurs during the beginning stage of cervical effacement,

where dilatation of the internal os results in protrusion of amniotic contents into the cervical canal. Funneling can be described by its appearance as the letters Y, V, and U (Figure 13-27).[54] As effacement progresses, the contour of the internal os progresses from a Y-shape to a V, and then to a U. Several criteria have been established that attempt to further quantify the degree of

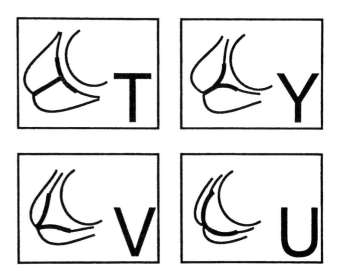

Figure 13-27. Diagram of funnel shapes described as T, Y V, U. As the cervix becomes progressively more affaced, funnel shape progresses from Y to V to U and cervical length decreases. (Reprinted with permission from Zilanti ZM, Azuaga A, Calderon F, et al. Monitoring the effacement of the uterine cervix by transperineal sonography: a new perspective. *J Ultrasound Med* 14:719, 1995)

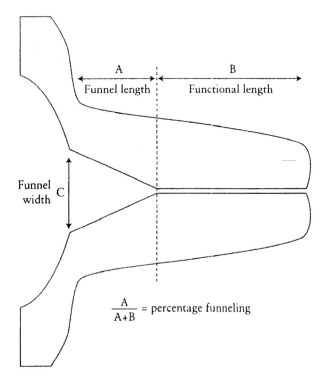

Figure 13-28. Percentage of funneling. Funnel length (A) divided by total cervical length (A + B) × 100. (Reprinted with permission from Berghella V, Tolosa JE, Kuhlman K, et al. Cervical ultrasonography compared with manual examination as a predictor of preterm delivery. *Am J Obstet Gynecol* 177:723, 1997)

funneling, including funnel length, width, and residual cervical length. The most often utilized value is the percentage of funneling, which is the ratio of the funnel length to total cervical length expressed as a percentage (Figure 13-28).[54]

NONOBSTETRICAL ABDOMINAL EMERGENCIES

The ultrasound findings associated with cholecystitis, appendicitis, and renal colic are discussed in Chapters 8, 9, and 10, respectively.

▶ COMMON VARIANTS AND SELECTED ABNORMALITIES

UTERINE RUPTURE

Uterine rupture is most likely to be diagnosed by ultrasound when it occurs in the setting of trauma.[11,29] Sonographic findings associated with uterine rupture include free intraperitoneal fluid, which may represent amniotic fluid or blood, and lack of fetal cardiac activity. In addition, the uterus may be empty, with the fetus dis-

covered in the peritoneal cavity. There are numerous case reports describing the use of sonography to diagnose uterine dehiscence during labor.[109,110] Sonographic findings include a visible defect in the uterine wall, fetal membranes intact and ballooning through the uterine wall, subchorionic hematoma adjacent to scar in the lower uterine segment, and evidence of blood layering within amniotic fluid. When uterine rupture during labor is strongly suspected on clinical grounds, an ultrasound examination is discouraged, as it may delay cesarean section.[15]

▶ PITFALLS

PLACENTA PREVIA

1. **Full bladder.** Although it provides an acoustic window, a full bladder may create a false impression of placenta previa by pushing the anterior wall of the lower uterine segment against the posterior wall, thereby shortening the distance between the artificially long cervix and the placenta (Figure 13-14).
2. **Myometrial contractions.** These contractions may lead to a false-positive diagnosis of placenta previa by thickening and shortening the lower uterine wall.
3. **Incomplete examination.** A false-negative diagnosis may result from failure to sweep the sonographic beam across the entire lower segment, thereby overlooking placental tissue that encroaches on the lateral aspect of the internal os.

PLACENTAL ABRUPTION

The diagnosis of abruption cannot be excluded solely by an ultrasound examination. The specificity of ultrasound is hampered by the common occurrence of prominent endometrial vessels, subchorionic cysts, and villous lakes. These are sonolucent or hyperechoic structures that may mimic the appearance of abruption but are of no clinical significance. Cardiotocographic monitoring is required for all patients when this diagnosis is considered.

CERVICAL LENGTH ASSESSMENT

1. **Full bladder.** A full bladder may create an artificially lengthened cervix by pushing the anterior wall of the lower uterine segment against the posterior wall (Figure 13-18).
2. **Pseudodilatation of the cervix.** A contracting lower uterine segment can produce pseudodilatation of the cervix. This can be distinguished

from true dilatation by the following findings: length of the cervix is >5 cm; the distal cervix is normal; there is thickened myometrium adjacent to the cervix; and the dilatation passes after the contraction ceases.[54]

3. **Other pitfalls.** Advanced dilatation is difficult to distinguish from total effacement. In the translabial examination, the bladder wall can be mistaken for the lower uterine segment.[59]

AMNIOTIC FLUID VOLUME

1. **Measurement errors.** Measurements may be deceptive if vertically long, but very narrow pockets are present (Figure 13-23).[69] This error may be avoided by using the two-diameter pocket method. Excessive pressure on the maternal abdomen may result in falsely low measurements of fluid depth.

2. **Improper gain settings.** Measuring a pocket containing mainly umbilical cord should be avoided. This can look like fluid, particularly when the gain is low or in an obese patient. Adjusting the gain upward or using Doppler may help identify the cord, particularly in an obese patient.

GESTATIONAL AGE ESTIMATE

The main pitfalls for gestational age estimation are failure to carefully follow the guidelines for measurement; failure to recognize the inherent variability of estimates; and measurement of femur length in an oblique plane relative to the long axis of the bone, which may result in a falsely short measurement.

▶ CASE STUDIES

CASE 1

Patient Presentation

A 31-year-old woman, who appeared to have a near-term pregnancy, presented to the emergency department after a high-speed motor vehicle crash. In the field, the paramedics had intubated the patient, obtained intravenous access, and reported a thready pulse. En route to the hospital, however, the woman became pulseless and cardiopulmonary resuscitation (CPR) with endotracheal intubation was initiated by the paramedics.

The physical examination revealed diminished breath sounds on the right lung field with ventilations, jugular venous distention, and tracheal deviation to the left. Femoral pulses were palpable only with chest compressions. There was a 6-cm scalp laceration over the right temporal area and obvious ecchymoses and abrasions over the chest wall and abdominal wall. The abdomen was tense and distended, and there appeared to be a gravid uterus.

Management Course

Needle decompression of the right-sided tension pneumothorax allowed the patient to regain a pulse (124 beats per minute) and blood pressure (105/75 mmHg). After needle decompression was completed, an ultrasound examination was performed to quickly assess for fetal viability since the patient's presenting vital signs indicated that an emergent perimortem cesarean section be considered. The patient's ultrasound examination revealed a normal uterus without evidence of a fetus; this finding was later confirmed by a negative pregnancy test. The patient's FAST examination was positive for free intraperitoneal fluid, but the patient's condition had stabilized allowing further diagnostic imaging. The patient's abdominal CT scan revealed a cirrhotic liver, a large amount of free fluid consistent with ascites, and no evidence for solid organ or intestinal injury. The patient was noted to have a left mid-shaft femur fracture. The patient was transferred to the surgical intensive care unit for orthopedic and neurosurgical consultation and further management of her injuries.

Commentary

In this case, a severely injured woman, who initially presented pulseless and appeared to be pregnant, would have been a candidate for an emergent perimortem cesarean section if there was a viable fetus of greater than 24 weeks of gestational age. The immediate use of a focused emergency ultrasound examination identified that the patient was, in fact, not pregnant and eliminated the possibility of emergent cesarean section. Free fluid from ascites is a potential pitfall for the FAST examination and is discussed further in Chapter 5 (Trauma).

CASE 2

Patient Presentation

A 30-year-old woman, G3P2, 34 weeks pregnant, presented to a small rural emergency department with severe abdominal pain and vaginal bleeding. She expressed that the pain was of sudden onset and did not feel like the contractions of her previous two pregnancies. On physical examination, her blood pressure was 140/90 mmHg, pulse was 115 beats per minute, and respirations 24 per minute. Perineal inspection revealed a moderate amount of frank blood on the sheet with no evidence of crowning.

Management Course

Intravenous access was obtained. The obstetrician was paged to come immediately to the hospital. Since digital cervical examination was contraindicated in this patient, the emergency physician performed an emergency ultrasound examination to assess the status of the fetus. Fetal cardiac activity was confirmed and measured to be 104 beats per minute. The placenta was seen in the posterior fundus and no evidence of placenta previa was visualized. The emergency physician immediately notified labor and delivery personnel to prepare for a crash cesarean section for presumed placental abruption while the patient was rapidly transported to the unit. Rapid evaluation by the obstetrician confirmed the findings, and immediate cesarean section was performed, resulting in the delivery of a live 34-week infant with Apgar scores of 5 and 8 at 1 and 5 minutes, respectively. Examination of the placenta demonstrated evidence of a severe abruption.

Commentary

In this case of a patient with third-trimester vaginal bleeding and abdominal pain, the emergency ultrasound examination revealed evidence of fetal distress and the absence of placenta previa, prompting a presumptive diagnosis of placental abruption. Advance notification to labor and delivery personnel during patient transportation saved crucial minutes from arrival to time of delivery, and likely contributed to the good outcome of the infant and mother. Cardiotocographic monitoring is also indicated and should be initiated as soon as possible when this diagnosis is considered and delivery is not immediate.

CASE 3

Patient Presentation

An 18-year-old pregnant woman presented to the emergency department with a severe asthma attack after smoking crack cocaine. The patient also complained of severe abdominal pain. She could provide only a limited history because of her respiratory distress. She had not received prenatal care and was unsure of her last menstrual period. On physical examination, the patient was lethargic and markedly diaphoretic. Her blood pressure was 150/105 mmHg, pulse was 136 beats per minute, respiratory rate 32 breaths per minute, and oxygen saturation 85% on a nonrebreather mask. She had markedly diminished air flow and faint expiratory wheezing on pulmonary examination. Her abdominal examination revealed a gravid uterus, with the fundus palpable in the mid-epigastric area. She had normal active bowel sounds, was diffusely tender throughout her abdomen,

and demonstrated no peritoneal signs. Perineal inspection revealed no vaginal bleeding, amniotic fluid, or signs of crowning.

Management Course

Intravenous access was obtained and a continuous albuterol nebulization was administered. Since the patient began to show signs of impending respiratory arrest, she was endotracheally intubated and placed on mechanical ventilation. The emergency physician performed an ultrasound examination to assess the status of the pregnancy and ordered cardiotocographic monitoring. She identified a fetus with a heart rate of 170 beats per minute and a biparietal diameter consistent with a 34-week gestation. No obvious placental abruption was seen and the cervical length was noted to be 3.5 cm without funneling. The emergency physician also did not note any signs of biliary disease. The patient was admitted to the medical intensive care unit for further treatment of her status asthmaticus and for continued cardiotocographic monitoring.

Commentary

After the airway was secured in this young pregnant woman and treatment for her status asthmaticus continued, emergency ultrasound allowed for the assessment of gestational age and fetal well-being. The focused ultrasound examination also was used to screen for potential causes of her abdominal pain, including cholecystitis and preterm labor. Transabdominal ultrasound demonstrated no evidence of cervical dilation; this information was critical for determining whether there was a need for emergent obstetrical intervention. Further evaluation by cardiotocographic monitoring was necessary in this patient to monitor for signs of fetal distress or development of uterine irritability that could have been indicative of fetal hypoxia, placental abruption, or preterm labor due to maternal cocaine abuse or respiratory failure.

► ACKNOWLEDGMENTS

We would like to acknowledge Dr. Katie Bakes and Dr. Eric Snoey for their work on the first edition of this chapter.

REFERENCES

1. Callen PW: The obstetric ultrasound examination, in Callen PW ed.: *Ultrasonography in Obstetrics and Gynecology*, 4th ed. Philadelphia, PA: W.B. Saunders, 2000:3.
2. Ewigman BG, Crane JP, Frigoletto FD, et al.: Effect of prenatal ultrasound screening on perinatal outcome. *N Eng J Med* 329:821–827, 1993.

3. Sanders RC: Legal problems related to obstetrical ultrasound. *Ann NY Acad Sci* 847:220–227, 1998.
4. Bioeffects Report Subcommittee: Bioeffects considerations for the safety of diagnostic ultrasound. *J Ultrasound Med* 7:s1–s38, 1998.
5. Stark CR, Orleans M, Haverkamp AD, et al.: Short and long-term risks after exposure to diagnostic ultrasound in utero. *Obstet Gyncecol* 63:194–200, 1984.
6. Salvensen KA, Bakketeig IS, Elk-Nes SH, et al.: Routine ultrasonography in utero and school performance at age 8–9 years. *Lancet* 62:339–342, 1992.
7. Kay HH, Spritzer CE: Preliminary experience with magnetic resonance imaging in patients with third trimester bleeding. *Obset Gynecol* 78:424, 1991.
8. Pearlman MD, Tintinalli JE, Lorenz RP: Blunt trauma in pregnancy. *N Eng J Med* 323:1609–1613, 1990.
9. Varner MW: Maternal mortality in Iowa from 1952–1986. *Surg Gynecol Obst* 168:555–562, 1989.
10. Agran PF, Dunkle DE, Winn DG, et al.: Fetal death in motor vehicle accidents. *Ann Emerg Med* 16:1355–1358, 1987.
11. Ma OJ, Mateer JR, DeBehnke DJ: Use of ultrasonography for the evaluation of pregnant trauma patients. *J Trauma* 40:665–668, 1996.
12. Pearlman MD, Tintinalli JE, Lorenz RP: A prospective controlled study of outcome after trauma during pregnancy. *Am J Obstet Gynecol* 162:1502–1510, 1990.
13. Van De Kerkhove K, Johnson TRB: Bleeding in the second half of pregnancy: Maternal and fetal assessment, In Pearlman MD, Tintinalli JE eds.: *Emergency Care of the Woman.* New York: McGraw-Hill, 1998:77–98.
14. Anderson HF: Emergency management of preterm labor, In Pearlman MD, Tintinalli JE eds.: *Emergency Care of the Woman.* New York: McGraw-Hill, 1998:113.
15. Katz VL, Dotters DJ, Droegemueller W: Perimortem cesarean delivery. *Obstet Gynecol* 68:571–576, 1986.
16. Filly RA, Hadlock FP: Sonographic determination of menstrual age, In Callen PW ed.: *Ultrasonography in Obstetrics and Gynecology,* 4th ed. Philadelphia, PA: W.B. Saunders Co., 2000:146–169.
17. Waldenstrom U, Axelsson O, Nilsson S: A comparison of the ability of a sonographically measured biparietal diameter and the last menstrual period to predict the spontaneous onset of labor. *Obstet Gynecol* 76:336–338, 1990.
18. Benson CB, Doubilet PM: Sonographic prediction of gestational age: Accuracy of second and third trimester fetal measurements. *AJR* 157:1275–1277, 1991.
19. Shepard M, Filly RA: A standardized plane for biparietal diameter measurement. *J Ultrasound Med* 1:145–150, 1982.
20. Smith RS, Bottoms SF: Ultrasound prediction of neonatal survival in extremely low birth weight infants. *Am J Obstet Gynecol* 169:490–493, 1993.
21. Wolfson RN, Peisner DB, Chik LL, et al.: Comparison of biparietal diameter and femur length in the third trimester: Effects of gestational age and variation in fetal growth. *J Ultrasound Med* 5:145–149, 1986.
22. Goldstein RB, Filly RA, Simpson G: Pitfalls in femur length measurements. *J Ultrasound Med* 6:203–207, 1987.
23. Mahony BS, Callen PW, Filly RA: The distal femoral epi-

physeal ossification center in the assessment of third-trimester menstrual age: Sonographic identification and measurement. *Radiology* 155:201–204, 1985.
24. Clark S: Placenta previa and abruptio placentae, In Creasy F, Resnick S eds. *Maternal–Fetal Medicine,* 4th ed. Philadelphia, PA: W.B. Saunders, 2000:616.
25. Curet MJ, Schermer CR, et al.: Predictors of outcome in trauma during pregnancy: Identification of patients who can be monitored for less than 6 hours. *J Trauma* 49:18, 2000.
26. Pearlman MD: Trauma in pregnancy, In Pearlman and Tintinalli eds.: *Emergency Care of the Woman.* New York: McGraw-Hill, 1998:69–76.
27. Kuhlman RS, Warsof S: Ultrasound of the placenta. *Clin Obstet and Gynecol* 39:519, 1996.
28. Towery R, English TP, Wisner D: Evaluation of the pregnant women after blunt injury. *J Trauma* 35:731, 1993.
29. Ripley D: Uterine emergencies: Atony, inversion and rupture. *Obstet Gynecol Clin* 26:419–434, 1999.
30. Scott J: Placenta previa and abruption, In Dansforth J ed.: *Obstetrics and Gynecology,* 8th ed. Philidelphia, PA: Lippincott Williams & Wilkins, 1999:407.
31. Baron F, Hill WH: Placenta previa, placenta abruptio. *Clin Obstet Gynecol* 41:527–532, 1998.
32. Ananth CV, Savitz DA, Luther ER: Maternal cigarette smoking as a risk factor for placental abruption, placenta previa and uterine bleeding in pregnancy. *Am J Epidemiol* 144:881–889, 1996.
33. Ajayi RA, Soothill PW, Campbell S, et al.: Antenatal testing to predict outcome in pregnancies with unexplained antepartum haemorrhage. *Br J Obstet Gynaecol* 99:122–125, 1992.
34. Lipitz S, Admon D, Menczer J, et al.: Midtrimester bleeding—variables which affect the outcome of pregnancy. *Gynecol Obstet Invest* 32:24–27, 1991.
35. Wexler P, Gottesfeld K: Early diagnosis of placenta previa. *Obstet Gynecol* 54:231–234, 1979.
36. Rizos N, Doran TA, Miskin M, et al.: Natural history of placenta previa ascertained by diagnostic ultrasound. *Am J Obstet Gynecol* 133:287–291, 1979.
37. Iyasu S, Saftlas AK, Rowley DL, et al.: The epidemiology of placenta previa in the United States, 1979 through 1987. *Am J Obstet Gynecol* 168:1424–1429, 1993.
38. Leerentveld RA, Gilberts EC, Marinua JCW, et al.: Accuracy and safety of transvaginal sonographic placental localization. *Obstet Gynecol* 76:759–762, 1990.
39. Harris RD, Alexander RD: Ultrasound of the placenta and umbilical cord, In Callen PW ed.: *Ultrasonography in Obstetrics and Gynecology,* 4th ed. Philadelphia, PA: W.B. Saunders Co., 2000:607–613.
40. Hertzberg BS, Bowie JD, Carroll BA, et al.: Diagnosis of placenta previa during the third trimester: Role of transperineal sonography. *AJR* 159:83–87, 1992.
41. Brown JE, Thieme GA, Shah DM, et al.: Transabdominal and transvaginal endosonography: Evaluation of the cervix and lower uterine segment in pregnancy. *Am J Obstet Gynecol* 155:721–726, 1986.
42. Farine D, Fox HE, Jakobson S, et al.: Vaginal ultrasound for diagnosis of placenta previa. *Am J Obstet Gynecol* 159:566–569, 1988.
43. Tan NH, Abu M, Woo JL, et al.: The role of transvaginal

sonography in the diagnosis of placenta praevia. *Aust NZ J Obstet Gynaecol* 35:42–45, 1995.

44. Oppenheimer LW, Farine D, Ritchie K, et al.: What is a low-lying placenta? *Am J Obstet Gynecol* 165:1036–1038, 1991.

45. Taipale P, Hiilesmaa V, Ylostalo P, et al.: Diagnosis of placenta previa by transvaginal sonographic screening at 12–16 weeks in a nonselected population. *Obstet Gynecol* 89:364–367, 1997.

46. Laurie MR, Smith RS, Treadwell CH, et al.: The use of second-trimester transvaginal sonography to predict placenta previa. *Ultrasound Obstet Gynecol* XX:337–340, 1996.

47. Doubilet PM, Benson CB: Emergency obstetrical ultrasonography. *Semin Roentgenol* 33:339–350, 1998.

48. Dawson WB, Dumas MD, Romano WM, et al.: Translabial ultrasonography and placenta previa: Does measurement of the os–placenta distance predict outcome? *J Ultrasound Med* 15:441–446, 1996.

49. Pritchard J, Mason R, Coley M, et al.: Genesis of severe placental abruption. *Am J Obstet Gynecol* 108:22, 1970.

50. Landy HJ, Hinson K: Placenta abruption associated with cocaine use. *Repro Toxicol* 1:203, 1987.

51. Ananth CV, Smulian JC, Vintileos AM: Incidence of placental abruption in relation to cigarette smoking and hypertensive disorders during pregnancy: A meta analysis of observational studies. *Obstet Gynecol* 93:622, 1999.

52. Cunningham FG, MacDonald PC, Leveno KJ, et al.: Parturition: Biomolecular and physiologic processes, In: Williams ed: *Obstetrics*, 19th ed. Norwalk, Appleton and Lange, 1993:297.

53. Berghella V, Tolosa JE, Kuhlman K, et al.: Cervical ultrasonography compared with manual examinationas a predictor of preterm delivery. *Am J Obstet Gynecol* 177(4):723, 1997.

54. Scheerer LJ, Bartolucci L: Ultrasound evaluation of the cervix, In: Callen PW ed: *Ultrasonography in Obstetrics and Gynecology*, 4th ed. Philadelphia, PA: W.B. Saunders Company, 2000:557.

55. Iams JE, Goldenberg RL, Meis PJ, et al.: The length of the cervix and the risk of spontaneous premature delivery. *N Engl J Med* 334:567, 1996.

56. Timor-Tritsch LE, Boozarjomehri F, Masakowski Y, et al.: Can a "snapshot" sagittal view of the cervix by transvaginal ultrasonography predict active preterm labor? *Am J Obsete Gynecol* 174:990, 1996.

57. Crane JM, Van Den Hof M, Armson BA, et al.: Transvaginal ultrasound in the prediction of preterm delivery: Singleton and twin gestations. *Obstet Gynecol* 90:357, 1997.

58. Anderson HF: Transvaginal and transabdominal ultrasonography of the uterine cervix during pregnancy. *J Clin Ultrasound* 19:77, 1991.

59. Mahony BS, Nyberg DA, Luthy DA, et al.: Translabial ultrasound of the third-trimester uterine cervix. *J Ultrasound Med* 9:717, 1990.

60. Berghella V, Kuhlman K, Weiner S, et al.: Cervical funneling: Sonographic criteria predictive of preterm delivery. *Ultrsound Obstet Gynecol* 10:161, 1997.

61. Mercer BM, Goldenberg RL, Meis PJ, et al.: The preterm prediction study: Prediction of preterm premature rupture of membranes through clinical findings and ancillary testing. The National Institute of Child Health and Human Development maternal–fetal medicine units network. *AM J Obstet Gynecol* 183(3):738, 2000.

62. Rageth JC, Kernen B, Saurenmann E, et al.: Premature contractions: Possible influence of sonographic measurement of cervical length on clinical management. *Ultrasound Obstet Gynecol* 9:183, 1997.

63. Fontenot T, Compbell B, Mitchell-Tutt E, et al.: Radiographic evaluation of breech presentation: Is it necessary? *Ultrasound Obstet Gynecol* 10:338, 1997.

64. Sanders RC, Miner NS: Uncertain dates, In: Sanders RC, Miner NS, eds: *Clinical Sonography: A Practical Guide*, 3rd ed. Philadelphia, PA: Lippincott, 1998:92.

65. Callen PW: The obstetric ultrasound examination, In: Callen PW ed.: *Ultrasonography in Obstetrics and Gynecology*, 4th ed. Philadelphia, PA: W.B. Saunders Co., 2000:8.

66. Benson CB, Doubilet PM: Sonography of multiple gestations. *Radiol Clin North Am* 28:149, 1990.

67. Magann EF, Martin JN: Amniotic fluid volume assessment in singleton and twin pregnancies. *Obstet Gynecol Clin North Am* 26:579, 1999.

68. Larmon JE, Ross BS: Clinical utility of amniotic fluid volume assessment. *Obstet Gynecol Clin North Am* 25:639, 1998.

69. McGrath-Ling M: Fetal well-being and fetal death, In: Sanders RC, Miner NS, eds: *Clinical Sonography: A Practical Guide*, 3rd ed. Philadelphia, PA: Lippincott, 1998:173.

70. Manning FA, Platt LD, Sipos L: Antepartum fetal evaluation: Development of fetal biophysical profile. *Am J Obstet Gynecol* 136:787, 1980.

71. Manning FA: Dynamic ultrasound-based fetal assessment: The fetal biophysical profile score. *Clin Obstet Gynecol* 38:26, 1995.

72. Walkinshaw SA: Fetal biophysical profile scoring. *Br J Hosp Med* 47:444, 1992.

73. Manning FA: Fetal biophysical profile. *Obstet Gynecol Clin North Am* 26(4):557, 1999.

74. Babbitt NE: Antepartum fetal surveillance. *SDJ Med* 49:403, 1996.

75. Garmel SH, D'Alton ME: Diagnostic ultrasound in pregnancy: An overview. *Seminars in Perinatol* 18(3):117, 1994.

76. Manning FA, Morrison I, Harman CR, et al.: Fetal assessment by fetal BPS: Experience in 19,221 referred high-risk pregnancies: The false negative rate by frequency and etiology. *AM J Obstet Gynecol* 157:880, 1987.

77. Alfirevic Z, Neilson JP: Biophysical profile for fetal assessment in high-risk pregnancies. *Cochrane Database Syst Rev* (2):CD000038, 2000.

78. Ghidine A, Salafia CM, Kirn V, et al.: Biophysical profile in predicting acute ascending infection in preterm rupture of membranes before 32 weeks. *Obstet Gynecol* 96:201, 2000.

79. Lewis DF, Adair CD, Weeks JW, et al.: A randomized clinical trial of daily nonstress testing versus biophysical profile in the management of preterm premature rupture of membranes. *Am J Obstet Gynecol* 181:1495, 1999.

80. Nathan L, Huddleston J: Acute abdominal pain in pregnancy. *Obstet Gynecol Clin North Am* 22:55, 1995.

81. Morrison LJ: Unique concerns of pregnancy, In: Rosen P,

Barken R eds.: *Emergency Medicine: Concepts and Clinical Practice*, 3rd ed. St. Louis, MO: Mosby, 1998:2327–2340.

82. Cunningham F, McCubbin J: Appendicitis complicating pregnancy. *Obstet Gynecol* 45:415, 1975.

83. Mann F, Nathens A, Langer S, et al.: Communicating with the family the risks of medical radiation to conceptuses in victims of major blunt-force trauma. *J Trauma* 48(2):354, 2000.

84. Abbott JT: Acute complications related to pregnancy, In: Rosen P, Barken R eds.: *Emergency Medicine: Concepts and Clinical Practice*, 3rd ed. St. Louis, MO: Mosby, 1998: 2342–2364.

85. Manas KJ: Hepatic hemorrhage without rupture in preeclampsia. *NEJM* 312:424, 1985.

86. Weingold AB: Appendicitis in pregnancy. *Clin Obstet Gynecol* 26:801, 1983.

87. Varner M: General medical and surgical diseases in pregnancy, In: Dansforth J ed: *Obstetrics and Gynecology*, 8th ed. Philidelphia, PA: Lippincott Williams & Wilkins, 1999: 427.

88. Lim HK, Bae SH, Seo GS: Diagnosis of acute appendicitis in pregnant women: Value of sonography. *AJR* 159:539, 1992.

89. Abu-Yousef MM, Bleichen JJ, Maher JW, et al.: High-resolution sonography of acute appendicitis *AJR*. 149:53, 1987.

90. Gomez A, Wood M: Acute appendicitis during pregnancy. *Am J Surg* 137:180, 1979.

91. Mahmoodian S: Appendicitis complicating pregnancy. *South Med J* 85:19, 1992.

92. Williamson S, Williamson M: Cholecystosonography in pregnancy. *J Ultrasound* 3:329, 1984.

93. Simon JA: Biliary tract disease and related surgical disorders during pregnancy. *Clin Obstet Gyneco* 26:810, 1983.

94. Duff P: Pyelonephritis in pregnancy. *Clin Obstet Gynecol* 29:17, 1984.

95. Fried A, Woodring J, Thompson D: Hydronephrosis of pregnancy: A prospective sequential study of the course of dilatation. *J Ultrasound Med* 2:255, 1983.

96. Harris RD, Alexander RD: Ultrasound of the placenta and umbilical cord, In: Callen PW ed.: *Ultrasonography in Obstetrics and Gynecology*, 4th ed. Philadelphia, PA: W.B. Saunders Co., 2000:597–615.

97. Hoddick W, Mahoney B, Collen P, et al.: Placental thickness. *J Ultrasound Med* 4:479, 1985.

98. Gilllieson MS, Winer-Muram HT, Muram D: Low-lying placenta. *Radiology* 144:577–580, 1982.

99. Sanders RC, Miner NS: Uncertain dates, In: Sanders RC, Miner NS, eds.: *Clinical Sonography: A Practical Guide*, 3rd ed. Philadelphia, PA: Lippincott, 1998:108.

100. Del Valle GO, Bateman L, Gaudier FL, et al.: Comparison of three types of ultrasound transducers in evaluating the amniotic fluid index. *J Reprod Med* 39:869, 1994.

101. Hill LM, Krohn M, Lazebnik N, et al.: The amniotic fluid index in normal twin pregnancies. *Am J Obstet Gynecol* 182:950, 2000.

102. Larmon JE, Ross BS: Clinical Utility of amniotic fluid volume assessment. *Obstet Gynecol Clin North Am* 25(3):639, 1998.

103. Walkinshaw SA: Fetal biophysical profile scoring. *Br J Hosp Med* 47:444, 1992.

104. Finberg HJ, Kurtz AB, Johnson RL, et al.: The biophysical profile: A literature review and reassessment of its usefulness in the evaluation of fetal well-being. *J Ultrasound Med* 9:583, 1990.

105. Gant N: Obstetrical hemorrhage, In: Cunningham FG, MacDonald PC, Gant NF, et al. eds.: *Williams Obstetrics*, 20th ed. Stamford, CT: Appleton & Lange, 1997:760.

106. Ananth CV, Berkowitz G, Savitz D, et al.: Placental abruption and adverse outcomes. *JAMA* 282:1646, 1999.

107. Nyberg DA, Mack LA, Benedetti TJ: Placental abruption and placental hemorrhage: Correlation of sonographic findings with fetal outcome. *Radiology* 358:357, 1987.

108. Nyberg DA, Cyr DR, Mack L: Sonographic spectrum of placental abruption. *AJR* 148:161, 1987.

109. Shrout AB, Kopelman JN: Ultrasonographic diagnosis of uterine dehiscence during pregnancy. *J Ultrasound Med* 14:399–402, 1995.

110. Gale JT, Mahony BS, Bowie JD: Sonographic features of rupture of the pregnant uterus. *J Ultrasound Med* 5:713–714, 1996.

CHAPTER 14

Gynecologic Concepts

J. Christian Fox and Michael J. Lambert

Female patients with lower abdominal pain presenting to the emergency department or acute care clinic may represent a diagnostic challenge. Faced with a large differential diagnosis (Table 14-1), their clinical work-up is often time and resource consuming. Bedside ultrasound is the diagnostic imaging modality of choice for the majority of cases. It provides real-time information that expedites patient care and disposition.

► CLINICAL CONSIDERATIONS

Imaging the pelvis is a crucial step in the evaluation of women with lower abdominal pain or pelvic pain. Accurate management is predicated on choosing the most effective diagnostic tool. Four diagnostic modalities are available for evaluating the pelvis: laparoscopy, computed tomography (CT), magnetic resonance imaging (MRI), and ultrasonography. Several clinical entities will be considered with regard to the advantages and disadvantages of each modality.

While CT is used routinely for the preoperative evaluation of masses that are suspicious for malignancy, it is generally considered a second-line imaging modality to ultrasound in the evaluation of pelvic pain. The advantage of CT is the ability to image the full extent of a large adnexal lesion that cannot be visualized in its entirety with sonography alone. Another advantage of CT is its usefulness in diagnosing gastrointestinal entities, such as

appendicitis and diverticulitis. A major disadvantage of CT is the cost involved in obtaining these readings. CT is not portable and is not immediately available at the bedside for serial examinations. Patients must be transported to the radiology suite, which expends personnel resources. CT exposes patients to radiation; if IV contrast is used, nephrotoxicity or severe allergies are potential side effects.

Although MRI is also considered a second-line imaging modality, it has several advantages over CT and ultrasound. MRI does not expose the patient to radiation and provides more detailed information for the detection of subtle tissue differentiation of pelvic organs. MRI has better tissue resolution than ultrasound, and is therefore more accurate in diagnosing pelvic inflammatory disease (PID) and pelvic masses. A 1999 study compared MRI with endovaginal ultrasound for the diagnosis of laparoscopy-proven PID. Of the 21 patients proven to have PID, MRI diagnosed 20 (95%) patients while endovaginal ultrasound correctly diagnosed 17 (81%) patients.[1] Many of the same disadvantages of CT—cost, availability, lack of portability—apply to MRI as well.

While laparoscopy remains the gold standard for the diagnosis of PID and pelvic masses, its use may not be readily available or justified in screening patients with vague symptoms. Laparoscopy is invasive, costly, time-consuming, results in scarring, and requires the small but measurable risk of general anesthesia. Furthermore, laparoscopy does not detect subtle signs of inflammation

▶ **TABLE 14-1. DIFFERENTIAL DIAGNOSIS OF LOWER ABDOMINAL PAIN IN FEMALE PATIENTS**

GASTROINTESTINAL
Appendicitis
Inflammatory bowel disease
Irritable bowel syndrome
Constipation
Gastroenteritis
Diverticulitis

URINARY TRACT
Cystitis
Pyelonephritis
Nephrolithiasis

REPRODUCTIVE
Ectopic pregnancy
Intrauterine pregnancy
Pelvic inflammatory disease
Tubo-ovarian abscess
Ovarian cyst
Hemorrhagic functional cysts
Ovarian torsion
Mittelschmerz
Dysmenorrhea
Endometriosis

within fallopian tubes or any findings consistent with endometritis.[2] The advantage of laparoscopy, however, is the ability to reveal other pathologic conditions that have been misdiagnosed as PID. In one study, 12% of patients diagnosed with PID revealed other pathologic findings during laparoscopy, such as appendicitis or endometriosis.[3] Another advantage of laparoscopy is the ability to intraoperatively intervene in a pathological process, such as the untwisting or resection of a torsed ovary, the drainage of an abscess, or appendectomy.

Ultrasound has proven to be a rapid, noninvasive, portable, repeatable, inexpensive, and accurate method for visualizing and diagnosing pathology within the pelvis. These advantages over CT, MRI, and laparoscopy have made ultrasound the first-line diagnostic imaging modality in patients with acute pelvic pain, PID, or pelvic masses. Ultrasound is immediately available to the physician at the bedside during the initial physical examination. This accessibility has far-reaching benefits to patient care by curtailing other diagnostic tests and pinpointing specific diseases within the differential diagnosis. Ultrasound does not expose patients to ionizing radiation. Since the clinician is at the bedside performing the ultrasound examination, patients perceive this as more time spent with their physician. This serves to improve patient satisfaction, provides them with more time to ask questions, and ultimately increases their confidence in their physician and understanding of their

condition. Another advantage unique to ultrasound is the ability of color flow Doppler sonography to evaluate pelvic organs for adequacy of blood flow.

The main disadvantage of ultrasound with respect to the other imaging modalities is its limited scope. Other imaging modalities, such as CT and MRI, may yield valuable information about other organ system pathology and the extent to which a disease process may have progressed. Sonograms occasionally may be of poor image quality due to interference from bowel gas.

▶ CLINICAL INDICATIONS

Clinical indications for performing pelvic ultrasound include

- acute pelvic pain,
- acute pelvic inflammatory disease, and
- evaluation of pelvic or adnexal masses.

▶ ACUTE PELVIC PAIN

Acute pelvic pain in women is a common complaint in the emergency or ambulatory care setting. The differential diagnosis is vast. Although life-threatening conditions such as ectopic pregnancy are in the differential, the majority of patients can be treated and discharged home. While the definitive evaluation of these patients ultimately may involve CT, pelvic sonography is the diagnostic imaging modality indicated in their initial evaluation.

OVARIAN TORSION

This entity should be considered in the differential diagnosis of any woman with lower abdominal pain (Table 14-2). Ovarian torsion is a gynecological emergency that can result in both reproductive and hormonal compromise if not promptly diagnosed and treated. Because the diagnosis is often elusive and sufficiently delayed, detorsion of the ovary is rarely an option. A twisting of the ovarian attachments through the utero-ovarian ligament to the uterus and through the infundibulopelvic

▶ **TABLE 14-2. DIFFERENTIAL DIAGNOSIS OF OVARIAN TORSION**

Appendicitis
Adnexal mass
Pelvic mass
Myoma
Ectopic Pregnancy
Tubo-ovarian abscess
Ruptured Viscus

ligament to the pelvic sidewall results in congestion of the ovarian parenchyma and eventual hemorrhagic infarction from decreased ovarian blood supply.[4] The "classic" symptoms of acute, severe, unilateral lower abdominal or pelvic pain are present only in approximately one third of the patients with confirmed ovarian torsion. Ovarian torsion is frequently missed on the preoperative diagnosis; the two most common incorrect preoperative diagnoses are tubo-ovarian abscess (TOA) and ruptured corpus luteum cyst.[5]

Torsion can occur in normal ovaries, but this would be an unusual occurrence. In general, for torsion to take place, the ovary or tube must be enlarged such as in the case of a mass or cyst as part of or immediately adjacent to the ovary or fallopian tube. These masses are thought to act as a fulcrum by which torsion can propagate. One study demonstrated that ovarian torsion was associated with palpable adnexal masses in over 90% of adults compared with only 50% of children.[6] Others reported that a unilaterally enlarged ovary with small peripherally located cysts (1–6 mm) was the most common finding (56%) in young and adolescent girls.[7] In 1985, it was reported that ovarian masses were associated with cases of torsion in only 50% of patients. Pregnancy appears to be a risk factor as well; 20% of all cases can been found to occur during pregnancy.[8]

Abnormal blood flow detected by Doppler sonography is highly predictive of ovarian torsion and is therefore useful in the diagnosis of ovarian torsion. Failure to identify arterial waveforms is highly suggestive of ovarian torsion. When normal flow is detected by Doppler sonography, it does not necessarily *exclude* ovarian torsion. In fact, ovarian torsion is missed in 60% of these cases, and time to diagnosis is therefore delayed. In patients undergoing hormonal therapy for ovarian stimulation, the sensitivity of Doppler for ovarian torsion increases to 75%.[9] Despite being intuitively similar to other organs, such as the testicle, lack of blood supply to the ovary cannot be adequately excluded using Doppler. The reason for this is twofold. First, Doppler flow may be present in one part of the ovary (peripheral or central) but not in the other due to the fact that the ovary has a dual blood supply. Second, thrombosis of venous structures produces the symptoms of ovarian torsion prior to the arterial system becoming occluded. While some authors have suggested that absent blood flow on spectral Doppler and color Doppler is specific for torsion,[10,11] others suggest that observing blood flow to the ovary should not be relied upon to definitively exclude this diagnosis.[12] Stark and Siegel reported that the presence of a Doppler signal was present in 9 of 14 patients ultimately proven to have ovarian torsion.[13]

Grayscale findings may be useful in diagnosing ovarian torsion by identifying a large ovary with enlarged follicles or an enlarged complex cystic adnexal mass. Conversely, it has been suggested that normal ovarian size and texture may be helpful in excluding this diagnosis. One study evaluated 41 patients suspected of having ovarian torsion who had undergone transabdominal ultrasound. Of the 11 patients who had ovarian torsion proven at surgery, 7 were correctly diagnosed by ultrasound. Ovarian enlargement was detected in all 11 patients. This study (albeit a very small sample size) yielded a positive predictive value of 87.5%. In the other 28 patients, sonography correctly excluded the diagnosis, yielding a specificity of 93%. All patients were followed for 63 months on an outpatient basis.[14]

VAGINAL CONDITIONS

Some gynecological procedures involve instrumentation that result in postoperative complications. These patients may present with vaginal bleeding, acute pelvic pain, and unstable vital signs. Ultrasound can play a crucial role in the timely diagnosis and management of these patients. For example, ultrasound can localize and diagnose a vaginal hematoma in a hypotensive patient who recently underwent a dilatation and curettage procedure. Typically, the ultrasound examination is performed transabdominally in an attempt to localize the hematoma within the vaginal tissue planes.

► ACUTE PELVIC INFLAMMATORY DISEASE

Acute PID, defined as an infection in the upper genital tract, represents a spectrum of disease entities, including any combination of endometritis, salpingitis, oophoritis, pelvic peritonitis, and TOA.[15] More than 1 million women are diagnosed with PID annually and 25% of them proceed to suffer at least one sequela of PID, which include infertility, ectopic pregnancy, or chronic abdominal pain.[16] The severity of clinical presentation corresponds poorly with the damage to the fallopian tubes. Many young women with PID have mild and vague symptoms.[17] Therefore, the diagnosis of PID on clinical grounds has been notoriously difficult and was shown to be only 66% accurate in one study.[18] It is not surprising that endovaginal ultrasound was demonstrated to be superior to bimanual examination alone in the diagnosis of findings consistent with PID.[19]

Early sonographic signs of PID are increased adnexal volume and periovarian inflammation with fluid collections. On ultrasound, this appears as structures that lack the distinct margins that are normally identified. Another sonographic sign of PID is the decreased ability of the ovary to slide smoothly in the adnexa (sliding organ sign) when the ultrasound probe is inserted and withdrawn from the vagina. This sign suggests that the ovary has been tethered to the fallopian tube by inflammatory adhesions. These sonographic findings were correlated with laparoscopic evidence of periovarian exudates and adhesions by Patten in 1990.[20] In 1992, it was demonstrated that sonographic evidence of free fluid had a sensitivity of 77% and specificity of 79% in culture-proven PID. Finally, the presence of "polycystic-like" ovaries containing increased stroma with several follicles scattered throughout the stroma has been found to be indicative of PID; Cacciatore demonstrated a sensitivity of 100% and a specificity of 71% for this finding.[21]

Another study evaluated four ultrasound markers to suggest evidence of PID: free fluid in the cul-de-sac, multicystic ovaries, visualization of fallopian tube or tubal fluid, and presence of an adnexal mass or TOA. These investigators found that in patient populations that have a high prevalence of PID, an endovaginal ultrasound examination positive for these markers is useful for suggesting the diagnosis of PID, and thus helping avoid laparoscopy. A negative ultrasound examination, however, should not be viewed by the clinician as being reliable for excluding the diagnosis of PID in a patient who appears clinically ill. In this subset of patients, laparoscopy may be required to make the diagnosis.[22]

▶ PELVIC AND ADNEXAL MASSES

HYDROSALPINX

Since hydrosalpinx is present only in abnormal conditions such as PID, TOA, or ectopic pregnancy, its finding should immediately raise a red flag. Fluid in the fallopian tube can be encountered after tubal ligation.

TUBO-OVARIAN ABSCESS

Women who present with a pelvic mass may have a TOA, tubo-ovarian complex, uterine fibroid, hydrosalpinx, ovarian cyst, or a variety of other complex adnexal masses. Clinicians cannot rely solely on their bimanual examination to accurately detect pelvic masses; 70% of pelvic masses found on ultrasound examination were initially missed during the bimanual examination.[23] A pelvic mass detected on physical examination is an indication for a pelvic ultrasound examination. If a cystic structure is found within the ovary, this may provide a finding for the clinician to explain the patient's symptoms and a clear disposition that often negates further work-up during that visit. The presence of a cystic structure on the ovary, however, is very common and does not exclude the presence of other concomitant pathology. Furthermore, if the cyst is large enough, typically over 3.5 cm, ovarian torsion may need to be considered.

Pelvic ultrasonography is indicated in cases of severe, recurrent PID with or without the presence of a mass on physical examination. It is critically important that a distinction be made between PID and TOA to direct specific treatment regimens. Since the same clinical diagnostic difficulties of PID apply to TOA, ultrasonography plays a crucial role in the diagnosis. Understanding that the development of a TOA occurs through a stepwise fashion will aid the sonologist with the ultrasound examination. The first stage involves inflammation of the tubal mucosa. The wall eventually thickens and purulent material fills the lumen and spills into the cul-de-sac. If either end of the fallopian tube becomes blocked, a pyosalpinx can occur. As the pressure within the lumen increases, the walls are stretched thin and the tube becomes distended. In some patients, the process stops at this stage, resulting in chronic hydrosalpinx. When the remnants of the endosalpingeal folds become fibrotic, they appear as spokes outlined by anechoic fluid ("cogwheel sign"). When interrogated using power Doppler, marked hyperemia is seen throughout this complex structure. As the acute inflammatory process continues to proceed, it erodes through the distended wall. If the ovary has a recent defect from the ruptured corpus luteum, it becomes exposed to this inflammation and purulent material enters this space. The final stage of abscess formation occurs when the pus walls itself off, fusing the tube and ovary together.

The incidence of PID developing into TOA has been reported to be between 4%[24] and 30%.[25] TOA requires a different treatment regimen than PID since it forms an abscess, tends to be polymicrobial, and consists of anaerobes.[26] Since the mid-1970s, ultrasonography has been shown to be an accurate, sensitive, and noninvasive imaging technique for diagnosing TOA.[27,28] Furthermore, serial ultrasound examinations have proven to be useful in following a TOA that is managed nonoperatively. Pelvic ultrasonography also assists in the selection of the most effective treatment regimen.[29,30] In a study of 106 patients with clinically suspected PID, ultrasound findings demonstrated 19 patients with pyosalpinx and 4 patients with hydrosalpinx. These 23 patients had their medical therapy directly altered as a result of the endovaginal ultrasound.[31]

UTERINE FIBROIDS

Uterine fibroids represent the most common gynecologic tumor. Leiomyomas start as a mass of smooth muscle proliferation in a whorled spherical configuration. Atrophy and vascular compromise eventually ensue, which result in necrosis and calcification. These patients can present with pelvic pain, dysuria, dysmenorrhea, constipation, or low back pain (from compression of lumbar plexus).

► ANATOMIC CONSIDERATIONS

To understand the pelvic anatomy, it may be helpful to think of the pelvis as two distinct regions: the true pelvis and false pelvis. The true pelvis has a basin-shaped contour and is bounded anteriorly by the pubic symphysis and pubic rami. It is bounded posteriorly by the sacrum and coccyx and inferiorly by the perineal musculature. The false pelvis is located superior to the true pelvis. The abdominal wall represents its anterior border, the iliac bones define its lateral border, and the sacral promontory outlines its posterior border. The empty bladder lies within the true pelvis and, when distended, enters the false pelvis (Figure 14-1).

The uterus is a thick-walled, muscular structure whose shape can vary with cyclical menstrual changes and distention of the bladder and rectum. Typically, the uterus is found in the anteverted position in its relationship with the bladder; in 25% of women, it is retroflexed. During the reproductive years, the uterus measures up to 7 cm × 4 cm × 5 cm. The postmenopausal uterus measures 7 cm in length and 1–2 cm in transverse. The endometrial thickness varies with the menstrual cycle from 6 mm to less than 1 mm following menstruation.

The ovaries are elliptical-shaped structures and are found in a range of positions in the parous woman. In the nulliparous woman, the ovaries are typically located on the posterolateral wall of the true pelvis, adjacent to the internal iliac vessels. The menstrual cycle is categorized into two phases: the proliferative phase, which culminates in ovulation, followed by the secretory phase, which ends in menstruation. Cystic follicles regularly occur during the proliferative phase and are not officially termed a "cyst" until they reach a diameter of 2.5 cm. A corpus luteum then forms at the site of ovulation during the secretory phase, but rarely exists for more than 6 weeks in the nonpregnant patient. Therefore, in the absence of ovulation, these cysts cannot occur. Once ruptured, the only evidence of their existence may be the presence of free fluid in the posterior cul-de-sac or near the ovary itself.[32]

The pouch of Douglas is a term that refers to the potential space in the posterior cul-de-sac of the pelvis. It consists of the peritoneal reflection posterior to the uterus and anterior to the rectosigmoid colon. Because this is the most dependent portion of the supine woman, a trace of free fluid is normally seen here, especially in 5 days prior to menstruation.[33] The anterior cul-de-sac lies between the bladder (anterior) and the uterus

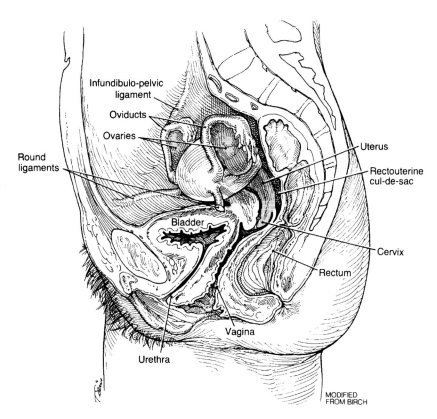

Figure 14-1. Normal pelvic anatomy. *(Reprinted with permission from Cunningham et al: Williams obstetrics, 21st ed. New York: McGraw-Hill, 36, 2001.)*

(posterior). Since this potential space is not dependent, it only contains free fluid when a significant amount is present in the pelvis.

▶ GETTING STARTED

Foremost in importance is patient positioning. Failure to allow for a full range of motion of the transducer handle will often result in inadequate imaging. Allowing the buttocks to come to the edge of a lithotomy table while the feet are securely placed in stirrups is the ideal position for endovaginal scanning. In lieu of an available gynecological gurney, one can elevate the patient's hips by placing several towels under the buttocks. This will allow for full transducer handle movement when attempting to view anterior structures. The second most important factor in endovaginal ultrasound is instructing the patient to empty her bladder. Even small amounts of urinary volume can cause significant artifact that make it difficult to discern pelvic contents. Conversely, scanning via the transabdominal route is facilitated by urinary bladder volume.

Endovaginal pelvic anatomy may at first seem confusing; however, using this higher frequency probe produces significantly superior images to the transabdominal approach (Figure 14-2). Despite these advantages, the ovaries are occasionally difficult to identify. Deeper insertion of the transducer and localization of the iliac vessels are the mainstays of ovarian localization. In perimenopausal women, the ovaries are often quite small in size and do not contain the characteristic follicular structures that make younger ovaries distinguishable.

The transducer orientation is different from the transverse and longitudinal positions of the abdomen. It may be helpful to imagine the patient standing on her head. As the endovaginal transducer is inserted into the vaginal vault, it will have the same orientation as the image on the screen, starting at the apex of the pie shaped image at the top and extending down (out) from there.

▶ TECHNIQUE AND NORMAL ULTRASOUND FINDINGS

TRANSABDOMINAL SONOGRAPHY

The advantage of transabdominal sonography is that it is rapid and noninvasive, and provides a good overall view of the pelvis. The disadvantage is that the pelvic organs are several centimeters away from the ultrasound transducer head and a lower frequency probe must be utilized.

Employing transabdominal sonography, the ultrasound probe is placed on the lower aspect of the midline abdominal wall just superior to the pubic symphysis. A low-frequency probe (3.5–5.0 MHz range) is advantageous to penetrate to the desired depth in the pelvis. Filling the bladder will likewise enhance the quality of sonographic images by displacing the air-filled bowel out of the true pelvis thereby aligning the solid organs perpendicular to the transducer. Overfilling the bladder should be avoided as the bladder can actually push the uterus and ovaries out of the way enough to make visualization difficult.

The transabdominal technique consists of two planes: longitudinal and transverse. In the longitudinal plane, the probe is placed vertically with the indicator toward the patient's head (Figure 14-3). In this plane, the bladder takes on a triangular, "tear drop" appearance. The uterus is pear-shaped and typically measures

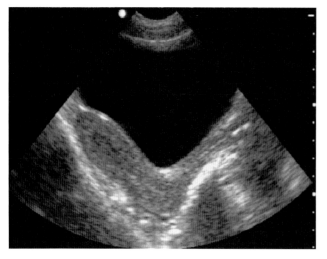

A

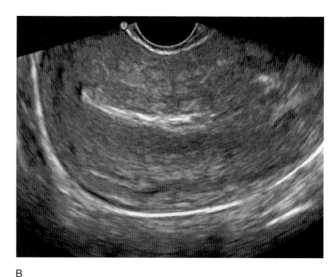

B

Figure 14-2. Comparison of ultrasound resolution of the uterus in the same patient using transabdominal (A) and endovaginal (B) longitudinal views.

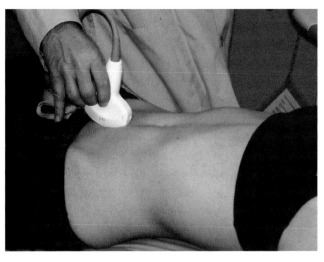

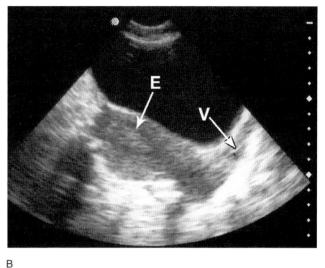

A

B

Figure 14-3. Transabdominal longitudinal view of the pelvis. Probe position (A) and ultrasound image (B). E = endometrial stripe, V = vaginal stripe. (Courtesy of James Mateer, MD)

5–7 cm in length in the menstruating female. One may need to rotate the probe in a slightly oblique fashion in women whose uterus is tilted off the midline or central axis. The endometrial stripe is a thin hyperechoic line running down the center of the uterus along its length, and it fluctuates with the menstrual cycle. It appears thin and less echogenic just following menses in the proliferative phase, and becomes thick and more echogenic following ovulation during the secretory phase. In this longitudinal plane, the endometrial stripe is visualized as the probe is fanned from left to right. The vaginal stripe that is unique to the transabdominal approach can be visualized in the longitudinal plane. It appears as a thin echo bright curved stripe seen posterior to the blad-

der. The cervix is visualized between the uterus and the vagina.

The majority of women have an anteverted uterus found angulated 90 degrees to the midline vaginal stripe when the bladder is empty. Filling the bladder straightens out the uterus so that it comes to lie in a more parallel alignment to the vaginal stripe. A retroverted uterus can be seen extending in an opposite direction to the bladder and appears linear when the bladder is full.

In the transverse view, the probe should be oriented horizontally with slight caudal angulation and with the indicator pointed toward the patient's right side (Figure 14-4). The ovaries are best viewed in this plane and are typically found posterior and lateral to the uterus. In the

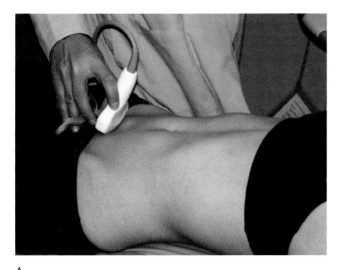

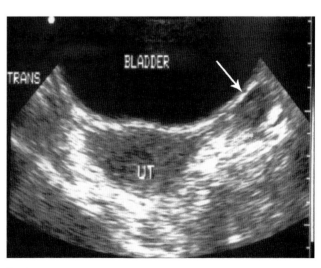

A

B

Figure 14-4. Transabdominal transverse view of the pelvis. Probe position (A) and ultrasound image (B). Ut = Uterus, Arrow = left ovary. (Courtesy of James Mateer, MD)

multiparous patient, ovaries may be found in a variety of positions, from as posterior as the pouch of Douglas to as anterior as the uterine fundus. Typical ovaries measure 2 cm × 2 cm × 3 cm in adults and are characterized by anechoic follicular structures in the periphery (cortex).

The uterus appears as an oval structure in the transverse plane. It is important to scan the uterus from the fundus to the cervix by fanning the ultrasound beam in superior to inferior movement. In this plane, the ovaries can be identified on either side of the uterus. Normal fallopian tubes generally cannot be visualized by transabdominal sonography unless surrounded by fluid.

ENDOVAGINAL SONOGRAPHY

The advantage of the endovaginal approach is that the probe is closer to the pelvic organs of interest, which enables the use of a higher frequency probe (4.0–9.0 MHz range). These higher frequency probes with their inherent enhanced resolution provide the sonologist with superior image quality when compared with transabdominal sonography. Most women report that the endovaginal technique is less uncomfortable than the transabdominal sonography technique. Even among adolescent patients undergoing evaluation for PID, 28% preferred the endovaginal route.[34] The advantage of not requiring patients to have a full bladder helps make the experience less uncomfortable.

The endovaginal technique initially involves disinfecting the probe with standard bactericidal agents between each usage. A proper acoustic medium should be applied on both sides of a protective sheath, typically a condom. Any air bubbles within the condom should be displaced to avoid beam scattering artifacts. In patients undergoing infertility therapy, the ultrasound gel should not contain any spermicidal agent; in these cases, tepid sterile water is suitable for lubrication.

There are two main types of endovaginal transducers (Figure 14-5). One type is referred to as an "end-fire" probe in which the handle and the shaft are in a straight line and the ultrasound waves exit the transducer surface along this line. The other type has an angulated handle and an ultrasound beam that fires askew. The authors will refer to these probe types as "end-fire" and "angulated" in the following discussion.

The patient should be placed in the lithotomy position. A gynecology table is preferable to elevation of hips on a stack of towels. In a systematic fashion, the entire pelvis should be scanned in both sagittal and coronal planes. With the handle of the endovaginal probe being held in a "pistol-grip" fashion, the endovaginal probe should be gently inserted with the indicator pointed toward the ceiling. While inserting the probe, it is important to confirm the bladder as a landmark anterior to

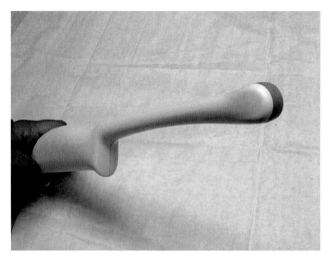

A

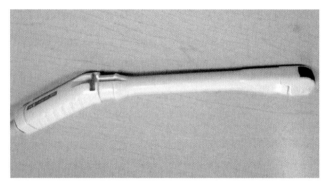

B

Figure 14-5. Endovaginal probes. End-fire type (A). Angulated type (B).

the uterus. It should be clearly discerned from any fluid collection in the anterior cul-de-sac. In a midline sagittal view of the uterus, the endometrial stripe should be clearly identified (Figure 14-6). Maintaining this sagittal plane, the entire uterus is evaluated. Lifting the handle toward the ceiling will direct the sound inferiorly enabling visualization of the cervix. By extending into both lateral projections, the boundaries of the uterus should be defined. To scan patients with a retroverted uterus, it may be necessary to slightly remove the probe and then severely angle the probe face posteriorly (handle toward the ceiling). This allows the beam to be directed in a posterior fashion, which permits sound waves to access the fundus. If the fundus still lies beyond the angle of the beam, and if the angulated transducer type is used, the handle may be rotated 180 degrees, reversing the on-screen direction of fundal image while allowing for adequate (and more comfortable) uterus evaluation.

From the midline sagittal plane, the probe is then rotated 90 degrees in a counterclockwise fashion (indicator toward the patient's right) to view structures in the

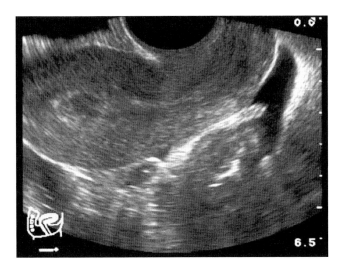

Figure 14-6. The endometrial stripe in a midline sagittal endovaginal view of the uterus. Endometrium is slightly thickened and irregular within the fundus in this example. Note also physiologic fluid in the cul-de-sac.

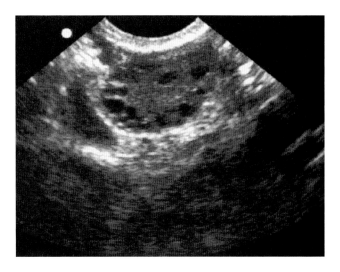

Figure 14-8. Endovaginal ultrasound of the left ovary containing normal follicles.

coronal plane. The coronal plane can also be thought of as axial, or transverse, and simply refers to the short-axis view of the uterus. Views are obtained by fanning through the entire uterus from cervix to fundus. The uterus and endometrial stripes assume a round appearance in this projection (Figure 14-7).

Ovaries are typically identified by the presence of circular hypoechoic follicles. These follicles can be confused with cross-sectional uterine vessels (arcuate arteries) that become tubular when the probe is rotated. Normal ovaries are mobile and may be found in differ-

ent positions during the same examination (Figure 14-8). To view the left ovary, the examiner should start in the sagittal plane with the top of the probe pointed toward the ceiling. Starting at the fundus, the examiner should scan until the iliac vessels are seen to stretch across the screen in their long axis. Then, this structure should be followed into the patient's left adnexa until the characteristic follicles of the left ovary are identified. The right ovary is similarly identified except the probe is turned toward the patient's right.

The fallopian tube is a poor sonic reflector, which makes it virtually impossible to scan in a transabdominal approach. Utilizing an endovaginal approach, the healthy fallopian tubes are easiest to locate by tracing them from their origin at the cornuate areas of the uterus. After ovulation, up to 10 mL of free fluid may be released from a functional ovarian cyst. Blood, ascites, or an exudative/infectious process producing free fluid in the pelvis will similarly enhance image acquisition. In addition, when the endovaginal probe is gently inserted further or removed slightly, it has the benefit of a third scanning plane along its own axis. This effectively moves the adnexa into various positions to enhance imaging. A clearly seen lumen of the fallopian tube should increase the suspicion of a pathological process. The tubal lumen is not normally visualized unless it is filled with fluid. Once the entire tubal lumen is filled, only then can the fimbriae be identified. In the longitudinal axis, the tortuous fallopian tube varies in length. Similarly the transverse axis may vary in width depending on the plane in which it is cut with the ultrasound beam. The width typically approximates 1 cm in normal individuals. The proximal (myometrial) portion of the fallopian tube may occasionally be visualized as a hyperechoic line as it enters the uterus.

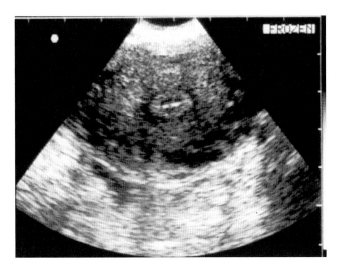

Figure 14-7. Transverse endovaginal ultrasound. Note prominent arcuate venous plexus in the peripheral myometrium. (Courtesy of James Mateer, MD)

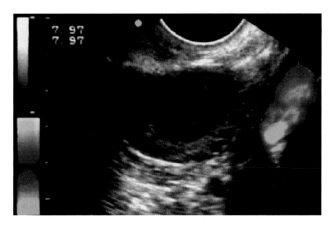

Figure 14-9. Follicular cyst. A 2.7-cm simple cyst is identified within the left ovary. The external iliac vein is identified with color Doppler.

► COMMON AND EMERGENT ABNORMALITIES

FUNCTIONAL SIMPLE CYSTS

These cysts are the most common ovarian masses in nonpregnant young women. Sonographically, they appear as thin-walled, unilocular anechoic spheres. Using specific criteria, a thin-walled, anechoic structure within the ovary is a physiologic cyst until it reaches a diameter greater than 2.5 cm. Follicular cysts can range from 2.5 cm to over 14 cm (Figure 14-9). As opposed to the anechoic interior of a simple cyst, cysts containing heterogenic variable echoes may be hemorrhagic (Figure 14-10). Typically unilateral, they may be found in both ovaries, as seen in polycystic ovarian disease.[35] Ovarian cysts contain heterogeneous tissue, with peripheral follicles frequently identified along its border. It is not un-

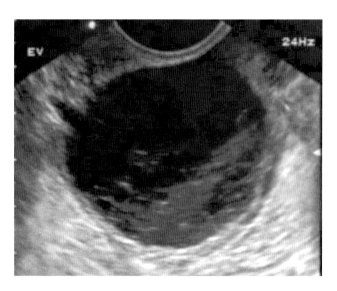

Figure 14-10. Hemorrhagic ovarian cyst.

common for these simple ovarian cysts to rupture. This event, however, is a clinical diagnosis and not a sonographic one. Regardless, clinical suspicion for a ruptured cyst should remain high in any patient who presents with severe lower abdominal pain and free fluid in the pelvis with or without an ovarian cyst (Figure 14-11).

CORPUS LUTEUM CYST

When a patient becomes pregnant, a corpus luteum cyst can persist up to 16 weeks' gestation and enlarge significantly because of failure to rupture or internal hemorrhage.[36] The corpus luteum cyst should not separate from the ovary on probing with the ultrasound transducer and abdominal palpation with the free hand. On the other hand, the vast majority of tubal rings will separate. The corpus luteum cyst can have a variety of appearances (Figure 14-12). Similar to a functional simple cyst of the ovary, corpus luteum cysts may also rupture resulting in severe abdominal pain.[37]

OVARIAN TORSION

The only specific grey-scale sonographic sign of ovarian torsion is demonstration of multiple follicles in the cortical part of a unilaterally enlarged ovary. Transudative fluid flows into the multiple follicles as the ovary becomes congested from circulatory impairment. Ovarian enlargement, when present, is relatively obvious. It has been reported that a torsed ovary is at least 34 times larger than the average *prepubescent* ovary and 8 times larger than the average *adult* ovary[38] (Figure 14-13).

Doppler can be helpful in making the diagnosis of ovarian torsion when there is complete absence or asymmetric blood flow to one ovary (Figure 14-14). To reduce operator error, it is important to scan in several different planes when examining the ovary for presence of blood flow. Optimizing power Doppler settings to detect slow flow is critical. While it is difficult to exclude ovarian torsion with power and pulse wave Doppler, torsion can be diagnosed when no flow is detected. By changing the scanning angle, the sonologist decreases the likelihood that the finding of absent blood flow is due to the angle at which the blood was moving in relation to the ultrasound beam.[39] Absence of ovarian enlargement due to a mass or cyst or effect from a nearby mass makes torsion very unlikely.

ACUTE PELVIC INFLAMMATORY DISEASE

Early sonographic signs of PID are increased adnexal volume and periovarian inflammation with fluid collections (Figure 14-15). On ultrasound, this appears as

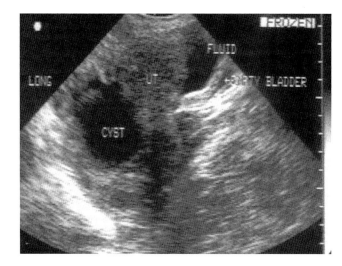

A

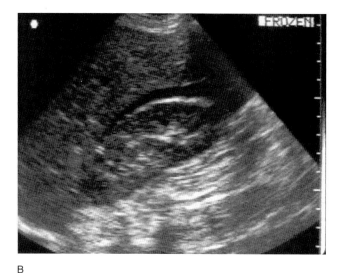

B

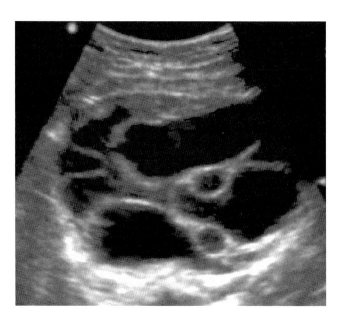

C

Figure 14-11. Ruptured corpus luteum cyst (A). Long-axis transabdominal image shows a collapsed bladder with fluid in the anterior cul-de-sac and a large cyst in the posterior cul-de-sac. (B) A small stripe of free fluid was noted in Morison's pouch. (C) Endovaginal ultrasound reveals a hemorrhagic cyst that has not fully collapsed. (Courtesy of James Mateer, MD)

structures that lack the distinct margins that are normally identified (Figure 14-16). Four ultrasound markers that suggest evidence of PID include (Figure 14-17) free fluid in the cul-de-sac, multicystic ovaries, visualization of fallopian tube or tubal fluid, and presence of an adnexal mass or TOA. An endovaginal ultrasound examination positive for these markers is useful for suggesting the diagnosis of PID, however, should not be considered reliable for excluding the diagnosis of PID in a patient who appears clinically ill.

TUBO-OVARIAN ABSCESS

Imaging the TOA has several caveats. First, the process of TOA formation usually occurs bilaterally, but not necessarily in step; therefore, bilateral TOA may appear "out of phase" with one another. Second, there often is absence of the sliding organ sign. Third, organisms producing gas

Figure 14-12. Echogenic, scalloped corpus luteum cyst.

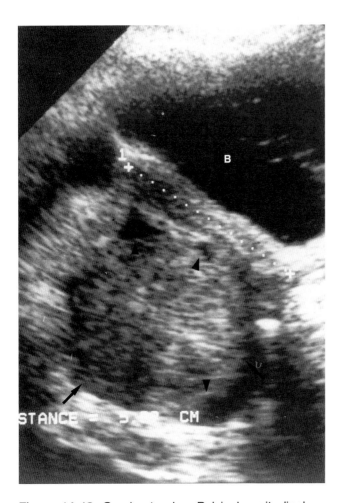

Figure 14-13. Ovarian torsion. Pelvis. Longitudinal plane. The uterus is marked off by measurement points. It is 5 cm in length. Posterior to it is a large solid mass (*arrows*) with a few peripheral cysts (*arrowheads*). This is a relatively classic image for ovarian torsion, although the echogenicity of the ultrasound image is related to the variable internal contents of the torsed ovary. This mass, which is the patient's torsed left adnexa, was much larger than the patient's normal right adnexa. B = bladder. (Reproduced from Cohen HL, Sivit CJ: *Fetal and pediatric ultrasound.* New York: McGraw-Hill, 516, 2001)

result in highly echogenic reflectors within the abscess. Finally, the fallopian tube surrounds the ovary causing it to lose the typical appearance of anechoic follicles in the periphery. This appears sonographically as an ovary connected to, or embraced by, the fluid-filled fallopian tube (tubo-ovarian complex).[40,41] (Figure 14-18). When interrogated using power Doppler, marked hyperemia is seen throughout this complex structure. As the acute inflammatory process continues to proceed, it erodes through the distended wall creating a localized or an expanding TOA (Figure 14-19).

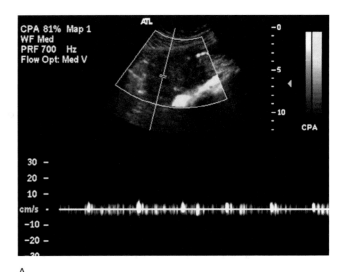

A

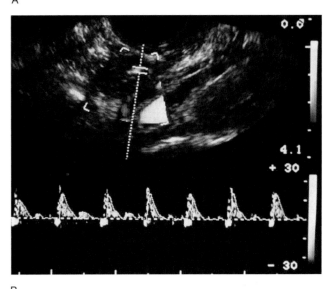

B

Figure 14-14. Inadequate ovarian arterial flow seen on spectral wave Doppler (A). Normal ovarian arterial flow seen on spectral wave Doppler (B).

UTERINE FIBROIDS

A uterus with multiple fibroids appears heterogeneous and globular, with discrete masses embedded in the uterine wall (Figure 14-20). They can be isoechoic, hyperechoic, or hypoechoic. Fibrotic changes and calcifications cause sonographic attenuation and loss of definite margins, which make size estimations problematic. Color Doppler can identify those fibroids containing a vascular supply, which may be responsive to hormonal therapy.[42] Because fibroids tend to reflect the sound waves, there is usually significant shadowing distal to the mass. In fact, the shadowing is often dense enough that it interferes with high-frequency imaging of the endovaginal approach. For this reason, patients with large or multiple fibroids may require a transabdominal, full

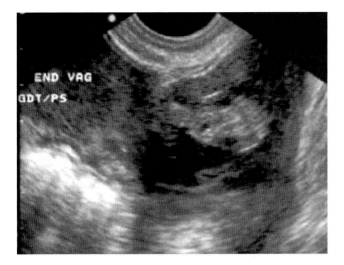

Figure 14-15. Endovaginal ultrasound demonstrating periovarian fliud collection.

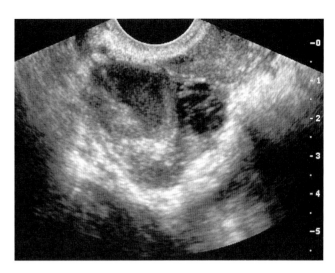

Figure 14-16. Endovaginal ultrasound demonstrating lack of distinct adnexal margins consistent with PID.

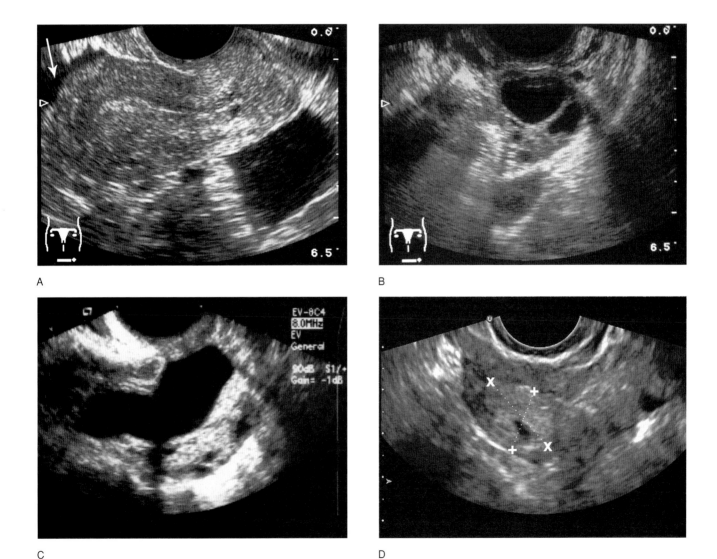

A

B

C

D

Figure 14-17. Four markers of PID. Endovaginal views. (1) Longitudinal ultrasound showing significant free fluid (A) in the posterior cul-de-sac (pouch of Douglas) and a small ammount of fluid in the anterior cul-de-sac (arrow); (2) endovaginal ultrasound demonstrating multicystic ovary (B); (3) hydrosalpinx (C) endovaginal ultrasound shows fluid-filled fallopian tube; (4) adnexal mass (D) is outlined by the measurement cursors.

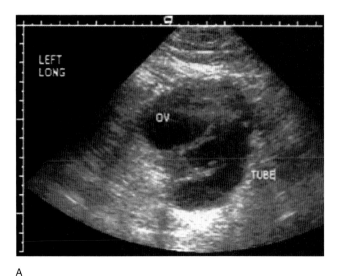

A

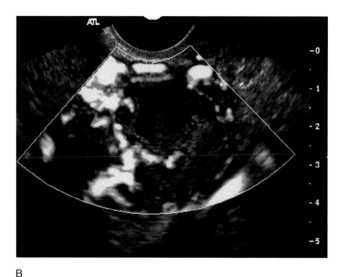

B

Figure 14-18. Tubo-ovarian complex. Endovaginal image of the left adnexa (A) shows a distorted ovary (OV) partially encircled by a fluid-filled hydrosalpinx (TUBE). Power Doppler (B) shows marked hyperemia throughout this similar complex structure.

bladder technique to obtain adequate images of the pelvic structures.

► COMMON VARIANTS AND SELECTED ABNORMALITIES

UTERINE CONDITIONS

Bicornate Uterus

One relatively common anatomic variant is the bicornate uterus. This can be very subtle ranging from a slight

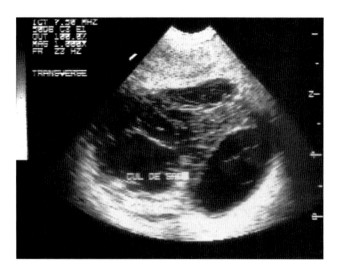

Figure 14-19. Tubo-ovarian abcess. Endovaginal transverse view of the cul-de-sac area shows a complex septated cystic mass 4 × 6 cm in size which proved to be a TOA. (Contributed by James Mateer, MD)

widening of the endometrial stripe to two separate entire uteruses each containing their own endometrial cavities (uterine didelphys). In the coronal plane, a partial bicornate uterus can be easily identified as having a widening of the fundus with separate endometrial stripes tracing away from each other in a Y-type of pattern (Figure 14-21A). For a complete bicornate uterus, as the sonologist fans the ultrasound beam from left to right, the uterine fundus will appear to "re-grow." It is important to note that in this longitudinal plane both fundi will not be visualized simultaneously, but rather in succession. Switching to the coronal plane makes it possible for both horns of the uterus to be examined simultaneously. As the sonologist fans anterior to posterior coronally, each horn is seen to grow and recede together including their respective endometrial stripes seen in short axis (Figure 14-21B).

Intrauterine Device

Occasionally, patients present to the emergency department or acute care clinic because of concerns that an intrauterine device (IUD) has been dislodged. This becomes further complicated when the string normally attached to the IUD has broken off or is missing. Sonographically, the IUD is strongly reflective and easily identified on endovaginal views unless located outside the uterus (Figure 14-22).[43] It is important to note that even though they represent a highly echoic structure, an IUD may not be distinguishable from the endometrial stripe using the transabdominal approach.

Endometritis

This condition is most often seen with PID, during postpartum or after instrumentation. The endometrial stripe

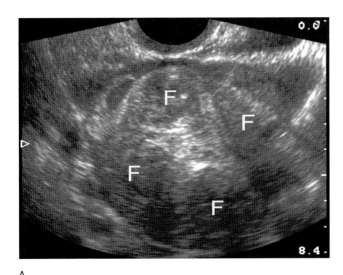
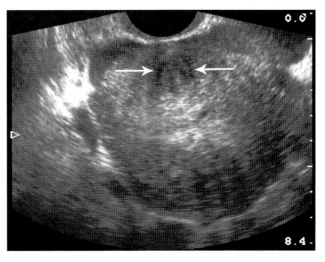

A   B

Figure 14-20. Fibroid Uterus. Endovaginal ultrasound reveals multiple isoechoic discrete masses embedded in the uterine wall (A). A single hypoechoic fibroid (B) is outlined (arrows). F = Fibroids.

appears prominent or irregularly shaped. Fluid, gas, or debris can often be visualized.

Endometriosis

This ectopic endometrial tissue is usually found in the cul-de-sac, ovaries, and fallopian tubes. During menses, this tissues hemorrhages, resulting in multiple small fluid collections (endometriomas) that generally are not easily visualized by ultrasound. An enlarged endometrioma (termed "chocolate cyst") appears on ultrasound as a cystic structures with thickened walls and containing mid-level echogenic centers.[44] The viscous-fluid center can be mistaken for a solid ultrasound mass, but is identified as a cyst by posterior acoustical enhancement distal to the structure.

Uterine Polyps

Uterine polyps, found in 10% of women, are pedunculated sections of endometrial tissue that can occur as a single lesion or as multiple lesions. They may become so large that they protrude through the cervical os. The endometrium is thickened with areas of focal echogenicity or endocavitary masses surrounded by fluid.

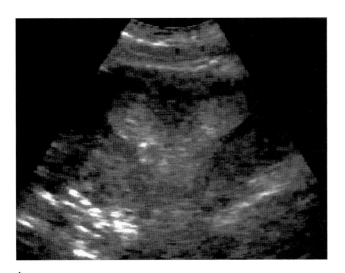
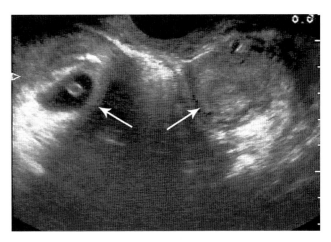

A   B

Figure 14-21. Bicornate uterus (partial). Endovaginal coronal view shows hyperechoic endometium with "Y" fundal projections (A). Bicornate uterus (complete). Transverse endovaginal view of uterine didelphys with each horn (arrows) separated by a loop of bowel (B). The patients right horn contains an early IUP and yolk sac.

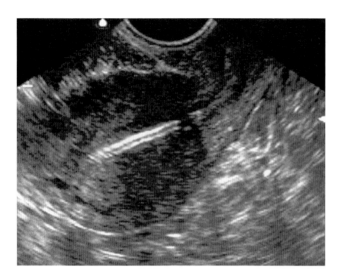

Figure 14-22. An IUD is strongly reflective and easily identified on endovaginal views.

Endometrial Hyperplasia

This condition results from the unopposed estrogen stimulation of endometrial proliferation without the shedding effects of progesterone. The sonographic findings are nonspecific but do suggest a thickened endometrial stripe often greater than 5 mm. Postmenopausal patients with greater than 1 cm of endometrial thickness usually indicates hyperplasia or carcinoma.[45]

Endometrial Neoplasm

These tumors range in echogenicity from hyper- to hypoechoic. Some tumors may simply stretch the endometrium without directly invading it, making them difficult to visualize on ultrasound. Tumors greater than 1 cm in anterior–posterior dimension or ones greater than 10 cc in volume may warrant endometrial biopsy. Hyperplasia, in general, is a known precursor to carcinoma.[46]

CERVICAL CONDITIONS

Nabothian Cysts

Nabothian cysts occur when the endocervical glands becomes obstructed and dilated. This is a benign condition that frequently occurs without symptoms and has no clinical or pathologic significance. They appear sonographically within the cervix as a thin-walled, anechoic cystic structure up to 1 cm in diameter (Figure 14-23).

Cervical Malignancy

The majority (90%) of cervical malignancies is squamous cell and appears as bulky heterogeneous material within the cervix. This entity is seen best in the sagittal view.

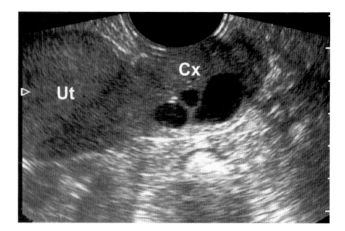

Figure 14-23. Longitudinal endovaginal ultrasound demonstrating benign nabothian cervical cysts. UT = Uterus, Cx = Cervix.

OVARIAN CONDITIONS

Ovarian cysts are common in all age groups, but especially in women of menstrual age. There exists a great deal of overlap in the sonographic appearances of the various masses found in the ovary and the adnexa. Their sonographic characteristics become even more similar when one considers the subset of masses with a complex morphology. It is the task of the clinician to sort through which findings require immediate diagnostic evaluation and which can be monitored on an outpatient basis.

Mucinous Cystadenomas

Mucinous cystadenomas are benign masses that represent the largest of the ovarian neoplasms. They are capable of growing to occupy the entire abdominal cavity such that patients appear gravid. They contain mucinous material, which appear sonographically as multiple fine, low-level echoes.[47]

Serous Cystadenomas

Serous cystadenomas, constituting approximately 20% of all benign neoplasms of the ovary, appear sonographically as a multilocular cystic mass containing few or no internal echoes. Septations are sufficiently thin so as to undulate with gentle transducer palpation. In the benign form, nodularity is typically absent; therefore, any solid tissue noted should raise concern for malignancy.

Cystadenocarcinoma

Ultrasound distinction between benign cystadenomas and malignant cystadenocarcinoma is difficult. Biopsy of the ovary has borderline histology 15% of the time.[48] Sonographic characteristics that suggest malignant histology include thick septa, increased mural nodularity, presence of solid tissue, and ascites. The presence of ascites was noted in over 50% of malignant epithelial neoplasms of the ovary and is completely absent with benign disease.[49]

Dermoid Cysts

Dermoid cysts, the second most common cause of ovarian masses, may contain hair, teeth, and fat. Calcified structures, such as teeth, produce strong shadows and are easily identified on plain films.[46]

Polycystic Ovaries

Represented as multiple immature follicles less than 1 cm packed along the periphery. Sometimes described as "beads on a string" morphology.[47] When stimulated with hormones, they have an exaggerated appearance resembling a stained glass window.

VAGINAL CONDITIONS

Ultrasound can be utilized to localize and diagnose a vaginal hematoma. Typically, the ultrasound examination is performed transabdominally in an attempt to localize the hematoma within the vaginal tissue planes (Figure 14-24).

▶ PITFALLS

1. **Presence of blood flow in the involved ovary does not necessarily exclude the diagnosis of ovarian torsion.** Absence of ovarian blood flow is helpful in diagnosing ovarian torsion. The converse has not been shown to be reliable for excluding ovarian torsion. In other words, in the correct clinical setting, the index of suspicion for ovarian torsion should be maintained even if blood flow is present in the involved ovary.

2. **The uterine vasculature may appear cystic on cross-sectional image planes and are frequently mistaken for follicles within an ovary.** The ovary can be confirmed by these cystic structures lacking blood flow. These structures should remain circular in different scanning planes when the transducer is rotated. Vascular structures contain blood flow and lengthen out when viewed in alternate scanning planes.

3. **Large ovarian follicles may be mistaken for fallopian tubes.** These ovarian follicles will change during the cycle and be localized within the ovary.

4. **Small ovarian cysts can falsely appear as a thin-walled hydrosalpinx.** The finding of ovarian tissue in the periphery helps exclude this diagnosis.

5. **Retained mucous secretions can imitate tumors by appearing to have endometrial thickening.**

6. **Other disease processes, such as tuberculosis and various gynecological malignancies, can cause peritoneal implantation to the uterine serosa.** These disease entities are easily identified sonographically when surrounded by fluid.

7. **Imaging the shrunken postmenopausal ovary is difficult because of its lack of follicles, decreased pelvic fluid, and decreased vaginal elasticity inhibiting probe movement.**

▶ CASE STUDIES

CASE 1

Patient Presentation

A 22-year-old nulliparous woman with a 1-day history of severe right lower quadrant abdominal pain and scant vaginal discharge presented to the emergency department. The patient was seen by her primary care physician 4 days previously and was treated for a urinary tract infection. She reported having unprotected sex with one sexual partner for the past several months. Her medical history and surgical history were unremarkable. Review of systems was significant for tactile fever and decreased oral intake.

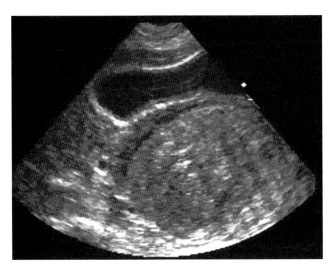

Figure 14-24. Vaginal hematoma. Transabdominal ultrasound view of a vaginal hematoma in patient who recently underwent a dilatation and curettage procedure.

On physical examination, the patient had a blood pressure, 110/70 mmHg; heart rate, 123 beats per minute; respiratory rate, 18 per minute; and temperature, 39.8°C. She appeared toxic. The abdominal examination revealed severe right lower quadrant tenderness slightly inferior to McBurney's point, no rebound or guarding, normoactive bowel sounds, and no costovertebral angle tenderness. The rectal examination lateralized tenderness to the right, and the stool was guaiac negative. Sterile speculum examination revealed a friable cervix with scant purulent discharge. Bimanual examination revealed right adnexal tenderness, cervical motion tenderness, but no evidence of fullness or masses. A urinalysis specimen was unremarkable, and the urine pregnancy test was negative. The white blood cell count was 15,000 with a left shift.

Management Course

At this stage in the work-up, acute appendicitis was suspected. A general surgeon ordered a CT scan of the abdomen and pelvis with triple contrast. This test was read as negative for appendicitis but did reveal a complex structure associated with the right ovary. A bedside endovaginal ultrasound revealed a cogwheel formation of the right ovary, absence of the sliding ovary sign, and heterogenic material within the right fallopian tube. A diagnosis of TOA was made, triple antibiotic therapy was initiated, and the gynecologist was consulted. The patient was taken to the operating room for laparoscopy with abscess drainage.

Commentary

Case 1 illustrated the diagnostic role that ultrasonography can have in the work-up of a young woman with lower abdominal pain. Ectopic pregnancy and urinary tract disease had been excluded by the urine sample. Appendicitis initially was at the top of the differential diagnosis. A negative CT scan, however, is not 100% accurate for excluding appendicitis, and the general surgeon continued to entertain thoughts of taking the patient to the operating room to perform an appendectomy. The pelvic ultrasound examination confirmed the diagnosis of TOA and the patient's care was expedited by having the gynecologist perform the laparoscopic procedure for abscess drainage.

CASE 2

Patient Presentation

A 16-year-old nulliparous woman presented to the emergency department with the sudden onset of severe left lower quadrant abdominal pain. The symptoms started 30 minutes before the arrival and were associated with nausea, three episodes of vomiting, and chills. The patient denied vaginal bleeding or discharge and any prior history of sexual intercourse. Medical history and surgical history were unremarkable.

On physical examination, the patient had a blood pressure, 120/70 mmHg; heart rate, 118 beats per minute; respiratory rate, 20 per minute; and temperature, 37.8°C. She appeared in severe distress secondary to the pain and nausea. Abdominal examination revealed moderate tenderness in left lower quadrant without rebound or guarding. Bowel sounds were normal. There were no masses or costovertebral tenderness. Rectal examination was nontender, and stool was guaiac negative. Sterile speculum examination was unremarkable and bimanual examination revealed left adnexal tenderness, cervical motion tenderness, normal right adnexa, and no masses or fullness. The white blood count was normal, and the urinalysis and urine pregnancy test were negative.

Management Course

The emergency physician's differential diagnosis included ovarian torsion, ruptured ovarian cyst with chemical peritonitis, and TOA. The physician's bedside endovaginal ultrasound examination showed no evidence of free fluid, ovarian mass, or TOA. There was, however, an enlarged left ovary with complete absence of any discernible blood flow despite evaluation in multiple planes. The right ovary had normal appearing blood flow. A gynecologist was immediately called to the bedside for suspected ovarian torsion, and she took the patient to the operating room for laparoscopy. Her ovary was immediately detorsed with intraoperative visual evidence of good perfusion.

Commentary

Case 2 was an example of a young woman who presented with acute ovarian torsion. This case illustrated that the pelvic ultrasound examination could be performed rapidly at the patient's bedside, which are two of the main advantages of ultrasonography. The emergency physician was able to expedite the patient's disposition to the operating room. This helped the gynecologist salvage the young woman's left ovary.

CASE 3

Patient Presentation

A 32-year-old, gravida 4, para 4 woman with worsening right lower quadrant abdominal pain over the past several days presented to the emergency department. She admitted that this pain felt like the same pain she has had in the past with her ovarian cysts. She denied vaginal discharge, vaginal bleeding, fever, chills, nausea, or vomiting. She had no medical history or surgical history.

On physical examination, the patient had a blood pressure, 110/70 mmHg; heart rate, 92 beats per minute; respiratory rate, 16 per minute; and temperature, 37.2°C. She appeared in mild distress secondary to abdominal pain. Abdominal examination revealed moderate tenderness to deep palpation in her right lower quadrant. No rebound or guarding was appreciated, and there were no masses or costovertebral tenderness. Rectal examination was nontender, and the stool was guaiac negative. Sterile speculum examination was unremarkable; however, bimanual examination revealed adnexal fullness on the right side with moderate tenderness. No cervical motion tenderness was elicited and the left adnexa was normal. The white blood cell count was normal, and the urinalysis and urine pregnancy test were negative.

Management Course

The differential diagnosis included appendicitis, ovarian torsion, PID, and TOA. The emergency physician performed a screening bedside endovaginal ultrasound examination that revealed a 4-cm right ovarian cyst and evidence of normal appearing blood flow to the surrounding ovarian tissue and trace free fluid in the posterior cul-de-sac. The patient's symptoms were alleviated with oral ibuprofen and she was discharged home. Arrangements were made with her gynecologist to schedule a repeat ultrasound examination later that week in her office. This follow-up ultrasound examination revealed resolution of the cyst with a moderate amount of free fluid in the posterior cul-de-sac.

Commentary

Case 3 demonstrated how utilization of bedside emergency ultrasound allowed the physician to avoid ordering expensive, time-consuming diagnostic tests for the evaluation of the patient's complaint. While the patient's differential diagnosis included several worrisome disease entities, the physician was able to match the patient's clinical picture to a finding on the ultrasound examination, and then initiated the appropriate therapy.

REFERENCES

1. Tukeva TA, Aronen HJ, Karjalainen PT, et al.: MR imaging in pelvic inflammatory disease: Comparison with laparoscopy and ultrasound. *Radiology* 210(1):209–16, 1999.
2. Centers for Disease Control and Prevention: 1998 Guidelines for treatment of sexually transmitted diseases. *MMWR* 47:79, 1998.
3. Jacobson L: Objectivized diagnosis of acute PID. *Am J Obstet Gynecol* 105:1088–1098, 1969.
4. Graif M, Itzchak Y: Sonographic evaluation of ovarian torsion in childhood and adolescence. *AJR* 150:647–649, 1988.
5. Hibbard L: Adnexal torsion. *Am J Obstet Gyn* 152:456–460, 1985.
6. Schultz LR, Newton WA, Clatoworthy HW: Torsion of previously normal tube and ovary in children. *N Engl J Med* 268:343–346, 1963.
7. Stark J, Siegel M: Ovarian torsion in prepubertal and pubertal girls: Sonographic findings. *AJR* 163:1479–1482, 1994.
8. Hibbard L: Adnexal torsion. *Am J Obstet Gyn* 152:456–460, 1985.
9. Pena JE: Usefulness of Doppler sonography in the diagnosis of ovarian torsion. *Fertil Steril* 73(5):1047–1050, 2000.
10. Surratt J, Siegel J: Imaging of pediatric ovarian masses. *RadioGraphics* 11:533–548, 1991.
11. Van Hoorhis B, Schwaiger J, Syrop C, et al.: Early diagnosis of ovarian torsion by color Doppler sonography. *Fertil Steril* 58:215–217, 1992.
12. Rosado W, Trambert M, Gosink B, et al.: Adnexal torsion: Diagnosis by using Doppler sonography. *AJR* 159:1251–1253, 1992.
13. Stark J, Siegel M: Ovarian torsion in prepubertal and pubertal girls: Sonographic findings. *AJR* 163:1479–1482, 1994.
14. Graif M, Itzchak Y: Sonographic evaluation of ovarian torsion in childhood and adolescence. *AJR* 150:647–649, 1988.
15. Centers for Disease Control and Prevention: 1998 guidelines for treatment of sexually transmitted diseases. *MMWR* 47:79, 1998.
16. Washington AE, Katz P: Cost of and payment source for pelvic inflammatory disease: Trends and projections, 1983 through 2000. *JAMA* 226:2565, 1991.
17. Lawson MA, Blythe MJ: Pelvic inflammatory disease in adolescents. *Pediatr Clin North Am* 46:4, 1999.
18. Jacobson L: Objectivized diagnosis of acute PID. *Am J Obstet Gynecol* 105:1088–1098, 1969.
19. Arbel-DeRowe Y, Tepper R, Rosn DJ, et al.: The contribution of pelvic ultrasonography to the diagnostic process in pediatric and adolescent gynecology. *J Pediatr Adolesc Gynecol* 10:3, 1997.
20. Patten RM: PID: Endovaginal sonography and laparoscopic correlation. *J Ultrasound Med* 9:681–689, 1990.
21. Cacciatore B, Leminen A, et al.: Transvaginal sonographic findings in ambulatory patients with suspected pelvic inflammatory disease. *Obstetr Gynecol* (80)6:912–916, 1992.
22. Boardman L, Peipert J, Brody J, et al.: Endovaginal sonography for the diagnosis of upper genital tract infection. *Endovagin Sonogr* 90:54–57, 1997.
23. Teisala K, Heinonen PK, Punnonen R, et al.: Transvaginal ultrasound in the diagnosis and treatment of tubo-ovarian abscess. *Br J Obstet Gynecol* 77:178–180, 1990.
24. Roberts W, Dockery JL: Management of tubo-ovarian abscess due to pelvic inflammatory disease. *S Med J* 77:7, 1984.
25. Reed S, Landers D, Sweet RL: Antibiotic treatment of tuboovarian abscess: Comparison of broad-spectrum beta-lactam agents versus clindamycin-containing regimens. *Am J Obstet Gynecol* 164:1556–1562, 1991.
26. Landers DV: Tubo-ovarian abscess complicating pelvic inflammatory disease, In: Landers DV, Sweet RL eds.: *Pelvic Inflammatory Disease.* New York: Springer Verlag, 1996: 94.

27. Taylor KJW, et al.: Accuracy of grey-scale ultrasound diagnosis of abdominal and pelvic abscesses in 220 patients. *Lancet* 1:83–84, 1978.

28. Uhrich PC, Sanders RC: Ultrasound characteristics of pelvic inflammatory masses. *Clin Ultrasound* 4:199–204, 1976.

29. Landers DV: Tubo-ovarian abscess complicating pelvic inflammatory disease, In: Landers DV, Sweet RL eds.: *Pelvic Inflammatory Disease*. New York: Springer Verlag, 1996: 94.

30. McNeeley SG: Medically sound, cost-effective treatment for pelvic inflammatory disease and tuboovarian abscess. *Am J Ob Gyn* 178:(6) 1272–1278, 1998.

31. Bulas DI, Ahlstrom PA, Sivit CJ, et al.: Pelvic inflammatory disease in the adolescent: Comparison of transabdominal and transvaginal sonographic evaluation. *Radiology* 183:435–439, 1992.

32. Holt SC, Levi CS, Lyons EA, et al.: Normal anatomy of the female pelvis, In: Callen P ed.: *Ultrasonography in Obstetrics and Gynecology*. St. Louis, MO: W.B. Saunders, 1993: 550–551.

33. Davis JA, Gosnick BB: Fluid in the female pelvis: Cyclic patterns. *J Ultrasound Med* 5:75–79, 1986.

34. Bulas DI, Ahlstrom PA, Sivit CJ, et al.: Pelvic inflammatory disease in the adolescent: Comparison of transabdominal and transvaginal sonographic evaluation. *Radiology* 183:435–439, 1992.

35. Holt SC, Levi CS, Lyons EA, et al.: Normal anatomy of the female pelvis, In: Callen P ed.: *Ultrasonography in Obstetrics and Gynecology*. St. Louis, MO: W.B. Saunders, 1993: 555.

36. Holt SC, Levi CS, Lyons EA, et al.: Normal anatomy of the female pelvis, In: Callen P ed.: *Ultrasonography in Obstetrics and Gynecology*. St. Louis, MO: W.B. Saunders, 1993: 561–562.

37. Rottem S, Timor-Tritsch I: Ovarian pathology, In: Timor-Trisch I, Rottem S eds.: *Transvaginal Sonography*. New York: Elsevier, 1991:156.

38. Graif M, Itzchak Y: Sonographic evaluation of ovarian torsion in childhood and adolescence. *AJR* 150:647–649, 1988.

39. Zagebski J: Doppler instrumentation, In: *Essentials of Ultrasound Physics*. St. Louis, MO: Mosby, 1996:90.

40. Rottem S, Timor-Tritsch I: Ovarian pathology, In: Timor-Trisch I, Rottem S eds.: *Transvaginal Sonography*. New York: Elsevier, 1991:155.

41. Cacciatore B, Leminen A, et al.: Transvaginal sonographic findings in ambulatory patients with suspected pelvic inflammatory disease. *Obstetr Gynecol* 80(6):912–916, 1992.

42. Rottem S, Timor-Tritsch I: Ovarian pathology, In: Timor-Trisch I, Rottem S eds.: *Transvaginal Sonography*. New York: Elsevier, 1991:155.

43. Comstock C: Ultrasonography of gynecologic disorders, In: Pearlman M, Tintinalli J eds.: *Emergency Care of the Woman*. New York: McGraw Hill, 1998:669.

44. Rottem S, Timor-Tritsch I: Ovarian pathology, In: Timor-Trisch I, Rottem S eds.: *Transvaginal Sonography*. New York: Elsevier, 1991:157.

45. Fleischer A, Kepple D, Entman A: Transvaginal sonography of uterine disorders, In: Timor-Trisch I, Rottem S eds.: *Transvaginal Sonography*. New York: Elsevier, 1991: 119.

46. Comstock C: Ultrasonography of gynecologic disorders, In: Pearlman M, Tintinalli J eds.: *Emergency Care of the Woman*. New York: McGraw Hill, 1998:671.

47. Rottem S, Timor-Tritsch I: Ovarian pathology, In: Timor-Trisch I, Rottem S eds.: *Transvaginal Sonography*. New York: Elsevier, 1991:155.

48. Mendelson EB, Bohm-Velez M, Joseph N, Neiman HL: Gynecologic imaging: Comparison of transabdominal and transvaginal sonography. *Radiology* 166:321–324, 1988.

49. Cramer DW, Welch WR: Determinants of ovarian cancer risk. Inferences regarding pathogenesis. *J Natl Cancer Inst* 71:717, 1983.

CHAPTER 15

Deep Venous Thrombosis

Michael Blaivas

In recent years, medicine has seen the spread of bedside ultrasonography beyond the traditional scope of practice employed by early emergency sonologists.[1–4] Many of the new applications adopted by emergency sonologists have resulted from a clinical need to improve efficiency of patient care. One such application has been ultrasonography for the detection of deep venous thrombosis (DVT).[5,6] This typically refers to lower extremity DVT, although the frequency of upper extremity DVTs encountered appears to be increasing.[7]

Approximately 260,000 cases of lower extremity DVT are diagnosed each year in the United States.[8] These, in turn, are thought to lead to as many as 50,000 deaths per year due to pulmonary embolism.[8] To avoid the potentially fatal sequelae of DVT, physicians in the United States order almost 500,000 lower extremity duplex ultrasound examinations per year.[9] Many vascular ultrasound laboratories find it difficult to maintain 24-hour coverage, 7 days per week, for emergency evaluation.[10] This has resulted largely from lack of funding and trained personnel. Many hospitals now have an absence of vascular laboratory services during off-hours. The result is that the emergency or primary care physician is compelled to empirically treat and often admit patients who may have a DVT.

Overcrowding in emergency departments has stretched resources to the breaking point, resulting in delays in obtaining a host of services for emergency department patients. Moreover, even though extremity ultrasonography may be available at a facility, it may take hours to obtain a result, thus delaying the patient in the emergency department unnecessarily. Emergency physicians choosing to perform ultrasound examinations of the lower extremity themselves have been shown to decrease the time to patient disposition by over 2 hours.[11]

▶ CLINICAL CONSIDERATIONS

The high incidence and considerable morbidity and mortality resulting from DVT, coupled with the potential difficulty encountered in trying to diagnose it, has made this a disease of significant importance.[12] The use of low-molecular-weight heparin makes it possible to send some patients home without obtaining a diagnostic study. The patient can then undergo an outpatient study the following day, which, if negative, would lead to termination of anticoagulation therapy.[13,14] However, there are some drawbacks to this strategy. Patients who are sent home require training in self-administration of low-molecular-weight heparin. This may be difficult to accomplish in a busy emergency department or outpatient setting. Furthermore, despite the relatively low incidence of bleeding with low-molecular-weight heparin, complications are occasionally encountered and can be severe. Another reality is that many primary care physicians still elect to admit their patients with actual or suspected DVT. Lastly, although rare, a fresh DVT can resolve rapidly with anticoagulation and it is possible that an ultrasound obtained 24 hour later may not demonstrate a DVT since it has already resolved—perhaps temporarily. This is a disservice to the patient who may not undergo a full evaluation for DVT or is at risk for recurrence.

It is not surprising that physicians have long sought a means of more accurately diagnosing or excluding DVT at the bedside. This is reflected by the many clinical decision rules that have been developed and the attempts made to integrate D-dimer assays into DVT evaluation.[15,16] The adoption of prediction rules has improved efficiency in choosing which patients are at a real risk for having a DVT. By excluding low-risk patients, those who would have required an ultrasound in the past can now be sent home without an imaging study. However, not all patients suspected for DVT are low risk and some will require evaluation by ultrasound.

Emergency ultrasound can within minutes diagnose or exclude DVT. With such rapid diagnosis available at the bedside, ultrasound examinations can be utilized routinely for diagnosis. In addition, physicians can perform follow-up examinations when patients are unable to obtain them as indicated. Although this is not ideal for treatment of DVT, it could reduce the frequency of patients lost to follow-up due to financial limitations or noncompliance.[17]

▶ CLINICAL INDICATIONS

The clinical indications for performing a venous ultrasound examination are as follows:

- Suspicion of lower extremity DVT
- Suspicion of upper extremity DVT

LOWER EXTREMITY DVT

An examination of the deep veins of the lower extremity is indicated whenever a proximal DVT is suspected. Proximal DVT is loosely defined as a clot or thrombus in the popliteal vein or higher in the leg. Its significance is that it is associated with a greater risk of embolization than a calf vein DVT.[18]

The complete duplex ultrasound examination performed by imaging specialists is somewhat lengthy, with one leg taking up to 37 minutes in one study.[19] In addition, it may or may not include an evaluation of the veins below the trifurcation of the popliteal vein distal to the knee. The complete study involves a slow, painstaking evaluation of each vein roughly one-probe width at a time. Each small segment of vein is visualized and checked for complete collapse under pressure from the transducer. Multiple blood flow measurements are taken using color and pulse wave Doppler. A difficult examination of the entire leg can take as much as an hour in some vascular laboratories. The main culprit for this extended period of time is the calf and its veins.

Several studies have shown that the traditional complete examination may not be necessary. An abbreviated approach may maintain high accuracy and patient safety while decreasing the time required for an examination. The abbreviated approach argues for spot checks of vein compressibility, usually at the junction of the common femoral, deep femoral, and superficial femoral veins and the popliteal vein. This allows for considerable time savings and increases patient comfort, and there is considerable evidence that this method is safe and effective.

One study evaluated 204 consecutive patients who had undergone elective, major lower extremity surgery.[20] These patients were part of a general screening for lower extremity DVT and were not specifically referred for testing. The investigators found that simply compressing the vein to assess its patency produced a sensitivity of 60% and a specificity of 96%. The addition of color Doppler did not improve the study results. In these patients, venous compression was performed over the entire leg, a time-consuming task. Perhaps the most important point here is that color Doppler did little to improve detection of proximal DVT.

In 1989, a group of investigators published their findings on a head-to-head comparison of contrast venography with B-mode ultrasonography in 220 consecutive patients.[21] The only criterion used to detect DVT with ultrasound was lack of compression in either the common femoral or popliteal veins. For proximal vein thrombosis, the study yielded a sensitivity of 100%. When patients with calf vein thrombi (located on venogram) were included, the sensitivity and specificity were 91% and 99%, respectively. The study showed that in comparison to the gold standard this simple method of DVT detection was highly accurate.

A number of other studies also confirmed high sensitivity and specificity for the detection of proximal lower extremity DVT without the utilization of color Doppler.[8,9,19,20] The studies noted considerable time savings when segmental checks were performed, which raised the question for the necessity of compressing every inch of vein in the proximal venous system. Proponents for compressing every inch of vein in the proximal venous system point out the potential for occurrence of segmental DVTs. These are venous thrombi that are limited to only one section of the deep venous system. For example, the popliteal vein may be without thrombus as well as most of the superficial femoral vein; however, a 3-inch section of the superficial femoral vein in the mid-thigh could contain thrombus. One study examined the incidence of a small isolated thrombus segment, such as in the iliac and popliteal veins, and found an incidence of 0 out of 195 legs studied.[22] Thus, the chance of missing evidence of segmental thrombi is minimal. Another study prospectively analyzed 72 patients for DVT using an abbreviated technique with only two compression sites per leg.[19] The two sites used were the saphenofemoral junction and the lower popliteal vein. For proximal DVT, the sensitivity and specificity of simple compression in these two sites were 100% and 98%, respectively. The authors addressed potential criticism of their abbreviated technique by noting that in a study of 491 patients found to be without DVT by compression ultrasonography, only 1.5% had a proximal DVT during the 6-month follow-up evaluation.[23]

In 1996, a study of 721 patients, on whom 755 examinations were performed, examined the safety of abbreviated studies for DVT.[24] All patients were referred to a vascular laboratory for suspicion of DVT. A complete examination was performed on each patient and the authors attempted to make retrospective inferences from the results. They concluded that DVT limited to a single vein occurs with enough frequency that the ultrasound survey for thrombosis should not be limited. However, the investigators failed to note that even the isolated thrombus segments in their study were within the area interrogated by the abbreviated approach and would have been detected.

In 1998, a large study evaluated the abbreviated compression approach in 405 consecutive outpatients suspected of having a first-time lower extremity DVT.[9] Each patient had his or her common femoral and popliteal veins assessed for compressibility. In those with normal results, testing was repeated in 5–7 days. Regardless of symptoms, patients with negative results on compression ultrasound did not receive anticoagulation. Follow-up was performed on all patients at 3 months after the initial negative study. Of the patients studied, 63 had DVT detected on initial ultrasound examination. Repeat ultrasound studies picked up 7 proximal DVTs that were not present on initial examination and may have propagated proximally from veins in the calf. None of the patients with normal results died of pulmonary embolism during the follow-up period.

The patency of lower extremity veins should be checked in any patient in whom a clinician suspects of having a lower extremity DVT. Patients with symptoms suggestive of DVT typically have calf swelling and pain posteriorly.[25] Redness of the posterior calf can also be suggestive. Although a number of studies have suggested that DVT is unlikely to be present without a minimum of a 2-cm difference in calf diameter between the affected and contralateral sides, in practice this is not always the case.[26] Debilitated patients or ones who are unable to communicate may require a lower threshold to image because of their inability to relate common symptoms of DVT.

The risk factors commonly described for the development of DVT include smoking, abdominal surgery, lower extremity injury, venous stasis, previous history of DVT, and congestive heart failure, among others.[27–29] Thus, any person who has a risk factor and presents with calf pain and swelling is a candidate for undergoing a study to exclude DVT. Despite a number of studies

that have suggested at least several risk factors must be present to warrant emergency evaluation for DVT, many physicians may feel obligated to exclude the presence of the disease for marginal indications.[27–29]

Bedside emergency ultrasound examination of lower extremity veins is of greatest use in facilities that lack vascular laboratory access at night or on weekends. Emergency or primary physicians often find themselves having to empirically treat patients they suspect of having a DVT. This typically involves either admission for heparin therapy or outpatient treatment with low-molecular-weight heparin therapy. The latter can be made difficult if expeditious follow-up cannot be arranged or if the local medical culture frowns on outpatient treatment of uncomplicated DVTs. The high accuracy that can be achieved with a modified lower extremity duplex will allow discharge without anticoagulant therapy for those patients found to have a negative study. It is imperative to keep in mind that moderate- and high-risk patients who require a lower extremity ultrasound to exclude a DVT should have a repeat scan in 5 to 7 days. This will allow for diagnosis of DVT if a distal thrombus (one in the calf itself) progresses proximally. This is expected to occur in not more than 20% of distal DVT cases.[9]

In general, bedside emergency ultrasonography is not recommended for diagnosing DVTs limited to the calf or ankle. Success rates can be as low as 40% even for experienced vascular technologists; if complicated by edema or large body habitus, success rates will be even lower.[30] Many vascular laboratories no longer scan below the calf and prefer to reexamine patients or perform venography if high suspicion of a calf DVT exists.

UPPER EXTREMITY DVT

Prior to the 1970s, upper extremity DVT was thought to account for less than 2% of all DVT cases.[31] Since that time, some studies have shown upper extremity DVTs to make up as much as 18% of all DVTs and 0.18% of adult hospital admissions.[32] The most common causes of this disease process include malignancy, central venous access lines, and pacemaker wires. Studies have demonstrated that as many as 7 to 9% of upper extremity DVTs will lead to an acute pulmonary embolism.[33,34]

While the gold standard test of venous compression works well in the lower extremities, the subclavian vein does not lend itself to easy compression. Excluding upper extremity DVT depends on indirect confirmation of vein patency in a major venous segment. Although not well studied, this suggests that ruling out an upper extremity DVT may be more difficult for the novice sonologist than in the lower extremities. The solution for some sonologists has been to rely on positive findings for an upper extremity DVT, but not on their negative findings. Patients who have a negative ultrasound examination may be referred to vascular laboratories or radiology for a formal examination. Essentially, since most sonologists are familiar with the appearance of thrombosed deep and peripheral veins, diagnosis of an upper extremity DVT will be highly reliable.

▶ ANATOMIC CONSIDERATIONS

The venous system of the lower extremity is quite simple in a proximal to distal examination until the calf is reached. Although many clinicians may feel they have a "sixth sense" for the location of the femoral vein and artery after several years of practice and the placement of numerous central lines, few clinicians are truly aware of the variations that can exist even at that level of the thigh. While physicians are taught that the femoral vein is located just medial to the pulse from the femoral artery, the novice sonographer quickly discovers that vein and artery may often lie on top of one another rather than side by side. When this happens, a typical arrangement is for the femoral artery to lie on top of the femoral vein.

Proceeding proximal to distal, the first segment after the external iliac vein is the common femoral vein. The common femoral vein then diverges into the deep femoral and superficial femoral veins (Figure 15-1). The nomenclature used here is deceptive and there have even been efforts to change the name of the superficial femoral vein as inexperienced clinicians have sometimes mistaken reports of thrombus in the superficial femoral vein as being outside of the deep venous system. The deep femoral vein travels deep into the thigh. The superficial femoral vein proceeds distally until it dives into the obturator canal. In this region, the vein is difficult to access until it emerges behind the knee as the popliteal vein.

The upper extremity deep veins include the radial and ulnar veins, which arise from the palmar venous plexus (Figure 15-2). The radial and ulnar veins run next to the radial and ulnar arteries and join in the antecubital area to form the brachial vein. The brachial vein runs superiorly, on either side of the brachial artery, and flows into the axillary vein approximately where it is joined by the basilic vein (superficial). The axillary vein flows into the thorax, changing into the subclavian vein. The subclavian vein is then joined by the internal jugular vein to form the brachiocephalic vein.

▶ GETTING STARTED

The ultrasound machine is traditionally parked on the right side of the patient. It should be turned on and allowed to boot up. Most modern ultrasound machines

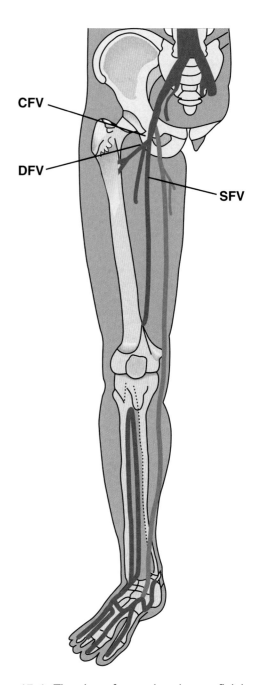

Figure 15-1. The deep femoral and superficial femoral veins are seen to come together, forming the common femoral vein. DFV: deep femoral vein; CFV: common femoral vein; SFV: superficial femoral vein.

will have specific settings that will optimize image processing for a lower extremity venous examination. Once these settings are selected, a linear transducer should be selected in the case of a multitransducer machine. In a machine with a single attached transducer, the linear one should be attached and activated. When possible, the lights in the examination area should be dimmed enough to optimize image visualization on the ultrasound screen while still being able to see transducer placement on the

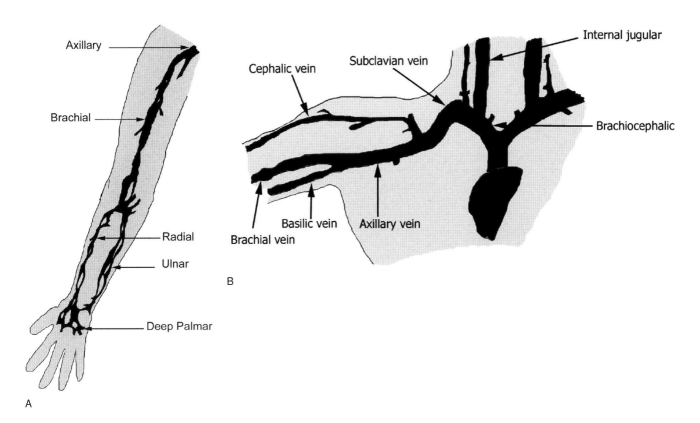

Figure 15-2. Deep veins of the arm (A). Deep veins of the proximal arm and thorax (B).

patient. In this chapter, linear probe or transducer refers to a transducer with a linear scanning format and one that is a linear array.

▶ TECHNIQUE AND NORMAL ULTRASOUND FINDINGS

LOWER EXTREMITY

To perform a lower extremity venous ultrasound examination, a high-resolution linear transducer is required. Most modern ultrasound systems found in emergency departments and clinician offices will have this capability. Color Doppler can be helpful, especially if vascular structures are difficult to distinguish because of poor visualization through soft tissue. Power Doppler, a more sensitive but nondirectional version of color Doppler, can be used as well and is even more likely to detect very slow blood flow, such as in veins.

Ideally, a patient is positioned as needed to maximally distend the leg veins. Many full-length protocols include having the patient dangle his or her leg over the edge of a bed or table (Figure 15-3). This kind of manipulation is not realistic for many clinicians, especially when dealing with acutely ill patients. That said, distended veins do make better targets and it is best

to have the head of the patient's bed up at least 30°, with 45° being preferable. This allows for blood to pool in the lower extremities and may make evaluation of the vein in question much easier. Alternatively, the bed can be put into reverse Trendelenburg position to have

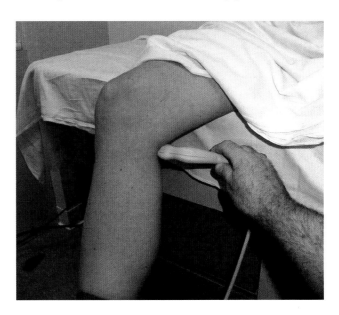

Figure 15-3. The leg is allowed to hang over the edge of the bed with the probe positioned in the popliteal fossa.

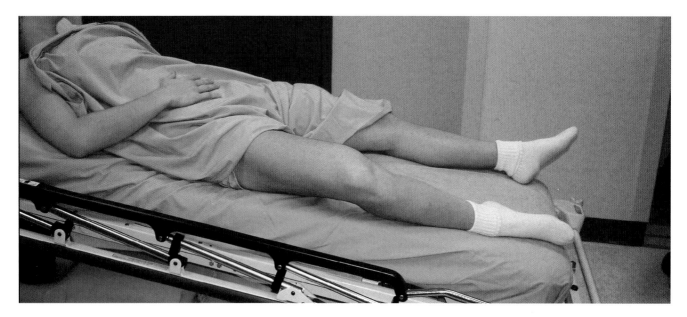

Figure 15-4. A bed angle of 30–45 degrees allows lower extremity veins to fill and makes them easier to locate. (Courtesy of James Mateer MD)

venous blood pool in the lower extremities (Figure 15-4). Vascular laboratories occasionally apply a tourniquet to the extremity to optimize vein engorgement.

An ultrasound transducer with appropriate resolution should be used. Thin patients may require a 7.5 to 10 MHz transducer while larger patients may need the increased penetration of a 5 MHz probe. All of these frequencies can often be obtained in a single broadband transducer. A probe should be utilized that will allow for adequate compression of underlying vascular structures (Figure 15-5). Transducers with a curved face can make it more difficult to achieve adequate compression of soft tissue to ensure collapse of a patent's vein or veins. If challenged by lack of adequate equipment, enterprising physicians can make due with a wide range of transducers, even an endovaginal probe, although the compression achieved may be poor.

The patient's leg may be bent at the knee and turned outward (Figure 15-6). This allows for greater access to the femoral vessels in the proximal thigh and the popliteal vein. However, too great a bend at the knee may actually hinder image acquisition by introducing additional soft tissue and skin between the transducer and vein. The proximal inner thigh and popliteal fossa should be well exposed. The femoral vein and artery are easiest to find with the transducer placed transverse to the long axis of the vessels (Figure 15-7).

An adequate amount of ultrasound gel should be placed on the area of skin where the transducer will be located. The examination starts as proximally as possible in the inguinal area; generally at this location the common femoral vein and artery are visualized in cross section. Ideally, the transducer should already be above the junction of the common femoral and saphenous veins,

but positioning may need to be adjusted more proximally. In some patients the pannus may need to be moved or lifted to expose the most proximal site. Firm pressure downward should be applied to the transducer at the junction of the saphenous and common femoral veins. Both veins should be observed to collapse, thus

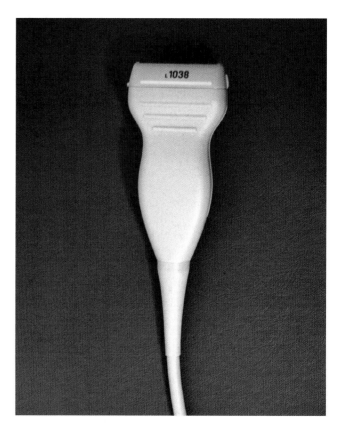

Figure 15-5. A linear array transducer is shown.

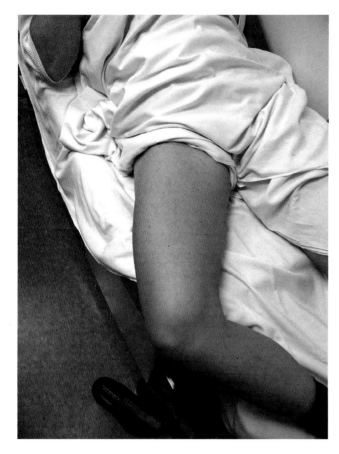

Figure 15-6. The leg is bent at the knee and rotated outward to allow best exposure of popliteal fossa as well as the junction of the common, deep, and superficial femoral veins.

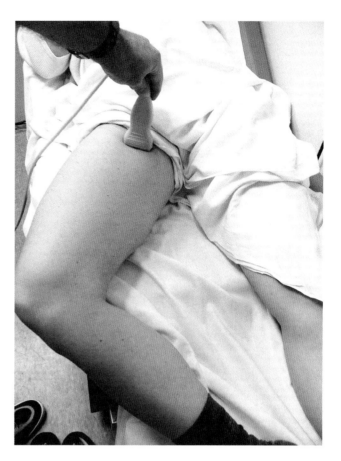

Figure 15-7. The approximate position of the linear probe is shown transversely over the common femoral vein. The probe handle is being held near the cord for demonstration.

ensuring patency. The transducer is then moved distally approximately 1 cm at a time and compression repeated. The examination proceeds through the junction of common femoral, superficial femoral, and deep femoral veins. At each point, firm compression should

be applied to achieve collapse of the vein (Figure 15-8). Although for purposes of demonstrating probe location, the sonologists here appear to be holding the transducer far from the scanning tip, actually doing this would make the scan difficult. The transducer is held close to the

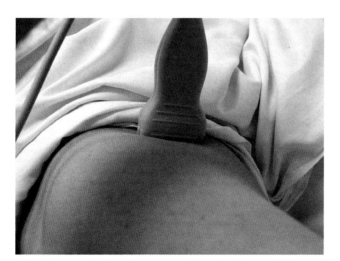

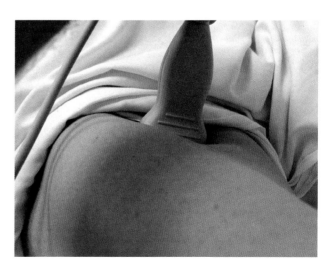

Figure 15-8. A moderate amount of pressure is applied to the leg as shown on the right in this figure. Inadequate pressure can lead to incomplete collapse of the vein.

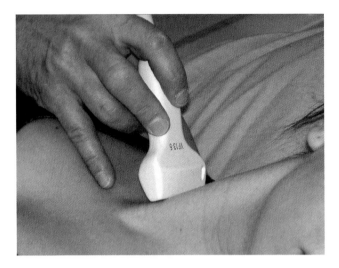

Figure 15-9. The transducer is held firmly and closer to the scanning tip for improved control. The edge of the hand and/or fingers are in contact with the skin to ensure stability and detection of transducer/hand sliding on the lubricated skin. (Courtesy of James Mateer MD)

scanning tip and a portion of the hand should touch the patient's skin to help anchor the transducer and keep it from sliding on the skin (Figure 15-9). In general, enough downward pressure has been applied when the artery is seen to deform. However, stiff venous walls that are resistant to compression in some patients can complicate this. The normal vein should collapse easily while the artery should remain largely intact (Figure 15-10). If there is any difficulty distinguishing artery from vein, color Doppler may be helpful. While both vein and artery may show color flow, the flow in the artery will usually appear more pulsatile than in the vein. The pulse repetition frequency (PRF) can be adjusted (increased) so that slower, and presumably venous, flow will not be picked up. The most reliable method to differentiate ve-

nous from arterial flow would be to activate pulse wave Doppler and compare waveforms between the vessels. The waveform seen in veins will tend to be continuous, with flow still noted in diastole. Arterial waveforms should have a peak and trough quality or a frank triphasic flow pattern. The deep femoral vein is often difficult to follow for more than 1 or 2 cm, but it is critical to ensure complete compression of the proximal segment as it drains into the common femoral vein (Figure 15-11). The total length of the upper leg segment scanned and sequentially compressed (includes the common femoral, saphenous, superficial, and deep femoral veins) is usually not more than 2 or 3 inches in length.

After ensuring patency of the common femoral, proximal great saphenous, common femoral, and deep femoral veins, the simplified approach calls for continuing on to the popliteal fossa. The proximal portion of the popliteal vein is found high in the popliteal fossa. The probe is placed behind the knee and the popliteal artery and vein are located (Figure 15-12). Again, firm pressure is applied to collapse popliteal vein. Applying counterpressure with the nonscanning hand on the outside of the knee may facilitate compression of the popliteal vein. The popliteal vein is traced down to its trifurcation, with compression and relaxation over every centimeter. The distance covered is usually less than 5 cm. It is useful to compress and ensure collapse of the very proximal portions of the calf veins just after trifurcation of the popliteal vein. A clot located in a proximal calf vein can easily extend in the popliteal and seed a proximal DVT. These patients should be treated as a typical proximal DVT. Duplication of the popliteal vein is possible and, if present, both should collapse completely. Complete collapse of the vein's lumen should be visualized, as described above for the femoral veins. Partial collapse can indicate the presence of a clot in the vein; however, poor collapse of the lumen may also be caused by inadequate compression of the vein. This

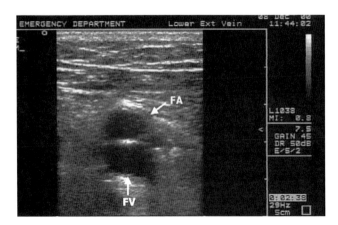
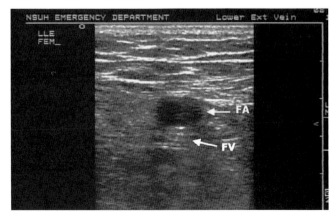

Figure 15-10. Pressure applied to the transducer results in complete collapse of the femoral vein. FV: femoral vein; FA: femoral artery.

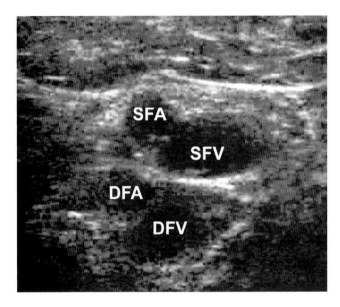
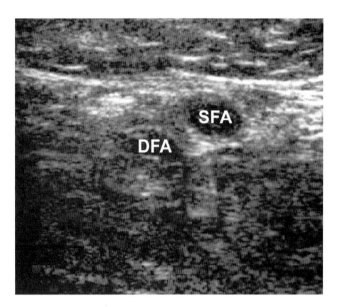

Figure 15-11. On the left side of the image, the transducer is positioned over the superficial and deep femoral arteries (SFA and DFA, respectively) and the superficial and deep femoral veins (SFV and DFV, respectively). On the right side, pressure has been applied and both veins have collapsed completely leaving only the two arteries visible.

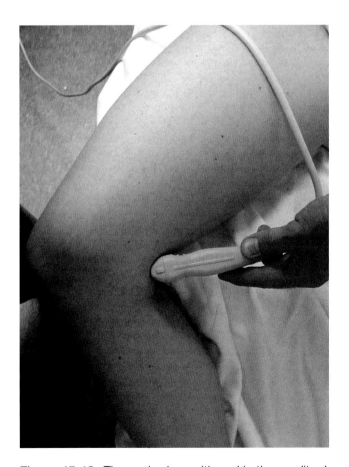

Figure 15-12. The probe is positioned in the popliteal fossa for visualization of the popliteal artery and vein.

can be improved by transducer adjustment or patient manipulation.

Opinions vary on whether or not the contralateral leg should be scanned on a routine basis. Two studies that looked at a combined 3202 patients concluded that in patients with unilateral leg symptoms scanning the contralateral leg was neither indicated nor cost-effective.[35,36] Others have argued that bilateral DVTs are not uncommon and scanning the contralateral leg is indicated.[37] However, this view fails to account for the fact that treatment of unilateral DVT is usually identical to treatment of bilateral DVT. Novice sonologists may find it helpful to compare the anatomy of the contralateral leg when it appears confusing on the extremity being investigated. Otherwise, routinely scanning the asymptomatic leg appears to be unnecessary.

When a DVT is diagnosed, locating the most proximal end of the thrombus may be helpful. Hence, if examination of the femoral vein is normal, but a DVT is found in the popliteal fossa, an effort should be made to track the clot proximally. Identifying the proximal end of the thrombus and noting it in the patient's chart may facilitate patient follow-up, especially if a repeat examination after anticoagulation identifies continued presence of thrombus. Longitudinal views of the vein may be helpful in outlining the shape and extent of the thrombus. Comparison with the position of the proximal end of the thrombus at the time of diagnosis will allow the treating physician to decide if therapy is failing and disease progression has occurred; this may result in more invasive interventions to safeguard the patient from embolization.

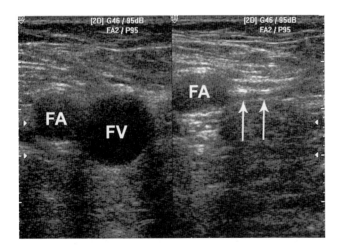

Figure 15-13. A split screen of the common femoral artery (FA) and common femoral vein (FV) with no compression on the left. On the right half, pressure has been applied to the transducer and the femoral vein has collapsed with its wall barely visible (arrows).

Documenting the results of the examination is required if formal reports are being issued. Still images have traditionally been used although physicians are also beginning to utilize video clips. When documenting still images in the medical record, a split screen feature is quite useful. The split screen allows the sonologist to show two images on the screen, with the view on the left being without compression and the one on the right with compression (Figure 15-13). Three standard thermal prints can be attached on one half of an 8.5 × 11 sheet of paper containing the written report on the other half of the same side. With split screen printouts, the sonologist can illustrate whether or not compression at the common femoral and saphenous junction resulted in vein collapse. The next split screen image can address vein lumen response of the proximal superficial femoral and deep femoral veins. The third and final one can show the response of the popliteal vein.

UPPER EXTREMITY

The patient should ideally be examined in the supine position to maximize venous distention. Sonologist preference varies for starting points. Some start at the internal jugular, as superior as possible (Figure 15-14). The jugular vein is located in cross section and lightly compressed. The carotid artery can be differentiated from the jugular vein based on pulse waveforms if the anatomy is not obvious. Gentle compression approximately every centimeter is employed as the jugular vein is traced proximally. Aggressive compression should be avoided in elderly persons. Furthermore, simply elevating the patient's torso will make many jugular veins disappear without any compression.

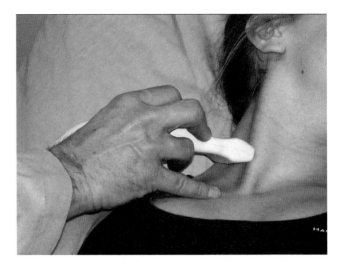

Figure 15-14. A linear transducer is held at the level of the internal jugular in transverse. The entire length of the jugular can be traced and evaluated for thrombus. Aggressive compression is avoided in this region, especially in elderly patients. Interrogation is started higher on the neck than shown here. (Courtesy of James Mateer MD)

The jugular vein can typically be visualized entering the brachiocephalic vein with the subclavian vein. Compression at this point is not possible and direct visualization of thrombus or lack of flow on color or power Doppler will be the best method for sonologists to diagnose a DVT. The subclavian vein is then traced toward the shoulder with Doppler interrogation wherever it is visible (Figure 15-15). Pulsed wave Doppler can differentiate between the subclavian artery and vein, if the anatomy is not obvious. The proximal portion of the axillary vein usually cannot be visualized because of overlying bone. Once in the axilla the axillary vein and the

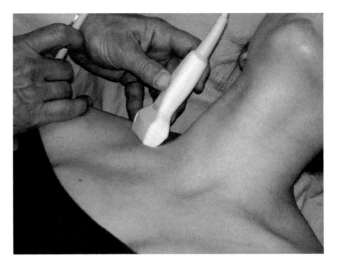

Figure 15-15. A linear transducer is held just above the clavicle, allowing a longitudinal view of the subclavian vein. (Courtesy of James Mateer MD)

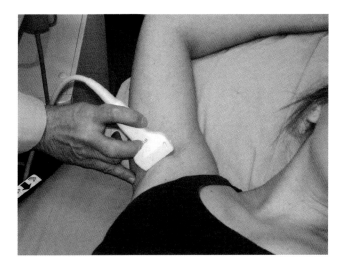

Figure 15-16. A linear transducer is held in the axilla. This allows transverse visualization of the vessels and compression. (Courtesy of James Mateer MD)

brachial vein can again be directly compressed to assure patency (Figure 15-16). Once the antecubital fossa has been reached the radial and ulnar veins split to either side of the forearm and are compressed one at a time.

► COMMON AND EMERGENT ABNORMALITIES

The inability to collapse a vein on ultrasound indicates the presence of thrombus within the vein (Figure 15-17). The same does not apply to arteries, which can be difficult to collapse. It is imperative to recognize that one must have adequate access to the vein to test collapsibility. Applying pressure at an angle or in an area where overlying structures may distribute pressure away from the vessel lumen might result in false-positive findings.

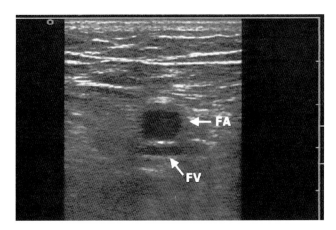

Figure 15-17. The femoral vein is not completely collapsed. If adequate pressure has been applied, a thrombus is likely present. FV: femoral vein; FA: femoral artery.

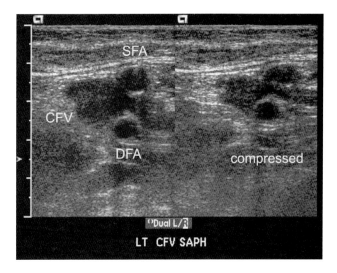

Figure 15-18. Split screen image of left common femoral vein (CFV) near saphenous junction. The superficial and deep branches of the femoral artery are labeled (DFA, SFA). The CFV contains echoes that represent clot, and does not fully collapse with compression (right image). (Courtesy of James Mateer, MD, Waukesha Memorial Hospital)

ACUTE DVT

The clot itself may be seen as an echogenicity within the lumen, and the vein will not collapse completely with compression (Figure 15-18). Longitudinal views of a vein may be helpful in outlining the shape and extent of thrombus (Figure 15-19). In many instances, especially with more primitive equipment, the only evidence of a DVT is the inability to compress the vein.

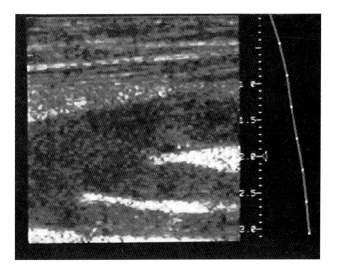

Figure 15-19. Longitudinal view of the common femoral vein reveals intralumenal clot also involving all of the branching vessels. (Courtesy of Lori Green, Gulfcoast Ultrasound)

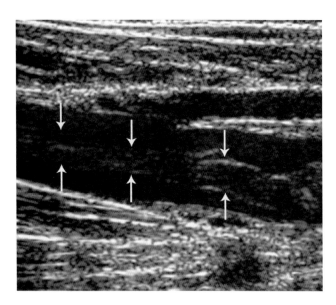

Figure 15-20. Arrows show a freely floating thrombus in the femoral vein. In this portion of the image the clot does not come in contact with the anterior or posterior wall of the vein.

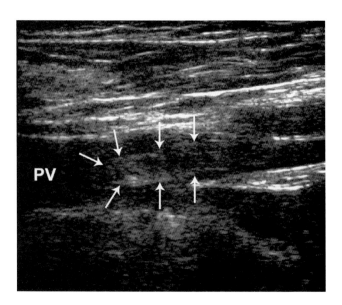

Figure 15-22. A longitudinal image of the popliteal vein (PV) on the left side of the image. On the right side the popliteal vein is splitting. Arrows outline a free floating thrombus coming out of a calf vein into the very distal portion of the popliteal. This clot would not have been caught if imaging had not included the proximal portion of popliteal trifurcation.

Near complete compression of the vein is not sufficient to exclude DVT (Figure 15-17). The lumen of the vessel must disappear completely to exclude the presence of a clot (Figure 15-10). An obvious thrombus that appears to be free floating, or not attached to the vessel walls, should not be unnecessarily compressed if the diagnosis is obvious (Figures 15-20 and 15-21). In such cases a longitudinal image of a floating clot will adequately relay

the diagnosis (Figure 15-22). While there have not been any reported cases of embolization caused by ultrasound evaluation, it is simply not necessary to compress an obvious floating thrombus. In addition, a floating thrombus has the highest chance of embolization.

CHRONIC DVT

This condition refers to the presence of an old clot within a vein that has recanulated and allowed venous flow around or through the clot. Complete collapse of the venous lumen will not be possible. Acute DVT may have a similar appearance and occlude only part of the vein. Acute clots tend to be less echogenic than chronic ones; however, this is not always reliable (Figure 15-23). Clots tend to recanalize centrally and may thus leave a channel of blood flow through the central area of the thrombus (Figure 15-24). Despite the fact that there may be historical indications that a clot is chronic, as well as echogenicity differences between acute and chronic clot, it may still be difficult to differentiate between the two in a newly diagnosed patient. Review of prior ultrasound studies is helpful when available. Interrogating the vein in long axis can also be helpful. The sonologist may be able to visualize thickened vessel walls resulting from scaring of the previous thrombus. This appearance differs from acute DVT enough to allow differentiation and correct diagnosis (Figure 15-25). The chronic

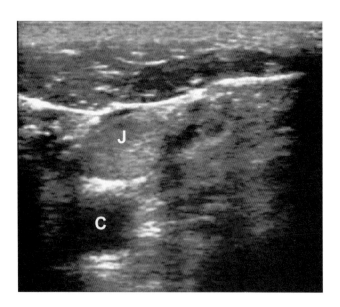

Figure 15-21. A transverse image shows a noticeable thrombus in this jugular vein (J), just superficial to the carotid artery (C). Compression was not necessary to verify that a DVT was present in this obvious case.

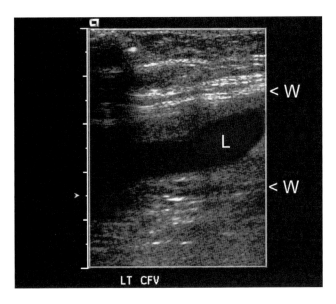

Figure 15-23. Longitudinal view of the common femoral vein shows chronic echogenic clot along the walls (W) with central recanulation of the lumen (L). (Courtesy of James Mateer, MD, Waukesha Memorial Hospital)

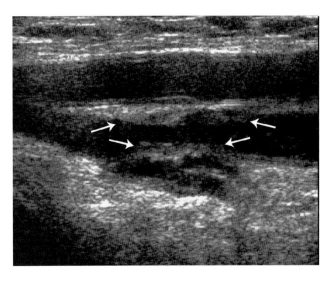

Figure 15-25. A chronic DVT is seen in this deep femoral vein. Arrows point to areas of scarring that are echogenic and lie along the walls of the vein. A channel is open for blood flow in between the two areas of scar or chronic DVT.

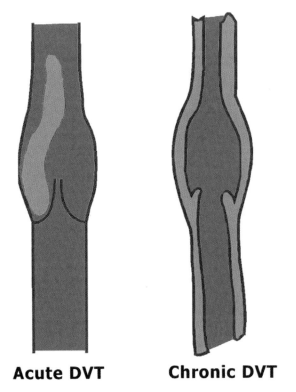

Acute DVT   Chronic DVT

Figure 15-24. The illustration on the right shows a recanalized, old thrombus. The left image demonstrates an early acute thrombus that can enlarge and obstruct flow completely.

thrombus will tend to be more irregular and will compress less. Collaterals are more likely to be present with a chronic DVT and should be sought. If the diagnosis remains uncertain at this point, it may be prudent to treat the patient for an acute DVT, with a formal ultrasound examination performed within 24 hours. This situation is infrequent, and the history and ultrasound examination will lead to a diagnosis in the majority of possible chronic DVT cases.

SUPERFICIAL VENOUS CLOT

The physician evaluating the source of focal leg pain and swelling may encounter a superficial venous clot. It is not uncommon to find a clot limited to the saphenous vein when investigating DVT in the thigh. Although recommendations for treatment of superficial clot, such as in the saphenous vein, differ from source to source, superficial venous thrombosis clearly does not pose the same degree of danger in most patients unless it is propagating into the saphenofemoral junction. Clot in the saphenous vein, near the entrance to the common femoral vein, should be considered a DVT since propagation and seeding of the common femoral vein is not unlikely. Similarly, superficial thrombi that have progressive symptoms may need to be reassessed to detect clot propagation (Figure 15-26). Findings of a propagating superficial thrombus may lead some clinicians to anticoagulate the patient or at least require close follow-up.

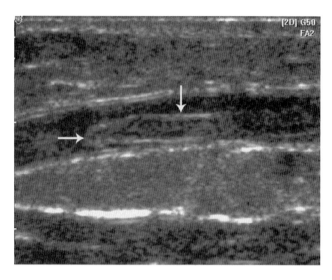

Figure 15-26. This thrombus (arrows) located in the great saphenous vein in the distal thigh was noted to travel to the upper thigh in just 2 days when the patient returned for follow-up.

► COMMON VARIANTS AND SELECTED ABNORMALITIES

When evaluating the lower extremity venous system, other cystic structures may be mistaken for normal and pathological findings. Lymph nodes may be encountered while studying the common femoral and femoral vein junction, especially in ill patients (Figure 15-27). An inflamed lymph node can be initially mistaken for a non-collapsing vein due to similar echogenicity and cross-sectional structure. Careful ultrasonographic evaluation of the structure will show its true shape to be spherical

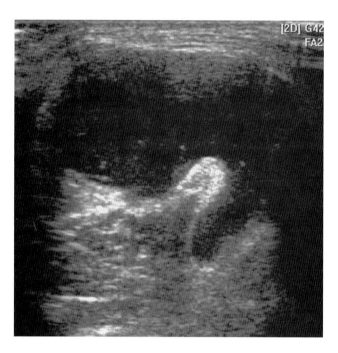

Figure 15-28. Longitudinal view of the posterior knee area demonstrates a large Baker's cyst.

rather than a tubular vessel. Duplication of vessels can occur, and it is important to identify any extra vessels and ensure their patency as well.

Findings in the popliteal fossa include Baker's cysts (Figure 15-28), which can be confusing when small in size (Figure 15-29). Careful examination of the structure should lead to its discrimination from the popliteal vein. Rupture of a Baker's cyst should be considered in any patient with calf swelling who has a history of chronic

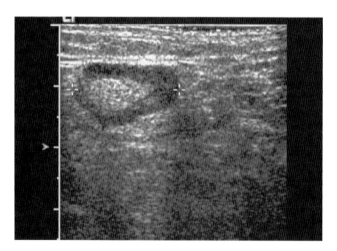

Figure 15-27. Typical appearance of an enlarged inguinal lymph node (2 cm). The thickened capsule is hypoechoic while the central hilum is echogenic. (Courtesy of James Mateer, MD, Waukesha Memorial Hospital)

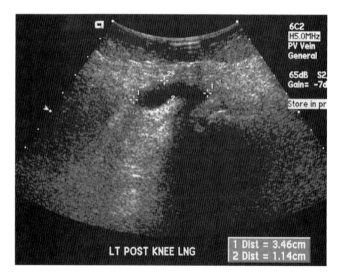

Figure 15-29. Longitudinal view of the posterior knee reveals a small Baker's cyst. (Courtesy of James Mateer, MD, Waukesha Memorial Hospital)

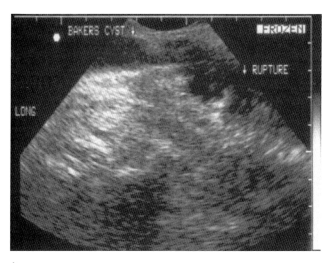
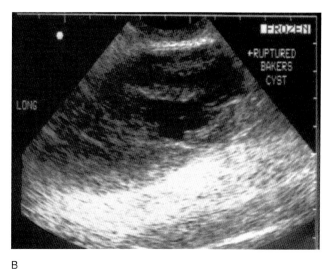

A

B

Figure 15-30. Ruptured Bakers's Cyst. (A) Longitudinal view of the posterior knee shows a Baker's cyst (left upper image) communicating with subcutaneous fluid in the upper calf. (B) Longitudinal view over the mid calf of the same patient shows a significant amount of subcutaneous fluid dissecting inferiorly. (Courtesy of James Mateer, MD)

arthritis or knee effusion. These can present with impressive swelling and pain and may reveal fluid, dissecting through soft tissue planes, posterior to and below the knee on ultrasound (Figure 15-30). Popliteal artery aneurysms are occasionally encountered and may make it harder to compress the popliteal vein in one location. Aneurysms over 2 cm can cause complications and should be followed closely.

▶ PITFALLS

1. **Contraindication.** There are no absolute contraindications to evaluating the deep venous system of the lower extremities. Patient comfort or level of cooperation may limit the examination. There have not been any documented cases of embolization as a result of DVT evaluation in a patient. An obvious free-floating clot, however, does not require compression.

2. **Imaging challenging subjects.** Patients who are morbidly obese or have severe lower extremity edema may be very difficult to image. The ultrasound beam greatly deteriorates with increased fat as well as distance. A variety of adjustments or changes can be made on some equipment to optimize imaging and the sonologist should be aware of what these are on the machine. Such helpful functions can include tissue harmonics, compound imaging, and other software or hardware functions.

3. **Segmental DVT.** One concern about this examination is the possibility of segmental DVT; for instance, a DVT potentially may span several centimeters of the femoral vein midthigh but cannot be found anywhere else. The true incidence of such an occurrence is not known, but evidence suggests that it is very rare. However, as is recommended for all moderate- and high-risk patients, a lower extremity ultrasound examination to exclude DVT should be repeated in 5–7 days to exclude propagation of an undetected calf thrombosis. Such a repeat examination would also catch a propagating segmental clot. If a patient is able to identify a specific area of localized pain or swelling on his or her thigh, evaluating that area for possible DVT is reasonable and may be reassuring.

4. **Misunderstanding the limitations of ultrasonography.** Although ultrasound is now the method of choice for detecting the presence of lower extremity thrombosis, the test is not 100% accurate. Practitioners should understand the limitation of this examination, especially when considering that the method described in this chapter does not attempt to evaluate veins in the calf. Furthermore, the use of ultrasound examination of bilateral lower extremities to exclude pulmonary embolism is fraught with potential danger if the physician does not keep in mind that only a positive finding if helpful. Specifically, as many as two thirds of all patients with a pulmonary embolisms will not have a proximal

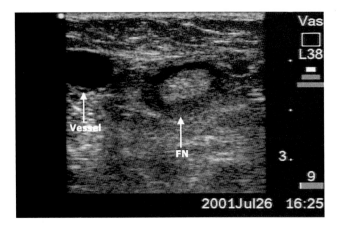

Figure 15-31. The femoral node next to the actual vein has an uncanny resemblance to a lumen filled with thrombus. FN: Femoral lymph node.

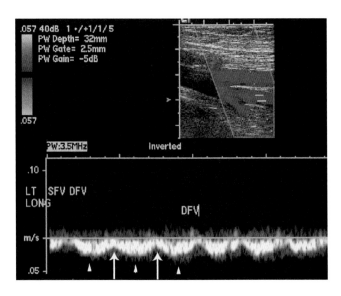

Figure 15-32. Respiratory variation in the venous flow pattern is seen in this tachypnaec patient. The venous tracing from the deep femoral vein has repeated peaks and troughs noted by arrow heads and arrows, respectively.

DVT found on ultrasound. This makes sense as the thrombus has probably embolized to the lungs.[38]

5. **Mistaking artery for vein.** While this is not a common pitfall, novice sonologists should be aware that in some cases an artery may be pliable enough to collapse under moderate transducer pressure while the vein lumen is held open by the presence of clot. If available, color and pulse wave Doppler may help simplify the identification of blood vessels.

6. **Femoral lymph nodes mistaken for a DVT.** Occasionally, lymph nodes encountered in the groin can be mistaken for an uncompressible deep vein. This is especially true for inflamed lymph nodes. Figure 15-31 shows an example of a large lymph node that was mistaken for a femoral DVT. The lymph node is a finite structure and moving the transducer proximally or distally will allow the sonologist to identify the edges of the lymph node. Rotating the probe will also frequently show the boundaries of the lymph node as well as its atypical appearance for a blood vessel. Lymph nodes tend to be more superficial or closer to the skin surface than deep vessels.

7. **Pelvic vein thrombosis.** Thrombosis of the pelvic veins, such as the external iliac, frequently occurs in combination with DVT of the common femoral and more distal venous segments. Thus, identification of clot in the external iliac vein is not as crucial when a common femoral DVT is located and the patient is anticoagulated. However, in a small percentage of cases, thrombosis of the pelvic veins is an isolated event.[39] Isolated pelvic vein thrombosis may be quite challenging to diagnose and poses a high risk of emboliza-

tion. Ultrasound interrogation of the external iliac, common iliac, and the proximal portion of the internal iliac vein is possible in some thin patients without interfering bowel gas. In a minority of patients, the external and common iliac can be seen and compressed. If suspicion for pelvic vein thrombosis exists and ultrasound will not provide adequate imaging, then other diagnostic measures such as computed tomography with venous angiography will have to be employed. Even if the iliac veins cannot be visualized, a DVT may be suspected if there is a lack of respiratory variation of the venous flow in the common iliac vein. Normally, variation is seen in the baseline venous flow with respiration (Figure 15-32). If this variation is absent, it is suggestive of a proximal obstruction, such as a thrombus in the external or common iliac ipsilaterally. Conversely, if respiratory variation is observed, then there is unlikely to be complete obstruction of proximal veins.

8. **Slow venous blood flow.** Occasionally blood flow in a vein segment may be slow enough that swirling of the blood is actually seen within the lumen. This can have the appearance of echogenic material in the vein and be mistaken for a thrombus. It is important not to make this mistake by moving too quickly through the examination. Compression of the vein segment will reveal complete collapse of the vein and disappearance of the vein lumen.

► CASE STUDIES

CASE 1

Patient Presentation

A 25-year-old woman presented to the emergency department with a complaint of right calf swelling and pain. The patient was a law school student who was studying for final examinations. She denied any strenuous activity and noted spending most of the last week sitting in the library. The patient is normally athletic and rides a stationary bicycle daily. She had an unremarkable medical history and did not smoke. She thought her older sister had a "blood clot" several years ago.

Physical examination revealed a healthy young woman with normal vital signs, including an oxygen saturation of 98% on room air. She had a moderately tender right calf without any visible erythema or palpable cord. The patient had moderate discomfort on manipulation of her foot at the ankle. Her right calf measures approximately 1.5 cm larger on the left, a fact the patient attributes to a left knee injury while playing soccer in college.

Management Course

The vascular laboratory was not open on Saturday and the on-call radiologist recommended that the patient be anticoagulated and admitted into the hospital until she could be imaged as the first case on Monday morning. The patient is originally from another state and did not have a primary care physician in the area. She insisted that she must study for her law school finals and, unless medically necessary, she would prefer to go home. She does voice concern regarding the possibility of a DVT as she noted her sister was "very sick" from her blood clot. The emergency physician performed an ultrasound examination of the patient's right leg. The common femoral and saphenous vein junction and the deep femoral and superficial femoral veins were located and complete obliteration of the lumen was seen with moderate compression. The popliteal vein was visualized behind the knee and also compresses normally. The patient was given appropriate instructions and was requested to follow up with the university's clinic Monday after her examinations. She was told that she should have a follow-up ultrasound evaluation in 5–7 days.

Commentary

Case 1 represents an example of a fairly low-risk patient who can still inspire considerable angst for the treating physician. With her suggestive symptoms and family history, the patient might present a medicolegal risk if she was discharged home without definitive diagnostic imaging. Conversely, if the patient were to be admitted to await an imaging study, she would spend the weekend in the hospital and miss her law school examinations. This scenario is quite realistic in many facilities. Staffing a vascular laboratory 24 hours a day, 7 days a week, can be too expensive, especially when coupled with a shortage of sonographers. Treating the patient with low-molecular-weight heparin as an outpatient may seem attractive, but has some limitations. The patient must be trained to administer the injections. Furthermore, while the risk of bleeding was low, it is present and could once again be a medicolegal issue for some physicians. In this case, the emergency physician was able to confidently exclude a proximal DVT and promptly discharge the patient. She could follow up in 2 days with the school's clinic and had a repeat ultrasound examination arranged to exclude propagation of a calf vein thrombosis.

CASE 2

Patient Presentation

A 60-year-old man with a history of chronic obstructive pulmonary disease, arthritis, coronary artery disease, and hypertension presented to the ED with complaints of vague pain in his left lower extremity. The patient noted that he typically had pain in either or both legs and requested a prescription for rofecoxib, which had helped with the pain in the past. He denied any new leg swelling and stated that they were both a little swollen all the time. The patient further denied chest pain or shortness of breath and gave no history of thrombosis in the past.

Physical examination revealed a comfortable appearing man. The patient's vital signs were within normal limits with an oxygen saturation of 96% on room air. The cardiac and lung examinations were remarkable for distant heart sounds and coarse breath sounds. The lower extremity examination revealed venous stasis changes on both lower legs as well as tenderness at both knees and ankles on range of motion. The patient appeared to complain of calf pain on both sides but more so on the left. There was mild nonpitting edema. No palpable cord was felt and no erythema was seen posteriorly.

Management Course

The vascular laboratory was contacted but was unable to perform the examination for several hours due to a backlog from the floor. The patient asked to be discharged, stating that this was just his arthritis and he would see his own physician when he was back from vacation next week. A bedside ultrasound examination was performed and showed normally collapsing femoral veins. However, the popliteal vein did not collapse completely with compression (Figure 15-33). The partner covering the

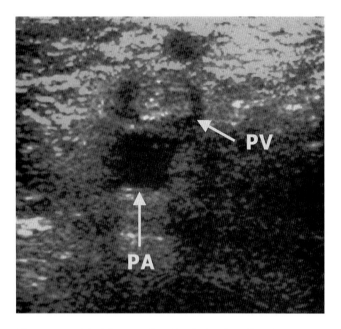

Figure 15-33. The popliteal vein is visualized above the popliteal artery and has a distinct echogenic thrombus within it. PV: popliteal vein; PA: popliteal artery.

patient's primary physician was contacted and agreed to see the patient in the office the next morning if a low-molecular-weight heparin injection could be administered to the patient. The patient received an injection and was discharged to be seen approximately 12 hours later by his physician.

Commentary

Case 2 illustrates the utility of focused compression venous ultrasound. The patient had several confounding issues such a chronic arthritic pain and lower extremity swelling. However, he deserved an ultrasound evaluation to exclude thrombosis. The vascular laboratory, busy as most are, was not able to perform the examination for several hours. A rapid examination of the proximal deep veins in the affected leg revealed a popliteal DVT. The patient was able to be treated with an injection of low-molecular-weight heparin and was discharged to follow up with his physician. The care of the patient was simplified and saved a considerable amount of time.

CASE 3

Patient Presentation

A 22-year-old woman with a history of sickle cell disease presents with a complaint of left lower leg swelling and pain. The patient states that she first began to notice discomfort in the leg 4 days ago and today notices swelling, redness, and increased pain. She denies any history of

trauma and states her typical sickle cell pain is higher in the leg and different from this episode.

Physical examination reveals normal vital signs with a temperature of 100.0°F. The examination is within normal limits except for the patient's lower left leg. She has erythema and increased temperature of the anterior shin as well as nonpitting edema. The area is sensitive to the touch. The calf is mildly tender and may be slightly swollen. The patient's ankle is also swollen but no deformity is noted. She had diffuse pain in the ankle and anterior shin with flexion and extension of the foot. Distal pulses are present and equal to the contralateral side.

Management Course

The patient is seen at night and no vascular laboratory testing is available. A bedside ultrasound examination of the left leg is performed and shows normally collapsing femoral and popliteal veins. With no proximal clot detected, the patient is given a dose of parenteral clindamycin and is discharged on oral clindamycin. The patient is scheduled for follow-up the next day with the primary care physician, who is advised to obtain a follow-up lower extremity Doppler examination in 5–7 days to rule out propagation of an undetectable distal venous clot.

Commentary

In case 3, the patient is once again at low risk, but cellulitis must be differentiated from a possible DVT. The clinician's ability to perform a bedside ultrasound examination provided accurate diagnosis and rapid disposition of the patient.

REFERENCES

1. Blaivas M, Sierzenski P, Lambert M: Emergency evaluation of patients presenting with acute scrotum using bedside ultrasonography. *Acad Emerg Med* 8:90–93, 2001.
2. Blaivas M: Bedside emergency department ultrasonography in the evaluation of ocular pathology. *Acad Emerg Med* 7:947–950, 2000.
3. Roy S, Dewitz A, Paul I: Ultrasound-assisted ankle arthrocentesis. *Am J Emerg Med* 17(3):300–301, 1999.
4. Hilty WM, Hudson PA, Levitt MA, Hall JB: Real-time ultrasound-guided femoral vein catheterization during cardiopulmonary resuscitation. *Ann Emerg Med* 29:331–337, 1997.
5. Frazee BW, Snoey ER, Levitt A: Emergency department compression ultrasound to diagnose proximal deep vein thrombosis. *J Emerg Med* 20:107–112, 2001.
6. Jolly BT, Massarin E, Pigman EC: Color Doppler ultrasonography by emergency physicians for the diagnosis of acute deep venous thrombosis. *Acad Emerg Med* 4:129–132, 1997.

7. Hendler MF, Meschengieser SS, Blanco AN, et al.: Primary upper-extremity deep vein thrombosis: High prevalence of thrombophilic defects. *Am J Hematol.* 76:330–337, 2004.

8. Trottier SJ, Todi S, Veremakis C: Validation of an inexpensive B-Mode ultrasound device for detection of deep vein thrombosis. *Chest* 110:1547–1550, 1996.

9. Birdwell BG, Raskob GE, Whitsett TL, et al.: The clinical validity of normal compression ultrasonography in outpatients suspected of having deep venous thrombosis. *Ann Inter Med* 128:1–7, 1998.

10. Blaivas M, Lambert M, Harwood R, Wood J, Konicki J: Lower extremity doppler for deep venous thrombosis: Can emergency physicians be accurate and fast? *Acad Emerg Med* 7:120–126, 2000.

11. Theodoro D, Blaivas M, Duggal S, Snyder G, Lucas M: Real-time B-mode ultrasound in the ED saves time in the diagnosis of deep vein thrombosis (DVT). *Am J Emerg Med* 22:197–200, 2004.

12. Chance JF, Abbitt PL, Tegtmeyer CJ, Powers RD: Real-time ultrasound for the detection of deep venous thrombosis. *Ann Emerg Med* 20:494–496, 1991.

13. Rydberg EJ, Westfall JM, Nicholas RA: Low-molecular-weight heparin in preventing and treating DVT. *Am Fam Physician* 59:1607–12, 1999.

14. Vinson DR, Berman DA: Outpatient treatment of deep venous thrombosis: A clinical care pathway managed by the emergency department. *Ann Emerg Med* 37:251–258, 2001.

15. Bates SM, Grand'Maison A, Johnston M, Naguit I, Kovacs MJ, Ginsberg JS: A latex D-dimer reliably excludes venous thromboembolism. *Arch Intern Med* 161:447–453, 2001.

16. Anderson DR, Wells PS, Stiell I, et al.: Management of patients with suspected deep vein thrombosis in the emergency department: combining use of a clinical diagnosis model with D-dimer testing. *J Emerg Med* 19:225–230, 2000.

17. McIlrath ST, Blaivas M, Lyon M: Patient follow-up after negative lower extremity bedside ultrasound for deep venous thrombosis in the ED. *Am J Emerg Med* 24(3):325–328, 2006.

18. Philbrick JT, Becker DM: Calf deep venous thrombosis. A wolf in sheep's clothing? *Arch Intern Med* 148:2131–2138, 1988.

19. Poppiti R, Papanicolaou G, Perese S, Weaver FA: Limited B-mode venous imaging versus complete color-flow duplex venous scanning for detection of proximal deep venous thrombosis. *J Vasc Surg* 22:553–557, 1995.

20. Lensing AWA, Doris CI, McGrath FP, et al.: A comparison of compression ultrasound with color Doppler ultrasound for the diagnosis of symptomless postoperative deep vein thrombosis. *Arch Intern Med* 157:765–768, 1997.

21. Lensing AWA, Prandoni P, Brandjes D, et al.: Detection of deep-vein thrombosis by real-time B-modee ultrasonography. *N Engl J Med* 320:342–345, 1989.

22. Lund F, Diener L, Ericsson JLE: Postmortem intraosseous phlebography as an aid in studies of venous thromboembolism. *Agiology* 20:155–176, 1969.

23. Heijboer H, Buller HR, Lensing AWA, Turpie AGG, Colly LP, Wouter TC: A comparison of real-time compression ultrasonography with impedance plethysmography for the diagnosis of deep-vein thrombosis in symptomatic outpatients. *N Engl J Med* 329:1365–1369, 1993.

24. Frederick MG, Hertzber BS, Kliewer MA, et al.: Can the US examination for lower extremity deep venous thrombosis be abbreviated? A prospective study of 755 examinations. *Radiology* 199:45–47, 1996.

25. Lennox AF, Delis KT, Serunkuma S, Zarka ZA, Daskalopoulou SE, Nicolaides AN: Combination of a clinical risk assessment score and rapid whole blood D-dimer testing in the diagnosis of deep vein thrombosis in symptomatic patients. *J Vasc Surg* 30:794–803, 1999.

26. Swarczinski C, Dijkers M: The value of serial leg measurements for monitoring deep vein thrombosis in spinal cord injury. *J Neurosci Nurs* 23:306–314, 1991.

27. Sellman JS, Holman RL: Thromboembolism during pregnancy. Risks, challenges, and recommendations. *Postgrad Med* 108:71–84, 2000.

28. Motykie GD, Caprini JA, Arcelus JI, et al.: Risk factor assessment in the management of patients with suspected deep venous thrombosis. *Int Angiol* 19:47–51, 2000.

29. Diamond PT, Macciocchi SN: Predictive power of clinical symptoms in patients with presumptive deep venous thrombosis. *Am J Phys Med Rehabil* 76:49–51, 1997.

30. Eskandari MK, Sugimoto H, Richardson T, Webster MW, Makaroun MS: Is color-flow duplex a good diagnostic test for detection of isolated calf vein thrombosis in high-risk patients? *Angiology* 51:705–710, 2000.

31. Tilney ML, Griffiths HJ, Edwards EA: Natural history of major venous thrombosis of the upper extremity. *Arch Surg* 101:792–796, 1970.

32. Mustafa S, Stein PD, Patel KC, Otten TR, Holmes R, Silbergleit A: Upper extremity deep venous thrombosis. *Chest* 123:1953–1956, 2003.

33. Becker DM, Philbrick JT, Walker FB IV: Axillary and subclavian venous thrombosis. Prognosis and treatment. *Arch Intern Med* 151:1934–1943, 1991.

34. Monreal M, Lafoz E, Ruiz J, Valls R, Alastrue A: Upper-extremity deep venous thrombosis and pulmonary embolism. A prospective study. *Chest* 99:280–283, 1991.

35. Sheiman RG, McArdle CR: Bilateral lower extremity US in the patient with unilateral symptoms of deep venous thrombosis: Assessment of need. *Radiology* 194:171–173, 1995.

36. Strothman G, Blebea J, Fowl RJ, Rosenthal G: Contralateral duplex scanning for deep venous thrombosis is unnecessary in patients with symptoms. *J Vasc Surg* 22:543–547, 1995.

37. Naidich JB, Torre JR, Pellerito JS, Smalberg IS, Kase DJ, Crystal KS: Suspected deep venous thrombosis: Is US of both legs necessary? *Radiology* 200:429–431, 1996.

38. Kluetz PG, White CS: Acute pulmonary embolism: imaging in the emergency department. *Radiol Clin North Am* 44:259–271, 2006.

39. Carpenter JP, Holland GA, Baum RA, Owen RS, Carpenter JT, Cope C: Magnetic resonance venography for the detection of deep venous thrombosis: Comparison with contrast venography and duplex Doppler ultrasonography. *J Vasc Surg* 18(5):734–741, 1993.

CHAPTER 16

Soft Tissue

Andreas Dewitz and Bradley W. Frazee

Beyond the well-known primary and secondary indications for emergency ultrasound lie a plethora of clinically useful soft tissue ultrasound applications. These offer the emergency care provider the ability to rapidly evaluate and better manage a wide array of common clinical problems. This chapter will focus on eight areas where the use of these soft tissue techniques can be of considerable value in the care of the emergency or ambulatory care patient. These include (1) evaluation of abdominal wall masses, (2) miscellaneous applications for the airway, (3) assessment of bony cortices for rapid fracture diagnosis, (4) foreign body localization, (5) imaging of tendons, joints, and muscles, (6) diagnosis of salivary gland disease, (7) bedside detection of maxillary sinusitis, and (8) evaluation of soft tissue infections, particularly for detection and accurate localization of subcutaneous abscesses prior to drainage.

▶ ABDOMINAL WALL

CLINICAL CONSIDERATIONS AND INDICATIONS

A surprisingly wide range of pathological processes can occur in the abdominal wall and a patient's abdominal pain may, on occasion, be discovered to be due to a lesion or defect within this anatomic region. Since the area of anatomic interest is quite superficial and free of shadowing artifacts, it is well suited to sonographic evaluation with a linear array transducer. When a palpable or indistinct abdominal wall mass is found on physical examination, or when a focal area of abdominal wall tenderness is encountered, a bedside ultrasound examination of the affected area may help provide immediate answers to a number of clinical questions. Is the region of tenderness due to a lesion within the abdominal wall itself or does it appear that an underlying structure (e.g., a metastatic lesion in the liver) is causing the discomfort? If a lesion is present, where is it and what are its sonographic characteristics? Is it solid, cystic, hypo, or hyperechoic, or is fluid collection present? Is a fascial defect present in the abdominal wall, and if so, is a loop of bowel seen passing through the defect? Armed with this additional anatomic knowledge, the site of the findings, and the history, the provider can then pursue a more targeted work-up of the abnormal process at hand.

Incisional hernias are said to occur as a delayed complication in up to 4% of abdominal surgeries[1] and ultrasound can sometimes detect the fascial defect early in its development. While many abdominal wall hernias are apparent on clinical examination alone and do not require sonographic evaluation for diagnosis, others can be difficult to diagnose because the fascial defect is small and difficult to appreciate clinically. The fascial defect in a Spigelian hernia (also known as an **interstitial hernia**) will always be found along the lateral border of the rectus muscle and a focal defect will be present in the aponeuroses of the transversus abdominus and internal oblique muscles but *not* in the aponeurosis of the external oblique muscle. Since the fascial defect lies beneath the external oblique aponeurosis, the defect may not be apparent on clinical examination. A Spigelian hernia will typically be found where the lateral rectus sheath intersects with the inferior margin of the rectus sheath at a region termed the arcuate line, located about halfway between the umbilicus and the pubis. Signs and symptoms of a Spigelian hernia can be nonspecific and the pain may be poorly localized. Peak incidence is said to occur at age 50, with men and women affected equally.[2]

The **femoral region** may be host to a wide range of pathologic and postoperative entities ranging from inguinal and femoral hernias, reactive and metastatic lymph nodes, lipomas, abscesses, hematomas, lymphomas, soft tissue sarcomas, vascular bypass grafts, and pseudoaneurysms.[3] Ultrasound examination of the groin can narrow the differential diagnosis and help differentiate among the many pathologic processes that occur in this anatomic region. Ultrasound has long been noted to be more effective at distinguishing adenopathy than clinical palpation alone.[1]

A patient's abdominal pain is sometimes discovered to be due to a spontaneous or posttraumatic **rectus sheath hematoma**, most frequently caused by sudden vigorous abdominal contractions in the setting of a seizure, a coughing or sneezing paroxysm, direct trauma, or recent surgery. Patients on anticoagulant therapy are most prone to this malady, and bleeding may occur because of rupture of an epigastric artery or vein or because of a tear of the rectus muscle fibers.[1] The resulting hematoma remains confined to the rectus sheath.

Abdominal wall endometriosis can occur at the site of a previous C-section or lapartomy and should be considered in the differential diagnosis of a women presenting with recurrent focal abdominal wall pain with menses. Although the sonographic finding of a hypoechoic mass within the region of the operative scar is nonspecific, this finding coupled with a characteristic history can help make the diagnosis.[4]

Finally, **other abdominal wall masses** such as lipomas, sebaceous cysts, subcutaneous abscesses, cutaneous metastases, a primary malignant melanoma, hemangiomas, and pseudoaneurysms of the epigastric artery may all occur in the abdominal wall and should also be included in the differential diagnosis of a palpable or tender abdominal wall mass. Ultrasound has also been used to help localize the injection port of an intrathecal drug delivery pump whose location in the abdominal wall could not be found clinically.[5]

ANATOMICAL CONSIDERATIONS

The abdominal wall is composed of skin, subcutaneous tissue of varying thickness depending on patient habitus, muscular layers that also vary in thickness with patient habitus and conditioning, and finally, a layer of extraperitoneal fat. The muscular layers are enclosed in fibrous fascial sheaths. The fascial sheaths or aponeuroses of the three lateral abdominal wall muscles (the external oblique, the internal oblique, and the transverses abdominus muscles) combine to form a thickened fascial layer known as the **Spigelian fascia** in the paramedian region just lateral to the paired midline rectus muscles. The region along the lateral border of the rectus muscles extending from the costal margin to the pubic bone is referred to as the linea semilunaris or Spigelius line. Moving medially, the Spigelian fascia divides into two layers to form the anterior and posterior rectus sheaths that surround the rectus muscles. In the midline, the anterior and posterior rectus sheaths from each rectus muscle combine and fuse into a single central fascial layer known as the **linea alba**. In long axis, the rectus muscles appear as paired bundles of muscle tissue with the muscle fibers aligned in a sagittal orientation, interrupted by three transversely oriented tendinous intersections. In cross section, the **rectus muscles** are ovoid in profile. Of note, the posterior layer of the each rectus sheath ends approximately midway between the umbilicus and the pubic symphysis. The thickened inferior edge of the rectus sheath at this level forms an anatomic region termed the arcuate line. Below the arcuate line the posterior layer of the rectus sheath is composed only of a thin layer of tissue known at the transversalis fascia.

The anatomy of the **inguinal region** is more complex and the region immediately adjacent to the inguinal ligament is the area of anatomic interest. The inguinal ligament represents the thickened inferior border of the aponeurosis of the external oblique muscle and is located between the anterior superior iliac spine and the pubic tubercle of the pelvis. Beneath the inguinal ligament lie three important bony prominences. Moving medially from the laterally situated anterior superior iliac spine, the next bony ridge encountered will be the anterior *inferior* iliac spine. Continuing further medially, the large curved bony ridge of the iliopubic eminence will be noted. This ridge corresponds to the anterior rim of the acetabulum. Medial to the iliopubic eminence lies the bony prominence of the pubic crest, about 1 cm medial to the pubic tubercle. The iliopsoas muscle runs beneath the inguinal ligament in the space between the anterior superior and inferior iliac spines and the iliopubic eminence. The femoral artery, vein, nerve, and lymph nodes are found just anterior to the iliopubic eminence. The deep inguinal ring lies superficial to the inguinal ligament in the region above the femoral vessels. From there, the inguinal canal courses medially and inferiorly toward the superficial inguinal ring that is found in close proximity to the pubic crest, still superficial to the inguinal ligament.

▶ TECHNIQUE AND NORMAL ULTRASOUND FINDINGS

The abdominal wall is divided into three sonographically distinct regions.[3] Since the anatomic structures of interest are all superficially located, a linear array transducer is most suited to this type of examination.

The **midline region** is best scanned in short axis. The linea alba (representing the midline confluence of the anterior and posterior fascial sheaths from each rectus muscle) appears beneath the skin and subcutaneous tissue of the midline abdomen as a horizontally oriented and somewhat hyperechoic and thickened line. The linea alba is surrounded on either side by the hypoechoic triangular medial portions of each rectus muscle. The rectus muscles appear hypoechoic and speckled in short axis and hypoechoic and striated in long axis. The anterior and posterior rectus sheaths appear as thin hyperechoic lines surrounding the muscle bundles. The underlying peritoneal interface will usually be apparent on real-time scanning. The adjacent bowel appears hyperechoic and gliding of the bowel is usually noted with respiration or with bowel peristalsis. Comet tail artifacts, or dirty shadowing arising from pockets of admixed air and fluid in the bowel loops may also be seen (Figures 16-1 and 16-2).

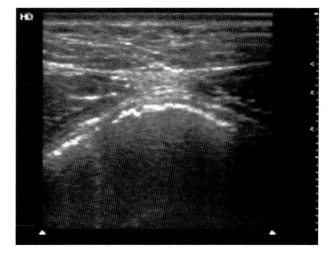

Figure 16-1. Transverse sonogram of the linea alba and adjacent rectus muscles. Skin and subcutaneous tissue are seen in the near field. The linea alba appears as a thickened, somewhat echogenic horizontal region in the midline. The hypoechoic triangular regions on either side of the linea alba represent the medial portions of the adjacent rectus muscles. The curved echogenic line beneath the linea alba and recti represent a loop of bowel adjacent to the peritoneum.

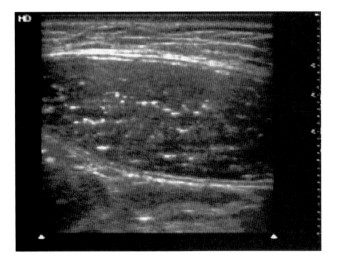

Figure 16-2. Transverse sonogram of a normal left rectus muscle above the umbilicus. The rectus muscle is seen as an ovoid, hypoechoic, and somewhat speckled structure in short-axis, outlined by the echogenic anterior and posterior layers of the rectus sheath. In long-axis, the muscle tissue would exhibit a more striated appearance.

In the **paramedian region**, the sonographic area of interest is at the lateral border of the rectus muscle at the confluence of the aponeuroses of the lateral abdominal wall muscles. This conjoined fascial layer is termed the Spigelian fascia. The hypoechoic lateral border of the rectus muscle serves as a localizing landmark for the region (Figures 16-3 and 16-4). The area of greatest

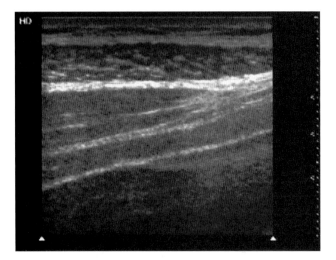

Figure 16-3. Oblique sonogram of the right paramedian abdominal wall just lateral to the rectus muscle. The external oblique, internal oblique, and transversus abdominus muscles appear as a succession of three hypoechoic layers surrounded by their respective hyperechoic fascial sheaths or aponeuroses. As they approach the rectus muscle, they taper to form the Spigelian fascia.

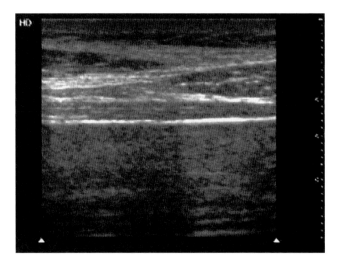

Figure 16-4. Transverse sonogram of the right Spigelian fascia. The tapered medial edge of the external oblique muscle is seen on the left near field of the image. The tapered lateral edge of the right rectus muscle is seen on the right near field of image. The hyperechoic aponeuroses of the muscles of the lateral abdominal wall combine, and then split to form the anterior and posterior rectus sheaths. The hyperechoic horizontal line in the mid field represents the peritoneal line.

sonographic interest will be in the region between the umbilicus and the pubic region where a Spigelian hernia is most likely to occur.

In the **inguinal region** the area of sonographic focus will be along an oblique plane between the palpable bony landmarks of the anterior superior iliac spine and the pubic crest. The region should be scanned in a series of successive parallel planes several centimeters above and below the inguinal ligament. In the normal patient, the hypoechoic psoas muscle will be seen occupying the region bounded by the anterior superior iliac spine laterally, the anterior inferior iliac spine below, and the edge of the iliopubic eminence medially. The hyperechoic curve of the iliopubic eminence will be noted beneath the anechoic femoral vessels (Figure 16-5).

► COMMON AND EMERGENT ABNORMALITIES

WOUND ABSCESS

As noted above, a wide range of pathology may occur in the abdominal wall. A postoperative wound abscess will appear as a hypoechoic fluid collection at the surgical site with clinical signs that suggest that a wound infection is present. A post-operative seroma, however, will manifest as an anechoic collection of easily compressible

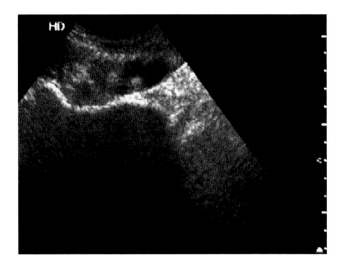

Figure 16-5. Oblique sonogram of the inguinal region with a curved array transducer. The scan plane is along the inguinal ligament. The curved hyperechoic line represents the shape of the bony pelvis beneath the inguinal ligament. The anterior superior iliac spine is not seen in this image and lies just beneath the skin off to the left of the sonogram. The first bony convexity seen on the left side of the image represents the anterior inferior iliac spine. The next convexity is somewhat shallower and more elongated, is seen on the right side of the sonogram, and represents the iliopubic eminence (corresponding to the anterior rim of the acetabulum). Posterior acoustic shadowing is seen beneath these bony ridges. The hypoechoic femoral vessels are seen in short-axis just above the curve of the iliopubic eminence. The iliopsoas muscle occupies the region to the left of the femoral vessels. The upsloping bony ridge that leads to the pubic tubercle is seen beneath the femoral vessels.

fluid with no associated clinical signs to suggest infection (Figure 16-6).

LYMPH NODE

A region of focal tenderness in the inguinal region may be discovered to be due to a reactive inguinal lymph node. A lymph node will appear as an elliptical structure in long axis, hypoechoic at the periphery with a variably hyperechoic fatty central hilum (Figure 16-7).

RECTUS SHEATH HEMATOMA

On occasion, a patient may present with a focal region of abdominal tenderness and swelling that is discovered to be due to a rectus sheath hematoma. Sonographically, the normally homogeneously hypoechoic rectus muscle will appear hyperechoic and a focal homogeneous

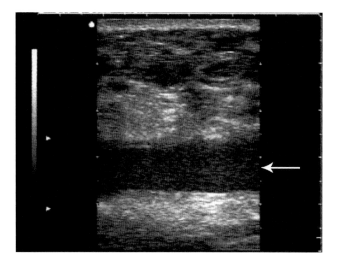

Figure 16-6. Transverse sonogram of an abdominal wall seroma in a patient several months after a hernia repair. A hypoechoic fluid collection (arrow) is seen beneath the subcutaneous tissues and is easily compressible. No clinical signs of infection were present.

collection consistent with a hematoma may be present (Figure 16-8).

HERNIA

A Spigelian hernia will appear as a hypoechoic fascial defect at or near the junction of the linea semilunaris and the arcuate line. A bowel loop may be seen extending laterally under the external oblique muscle. A small epigastric hernia will appear as a hypoechoic fascial defect

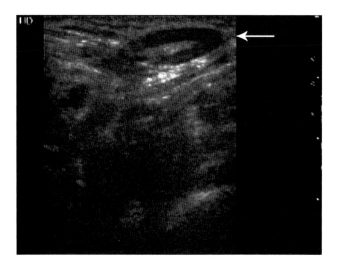

Figure 16-7. Long-axis sonogram of an inguinal lymph node. The lymph node (arrow) appears hypoechoic at its periphery and echogenic at its fatty hilum. This patient's groin tenderness was attributable to a reactive adenopathy and not a hernia.

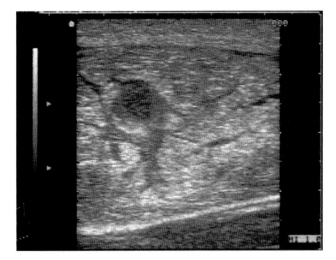

Figure 16-8. Transverse sonogram of a rectus sheath hematoma. The normally hypoechoic rectus muscle appears hyperechoic and quite thick in this patient. In the center there is a hypoechoic region consistent with an inferior epigastric artery aneurysm. The hemorrhage dissects through the muscle tissue but is contained within the rectus sheath.

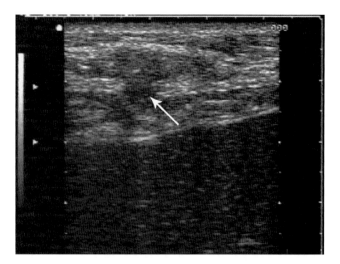

Figure 16-9. Transverse sonogram of an epigastric hernia. The patient had localized tenderness of the midline abdominal wall in the epigastric region but no fascial defect was appreciated clinically. A hypoechoic fascial defect (arrow) is seen on the sonogram in the otherwise echogenic linea alba. The hypoechoic mushroom-shaped region around and above the lesion represents a loop of small bowel that has herniated through the defect. On real-time imaging peristalsis of the bowel loop was appreciated.

in the linea alba; visualization of peristaltic movements in the herniated bowel loop during real-time scanning will help confirm that a hernia is indeed present (Figure 16-9). Seen in cross section, a herniated loop of small bowel will have a rounded target-like appearance with a hypoechoic outer muscular layer, followed by a hyperechoic mucosal layer and, on occasion, strongly reflec-

tive central echoes that arise from admixtures of air and fluid in the bowel lumen (Figure 16-10A). In long axis, a linear region of "dirty shadowing" and reverberation artifacts will be seen (Figure 16-10B). When obstructed, small bowel loops will appear as hypoechoic tubular

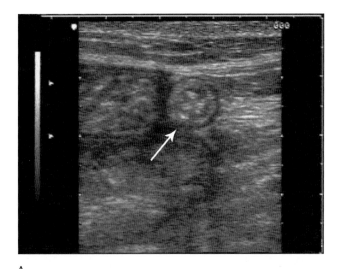

A

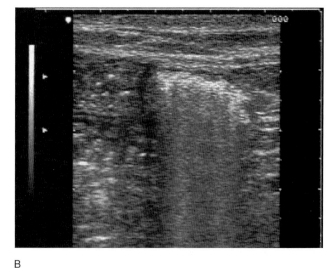

B

Figure 16-10. Transverse (A) and sagittal (B) sonograms of a small ventral hernia. A herniated loop of small bowel is seen within the abdominal wall between a fascial defect in the linea alba (to the right of the image) and the medial border of the rectus muscle (to the left). In short-axis, the bowel segment has a characteristic circular and target-like appearance (arrow). In long-axis, the sonographic pattern is one of "dirty shadowing" and reverberation artifacts.

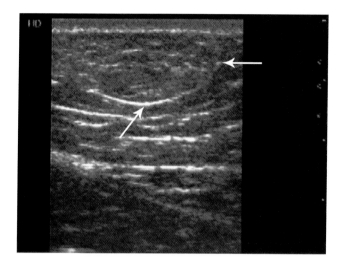

Figure 16-11. Transverse sonogram of an abdominal wall lipoma. A firm and somewhat tender mass was appreciated clinically but its etiology was unclear. The subtle hyperechoic curved outline of an ovoid structure is seen occupying most of the near field of the image. The echogenicity of the lesion is identical to that of the soft tissues, consistent with the sonographic appearance of a lipoma.

fluid-filled structures with prominent hyperechoic valvuli conniventes.

LIPOMA

These masses will appear as rounded or ovoid structure similar in echotexture to the surrounding subcutaneous tissue. Palpation of the lesion will guide the clinician to the region of sonographic interest. On the sonogram, a subtle curved region of echogenicity will outline the border of the lipoma in what otherwise appears to be a homogenous layer of subcutaneous tissue (Figure 16-11.)

▶ COMMON VARIANTS AND SELECTED ABNORMALITIES

An abdominal wall **endometrioma** will be found at the site of a prior caesarean section or laparotomy and will appear as a solid hypoechoic mass with sharply defined borders and scattered internal echoes similar to the endometriomas that occur in the abdominal cavity.[4] An undescended testicle will appear as a homogenous mass smaller in size but similar in echotexture to a normal testicle, with its long axis parallel to the inguinal canal.

A **pseudoaneurysm** represents an area of fibrous encapsulation around a pulsatile and expansile hematoma that occurs from arterial bleeding into adjacent soft tissue. Because there is a persistent communication between the vessel and the fluid space, to and fro flow will be noted between the mass and the adjacent artery and characteristic echogenic swirls will be seen on color Doppler examination. In contradistinction to a true aneurysm, the neck of a pseudoaneurysm is narrow.

▶ PITFALLS

The major sonographic pitfalls of abdominal wall imaging are failure to consider a malignant etiology for any homogeneously hypoechoic solid lesion, especially in the groin, and failure to consider a vascular etiology for an anechoic lesion, particularly if aspiration is considered.

▶ AIRWAY

CLINICAL CONSIDERATIONS AND INDICATIONS

The anatomic structures of the larynx and upper airway are superficially located and well suited for bedside sonographic assessment. The sonographer may thereby (1) obtain precise knowledge of the location of the thyroid, cricoid, and tracheal cartilages if landmarks are difficult to palpate and a surgical airway is planned, (2) visualize motion of the vocal cords and arytenoids when there is a question of a vocal cord palsy, or (3) visualize the real-time passage of an endotracheal tube to ascertain whether it is in the airway or esophagus, and confirm cuff location within the trachea. Ultrasound may also be used to assess for diaphragmatic movement or pleural gliding during the phases of respiration and can thereby provide indirect evidence of endotracheal, endobronchial, or esophageal intubation. A brief review of these airway-related ultrasound applications follows.

The distinctive ultrasound images that are obtained from **endotracheal intubation** compared were esophageal intubation were described in one report[6]; recognition of these characteristic sonographic patterns on a transverse view of the trachea can be of value for rapid identification of an inadvertent esophageal intubation. In a related report, real-time imaging of the trachea on a transverse view at the level of the cricothyroid membrane was reported to be 99.7% sensitive and 97% specific for detection of endotracheal intubation. Of note, real-time imaging during the intubation was found to be superior to a static imaging technique performed after the intubation. Evaluation of the static imaging technique alone revealed notably improved test characteristics when images were obtained at a suprasternal location (97% sensitivity and specificity) instead of at the cricothyroid membrane (73% sensitivity and 56% specificity).[7] Because of the large acoustic impedance mismatch between soft tissue and the air-filled trachea, visualization of an endotracheal tube within the airway may be difficult unless it is in direct contact with the tracheal wall. When a saline or foam-filled endotracheal tube cuff is utilized, the cuff will be in contact with the trachea and will exhibit a distinct sonographic pattern that assists in its identification. This technique was investigated in a series of 24 intubated patients and reached the following conclusions: (1) the saline or foam-filled cuff was best visualized in a long-axis view, (2) a slight longitudinal to and fro motion of the endotracheal tube further enhanced visualization of the cuff, and (3) when the cuff was visualized at the level of the suprasternal notch, the endotracheal tube was usually ideally situated midway between the vocal cords and the carina. The authors concluded that this sonographic technique could be clinically useful for rapid assessment of endotracheal tube position in any situation where tube movement, near extubation, or endobronchial intubation might have occurred.[8]

In addition, ultrasound may be used for secondary **confirmation of endotracheal tube position** either by direct observation of diaphragm motion during ventilation or by evaluation for lung sliding. A study of 59 emergently intubated patients ranging from newborn to 17 years of age utilized real-time B and M-mode ultrasound and a subxiphoid window to evaluate diaphragm motion during ventilation. Of the 59 intubations, all correct tube placements, both esophageal placements, and all 8 right mainstem placements were correctly identified with ultrasound. The authors concluded that ultrasound imaging of diaphragm motion was a "useful, quick, noninvasive, portable, and direct anatomic method for assessment of endotracheal tube position."[9] Using a cadaver model and a 4–2 MHz microconvex transducer, the performance of the lung sliding sign as a predictor of endotracheal tube placement was evaluated in 68 intubations in 9 cadavers.[10] For differentiating esophageal vs. tracheal intubation sensitivity ranged from 95 to 100% and specificity was 100%.

A real-time image of the vestibular folds (the false vocal cords), the vocal folds (the true vocal cords), and the arytenoids can be obtained by scanning transversely though the thyroid cartilage. Ultrasound has been found to be a useful tool for evaluation of **vocal cord function** by a number of investigators.[11–13] Ultrasound has also been evaluated to assess the anteroposterior **thickness of the epiglottis**. One study examined 100 subjects, using a subhyoid window and a transverse scan plane, and the epiglottis was visualized in all cases. There is apparently little variation in the AP diameter of the normal adult epiglottis with an average AP dimension of 2.39 ± 0.15 mm in this report.[14] Its application for rapid bedside airway assessment of a patient with suspected epiglottitis is as of yet unclear.

ANATOMICAL CONSIDERATIONS

The **thyroid and cricoid cartilages**, the cricothyroid membrane, and the upper trachea are located within the superficial subcutaneous tissues of the anterior midline neck. The thyroid cartilage is composed of two broad rectangular laminae that meet in the anterior midline at about a 90 degree angle. Superiorly, the thyroid cartilage attaches to the hyoid bone via the thyrohyoid membrane. Posteriorly, the superior and inferior horns of the thyroid cartilage connect the thyroid cartilage with the hyoid bone and cricoid cartilages, respectively. Inferiorly and anteriorly, the thyroid cartilage connects to the cricoid ring via the cricothyroid ligament or membrane; in an adult, it averages about 2×1 cm in size. A V-shaped gap separates the upper aspects of the thyroid laminae in the midline and the base of this gap forms the superior thyroid notch or the laryngeal prominence. The strap muscles (the sternohyoid, omohyoid, and thyrohyoid muscles) lie just anterior to the thyroid cartilage. The cricothyroid muscles extend from the lower border of the thyroid cartilage to the lower aspect of the cricoid ring and surround the anterolateral portions of the cricothyroid membrane and cricoid cartilage. The thyroid gland surrounds the lateral portions of the cricoid ring, and extends superiorly to the lower border of the thyroid cartilage and anteriorly over the upper tracheal cartilages. The narrow rectangular midline segment of the thyroid gland is known as the thyroid isthmus.

The **vestibular folds** (also known as the false vocal cords or ventricular folds) are composed of a thick fold of mucous membrane and connective tissue. They lie just above and protect the more delicate **vocal cords** below. The vocal folds (or true vocal cords) are composed of the vocal ligaments medially and the laterally adjacent vocalis and thyroarytenoid muscles. They are covered by a mucous membrane and extend from the level of the mid thyroid cartilage anteriorly to the paired arytenoids cartilages posteriorly. The arytenoids rest on the broad posterior cricoid ring and are attached to the thyroarytenoid muscles that adduct the vocal folds. The midline gap between the vocal ligaments is referred to as the rima glottidis.

The base of the **epiglottis** attaches to the upper border of the thyroid cartilage via the thyroepiglottic ligament; more superiorly the hyoepiglottic ligament provides the anterior support for the epiglottis. A preepiglottic fat pad separates the epiglottis from the thyrohyoid membrane. The epiglottis approaches its widest dimension just below the level of the hyoid bone.

The cricoid cartilage attaches distally to the first **tracheal ring** via the cricotracheal ligament. The upper five or six tracheal rings of the trachea lie just beneath the skin in the region between the cricoid cartilage and the lower aspect of the suprasternal notch.

► TECHNIQUE AND NORMAL ULTRASOUND FINDINGS

TRANSDUCERS

The upper airway is best imaged with a 5–10 MHz linear array transducer. Long- and short-axis midline views may be used, depending upon the airway application being performed. The length of the transducer face may limit its utilization in long axis if the neck is short or the transducer is long. A stand-off pad may be helpful if a lower frequency transducer is being used. Copious use of gel may help with obtaining images at the suprasternal notch.

THYROID CARTILAGE

The thyroid cartilage is best imaged in a transverse scan plane in the upper neck with the neck slightly extended. Beneath the skin and subcutaneous tissues the thyroid cartilage appears as an inverted V-shaped structure that exhibits a range of echogenic appearances, from hyperechoic to nearly isoechoic with the adjacent strap muscles. When hyperechoic, the region beneath appears nearly anechoic (Figure 16-12); when isoechoic with the surrounding muscles, the laryngeal structures beneath are more readily identified (Figure 16-13). When scanning just above the superior thyroid notch, the anterior por-

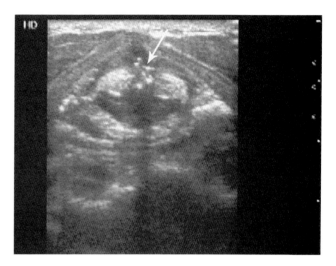

Figure 16-13. Short-axis sonogram of the thyroid cartilage. Here the thyroid cartilage is nearly isoechoic with the strap muscles on either side. The inverted V shape is again apparent and visualization of the inner structures of the larynx is excellent. Seen here are the arytenoids (hyperechoic and rounded structures near the midline), the glottic opening (arrow) (echogenic anteriorly with posterior shadowing), and the posterior portion of the cricoid cartilage (moderately echoic curved structure deep to the arytenoids).

tion of the inverted V will always appear hypoechoic; a thin echogenic line that corresponds to the anterior portion of the thyrohyoid ligament may be noted (Figure 16-14). The hypoechoic strap muscles are seen overlying the laminae on each side of the thyroid cartilage.

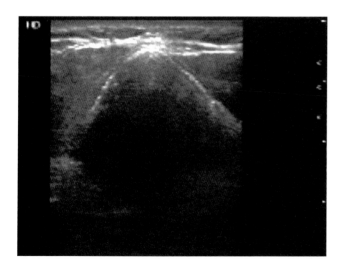

Figure 16-12. Short-axis sonogram of the thyroid cartilage below the level of the thyroid notch. Beneath a thin layer of skin and subcutaneous tissue, the two laminae of the thyroid cartilage meet in the anterior midline at about a 90 degree angle and appear as an inverted V shape. In some subjects, as in this example, the cartilage will appear hyperechoic and the region beneath anechoic. The hypoechoic structures on either side of the cartilage are the strap muscles.

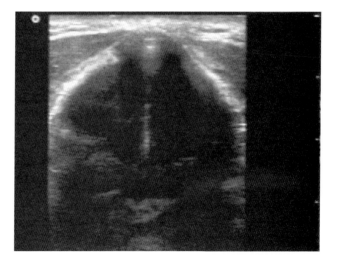

Figure 16-14. Short-axis sonogram of the thyroid cartilage *above* the level of the superior thyroid notch. A hypoechoic gap is seen in the space between the two laminae of the thyroid cartilage. The thin echogenic line in the center of the image corresponds to the vocal ligaments.

CRICOID CARTILAGE AND CRICOTHYROID MEMBRANE

As the transversely oriented transducer slides down the length of the thyroid cartilage, the inverted V-shape of the thyroid cartilage suddenly disappears, and the airway takes on a more rounded appearance. A prominent area of hyperechogenicity will be noted in the anterior midline at the level of the cricothyroid membrane. When the insonating beam suddenly encounters the air-filled lumen of the airway, the large acoustic impedance mismatch gives rise to an echogenic periodic resonance artifact that makes identification of the cricothyroid membrane simple (Figure 16-15). The cricothyroid muscles surround the cricoid cartilage at this level and appear as anechoic crescents on either side of the somewhat echogenic outline of the cricoid ring. The cricoid ring is the only complete ring in the airway, is round in its transverse profile, wedge-shaped in a lateral profile, and becomes progressively taller as one moves laterally and posteriorly. The cricoid ring appears as a smaller circular structure in the center of the sonogram. The thyroid isthmus may be seen overlying the cricothyroid membrane and exhibits a homogenous grey echotexture. When scanning the airway in long axis, the cricoid cartilage typically appears hypoechoic and ovoid in shape, and may contain some internal areas of calcification that

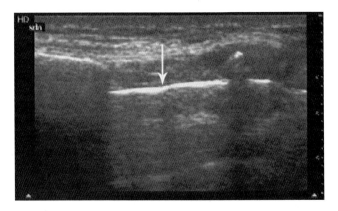

Figure 16-16. Long-axis sonogram of the anterior larynx over the cricothyroid ligament. To the upper left is a somewhat echogenic line that slants down toward the center of the image and corresponds to the anterior surface of the larynx. The echogenic horizontal line in the center of the image corresponds to the cricothyroid membrane (arrow). The hypoechoic ovoid structure to the upper right corresponds to the anterior cricoid ring in cross section. Some internal calcifications are seen within the cricoid with some associated posterior acoustic shadowing.

appear echogenic. The cricothyroid membrane appears as a hyperechoic horizontal line located between the downward slanting thyroid cartilage on the left of the image, and the ovoid hypoechoic cross section of the cricoid cartilage on the right (Figure 16-16). Either long- or short-axis views can be used for rapid localization of the cricothyroid membrane.

Vocal Cords

The patient can be seated or supine with the neck in a relaxed neutral position. The vocal cords are imaged with a linear array transducer in a transverse scan plane either through the thyroid cartilage itself if it is not echogenic or through the membranous portion of the thyrohyoid ligament immediately above the superior thyroid notch. The arytenoids appear as rounded echogenic structures that are easily identified by their posterior midline location within the larynx and their movements on abduction and adduction (Figure 16-17).

Trachea

In long-axis orientation the tracheal rings are identified as small hypoechoic rectangular structures that appear like a string of beads in the midline near field. They may be either completely hypoechoic (in which case no shadowing will be seen) or somewhat calcified and have an echogenic surface that is associated posterior acoustic

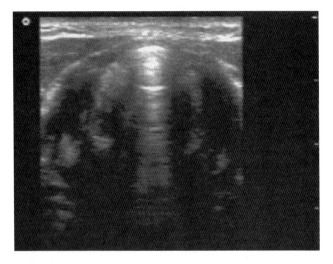

Figure 16-15. Short-axis sonogram at the level of the cricothyroid ligament or membrane. The airway has transitioned from an inverted V shape to a more ovoid shape. In the center of the image a prominent echo is seen with an associated periodic resonance artifact corresponding to the cricothyroid membrane and the air-filled tracheal lumen. The anechoic crescents on either side of the oval correspond with the cricothyroid muscles. A slightly echogenic circular structure is seen in the central half of the image and represents the cartilaginous cricoid ring.

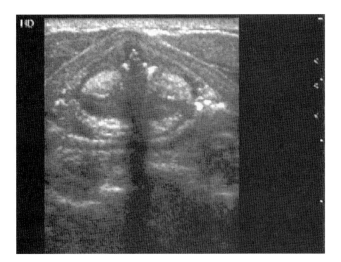

Figure 16-17. Short-axis sonogram through the lower larynx demonstrating the rima glottidis in normal respiration. The appearance is triangular anteriorly with posterior acoustic shadowing from the vocal ligaments. The rounded arytenoids appear on either side of the glottic opening and the posterior cricoid ring is seen as a curved somewhat echogenic structure below.

shadowing. The tracheal lumen appears as a brightly echogenic line immediately beneath the cartilages (Figures 16-18 and 16-19). The cricoid cartilage can be identified by its larger size and more ovoid profile allowing for accurate identification and numbering of the tracheal rings if needed.

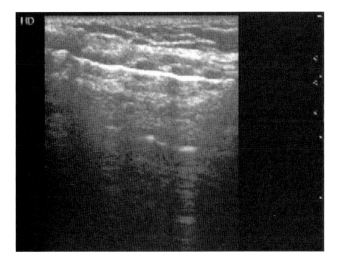

Figure 16-18. Long-axis midline sonogram of the upper tracheal cartilages in the neck. In this image, the tracheal cartilages appear hypoechoic in cross section and resemble a string of beads. A periodic resonance artifact is seen beneath some of the cartilages.

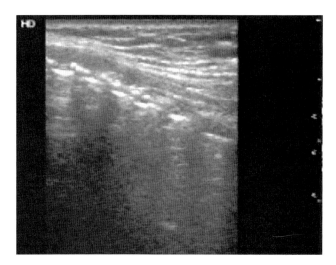

Figure 16-19. Long-axis midline sonogram of the upper tracheal cartilages in the neck. The tracheal cartilages appear more echogenic in this image and posterior acoustic shadowing is seen beneath each cartilage.

CONFIRMATION OF ENDOTRACHEAL INTUBATION

For evaluation of endotracheal tube location and cuff position, both transverse and long-axis views may be utilized. A long-axis view is best for visualizing the passage of the endotracheal tube into the trachea at the time of intubation and slight to and fro motion of the endotracheal tube will further enhance its visualization (Figure 16-20). A foam filled cuff or 8–10 mL of saline within the cuff can also enhance cuff visualization and assist with its accurate placement in the suprasternal notch (typically located midway between the vocal cords and the carina). The portion of the endotracheal tube that is in contact with the tracheal wall will be seen as two parallel echogenic lines (curved in short axis and linear in long axis) that represent the inner and outer surfaces of the endotracheal tube. The tube will typically demonstrate a distinct comet-tail or reverberation artifact in contradistinction to the periodic resonance artifact of the unintubated airway. Although less distinct than a fluid-filled cuff, an air-filled cuff may be apparent by its curved profile and associated comet tail artifacts (Figures 16-21, 16-22, and 16-23). One recommended technique is to start in transverse orientation at the level of the cricothyroid membrane to quickly confirm that the endotracheal tube is not in the esophagus, after which the transducer is rotated to a long-axis orientation to confirm mid-tracheal cuff placement with a gentle to and fro movement of the tube. This technique has been touted as good for supervising resident intubations and can be used as a rapid

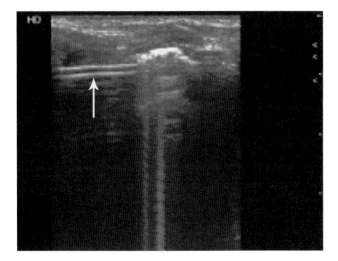

Figure 16-20. Long-axis sonogram of an endotracheal tube within the airway. The endotracheal tube appears as two closely spaced echogenic parallel lines with an associated reverberation artifact below (arrow). The air-filled cuff appears as a distinctly different, somewhat curved and brightly echogenic structure with associated comet tail artifacts. The hypoechoic thyroid cartilage is seen slanting down on the left near field and the cricoid cartilage is seen in cross section to the right of the image just above the endotracheal tube cuff. The cuff needs to be moved further toward the suprasternal notch where cuff placement will typically result in the tube being in an ideal mid tracheal position.

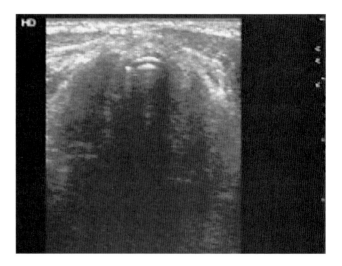

Figure 16-22. Short-axis sonogram of an intubated trachea about 1 cm below the cricoid cartilage. Two parallel curved echogenic lines are again present in the anterior airway.

confirmatory test in a postarrest situation in which capnography may not be useful.

SECONDARY CONFIRMATION OF ENDOTRACHEAL TUBE PLACEMENT

Diaphragmatic movement may be observed real-time from a subxiphoid window using a standard curved array abdominal transducer. A wide sector angle should be used so that both diaphragms may be easily visualized

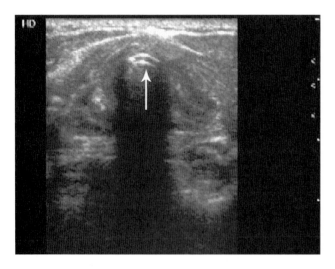

Figure 16-21. Short-axis sonogram of an intubated trachea at the level of the thyroid cartilage. The endotracheal tube is seen in the anterior airway as two parallel curved echogenic lines (arrow). Prominent posterior acoustic shadowing is present in this image.

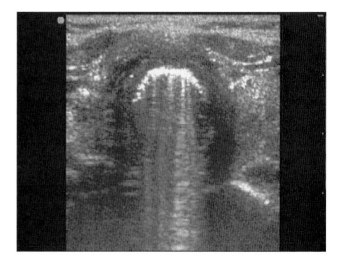

Figure 16-23. Short-axis sonogram of an intubated trachea at the level of the air-filled cuff. The hyperechoic signature of the air-filled endotracheal tube cuff appears different from that of the endotracheal tube: the cuff surface appears echogenic but irregular in contour and comet-tail artifacts are prominent.

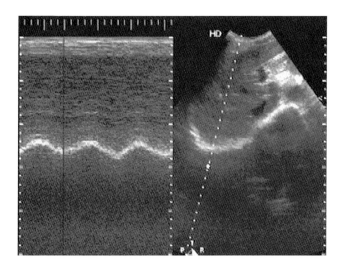

Figure 16-24. Combined B and M-mode subxiphoid view of the right diaphragm with a curved array transducer during quiet respirations. The echogenic diaphragm moves toward the transducer during inspiration and the M-mode image traces the excursions during the respiratory cycle. With an esophageal intubation, the diaphragm will move away from the transducer during ventilation. Asymmetric movement of the left and right diaphragms is indicative of a mainstem intubation.

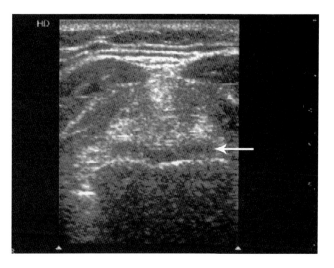

Figure 16-25. Short-axis sonogram of the upper neck just below the hyoid bone. The sonogram has the appearance of a face or mask. The ovoid "eyes" represent the sternohyoid muscles in cross section. The hyperechoic "nose" represents the pre-epiglottic fat pad beneath the thyrohyoid membrane. The hypoechoic "mouth" is the sonographic representation of the epiglottis (arrow) in cross section. The hyperechoic line beneath the mouth occurs because of the impedance mismatch between the epiglottis and the airway beneath.

from a single scanning plane. When this is not feasible, a sagittal right or left chest view from the anterior to mid axillary line may be employed. A combined B- and M-mode image may be obtained and the direction and depth of diaphragm motion observed and in real-time and recorded. With normal respirations or ventilation, the echogenic line that represents the diaphragm on the M-mode tracing will be seen to move toward the transducer with inspiration and away with expiration (Figure 16-24). With correct endotracheal tube placement, symmetrical movement toward the transducer should be seen with a delivered breath at both diaphragms. With esophageal intubation, the air-filled stomach will push the diaphragm away from the transducer during inspiration. Asymmetry of movement of the two diaphragms is seen with inadvertent right mainstem intubation. In an analogous fashion, evaluation of pleural gliding may similarly be used to assess for correct tube placement. Absence of a gliding implies that the hemithorax being assessed is not being ventilated or that on pneumothorax is present.

Epiglottis

The epiglottis is reliably imaged from a subhyoid window in transverse orientation. The appearance of the sonogram is that of a face or mask; two ovoid hypoechoic "eyes" represent the sternohyoid muscle in cross section; the hyperechoic "nose" correlates with the fat

pat beneath the thyrohyoid ligament, and the hypoechoic "mouth," somewhat downturned in the center with a hyperechoic inferior border, represents the epiglottis in cross section (Figure 16-25). As noted above, the average AP diameter of the epiglottis in a series of 100 normal subjects was of 2.39 ± 0.15 mm.[14]

▶ COMMON AND EMERGENT ABNORMALITIES

ESOPHAGEAL INTUBATION

With an esophageal intubation, the otherwise flaccid and normally flattened esophagus will be stented open by the endotracheal tube. On a short-axis view, the endotracheal tube will appear as a series of parallel curved echogenic lines anteriorly with posterior acoustic shadowing. It may be seen either behind the posterolateral edge of the thyroid cartilage or lateral to the trachea at a level below the cricothyroid membrane. The lumen of the airway will not show evidence of endotracheal tube presence. Best visualization is reported to occur about 1 cm below the cricoid ring (Figure 16-26). A nasogastric tube will similarly stent open the normally flaccid and flattened esophagus and will be apparent on the sonogram as an additional hypoechoic circle with posterior acoustic shadowing adjacent to the airway (Figure 16-27).

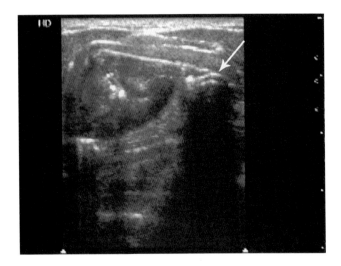

Figure 16-26. A somewhat-tilted transverse sonogram of an esophageal intubation seen at the level of the thyroid cartilage. The inverted V of the thyroid cartilage is apparent in the near field and the vocal cords are adducted. The endotracheal tube (arrow) is seen lateral and posterior to the glottis and is recognizable by the paired parallel curved echoes anteriorly with posterior acoustic shadowing.

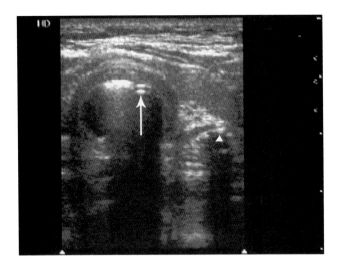

Figure 16-27. Short-axis sonogram of an intubated trachea at the level of the tracheal cartilages. A portion of the thyroid gland appears as a region of homogeneous mid-gray echogenicity anterior and lateral to the tracheal cartilage. The tracheal cartilage appears as a hypoechoic C that is open posteriorly. The signature double echo of the plastic wall of the endotracheal tube (arrow) is apparent adjacent to the tracheal ring; the adjacent echo from the cuff is less distinct and exhibits comet-tail artifacts. A simultaneously placed nasogastric tube (arrowhead) demonstrates the lateral and somewhat posterior location of the esophagus relative to the airway. Both endotracheal and nasogastric tubes exhibit strong posterior acoustic shadowing.

VOCAL CORD PALSY

Prolonged vocalization of a single vowel (such as "e") will enhance visualization of both asymmetric vocal cord motion and abnormal arytenoid movement and should be apparent on a real-time examination. The affected vocal cord will appear shorter and in a lower position on the sonogram with anterior bowing of the flaccid vocal cord.[11]

▶ PITFALLS

Subcutaneous emphysema, significant neck edema or hemorrhage from trauma or recent surgery, or an open wound over the anterior neck can make sonographic imaging of the upper airway difficult to impossible. Significant neck flexion may also impair adequate imaging by making it difficult to place the transducer (especially in a long-axis orientation) on the anterior surface of the neck. A deep suprasternal notch may be difficult to image because of poor transducer skin contact; copious use of gel and an acoustic stand-off pad may help in this latter situation. An endotracheal tube cuff may be difficult to visualize if a large amount of bubbles have entered along with the saline. Real-time imaging during intubation can be difficult in a patient with a short neck and could interfere with unobstructed use of the laryngoscope handle.

▶ BONY FRACTURE EVALUATION

CLINICAL CONSIDERATIONS AND INDICATIONS

Ultrasound excels at identifying the interface between soft tissue and bone due to the large difference in acoustic impedance between the two tissues. When perpendicular to a given bony surface, most of the incident ultrasound beam will be reflected back to the transducer and the interface will be represented by a brightly echogenic line that follows the contour of bony cortex being imaged. These cortical outlines on the sonogram can be used to identify precise locations for arthrocentesis or even for finding landmarks for ultrasound-guided lumbar puncture. With the bony cortex so readily visible, sometimes to less than a millimeter resolution, sonography also provides us with a rapid and portable means to assess for bony fractures. This section will focus on the identification of selected fractures in the ED, specifically, rib and sternal fractures, long bone fractures in the trauma patient, nasal bone fractures, and zygomatic arch fractures.

Ultrasound has long been known to be considerably more sensitive for diagnosing **rib fractures** than standard chest radiography.[15-17] In one series of 50 patients with suspected rib fractures, sonography detected fractures in six times as many patients as radiography (using a standard PA chest radiograph and a single oblique view) and was found to detect 10 times as many fractures as radiography.[15] In another review of 103 patients with suspected rib injury, rib fractures were diagnosed about twice as often with ultrasound when compared to standard chest radiography.[16] Ultrasound was also found to be useful for detecting coexisting small pleural effusions that were not demonstrated on the chest radiograph. The authors of this latter report opined that the ability to provide a definitive diagnosis of rib fracture (and thus better estimate the duration of work disability) was an important advantage that supported the use of ultrasound in this clinical setting.

The time-consuming nature of the examination (from 10 to 15 minutes/patient reported in one study) and the inability to visualize retroscapular and infraclavicular rib injuries are some of the disadvantages reported for this particular ultrasound application, however.[15] Nevertheless, the potential utility of this rapid, bedside application for the workup of the ambulatory patient with a suspected cough fracture or isolated rib injury is undeniable.

Although the diagnostic sensitivity of chest radiography and ultrasound for suspected **sternal fracture** is similar, the time required to make this diagnosis can be considerably shortened with the use of bedside ultrasound. In one report on 16 patients with radiographically documented sternal fractures, an examiner unfamiliar with the chest radiograph results was able to locate and diagnose the sternal fracture with ultrasound in each of the 16 patients within 1 minute.[18]

A number of authors have commented that ultrasound may be useful for diagnosis of **bony fractures in "austere" environments** where power, weight, and space requirements make conventional radiography impractical (e.g., battlefield or military settings, on a spacecraft or submarine, or in rural or wilderness medicine settings).[19-21] In an effort to evaluate the test characteristics of ultrasound for fracture diagnosis, investigators trained cast technicians to assess ED patients for fractures after a 2-hour training program. One hundred fifty-eight ultrasound examinations were performed in 95 patients; the diagnostic accuracy was found to be greater in midshaft locations and least in the metacarpals, metatarsals, proximal femur, and hip. Leg and forearm fractures were found to be easy to diagnose with no missed injuries in patients with midshaft fractures of the radius, ulna, humerus, femur, tibia, or fibula. Of added note, no false positives were reported in any location. The authors suggested that the FAST examination could be expanded to include both *Extremity* assessment for fractures as well as *Respiratory* assessment for pneumothorax, coining an alternate acronym: the "FASTER" examination.[19] Requir-

ing little added time to perform, such an extension of the FAST examination might provide useful and timely diagnostic information in the ED trauma room setting.

The accuracy of physician-performed ultrasound in the detection of **long bone fractures** was investigated. With only 1 hour of training, physicians with minimal ultrasound experience evaluated 58 ED patients with bedside ultrasound and results were compared to plain films or CT as the gold standard. US provided improved sensitivity with less specificity compared with physical examination. For detecting humerus and midshaft femur fractures ultrasound was found to be 100% sensitive. Ultrasound was found to be limited in detection of fractures at or above the intertrochanteric line of the hip, however, with five false-positive readings reported in this subset of patients.[20]

The past decade has also seen ultrasound employed as a diagnostic tool in the assessment of patients with **nasal trauma**. In a report on 63 patients seen in an ENT clinic with clinical signs of a nasal bone fracture, standard radiography employing lateral and occipitomental views was compared with ultrasound. A 10 MHz linear array probe was used, and images were obtained in three locations: on the left and right lateral nasal walls (for evaluation of the frontal processes of the maxillary bone), and on the nasal dorsum (for evaluation of the nasal bones). Of the 63 patients evaluated, 42 (67%) were diagnosed with nasal fractures. Ultrasound was found to be statistically superior to radiography for assessment of the lateral nasal walls, and conventional radiography superior for evaluation of the nasal dorsum.[22] Scanheads (20 MHz) normally used for evaluation of skin tumors and skin thickness assessment have also been utilized for evaluation of nasal bone fractures.[23]

Additional diagnostic applications reported in the ultrasound literature are many and include intraoperative postreduction confirmation of the position of zygomatic arch fracture fragments,[24] diagnosis of infant hip dislocation, diagnosis of infant posterior shoulder dislocation,[25] diagnosis of posterior sternoclavicular dislocation,[26,27] diagnosis of subtle fractures of the clavicle and femur in infants,[28] and finally, use of ultrasound as a procedural aid for closed reduction of displaced extra-articular distal radius fractures[29] or pediatric forearm fractures.[29] For each of these applications, it is the identification of the bright bony cortical echo on the sonogram that allows the provider to assess whether the bone being imaged and its relationship to surrounding structures are normal or abnormal.

ANATOMICAL CONSIDERATIONS

The location for ultrasound of the **ribs** is usually guided by the patient's complaint of pain; the rib segment in question will be found beneath skin, subcutaneous tissue, and the relevant chest wall musculature at the site being investigated. It is important to remember the curved course of the ribs when scanning. The **sternum** is superficially located beneath skin, subcutaneous tissue, and the medial portions of the pectoralis major muscles, and is composed of two flat bones, the manubrium superiorly and the sternal body inferiorly. The first through the seventh ribs articulate with the manubrium and sternum laterally, and the manubrium articulates with the sternum at the sternal angle. The shafts of the **long bones** (humerus, radius, femur, and tibia) are fairly rounded in cross-sectional profile and become wider and flatter on their distal aspects. The bony supports of the external nose are composed of two **nasal bones** along the dorsum of the nose and the frontal processes of the maxilla laterally. The nasal bones are contiguous with the frontal bone above via the nasofrontal suture and the maxillae laterally via the nasomaxillary sutures (Figures 16-28 and 16-29). The frontal processes of the maxillae are contiguous with the frontal bone via the frontomaxillary sutures. The bony **zygomatic arch** sits beneath skin and subcutaneous tissue and is formed anteriorly by the temporal process of the zygoma and posteriorly by the zygomatic process of the temporal bone. The masseter muscle originates from the edge of the zygomatic arch and inserts on the ramus of the mandible below.

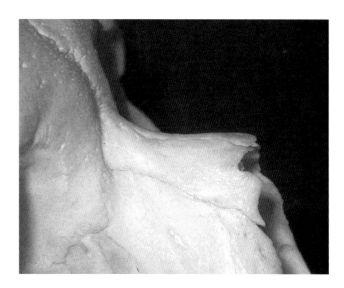

Figure 16-29. Lateral view of the right nasal bone, the nasomaxillary suture, and the right frontal process of the maxilla.

▶ TECHNIQUE AND NORMAL ULTRASOUND FINDINGS

Evaluation of **rib and costochondral cartilage** fractures is usually undertaken with linear array transducers in the 7.5–12 MHz range. In short-axis orientation, a rib will be seen casting a dense posterior acoustic shadow beneath its echogenic superficial cortical surface (Figure 16-30). Slightly below the rib, the pleura will be seen as a brightly echogenic horizontal line. Pleural gliding

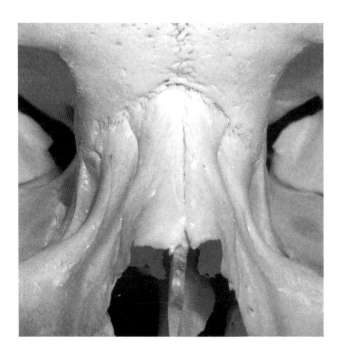

Figure 16-28. Frontal view of the nasal bones and nasal pyramid on a skull. The paired nasal bones are in the midline. The frontal processes of the maxillae make up the lateral walls of the nasal pyramid on either side. The frontomaxillary and nasofrontal sutures are seen at the top of the nasal pyramid.

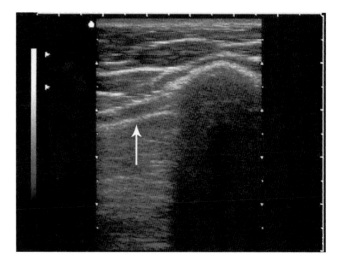

Figure 16-30. Short-axis sonogram of a rib. The curved echogenic surface of the rib appears on the right with dense posterior acoustic shadowing. The pleural line is seen as a horizontal echogenic line in the left mid portion of the image; it lies about 1 cm deep to the most superficial aspect of the rib (arrow).

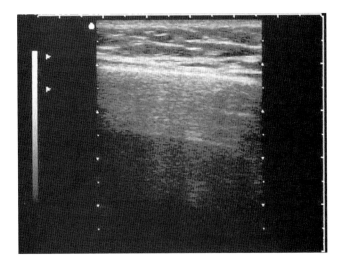

Figure 16-31. Long-axis sonogram of a rib. The cortical surface of the rib is seen as a thin, echogenic, superficially located horizontal line just beneath the skin and subcutaneous tissue in this image.

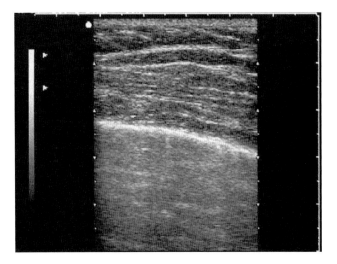

Figure 16-32. Long-axis sonogram of a rib interspace. The pleural line appears as a somewhat deeper, thicker, and more echogenic horizontal line beneath the skin, subcutaneous tissue, and intercostal muscle. Comet-tail artifacts and a positive gliding sign are typically seen when scanning this interface in real-time.

and comet-tail artifacts will usually be seen at this interface on real-time scanning. At the site of maximal tenderness, the rib being evaluated should first be aligned in short-axis orientation in the center of the image. The transducer should then be turned parallel to the long axis of the rib. The superficial cortex of the normal rib and costal cartilage will appear as a thin echogenic line on the sonogram (Figure 16-31). Care should be taken to remain directly over the long axis of the rib since the pleural line will also appear as a horizontal echogenic line on the sonogram, albeit deeper and with pleural gliding and comet-tail artifacts usually apparent (Figure 16-32).

A 5.0–10 MHz linear array scanner is recommended for evaluation of a suspected sternal fracture. The sternum should be imaged in both long- and short-axis views, although the long-axis view is reported to be the most fruitful for fracture detection. The sternal surface will appear as a horizontal echogenic line with a slight elevation in the cortical surface noted at the level of the sternomanubrial junction. As with evaluation for suspected rib fractures, scanning at the area of maximal tenderness can help locate the fracture site quickly. An acoustic stand-off pad may be useful to bring the sternal surface into an optimal focal zone.

Imaging of **long bones** in the trauma setting can be undertaken with the transducer used for the FAST examination. A transverse orientation on the limb being scanned is best for quickly establishing the location and depth of the bone being examined (Figure 16-33). Once the lower end of the relevant bone has been located, the transducer is oriented sagittally and the transducer can be slid up the extremity to evaluate for any cortical

irregularities along the shaft (Figure 16-34). Again, the cortical surface of the bone closest to the transducer will be seen as a brightly echogenic line on the sonogram.

For sonography of the **nasal pyramid**, a 10 MHz or higher frequency linear array transducer is typically utilized. It is placed along each side of the nose aiming

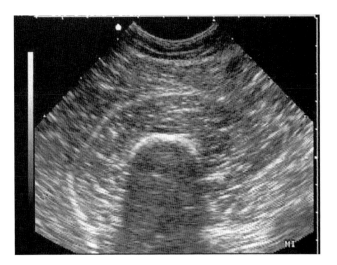

Figure 16-33. Short-axis sonogram of the proximal thigh. The hypoechoic and speckled appearing vastus muscles (vastus lateralis, intermedius, and medialis) are seen in cross section lateral, anterior, and medial to the femur. The anterior surface of the femur is seen in the center of the image as a brightly echogenic curved line with a prominent posterior acoustic shadow.

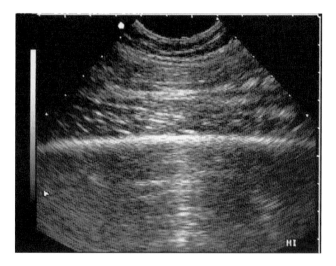

Figure 16-34. Long-axis sonogram of a normal femur. The anterior cortical surface of the femur appears as a smooth and regular echogenic line beneath the hypoechoic thigh muscles; a slight curvature of the image occurs when a curved array transducer is used.

superomedially along the lateral nasal pyramid to assess both the frontal process of the maxilla and ipsilateral proximal nasal bone, and along the left and right paramedian midline to assess the full length of the nasal bones proper (Figures 16-35 and 16-36). Imaging depth is typically set to 3 cm and, as with all bone imaging, the electronic focus should be adjusted to maximize resolution at the level of the cortex. Using transducers and settings similar to those used for nasal bone imaging, the zygomatic arch can be readily visualized with ultrasound by scanning the upper lateral cheek in a horizontal scan plane (Figure 16-37).

The same imaging techniques apply when ultrasound is used for **reducing fractures** (distal radius and forearm).

▶ COMMON AND EMERGENT ABNORMALITIES

RIB FRACTURES

Fractures of the rib or costochondral junction will be recognized by a clear discontinuity of the anterior cortical

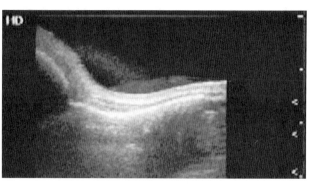

A

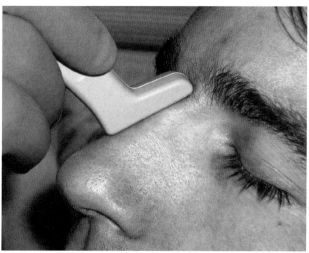

C

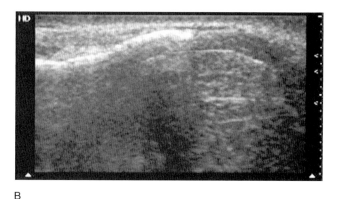

B

Figure 16-35. This image shows the anterior location where the ultrasound transducer should be placed when assessing the nasal pyramid for a fracture (A). Although a linear array transducer may also be used for this application, these images will be more easily obtained if a small parts (and hence, small footprint) transducer is used. Sonogram of a normal nasal bone (B). The nasofrontal border is not visualized in this image because the edge of a standard linear array transducer does not easily fit on the superior nasal bridge. Sonogram of the normal nasal bone and a portion of the frontal bone (C). A copious amount of gel was placed on the nasal bridge and the image now includes a portion of the frontal bone on the left, the nasofrontal suture, and the nasal bone proper.

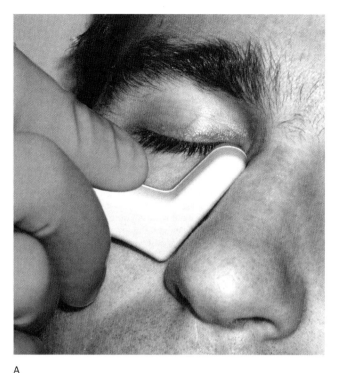

A

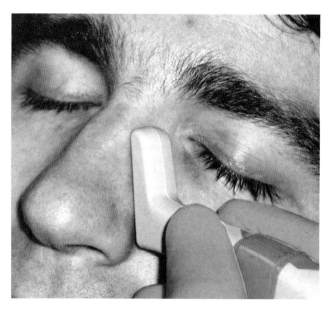

B

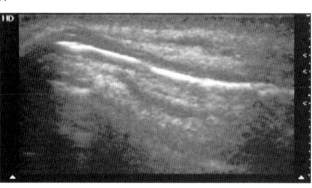

C

Figure 16-36. This sequence of images shows the two additional locations where the ultrasound transducer should be placed when assessing the nasal pyramid for a fracture (A, B). Sonogram of the normal lateral nasal pyramid (C). The echogenic surface of the nasal bone, the slightly hypoechoic nasomaxillary suture, and the frontal process of the maxilla are all seen on this sonogram of the lateral nasal wall.

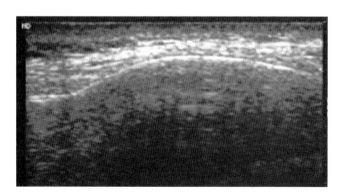

Figure 16-37. Sonogram of the bony contour of the normal zygomatic arch; the arch is seen as a thin echogenic line several millimeters below the skin surface.

echo of the rib, costochondral junction, or costal cartilage being scanned (Figure 16-38), or by real-time visualization of widening of the fracture line with local transducer pressure. Comet-tail artifacts may be noted to emanate posteriorly from the mobile fracture site (Figure 16-39) and a hypoechoic fracture hematoma may be noted adjacent to the fracture.

STERNAL FRACTURES

A sternal fracture will appear as a disruption in the cortical echo of the anterior sternum; movement of the sternum fracture fragments with respiration may be noted during real-time scanning. A hypoechoic fracture

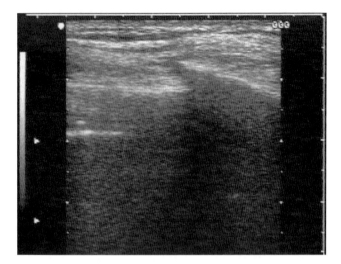

Figure 16-38. Long-axis sonogram of rib fracture with some bony displacement. Comet-tail artifacts were seen at the fracture site on real-time imaging.

hematoma may be seen adjacent to the fracture site (Figure 16-40).

LONG BONES

Fractures of the femur, tibia, and humerus are best appreciated with a long-axis scanning technique and will be apparent as an obvious disruption in the echogenic line that corresponds to the cortical surface of the bone being imaged. Examples of common long bone fractures are demonstrated in Figures 16-41, 16-42, and 16-43.

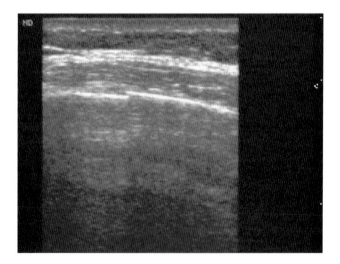

Figure 16-39. Long-axis sonogram of a rib fracture. Skin, subcutaneous tissue, fascia, and chest wall musculature are seen as distinct layers just above the thin echogenic rib surface. Even though the step-off at the fracture line is less than a millimeter, it is readily apparent on the sonogram.

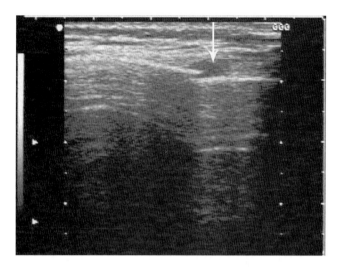

Figure 16-40. Long-axis sonogram of a sternal body fracture. There is an area of cortical discontinuity in the near field to the right of the image and there is a small associated hypoechoic fracture hematoma (arrow).

NASAL BONES

A nasal bone fracture is clearly demonstrated by the large hypoechoic gap in the normally echogenic cortical surface in Figure 16-44.

ZYGOMATIC ARCH

The normal contour of the zygomatic arch is clearly disrupted in Figure 16-45, and a prominent hypoechoic fracture hematoma is present.

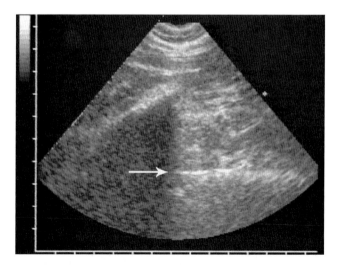

Figure 16-41. Long-axis sonogram of the proximal femoral shaft in a patient with femur fracture. The proximal fragment is seen to angulate anteriorly and there is a prominent posterior acoustic shadow. The distal femur is seen as a horizontal echogenic line (arrow) about 4 cm deep to the anterior fragment.

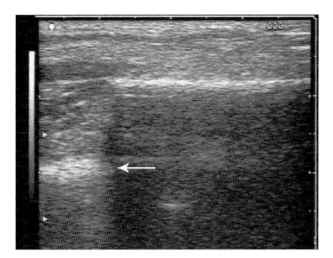

Figure 16-42. Long-axis sonogram of a tibial shaft fracture. About a centimeter of bony displacement is seen between the proximal (arrow) and distal fracture fragments in this image.

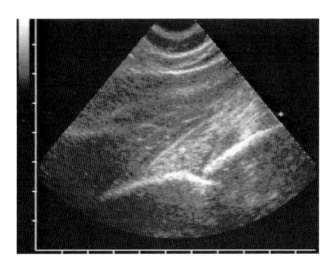

Figure 16-43. Long-axis sonogram of a humerus fracture. There is obvious disruption of the cortical surface in this image.

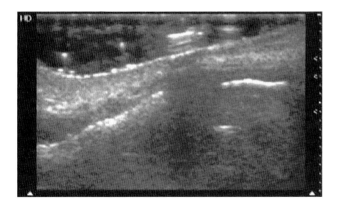

Figure 16-44. Sonogram of a nasal bone fracture. There is a region of obvious cortical discontinuity and a large gap is seen between the proximal nasal bone and the displaced distal fragment.

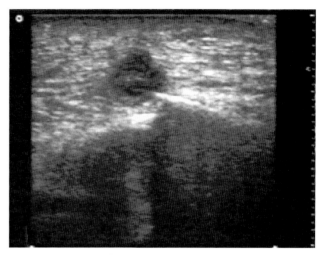

A

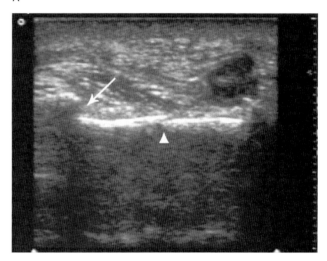

B

Figure 16-45. Sonogram of a right zygomatic arch fracture. This image was taken near the zygomaticotemporal suture (A). The normally smooth contour of the cortical surface of the zygomatic arch has been disrupted and a hypoechoic fracture hematoma is seen at the fracture site. The overlying soft tissues are notably thicker than normal. The next image was taken over the zygomatic process of the temporal bone or the zygomatic arch proper (B). A depressed zygomatic arch fracture is apparent (arrow) and a fracture line is seen in the mid arch (arrowhead). The hypoechoic fracture hematoma in the area of the zygomaticotemporal suture is now seen to the right of the image.

▶ PITFALLS

1. **General pitfalls**. An important pitfall of fracture sonography was illuminated in an experimental study examining the sonographic profile of fractured cadaver bones. It was observed that fractures and bony defects were not well visualized when the transducer was oriented parallel to the fracture line or zone of bony impaction. Optimal imaging of a fracture and any associated bony displacement requires that the ultrasound transducer be oriented axially along the bone and, ideally, perpendicular to the fracture line.[30] Characteristically, an interruption of the normal cortical echo reflection and its associated posterior acoustic shadow will be noted; additionally, a dorsal band of comet-tail echoes may be seen at the fracture site.[31]

2. **Rib imaging pitfalls**. The **pseudofracture**. If the transducer is located partly over the rib and partly over an intercostal space (or over a portion of the scapula), the image obtained on the sonogram may be interpreted as representing a fracture when in fact none is present. Costal cartilage calcifications may also give rise to this "pseudofracture" phenomenon.

    Misidentifying pleura for a rib. The brightly echogenic pleural surface (seen when scanning along the long-axis of an intercostal space) should not be mistaken for the cortex of the rib. The rib in question should first be scanned in short-axis orientation and can be easily identified by its characteristic posterior acoustic shadowing. Note should be taken of the location of the superficial surface of the rib and its depth within the soft tissues of the chest wall. When the transducer is subsequently rotated into a long-axis orientation to assess the rib for the presence of a fracture, the sonographer will then be aware of the expected depth of the rib surface. The brightly echogenic pleural line will usually be seen about a centimeter deep to the superficial surface of the rib. Careful observation during real-time scanning will typically reveal the to-and-fro gliding movements (the "gliding sign") of the brightly echogenic pleural interface. Gliding comet-tail artifacts (arising from the visceral pleural surface and the adjacent air-filled alveoli) are also usually apparent at this location and can aid in its identification as pleura and not rib. Both these findings will be absent if a coexistent pneumothorax is present, however, and it may be the depth of this echogenic line alone that identifies the structure.

3. **Sternum fracture pitfalls**. The hypoechoic sternomanubrial junction may be confused with a fracture on the long-axis view. In general, a fracture of the sternum will appear as a sharply defined area of cortical discontinuity, whereas the sternomanubrial junction will appear as a gentle and smoothly edged ridge with a small hypoechoic joint space in between. Another reported pitfall, when imaging the sternum with ultrasound, is mistaking the hypoechoic pectoralis muscles for a hematoma on a short-axis view.[18]

4. **Long bone fracture pitfalls**. While generally excellent for diagnosing midshaft fractures of the long bones, diagnostic accuracy for fracture detection with ultrasound is limited by a number of factors. Diagnostic accuracy is notably poorer in the metacarpals, metatarsals, with small avulsion injuries and injuries involving the joint space. Notably, imaging "at or above the intertrochanteric line of the femur" is felt to be fraught with difficulty, with a propensity for false positive studies to occur in this area.[20] These areas of poorer diagnostic accuracy are generally more challenging to image and interpret, likely due to the many irregular bony acoustic interfaces present. Subcutaneous air around an open fracture may also adversely affect image quality and therefore diagnostic accuracy.

5. **Nasal bone fractures pitfalls.** A large probe head may be difficult to place on a small nose. In such cases, copious use of gel or an acoustic stand-off such as a gel-filled portion of a rubber glove or a piece of a commercially available gel pad may prove helpful for obtaining an adequate image.

6. **Zygomatic arch fracture pitfalls**. The zygomatic arch is wide and narrow and the transducer needs to be accurately aligned to image the arch fully. The length of the full contour of the arch may exceed the length of the transducer, and several images may be required to fully assess the arch for a fracture.

▶ FOREIGN BODY LOCALIZATION

CLINICAL CONSIDERATIONS

Correctly diagnosing and managing a wound that harbors a soft tissue foreign body can be challenging, especially when the foreign body is radiolucent. To further complicate matters, wounds that harbor foreign bodies often occur in the hand or foot where the likelihood of iatrogenic injury from blind wound exploration and the potential for subsequent infectious complications is high. Although usually located in superficial soft tissues, foreign bodies may cause no symptoms initially and can easily be overlooked. In a retrospective review of 200 patients referred for retained foreign bodies, 38% were misdiagnosed on the index visit.[32] Even with a high index of suspicion, liberal use of radiography, and exploration, a soft tissue foreign body can be missed. The possible infectious and medico-legal consequences of this missed diagnosis can be unfortunate for the patient and the provider alike. Missed foreign bodies have been reported to be one of the most common causes of malpractice claims against emergency physicians.[33]

While metal and glass are radio-opaque and usually apparent on standard two-view radiographs, other commonly encountered foreign bodies, particularly organic material such as wood or thorns, are nearly always radiolucent. Plastic also is frequently radiolucent. CT or MRI may be useful in the assessment of suspected foreign bodies, but these modalities are expensive, time-consuming, and not always readily obtainable. Furthermore, the sensitivity of CT for the detection of wooden foreign bodies is low, reported to range from 0 to 60%.[34,35] Ultrasound offers some decided advantages in this setting. For detecting wooden foreign bodies—nearly always missed with plain radiography—ultrasound is 79–95% sensitive, and 86–97% specific.[34,36,37] In a case where a radiolucent foreign body is suspected, ultrasound equipment can be brought to the bedside at the time of the examination, functioning as an extension of the physical examination. With ultrasound equipment now readily available in many emergency departments, bedside sonographic assessment of wounds suspected of harboring a radiolucent foreign body should become increasingly common.

Whether radio-opaque or radiolucent, once a soft tissue foreign body has been identified, the next issue faced by the clinician is how best to remove it. As most experienced clinicians will confirm, removal of a subcutaneous foreign body can be enormously frustrating. Ultrasound can additionally be used to provide precise preoperative localization of the foreign body, or, if desired, the foreign body may be retrieved under direct sonographic guidance.

CLINICAL INDICATIONS

The clinical indications for the use of ultrasound in the management of a suspected soft tissue foreign body include

- detection of a radiolucent foreign body,
- localization of a radiolucent or radio-opaque foreign body, and
- foreign body removal.

The literature on sonographic detection of soft tissue foreign bodies encompasses a wide range of specialties and methodologies.[34,36−49] The types of foreign

bodies that have been studied include metal, wood, plastic, gravel, sand, and thorns or cactus spines. Sonographers with varying levels of skill perform the ultrasound examinations in these studies, ranging from emergency physicians with no prior formal training, credentialed sonographers, and radiologists specially trained in musculoskeletal ultrasound. The ultrasound machines and transducers are different in nearly every study. While this literature is therefore somewhat difficult to synthesize, a number of useful conclusions can be drawn.

Success in detecting foreign bodies varies widely in the experimental literature, depending in part on the tissue model employed and foreign body type. Using a homogenous beef cube as a tissue model, ultrasound was 98% sensitive and specific in identifying a variety of embedded foreign bodies in one report,[39] whereas another study using a chicken thigh model (a model that more closely mimics the human hand) reported an overall sensitivity of only 79% for detecting a wooden foreign body.[36] In studies involving "freshly thawed" cadaver feet and hands, diagnostic sensitivities and specificities ranged from 90 to 94% and from 90 to 97%, respectively.[42,47] In contrast to such excellent results, another investigation that used ultrasound for detecting foreign bodies in chicken thighs reported an overall sensitivity and specificity of only 43% and 70%, respectively, with a sensitivity of only 50% for detecting a 1-cm-long piece of wood.[41] Review of the methods employed in this study revealed that the chicken thighs were incised and systematically opened with a hemostat prior to foreign body placement. Such tissue disruption with the likely introduction of subcutaneous air probably exceeds that which occurs in natural wounding and may have made subsequent sonography difficult. Of note, vigorous wound irrigation itself can introduce subcutaneous gas bubbles that interfere with subsequent attempts to locate small glass fragments with ultrasound. However, in another study in which air was purposely injected into turkey breasts containing glass, metal, and bone, the soft tissue gas did not appear to diminish the ability to locate the foreign bodies.[50]

Success in soft tissue foreign body detection also depends on foreign body size. The test characteristics of ultrasound reported among various studies must therefore be interpreted with an awareness of the size of the experimental foreign body being imaged. Small glass fragments and cactus thorns were difficult to detect in one report, and may have exceeded the limits of the ultrasound transducer's resolution.[39] Variations in detection rates with two differing lengths of wooden toothpicks inserted into freshly thawed cadaver feet were reported. Sensitivity decreased from 93% for detecting a 5.0-mm-long fragment to 87% for detecting one that was 2.5 mm long.[42] Specificities were uniformly high across studies, indicating that it is uncommon to falsely identify a foreign body when none is present.

While it might appear intuitive that sonographer experience and expertise would be a crucial determinant of success for foreign body localization, there is little experimental evidence to support this assumption. Only one study directly compared the ability of various types of sonographers to locate foreign bodies with ultrasound.[36] It found no statistically significant difference in accuracy between a board-certified radiologist whose practice was limited to ultrasonography, two ultrasound technologists, and three emergency medicine residents. Sensitivity was 74% in the hands of the emergency physicians compared to 83% and 85%, respectively, for the radiologist and technologists.

In clinical case series, wood is the most common radiolucent material reported, hand and foot injuries predominate, and most foreign bodies are found to be superficial in location.[34,37,51] One series of 50 patients evaluated for radiolucent foreign bodies noted that 45 of the 50 injuries involved the hand or foot.[37] All of the 21 foreign bodies retrieved at surgery were found less than 2 cm from the skin surface in this report. In another case series of patients evaluated for suspected wooden foreign bodies in the feet, all 10 of the wooden foreign bodies discovered with ultrasound were located between 0.4 and 1.4 cm from the skin surface.[34]

ANATOMIC CONSIDERATIONS

Since hand and foot wounds are the most common injuries that may harbor a subcutaneous foreign body, a thorough familiarity with the anatomy of the hands and feet is essential for the clinician scanning these regions. Given the relatively shallow depth of the soft tissues in these anatomically intricate regions and the multiple acoustic interfaces present, clinicians should practice scanning on normal hands and feet to gain familiarity with the normal sonographic appearance of these commonly injured areas. The utility of examining the contralateral, uninjured extremity for comparison when a confusing sonographic finding is encountered cannot be overemphasized.

▶ TECHNIQUE AND NORMAL ULTRASOUND FINDINGS

The **highest frequency linear array transducer** available should be used when searching for subcutaneous foreign bodies since most will be found located within 2 cm of the skin surface. A linear array transducer in the 7.5–10.0 MHz range is generally recommended. A 7.5 MHz curvilinear transducer, such as an endocavitary probe, may also function adequately for this application and has the added advantage of a smaller, rounded

skin contact footprint for scanning in web spaces.[38,52] A 5.0 MHz transducer may be useful when searching for a deep foreign body. Higher frequency small parts transducers (typically in the 10–13.0 MHz range) offer the ability to discern very small foreign bodies; a 12.0 MHz transducer can reportedly detect a 1–2 mm foreign body. In recent years, small parts transducers have become a more common addition to ultrasound equipment purchased for use in the ED. The combination of high-image resolution and a small skin contact footprint make these transducers useful for imaging digits and Web spaces for foreign bodies, in addition to ocular imaging, and selected procedural and musculoskeletal applications.

Use of an **acoustic stand-off pad** may be necessary with some transducers to adequately image the superficial soft tissues. Stand-off pads provide a sonolucent acoustic window, raise the transducer 1–2 cm above the skin surface, and move the subcutaneous region of interest beyond the extreme near field (and beyond the transducer's "dead zone") into a more suitable focal zone. Although incorporating the use of a stand-off pad into the ultrasound examination requires additional technical agility and some practice, the effort can be amply rewarded with improved near-field image quality. Inexpensive, commercially available gel pads are available just for this purpose and smaller chunks can be cut off for single patient use and then discarded. Other options include the use of a water- or gel-filled glove or glove finger. When using a water-filled glove, it is essential to exclude any air bubbles that may impede subsequent imaging. In the case of a large or gaping wound, copious sterile surgical gel can be applied onto the wound; after the ultrasound examination is completed, the wound should be thoroughly irrigated. A **water bath technique**, in which the affected extremity is submerged in a basin of water during scanning, represents an alternative to the use of a stand-off pad or the copious use of gel. Compared to direct contact with gel, the water-bath technique was easier to perform and provided superior images of tendons and foreign bodies in one report.[53,54] The water bath technique is also reported to cause less patient discomfort, since images may be obtained without direct contact between the patient and the transducer.[55] The sonographer should ensure that only sealed portions of a transducer are immersed in the water bath.

Optimizing depth and focus settings is particularly important when using ultrasound to search for a small, subcutaneous foreign body. The transducer should be held perpendicular to the skin surface and area of interest systematically scanned in two orthogonal imaging planes. Best visualization of a foreign body will occur when the transducer is aligned such that the long-axis of the ultrasound beam is parallel to the long-axis of the foreign body. Small objects can easily be missed when scanned in short-axis orientation alone. With a small wooden foreign body, however, it is sometimes the prominent posterior acoustic shadow on the *short-axis view* that alerts the sonographer to its presence. Because wounds containing foreign bodies can occur on any part of the body, a wide array of **normal sonographic findings** is therefore possible depending on the anatomic region being scanned. Most wounds suspected of harboring a foreign body occur in the hands and feet, however, where numerous anatomic structures and interfaces, each with a distinct sonographic appearance, will be encountered. The **skin** surface is the most superficial echogenic structure encountered, and is seen adjacent to the transducer surface (or, if an acoustic stand-off is used, adjacent to the distant side of the anechoic stand-off pad). In the hands and especially the feet, this layer is notably thicker than elsewhere on the body. **Subcutaneous fat** appears hypoechoic with a reticular pattern of echogenic connective tissue seen between the fat lobules. The thickness of this layer varies considerably with body location and habitus. **Fascial planes** appear as thin, echogenic, usually horizontal lines above the muscle layer immediately below. **Muscle tissue** appears relatively hypoechoic with regular internal striations (linear or pennate in long-axis, speckled in short-axis relative to the orientation of the muscle fibers). **Tendons** are moderately echogenic, appear ovoid and finely speckled in short-axis, and rectangular with a characteristic fibrillar sonographic pattern in long-axis orientation. Interestingly, tendons will appear considerably more hypoechoic when imaged obliquely; this characteristic of tendon imaging is known as anisotropy and is discussed in greater detail in the musculotendon portion of this chapter. Tendon movement can be observed real-time when the corresponding joints are moved. **Bone** appears brightly echogenic on the cortical surface closest to the transducer, with prominent posterior acoustic shadowing. **Joint spaces** can be readily identified by a V-shaped discontinuity in the bright cortical echo of adjacent bones. **Blood vessels** are anechoic and have a circular or tubular profile when scanned in short or long-axis, respectively. They can be further characterized with color flow Doppler, if necessary. In general, veins will compress easily with transducer pressure whereas arteries will remain pulsatile. Sonograms of the thenar eminence of a normal hand and a chicken thigh (commonly used as a tissue model for foreign body imaging) are shown in Figures 16-46 and 16-47.

▶ COMMON AND EMERGENT ABNORMALITIES

Soft tissue foreign bodies exhibit a variety of sonographic patterns depending on the material involved, the size of the foreign body, and the length of time the foreign body

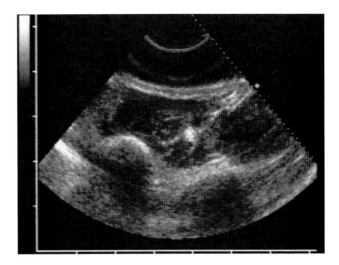

Figure 16-46. Sonogram of the thenar eminence of a normal hand using a 7.5 MHz annular array transducer and an acoustic stand-off pad. The anechoic stand-off appears first, then the hyperechoic skin surface, followed by the hypoechoic thenar eminence muscles below. The flexor pollicis longus tendon is seen in cross section as a hyperechoic circle in the middle of the image. The hyperechoic surfaces of the first and second metacarpals are seen in the far field with associated posterior acoustic shadowing.

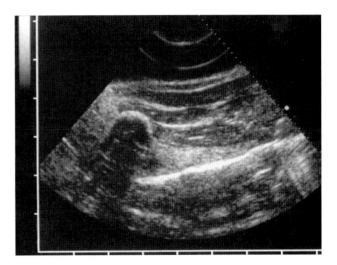

Figure 16-47. Sonogram of a chicken thigh using a 7.5 MHz annular array transducer and an acoustic stand-off pad (a similar technique is used for all the experimental foreign body images that follow). Note the tissue thickness and appearance is similar to that of the hand. The skin has been removed, thigh muscle tissue appears hypoechoic, the thigh bone on the left of the image appears hyperechoic with posterior acoustic shadowing, and an echogenic horizontally oriented fascial plane is seen in the far field.

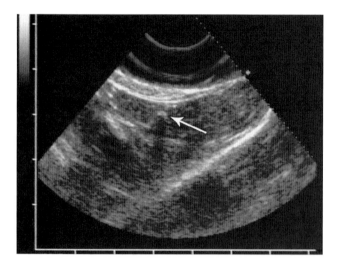

Figure 16-48. Short-axis sonogram of a wooden toothpick embedded in a chicken thigh. The hyperechoic wood fragment is seen in the near field. The posterior acoustic shadow draws the eye up to the location of the foreign body (arrow).

has been present in the tissue. Common materials such as wood, glass, metal, plastic, and gravel will generally appear **hyperechoic** with variable amounts of posterior acoustic shadowing and associated artifacts that are material and shape dependent. A wooden foreign body typically casts a **hypoechoic** posterior acoustic shadow that often facilitates its discovery (Figures 16-48, 16-49, 16-50, and 16-51). Linear metallic foreign bodies will typically display a **reverberation artifact** with bright,

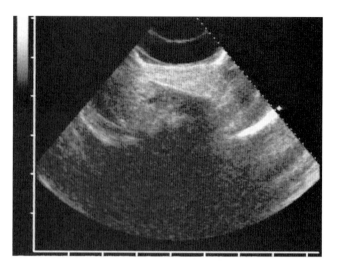

Figure 16-50. Long-axis sonogram of a wooden foreign body in a patient's foot. A 7.5 MHz annular array transducer and an acoustic stand-off pad were used to obtain the image; the skin surface and immediate subcutaneous tissue appear hyperechoic. The wood fragment appears in the near field as a hyperechoic linear structure that slants to the right; a prominent posterior acoustic shadow is seen beneath the wood fragment.

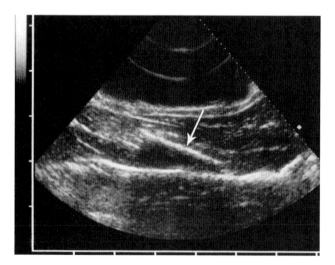

Figure 16-49. Long-axis sonogram of a wooden toothpick in a chicken thigh. The hyperechoic surface of the 2-cm wood fragment is seen in the near field in the center of the image (arrow points to center of toothpick); a posterior acoustic shadow is seen below.

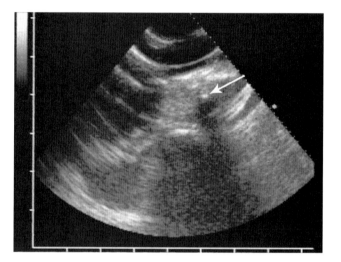

Figure 16-51. Short-axis sonogram of the wooden foreign body in Figure 5. The hyperechoic wood fragment appears in the near field on the right side of the image (arrow). The transducer is no longer entirely in contact with the foot because of the location being scanned. A prominent posterior acoustic shadow is again seen beneath the foreign body. More distally and in the center of the sonogram, the first metatarsal bone and its posterior acoustic shadow are seen in cross section.

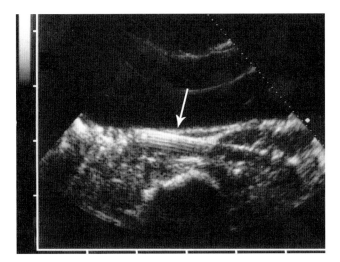

Figure 16-52. Long-axis sonogram of a needle in a chicken thigh. The needle appears hyperechoic (arrow) with a characteristic reverberation artifact seen below.

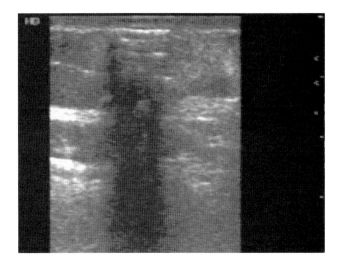

Figure 16-54. Clinically stable appearing victim of a gunshot wound to the right chest with a bullet seen on the *left* side in the chest radiograph. A mass was palpable beneath the skin on the left chest wall. A sonogram of the mass (the bullet) is notable for a reverberation artifact and posterior acoustic shadowing. The bullet was superficial in location and outside of the chest cavity (confirmed by CT).

regularly spaced parallel lines seen distal to the actual object (Figures 16-52, 16-53, and 16-54). Metal objects that are small, or rounded, may display a **comet-tail artifact** (Figure 16-55). The acoustic profile of glass is less consistent, however, and acoustic shadowing, reverberation artifact, or diffuse beam scattering may

all be encountered during scanning (Figures 16-56 and 16-57). Foreign bodies retained for longer than 24 hours are frequently surrounded by a **hypoechoic "halo"** resulting from edema, pus, or granulation tissue. This hypoechoic region around the foreign body facilitates

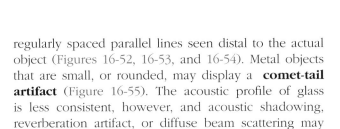
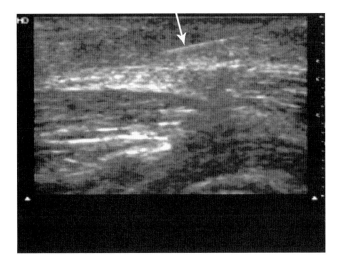

Figure 16-53. Long-axis sonogram of a broken needle fragment in the arm of an injection drug user. The needle appears hyperechoic (arrow). Although not appreciated on the sonogram, a fine reverberation artifact was seen on real-time imaging.

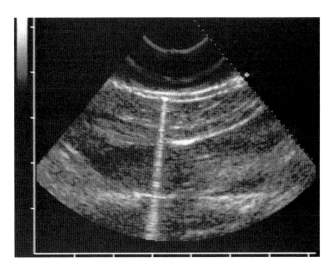

Figure 16-55. Sonogram of a BB in a chicken thigh. A prominent comet-tail artifact is seen.

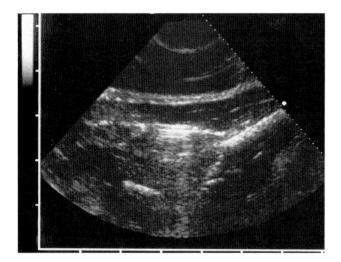

Figure 16-56. Sonogram of a linear glass shard embedded in a chicken thigh. The glass fragment in the center or the image appears hyperechoic with an associated reverberation artifact.

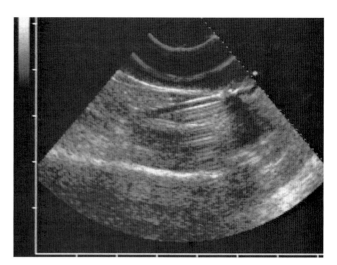

Figure 16-58. Long-axis sonogram of a plastic toothpick in a chicken thigh. The plastic surface of the toothpick appears hyperechoic with a prominent reverberation artifact seen below.

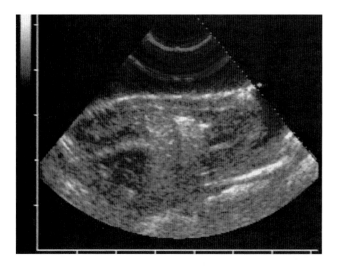

Figure 16-57. Sonogram of a piece of a broken glass bottle embedded in a chicken thigh. Although hyperechoic, the glass fragment in this image is indistinct with some dirty shadowing possibly due to air pockets surrounding the fragment.

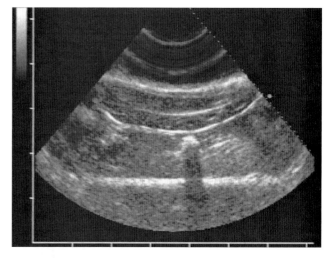

Figure 16-59. Sonogram of a piece of gravel in a chicken thigh. A prominent posterior acoustic shadow is seen beneath the hyperechoic surface of the gravel fragment.

► COMMON VARIANTS AND SELECTED ABNORMALITIES

identification and localization of the foreign body (see Case Study). In a similar fashion, a local anesthetic injected adjacent to a foreign body may improve the ability to visualize it. Finally, sonograms of less commonly encountered foreign bodies such as plastic (with a prominent reverberation artifact) and gravel (with a prominent posterior acoustic shadow similar to a gallstone) are seen in Figures 16-58 and 16-59.

Various wound characteristics can complicate sonographic evaluation for a soft tissue foreign body. Air introduced into the wound by the injury itself, from the process of wound exploration or wound irrigation, or from bubbles inadvertently administered with the anesthetic agent can cause imaging difficulties. Air bubbles and associated artifacts may obscure the foreign body or may be mistaken for a foreign body when none is actually present. Air bubbles introduced during wound irrigation can complicate subsequent attempts to locate small glass fragments. Air pockets can sometimes be obliterated by compression with the transducer, thereby improving image quality. Ultrasound examination of large open wounds may be difficult because of bleeding, associated tissue distortion, or patient discomfort.

▶ PITFALLS

1. **Inadequate knowledge of the regional sonographic anatomy.** Lack of familiarity with normal sonographic anatomy, particularly of the hand and foot, can make correct interpretation of the ultrasound image difficult. Normal acoustic shadows from bone, brightly echogenic tissue interfaces and fascia, and artifacts arising from vascular calcifications, can all lead to misinterpretation of the image. Sesamoid bones may be falsely interpreted as a foreign body. Bony shadowing of the multiple carpal and metacarpal bones (or tarsal and metatarsal bones) and phalanges should not be confused with a foreign body.

2. **Failure to take necessary steps to optimize scanning of small, superficial objects.** Scanning for subcutaneous foreign bodies, particularly in hands and feet, requires a significant investment in time, patience, and attention to certain scanning principles. A stand-off pad or water bath may be required. Attention to transducer frequency, depth, and focus adjustment is crucial. In addition, the location of the wound and the transducer's skin contact footprint may make adequate imaging technically difficult. Scanning small curvilinear regions, such as a Web space, may require a small parts transducer or an endocavitary probe, as well as stand-off pad *and* the help of an assistant.

3. **Other pitfalls.** Small foreign bodies may exceed the limits of the transducer's resolution. Tissue interfaces in close proximity to one another may distort the image. A small foreign body adjacent to a bone may be hidden by the bone's posterior acoustic shadow. Scar tissue, air, ossified cartilage, and keratin plugs may all appear as small hyperechoic structures and be mistaken for foreign bodies.

4. **Foreign body removal.** Once a soft tissue foreign body has been located, an important clinical decision must be made as to whether retrieval is appropriate or even technically feasible. Various factors to consider include the skill of the operator, the body part injured, the time available, and the size and type of foreign body involved.

In the case of a deep wound, a poorly accessible foreign body or closely adjacent neurovascular structures, consultation or referral to an appropriate surgical specialist is recommended.

▶ CASE STUDY

Patient Presentation

A 42-year-old man presented with a 10-day-old puncture wound of the finger with associated soft tissue swelling. The patient reported getting a splinter in his hand while sitting on a park bench. He thought he had removed the entire splinter at the time of the injury.

On physical examination there was swelling over the volar proximal third phalanx area but no definite fluctuance (Figure 16-58a). Distal neurocirculatory examination was intact, and there were no signs of lymphangitis or tenosynovitis.

Management

A radiograph of the affected digit was obtained and notable only for some soft tissue swelling (Figure 16-58b). An ultrasound was performed using a 7.5 MHz annular array transducer and an acoustic stand-off to obtain the images in both longitudinal (Figure 16-58c) and transverse (Figure 16-58d) planes. A hyperechoic foreign body with an associated hypoechoic surrounding inflammatory response was seen above the PIP joint. The wood fragment was easily removed in toto with a superficial skin incision along the PIP crease (Figure 16-58e).

Commentary

This case emphasizes the advantage of sonography over plain radiography for identification of wooden (and other) foreign bodies. Foreign bodies retained for longer than 24 hours are frequently surrounded by a hypoechoic "halo" resulting from edema, or early infection around the foreign body. This "halo" can facilitate identification and successful removal of a foreign body.

▶ MUSCULOTENDINOUS APPLICATIONS

CLINICAL CONSIDERATIONS

Technological advancements over the past decade have led to the increased use of diagnostic ultrasound for the evaluation of a wide range of musculotendinous and rheumatologic conditions. Smaller, more portable ultrasound units, high-frequency small parts transducers with resolutions to a fraction of a millimeter, tissue harmonics,

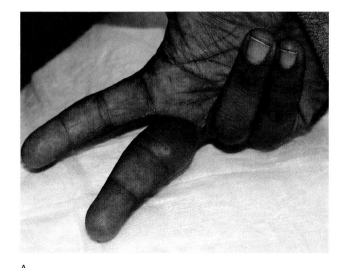

A

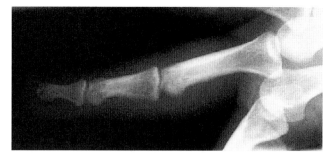

B

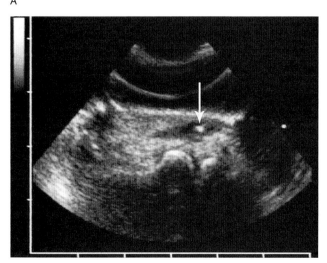

C

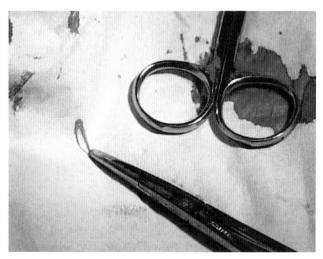

D

E

Figure 16-60. Case study. Photo of swollen digit (A). Radiograph of the affected digit is notable only for some soft tissue swelling (B). Longitudinal sonogram on the volar surface of the third digit over the PIP joint shows a hyperechoic foreign body (arrow) in cross section (C). Note associated hypoechoic surrounding inflammatory response. Long-axis view of 1-cm splinter (arrow) (D). Wood fragment removed (E).

compound imaging technology, and extended field of view features have helped promote ultrasound as a diagnostic tool for evaluating musculotendinous complaints, whether in the hands of radiologists, rheumatologists, or emergency physicians. Ultrasound has emerged as "a powerful extension of the physical examination"[56] and nowhere more so than in the realm of musculotendinous assessment. Imaging of tendons, joints, and muscles can help the provider make a correct diagnosis for a host of painful musculoskeletal conditions; armed with this knowledge, optimal treatment and management can follow. Self-teaching programs in musculoskeletal ultrasound have been promulgated for rheumatologists with excellent results reported after 24 hours of active scanning and 8–9 hours reviewing images with tutors.[57]

A myriad of musculoskeletal applications for diagnostic ultrasound have been described in the ultrasound literature. These include (1) evaluation of suspected partial or complete tendon tears (rotator cuff, triceps tendon, distal biceps tendon, Achilles tendon, quadriceps tendon, patellar ligament, and flexor tendons of the hand), (2) evaluation for muscle tears (specifically, the rectus femoris and gastrocnemius muscles), (3) diagnosis of occult ganglion cysts[58] (wrist or fingers), (4) dynamic evaluation of flexor tendons of the hand (for evaluation of annular pulley ligament disruption or assessment of tendon location after flexor tendon avulsion), and (5) assessment of selected nerves for suspected entrapment or compression (e.g., the ulnar and median nerves in cubital and carpal tunnel syndromes). Some of these applications require expertise in ultrasound beyond that of most sonographers, or they may require specialized transducers that are not generally available in the emergency or urgent care settings. With the now common presence of linear array transducers available for compact ultrasound units, however, and the increasing appearance of small parts transducers available on newer equipment packages, a host of selected musculotendinous applications can easily be added to the diagnostic armamentarium of the emergency sonographer.

▶ CLINICAL INDICATIONS

Clinical indications for performing a musculotendinous ultrasound examination may include

- assessment of suspected partial or complete tendon tears,
- evaluation of suspected tenosynovitis and selected tendinopathies,
- assessment of joint involvement in chronic arthritis, and
- precise guidance for aspiration and soft tissue injection procedures involving tendons and bursae.

A number of clinical studies have investigated the use of ultrasound to image rotator cuff tears with variable success.[59–61] In an attempt to explain the wide range of reported accuracy for diagnosing rotator cuff tears with ultrasound (60–95%), a number of contributing factors were identified. The technical difficulty involved, the considerable experience required to perform the examination, the complex anatomy of the shoulder, and the occurrence of prominent beam propagation artifacts in the shoulder all combine to make sonographic evaluation of rotator cuff injuries a challenge.[62] Because of these difficulties, only a few centers routinely use ultrasound to evaluate the shoulder for a suspected rotator cuff injury. MRI, with its excellent image quality and lack of operator dependence, has become the diagnostic imaging technique most commonly used for these injuries. In general, sonography of the rotator cuff has little utility for the emergency evaluation of a shoulder injury since the clinical examination and radiography will usually adequately guide the direction of clinical care. Similarly, ultrasound is generally considered unsuitable for evaluation of meniscal or other ligamentous injuries of the knee; MRI has become the imaging technique of choice for these injuries as well.

Complete disruptions of the rotator cuff, the biceps, triceps, quadriceps, or Achilles tendons are usually reliably diagnosed clinically and imaging is usually not required. If desired, however, sonography *can* be used to rapidly demonstrate the site of the specific tendon disruption at the bedside. **Partial tendon tears** present more of a diagnostic challenge. These may be difficult to diagnose on clinical grounds alone, and may therefore be misdiagnosed altogether. It is in this clinical scenario that ultrasound can ably assist the provider and help clarify the nature and extent of the suspected tendon injury. The Achilles tendon, quadriceps tendon, patellar ligament, and the triceps tendon all lend themselves to ready sonographic evaluation when a partial tendon tear is being considered. Each of these tendons is located in the superficial soft tissues and can therefore be examined in detail with a high-frequency transducer. The ability to both visualize the substance of the tendon and perform dynamic assessment of its function and integrity in real-time can offer important diagnostic information that may not be appreciated on physical examination or with plain radiography alone.

Tenosynovitis is also readily diagnosed with bedside ultrasound and its characteristic sonographic signature (hypoechoic fluid surrounding the tendon or tendons) makes arriving at this diagnosis simple. In a patient with a swollen and painful hand or foot, the ability to rapidly and confidently make a diagnosis of tenosynovitis improves patient care and assists with the implementation appropriate therapy. Similarly, selected **tendinopathies** can be diagnosed with a sonographic evaluation that reveals a characteristic focal area of hypoechogenicity of the tendon being assessed. A suspected ganglion cyst can similarly be quickly diagnosed with the visualization of an anechoic sac-like structure with a thin pedicle connecting it to a joint space or a tendon sheath. Use of ultrasound for the assessment of a host of painful arthritic joint conditions is discussed in detail in the section on ultrasound guided arthrocentesis (Chapter 20).

Finally, ultrasound guidance may be used to advantage for precise **percutaneous injections of painful conditions** of the musculotendinous system, specifically, injections of tendon sheaths, joints, bursae, and peri-fascial injections for the treatment of common tendinopathies, bursitidies, arthritidies, and fasciitis.[63] Inadvertent administration of corticosteroids within the substance of a tendon has long been known to put the patient at risk of tendon rupture. Real-time ultrasound imaging allows for continuous observation of both needle placement and medication delivery and is therefore ideally suited for precise deposition of corticosteroids and local anesthesia used for treating these conditions. A specific example is the improved management of patients with subacromial bursitis. In a report investigating the treatment effectiveness of ultrasound-guided injections, a group of 40 patients with sonographically confirmed subacromial bursitis were divided into standard blind injection and ultrasound-guided injection groups.[64] The outcome measure assessed was shoulder abduction range of motion preinjection compared with 1-week postinjection. No statistical differences were noted in shoulder range of motion at 1 week in the blind injection group, whereas a statistically significant difference was reported in the group that received the ultrasound-guided injections. The study authors concluded that ultrasound could be used to advantage in guiding the injection needle accurately into the inflamed synovial bursa with significant therapeutic benefits as a result.

▶ ANATOMICAL CONSIDERATIONS

Nearly all of the tendinous structures that are likely to be evaluated in an ED setting are superficial in location. Tendons consist of parallel fascicles of collagen fibers and may form a single homogenous bundle, or they may be composed of multiple bundles or laminae in which case they are referred to as complex tendons. A thin layer of connective tissue, the peritenon, surrounds all tendons. A peritendinous synovial sheath usually surrounds tendons that take a more curvilinear course. This sheath contains a thin film of synovial fluid that helps reduce tendon friction and abrasions. Peritendinous bursae may additionally reduce friction between a tendon and adjacent bones during movements. Tendons are sparsely vascularized and receive their nourishment primarily from segmental vessels arising from the surrounding peritenon or through vinculae.[65]

▶ TECHNIQUE AND NORMAL ULTRASOUND FINDINGS

Musculotendinous ultrasound imaging should, in general, be performed with high-frequency linear array or small parts transducers in the 7.5–13.0 MHz range. Sector transducers are generally not recommended for this application because the diverging beam of sector transducers can create undesirable beam scattering artifacts that leave only a small central portion of the image unaffected.[62] This drawback can be somewhat compensated for by narrowing the sector angle and using a stand-off pad. When imaging very superficial structures, such as the Achilles tendon, patellar ligament, or structures within the finger, the use of an acoustic stand-off pad may be helpful. Attention should be paid to proper frequency, focus, and depth settings to obtain optimal images. A split screen set up may be useful for comparing corresponding images from each side of the body.

Skin is typically seen as a thin, hyperechoic layer adjacent to the transducer or stand-off pad. **Subcutaneous tissue** appears hypoechoic, is of variable thickness depending on body location and habitus, and has a somewhat hyperechoic reticular pattern of connective tissue between the fat lobules. **Skeletal muscle** is readily identified by its characteristic hypoechoic echotexture with echogenic internal striations that appear linear or pennate (feather-like) in long-axis and speckled in short-axis. **Fascial planes** are brightly echogenic and follow the surface contour of the muscle being imaged. Muscle fiber movement is often visible with muscle contraction in real time. In long-axis, **tendons** appear as hyperechoic rectangular or linear structures that generally track on a parallel course with the skin surface. The tightly packed parallel echoes emanating from the collagen fibrils within the substance of the tendon give rise to a tendon's characteristic fibrillar echotexture. In short-axis, tendons appear round, ovoid, or flat, and will usually appear as a cluster of multiple small echogenic dots. A subtle anechoic rim will be seen in tendons with a tendon sheath. Commonly imaged normal tendons are seen in Figures 16-61 through 16-65.

Tendons exhibit an optical phenomenon known as *anisotropy* (i.e., the image obtained from the tendon is directionally dependent on the angle of the ultrasound beam) and a thorough understanding of this concept is essential for anyone engaged in musculotendinous imaging. A tendon will appear hyperechoic only when the insonating beam is precisely perpendicular to the tendon fibers. At all other angles, there is a significant reduction in the percentage of the ultrasound beam that is reflected back to the transducer and the tendon will therefore appear hypoechoic. Anisotropy is important because if a tendon is not properly imaged its internal structure cannot be adequately assessed.[65] It should be noted that most significant tendon pathology manifests

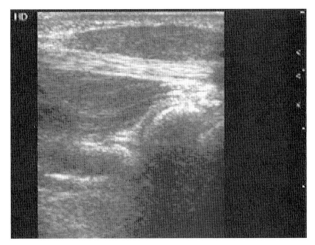

A

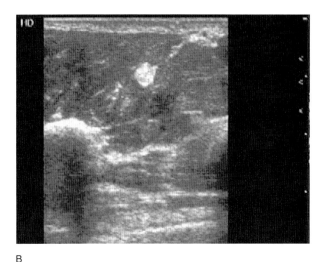

B

Figure 16-61. Long-axis sonogram of the flexor pollicis longus (FPL) tendon in the thenar eminence of the hand (A). Somewhat hyperechoic skin and hypoechoic thenar muscles appear in the near field. Immediately beneath is the FPL tendon notable for its moderately echogenic and fibrillar appearance. The hypoechogenic region at the far right edge of the tendon is due to anisotropy. Tendon motion within the tendon sheath can be observed with real-time imaging. The curved echogenic surface of the first metacarpal bone and its acoustic shadow are seen in the right mid field of the image. Short-axis sonogram of the FPL tendon (B). Skin appears in the near field and the thenar muscles appear hypoechoic with some linear echoes that represent fascial planes. The FPL tendon appears round and echogenic with multiple small dots making up the substance of the tendon. The echogenic first metacarpal and its associated posterior acoustic shadow are seen in the left mid field of the image.

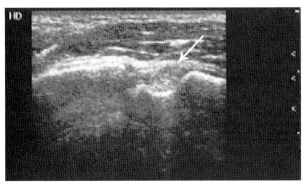

A

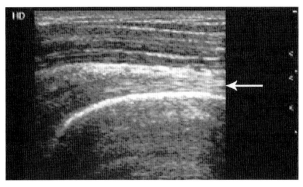

B

Figure 16-62. Short-axis sonogram of the biceps tendon (A). Skin and deltoid muscle appear in the near field. The anterior humeral head is seen in cross section as an echogenic line with a U-shaped depression known as the bicipital groove. The moderately echogenic biceps tendon (arrow) is located within the bicipital groove. Long-axis sonogram of the biceps tendon (B). Successive layers seen in this image are skin, hypoechoic deltoid muscle scanned along the long-axis of its muscle fibers, the hyperechoic and fibrillar appearing biceps tendon (arrow), and the brightly echogenic surface of the anterior humerus.

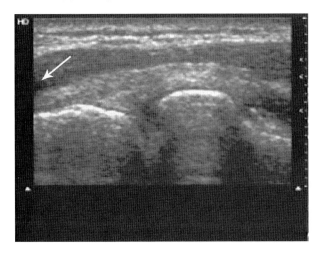

Figure 16-63. Sonogram of the lateral epicondyle of the elbow. The common extensor tendon appears somewhat hypoechoic beneath the skin and subcutaneous tissue. The radial collateral ligament is somewhat more hyperechoic in this image and connects the lateral epicondyle on the left with the radial head on the right of the image. The origin of the common extensor tendon is located somewhat higher up on the lateral epicondyle to the left of this image (arrow).

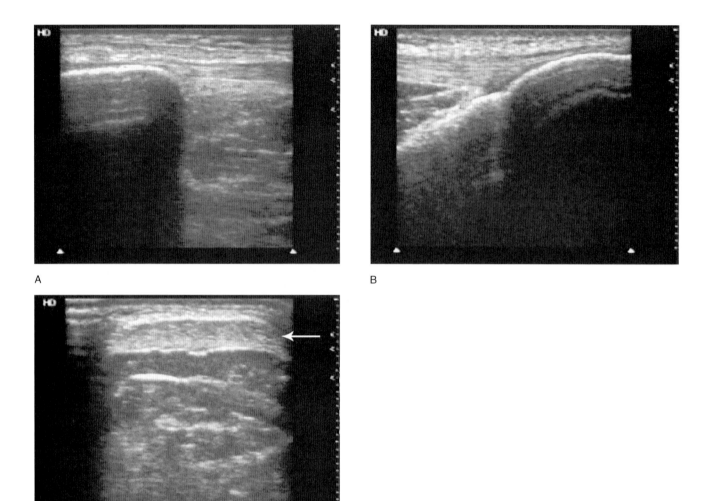

A

B

C

Figure 16-64. Sonogram of the patellar ligament. Long-axis view of the proximal aspect (A). The echogenic surface of the patella is seen on the left of the image with a sharply demarcated posterior acoustic shadow. The proximal portion of the patellar ligament is seen as a 3–4 mm thick, horizontal, and somewhat fibrillar appearing band coming off the inferior pole of the patella. Hoffa's fat pad lies beneath the ligament. Long-axis view of the distal portion of the patellar ligament (B). The fibrillar ligament is seen inserting on the tibial tuberosity to the right near field of the image. A small portion of Hoffa's fat pad is seen beneath the ligament on the left. An extended field of view feature or a longer linear array transducer would allow the entire ligament to be demonstrated on one image. Short-axis view of the proximal patellar ligament (C). The ligament (arrow) is seen to be thick and generally rectangular in configuration with slightly curved edges. It sits immediately beneath the skin, extends almost the entire width of the image, and is hyperechoic relative to the hypoechoic fat pad below.

itself sonographically as a hypoechogenic defect. If inadequate attention is paid to the imaging technique, a focal area of false hypoechogenicity may be interpreted as representing evidence of tendinosis or tendon rupture when, in fact, the hypoechogenicity is simply due to the insonating beam not being perfectly parallel with the tendon fibers at that region. A heel–toe imaging technique helps avoid this pitfall; the transducer is gently rocked in its long-axis plane from one end to the other while scanning long-axis over a tendon. A focal area of hypoechogenicity that disappears with this technique is due to anisotropy; a defect that persists throughout changes in the angle of insonation likely represents true tendon pathology. Anisotropy is present in both long- and short-axis planes, although it is more apparent when scanning the tendon in long-axis.

SPECIFIC IMAGING TECHNIQUES

The **biceps tendon** is most easily found by scanning the upper arm in short-axis just above the level of the

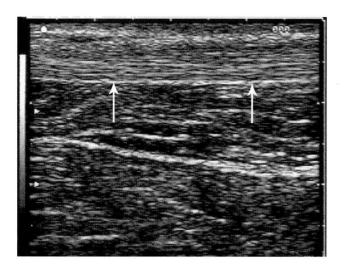

Figure 16-65. Long-axis sonogram of the Achilles tendon. The tendon is seen immediately beneath the skin, appears about 5 mm in thickness, and has a fibrillar appearance in this long-axis view (above arrows). Posterior compartment muscles lie beneath the tendon. The calcaneus lies to the right but is not seen in this image. An acoustic stand-off might help bring the tendon into a more optimal focal zone.

axillary crease with the arm slightly externally rotated. The normal biceps tendon will be seen as a hyperechoic circular structure resting within the echogenic bicipital groove of the proximal humerus. Once located in short-axis, a long-axis view can easily be obtained by simply rotating the transducer.

The **triceps tendon** is best imaged from behind the patient with the transducer oriented in a midline long-axis orientation just above the olecranon process. This view is similar to that used when evaluating the elbow joint for an effusion. The triceps tendon will be seen in the near field as a moderately echogenic fibrillar structure that inserts on the echogenic olecranon process. The hypoechoic posterior fat pad and the echogenic outline of the posterior humerus, olecranon fossa, and olecranon will be seen in the far field of the image.

The **lateral and medial epicondyles** of the elbow are best imaged in long-axis across the joint line with the arm and elbow in full extension, and the hand in either a "thumbs up" position for lateral epicondyle imaging or in a hypersupinated position for medial epicondyle imaging. The bony outlines of the respective epicondyles and either the radial head (lateral) or coronoid process (medial) will be noted on the sonogram. The radial and ulnar collateral ligaments are thin structures found adjacent to and crossing the joint line. The common extensor or flexor tendons will be seen lying superior to the collateral ligaments and their point of origin lies several centimeters above the joint line on their respective epicondyles.

Hand and foot tendons are quickly assessed for tenosynovitis by placing the transducer in the region of clinical interest in a short-axis orientation relative to the direction of the tendon. Individual tendons are best examined in long-axis when evaluating for tendon disruption.

The **patellar ligament** should be scanned in longitudinal and transverse scan planes with the knee held in 30 degrees of flexion to avoid the "false hypoechogenicity" artifact that can occur in this location. This phenomenon is due to tendon anisotropy in the region adjacent to the patella. The contralateral knee should always be scanned for comparison.[62]

The **Achilles tendon** is best evaluated with the patient prone with the foot hanging over the edge of the examining table. Use of a stand-off pad can be helpful, and the foot should be plantarflexed and dorsiflexed to observe dynamic tendon movement.

Soft tissue injection techniques. Ultrasound imaging can provide real-time guidance for delivery of therapeutic injections of corticosteroids. A free-hand technique is most commonly used for injection of tendon sheaths, joints, and bursae. The guiding principle is that the medication delivery needle (typically a 1 1/2″ 20–25 G spinal needle) should be oriented as perpendicular to the insonating beam as possible in order that the needle will appear maximally reflective. The needle's position will be apparent by its strong reverberation or ring-down artifact and its position can be further fine-tuned by injecting a small amount of anesthetic solution and observing the corresponding echoes. When a soft tissue injection procedure is undertaken, the tendons should be oriented so that they display maximal anisotropy for best visualization. A short-axis orientation over the tendon and a long-axis orientation over the injection needle are recommended for avoiding intratendinous injections.[63]

▶ COMMON AND EMERGENT ABNORMALITIES

GENERAL ULTRASOUND FINDINGS

Partial tendon tears are usually seen on ultrasound as hypoechoic to anechoic regions within the substance of the tendon. Complete tendon tears will demonstrate obvious tendon discontinuity during real-time scanning and the tendon sheath may be seen to be filled with a hypoechoic hematoma at the site of disruption. *Tenosynovitis* will sonographically manifest as tendon thickening, tendon sheath widening, and loss of the tendon's normal fibrillar echotexture. An associated anechoic collection of inflammatory synovial fluid will be seen surrounding the tendon. Synovial fluid is typically anechoic in acute inflammatory processes. *Tendonitis* or *tendinosis* usually manifests as areas of patchy hypoechogenicity and loss of fibrillar echotexture within the tendon. Tendons without a sheath will show thickening and altered echogenicity that varies according to the duration of the process.

SPECIFIC CLINICAL SCENARIOS

Tenosynovitis

DeQuervain's disease is an overuse injury involving the first dorsal compartment or the hand (specifically, the abductor pollicis longus and extensor pollicis brevis tendons). Although a positive Finkelstein's sign usually confirms the diagnosis, the tendon can be rapidly imaged in short-axis to confirm the diagnosis in ambiguous cases. Fluid within the tendon sheath, tendon thickening, and pain on "sonographic palpation" are typical (Figure 16-66). Septic or reactive tenosynovitis may be encountered in the hands or feet, most commonly in injection drug users. The affected tendons in both entities typically appear thickened and hyperechoic with variable amounts of surrounding inflammatory synovial fluid (Figure 16-67).

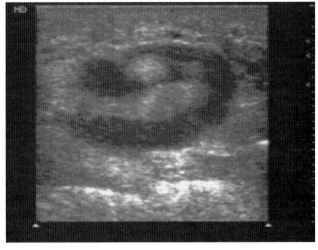

Figure 16-66. Short-axis sonogram of a patient with tenosynovitis of the first dorsal compartment of the hand (DeQuervain's disease). The combined abductor pollicis longus and extensor pollicis brevis tendons appear hyperechoic and thickened and fluid is seen surrounding the tendon. An adjacent vein is seen to the left of the tendon sheath. There is no skin contact with the transducer on the right because the footprint of the transducer exceeds the relatively narrow curved surface of the radial wrist. Tenderness was present on "sonographic palpation."

Tendinopathies

Ultrasound can play a useful role in the evaluation of the athlete with chronic localized knee pain suggestive of tendinopathy of the proximal patellar ligament ("jumper's knee"). In a review of 25 surgically proven cases of "jumper's knee," ultrasound correctly identified the lesion in all patients. The authors advocated the use of ultrasound as "the method of choice for the evaluation of jumper's knee, as it is cheap, noninvasive, repeatable and accurate."[66] Sonographically, the lesion

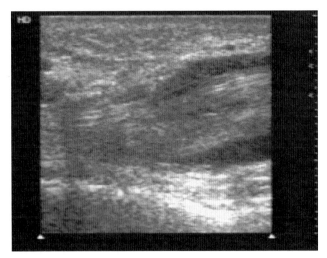

A

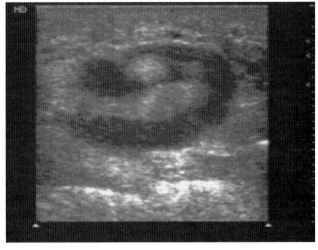

B

Figure 16-67. Long-axis sonogram of the thenar region in an injection drug user with a palmar tenosynovitis (A). The fibrillar flexor tendons of the hand are seen surrounded by a large amount of hypoechoic fluid. Short-axis sonogram of the same case in (B). Multiple flexor tendons are seen in cross section and a large amount of surrounding hypoechoic inflammatory fluid is noted.

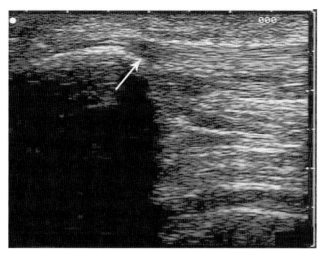 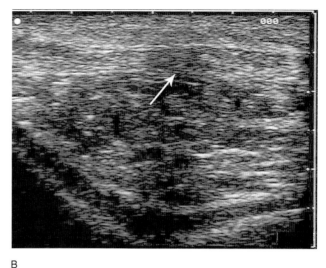

A   B

Figure 16-68. Long-axis sonogram of the proximal patellar ligament showing a hypoechoic tendon defect near the origin of the patellar tendon (A). The remainder of the tendon appears fibrillar and echogenic. A heel–toe insonating technique confirmed that a hypoechoic defect was present and that a tendinopathy ("jumper's knee") was present. Short-axis sonogram of the same patellar ligament (B). The ligament is seen as a somewhat echogenic horizontal structure about 5 mm beneath the skin surface and about 4 mm in width. In the central portion of the tendon there is a focal area of hypoechogenicity that persists with careful imaging. This is the classic location and appearance of a "jumper's knee" or tendinopathy of the proximal patellar tendon.

appears as a localized area of hypoechogenicity in the central portion of the patellar ligament near its insertion on the patella. The patient usually has exquisite tenderness with palpation at this site (Figure 16-68). Diagnosis and injection therapy of another common tendinopathy, lateral epicondylitis or "tennis elbow," is discussed in detail below.

Partial and Complete Tendon Tears

The final common pathway for each of these lesions is excessive stress placed on the actively contracting muscle in question. Partial rupture of the proximal *patellar ligament* is apparent sonographically as a characteristic cone-shaped hypoechoic lesion, exceeding 0.5 cm in length, and found close to the origin of the patellar tendon at the inferior border of the patella. This hypoechoic lesion represents a focal discontinuity of the ligament in that anatomic area and an associated hematoma. An underlying tendonitis ("jumper's knee," above) is often associated with this injury and is identified by thickening of the tendon and overall hypoechogenicity in the area of inflammation. A complete tear of the patellar ligament is usually clinically obvious. The disruption usually occurs at the point of attachment to the patella. On sonography the discontinuity between the patellar ligament and the patella will be apparent. An associated avulsion fracture fragment originating from the inferior pole of

the patella may be seen attached to the proximal end of the ligament (Figure 16-69). A partial tear of the *triceps tendon* will appear as a focal area of hypoechogenicity seen along the anterior insertion of the triceps tendon

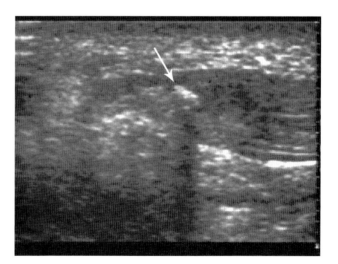

Figure 16-69. Long-axis sonogram of a patellar ligament rupture. The ligament is retracted and thickened with a hyperechoic avulsion fracture fragment attached to its proximal end (arrow). A high riding patella sits out of the field to the left of the image. The ligament has completely torn from its attachment at the lower pole of the patella.

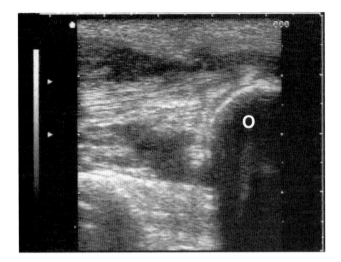

Figure 16-70. Long-axis posterior sonogram of the elbow in a patient with painful ROM after a fall on an outstretched arm. Plain radiographs were normal. The insertion of the triceps tendon onto the olecranon (O) reveals a large hypoechoic defect in the substance of the triceps tendon. Hypoechoic hematoma is seen extending around the tendon posteriorly. The hyperechoic posterior fat pad is seen below the partial tendon tear; no joint effusion was detectable in the posterior recess.

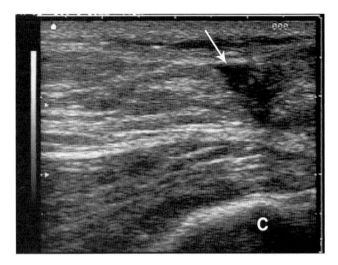

Figure 16-71. Long-axis posterior sonogram of an "ankle sprain." The lower end of the Achilles tendon is seen in the near field about 5 mm beneath the skin. A large hypoechoic defect in the substance of the tendon is apparent (arrow), and on dynamic scanning the hypoechoic gap could be seen to widen. On short-axis views, some of the tendon was noted to still be intact. The hyperechoic curve of the posterior surface of the calcaneus (C) is seen in the right far field of the image.

on the olecranon process. The hypoechoic defect represents both torn tendon and an associated hematoma (Figure 16-70). Similarly, a partial tear of the Achilles tendon will appear as an obvious hypoechoic region of tendon discontinuity and hematoma. Dynamic imaging can help further clarify the extent and location of the tendon disruption (Figure 16-71).

Bursopathies

The Achilles tendon is surrounded anteriorly and posteriorly by two bursae near its point of insertion on the calcaneus. The superficial calcaneal bursa lies in the subcutaneous tissue posterior to the Achilles tendon, and the retrocalcaneal bursa is found between the distal Achilles tendon and the calcaneus. These bursae are not typically seen in normal subjects and a sign of bursitis is that the bursae are demonstrable by ultrasound at all (Figure 16-72).[69] Injection of the retrocalcaneal bursa is sometimes performed to relieve the pain of a chronic Achilles tendon bursitis. The patient is scanned prone with the tendon and bursa in a transverse scan plane using a 7.5 or higher MHz transducer. Needle placement and steroid injection into the bursa are best accomplished with a lateral approach.

► COMMON VARIANTS AND SELECTED ABNORMALITIES

GANGLION CYSTS

A patient with a palpable mass in the hand, wrist, or digit may be assessed with ultrasound for the presence of a ganglion cyst. Ganglion cysts reportedly represent 50–75% of all soft tissue masses of the hand; they commonly appear as a sonolucent cystic or ovoid structure adjacent to a tendon sheath or the wrist joint. Typically, an anechoic linear duct will be seen extending from the ganglion cyst to the tendon sheath or joint giving the structure a "tadpole" appearance (Figure 16-73).[67]

ULTRASOUND-GUIDED STEROID INJECTIONS

The techniques employed for ultrasound-guided soft tissue injection therapy have been reviewed above. Injection of a common tendinopathy, *lateral epicondylitis*, is demonstrated in Figure 16-74. Medial or lateral epicondylitis is thought to occur as a result of chronic repetitive stress and microtrauma of the common flexor or common extensor tendons, respectively.[68,70] Sonographically, there may be some swelling of the extensor or flexor tendon near its origin on the epicondyle. With lateral epicondylitis, there is a reported predilection for

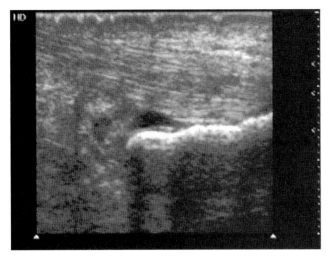

A

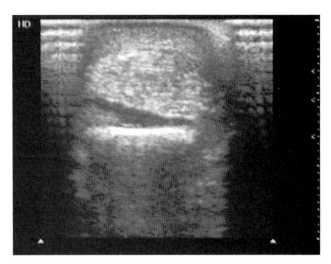

B

Figure 16-72. Long-axis sonogram of the posterior heel in a patient with chronic heel pain (A). The Achilles tendon is seen in the near field as a thick fibrillar structure just beneath the skin. The echogenic line beneath the tendon represents the posterior surface of the calcaneus and the site of the Achilles tendon insertion. Between the Achilles tendon and the upper border of the calcaneus is a hypoechoic sac-like structure that represents the retrocalcaneal bursa. The bursal sac extends somewhat above and around the superior edge of the calcaneus and contains some echogenic debris within it, likely thickened synovium. Light probe pressure is required to avoid collapsing the bursa. Short-axis sonogram of retrocalcaneal bursitis in the same patient (B). This is the orientation that should be used for an intrabursal injection. The retrocalcaneal bursa is again seen as a hypoechoic sac just above the echogenic posterior calcaneal surface. Echogenic thickened synovium is seen on the left side of the bursal cavity. The Achilles tendon appears somewhat ovoid in this orientation, and the tendon fibers appear as multiple echogenic dots in short-axis. The injection needle should be inserted from the lateral aspect of the ankle and the needle directed into the bursal sac under real-time guidance. The injection needle should be maximally reflective in this orientation since it will be nearly perpendicular to the insonating beam.

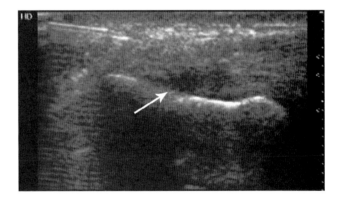

Figure 16-74. Long-axis sonogram over the lateral epicondyle in a patient with a clinical diagnosis of lateral epicondylitis. An ultrasound-guided steroid injection was performed at the site of maximal tenderness, several centimeters above the joint line (the joint line appears on the far right of the image, adjacent to the curve of the distal lateral epicondyle). The injection needle (located on upper left corner of image) is passed as perpendicular to the insonating beam as possible for maximal reflectivity and is readily identified by its reverberation artifact. The injection site is immediately above the common extensor tendon to avoid intratendinous adminis-tration of steroids that can lead to tendon rupture. The deeper fibers adjacent to the bony epicondyle (arrow) reveal a focal area of hypoechogenicity that is typical for lateral epicondylitis.

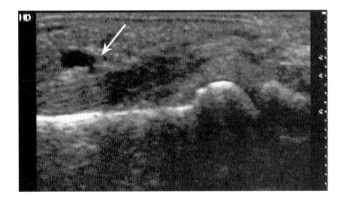

Figure 16-73. Long-axis sonogram of a volar index finger in a patient with atraumatic finger pain. The bony outline of the proximal phalanx and the PIP joint are apparent. The flexor tendons reveal a finely fibrillar echotexture with a focal region of hypoechogenicity that persisted even with a heel–toe imaging technique to exclude anisotropy as the cause. A small hypoechoic ganglion cyst (arrow) is seen adjacent to this focal area of tendonitis and appears as a hypoechoic sac with a thin neck connecting it to the synovial sheath.

deep tendon fiber injury. Intratendinous hyperemia may additionally be noted with color flow assessment.

Ultrasound may also play a useful role in the management of patients with *subacromial bursitis*. On a subacromial scanning window (patient seated, arm behind the back with the elbow flexed), subacromial bursitis will appear as a hypoechoic fluid collection between the deltoid muscle and the supraspinatus tendon.

Other Musculotendinous Sonographic Findings

With biceps femoris, rectus femoris or gastrocnemius muscle tears, a "clapper in the bell" sign may be seen on the sonogram where the retracted, ruptured upper portion of the muscle (the clapper) is surrounded by a hypoechoic hematoma (the bell). Gouty tophi will demonstrate posterior acoustic shadowing, much like gallstones. Inflamed bursae (also discussed in the Arthrocentesis section) will appear as superficial hypoechoic fluid collections. Care should be taken to limit transducer pressure on smaller bursae to avoid causing them to collapse and thereby displacing the bursal fluid out of the field of view.

▶ PITFALLS

The most important potentially misleading artifact in tendon sonography is the false hypoechogenicity that results from the slightest obliquity of the ultrasound beam in relation to the tendon fibers.[62] Since areas of hypoechogenicity are the sonographic clues to tendon pathology (specifically, tendon disruption and tendonitis), optimal tendon imaging is paramount. The angle of insonation should ideally be as parallel to the course of the tendon fibers as possible to avoid this significant pitfall. Where areas of tendon hypoechogenicity are encountered, a heel–toe scanning technique should be employed to further clarify the true sonographic character of the area in question.

▶ SALIVARY GLANDS

CLINICAL CONSIDERATIONS AND INDICATIONS

When evaluating a patient with preauricular or submandibular swelling or tenderness, a bedside ultrasound examination of the area can rapidly clarify if the source of the problem lies within the parotid or submandibular gland. Although CT is the traditional imaging modality of choice for parotid and submandibular inflammatory conditions, and MR is considered the modality of choice for evaluation of parotid and submandibular tumors, ultrasound is considered by some to be the initial imaging modality of choice for assessment of any palpable abnormalities of the parotid gland.[71] Ultrasound can clarify if an intra- or extraglandular lesion is present, provides information as to whether a focal process or diffuse glandular involvement is present, and can help guide aspiration if an abscess is found in a case of acute bacterial sialadenitis. Ultrasound is particularly useful in the evaluation of suspected sialolithiasis where it has a reported 96% diagnostic accuracy.[72] Given the somewhat questionable reliability of the clinical examination (one report notes that 30% of a series of 38 preauricular masses were not intraparotid in location[73]) and the ready availability of portable ultrasound equipment in many emergency departments, ultrasound examination of the region of facial swelling or tenderness should be considered to be part of the bedside workup of any patient with suspected salivary gland disease in the ED.

Salivary gland disease can be broadly classified into four categories: acute sialadenitis (with viral and bacterial etiologies), chronic sialadenitis (with infective and noninfective etiologies), sialolithiasis, and tumors (benign and malignant). The sonographic features of these diseases will be discussed in further detail below. The majority of parotid tumors (85–90%) are benign pleiomorphic adenomas. They are slow growing, painless masses seen most commonly in middle-aged patients and are usually found in the superficial lobe of the parotid gland. By contrast, 50% of tumors in the submandibular gland are found to be malignant. Salivary gland calculi may occur in the parotid gland, but they are most commonly found in the submandibular gland, presumably because of the more mucinous content of submandibular gland secretions. Most salivary gland calculi occur in the submandibular duct; the remainder are found within the gland or in the ductal hilum. Multiple stones are found in 25% of patients.[72]

ANATOMICAL CONSIDERATIONS

The body of the **parotid gland** lies in a preauricular location, its uppermost portion roughly in line with the external acoustic meatus and from there the gland extends inferiorly and posteriorly to the angle of the jaw. The parotid duct (Stenson's duct) arises from the anterior border of the gland, lies superficial to the masseter muscle and about 1–2 cm below the zygomatic arch, courses horizontally at earlobe level through the buccal fat pad, and pierces the buccinator muscle to enter the mouth at the parotid papilla opposite the upper 2nd molar. The normal duct is approximately 2–3 mm in diameter and 4–6 cm in length. On occasion, an accessory parotid gland may be seen lying anterior to and following the course of the parotid duct. The gland is broad and flattened superficially and wedge-shaped on its posterior and deep aspects. The bulk of the gland overlies the masseter and mandible. The facial nerve, the retro-mandibular vein, and the external carotid artery lie in a vertical orientation immediately deep to the gland. Lymph nodes may be found within the substance of the parotid gland.

The **submandibular glands** are found beneath the superficial subcutaneous tissues of the submandibular triangle, lateral to the anterior belly of the digastric muscle. The much larger superficial lobe and the much smaller and more posterior deep lobe are C-shaped in long-axis profile and connect where they wrap around the lateral border of the mylohyoid muscle. Intraglandular ducts drain into the submandibular (or Wharton's) duct that emerges from the hilum of the submandibular gland. The submandibular duct passes medially, then up and over the lateral border of the mylohyoid muscle where it then courses medial to the sublingual gland to a papilla adjacent to the lingual frenulum in the anterior floor of the mouth. The duct is about 5 cm in length. Unlike the parotids, no intraglandular lymph nodes are found within the submandibular gland. The named Küttner lymph node is reliably found in the space between the posterior border of the submandibular gland and the anterior border of the inferior aspect of the parotid gland.[72]

Sublingual glands are located below the mucous membranes of the floor of the mouth adjacent to the mandible and the genioglossus muscle. They drain via numerous small caliber ducts either directly into the floor of the mouth or into the submandibular duct.

▶ TECHNIQUE AND NORMAL ULTRASOUND FINDINGS

The parotid and submandibular glands are best imaged with a 7.5–12 MHz linear array transducer. The **parotid gland** is scanned in long-axis in a vertical scan plane in front of the lower ear. The superior portion of the transducer will need to be angulated somewhat anteriorly, however, to evaluate the portion of the gland that lies inferior to the ear at the angle of the jaw. The gland is predominantly superficial in location with some deeper portions of the gland hidden by the mandible. When evaluating the parotid duct in its long-axis, a transverse scan plane is employed where transducer orientation is nearly horizontal from mid earlobe level to the mid cheek. The parotid duct appears as two closely spaced parallel echogenic lines with a thin region of lucency between them, and is found superficial to the masseter muscle. Because of the fatty glandular tissue composition of the gland, the normal parotid appears fairly homogeneous with a fine granular echotexture that appears similar to a fatty liver (Figures 16-75 and 16-76). Intraparotid ducts appear as echogenic linear structures within the substance of the gland. Intraparotid nodes

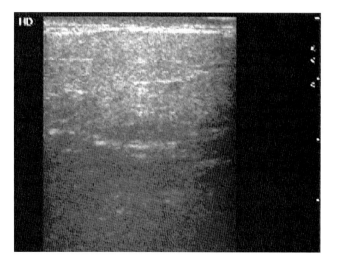

Figure 16-75. Long-axis sonogram of a normal parotid gland. The gland demonstrates a fine homogeneous mid gray echo texture that appears similar to a fatty liver. Immediately beneath the gland lies the retromandibular vein and beneath it, the external carotid artery. Their locations are best appreciated with the use of color Doppler imaging.

are common, most commonly in a preauricular location. Lymph nodes are typically elliptical in shape with a hypoechoic periphery and a hyperechoic fatty central hilum. When scanning the parotid in a long-axis orientation, the retromandibular vein and the external carotid artery will appear as two parallel hypoechoic channels beneath the gland; they are best appreciated with the

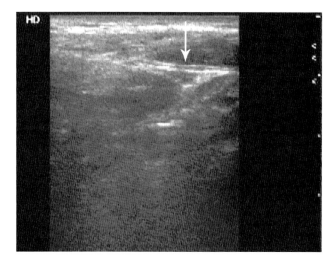

Figure 16-76. Transverse sonogram of a portion of the parotid duct. The normal parotid duct (arrow) appears as two narrowly spaced echogenic lines in the near field with the masseter muscle in cross section below (seen on the left half of the image). The transducer is placed just in front of the ear in a horizontal orientation at the level of the mid earlobe.

use of color Doppler imaging. The facial nerve may be seen as a thin fibrillar structure overlying the more superficially located vein.

When scanning the **submandibular gland**, the transducer should be placed in the submental region just medial to the mandible aiming toward the middle of the chin. From whatever side is being imaged, the orientation marker should always face left. By so doing, the chin will appear on the right side of the image when scanning the right submandibular gland, and on the left side of the image when scanning the left submandibular gland. The bulk of the gland appears posterolateral to the mylohyoid muscle and appears as a rounded and somewhat lobular structure with a finely granular echotexture identical to that of the parotid gland. The Küttner lymph node may be seen posterior and adjacent to the submandibular gland. The mylohyoid muscle appears as a horizontally oriented and somewhat striated appearing rectangular region of hypoechogenity in the near field of the image; the muscle tapers as it approaches its insertion on the symphysis menti. The inferior aspect of the symphysis menti appears as a slightly curved region of hyperechogenicity in the near field with a dense posterior acoustic shadowing beneath. The submandibular duct is somewhat narrower in caliber than the parotid duct, has a similar hyperechoic tubular appearance, and is best visualized when it is pathologically dilated. When scanning the submental region, it is important to remember that the patient's anatomy on the sonogram appears upside down; the image obtained represents a somewhat oblique sagittal section of a patient standing on his or her head.

► COMMON AND EMERGENT ABNORMALITIES

SIALADENITIS

A variety of sonographic patterns may be encountered with parotid and submandibular gland disease. With acute **viral sialadenitis** (most commonly caused by mumps) and acute bacterial sialadenitis (most commonly caused by *Staphylococcus aureus* and *Streptococcus viridans*) the gland appears enlarged, hypoechoic, and of heterogenous echotexture. With **bacterial sialadenitis**, air may be present within the intraglandular ducts and small hyperechoic foci with associated comet tail artifacts may be seen. If an abscess has formed, it will usually appear hypoechoic or anechoic and demonstrate posterior acoustic enhancement similar to a subcutaneous abscess. **Chronic sialadenitis** may occur as a result of infective or noninfective causes and has a sonographic appearance that varies with the type and stage of the disease.

MASSES

Solid lesions will typically appear hypoechoic and demonstrate posterior acoustic enhancement. Cystic lesions will typically appear anechoic. A pleiomorphic adenoma is the most common benign solid parotid tumor encountered and comprises 85–90% of parotid tumors. Sonographically it appears rounded or lobular in shape, well circumscribed, and is homogeneously hypoechoic with posterior acoustic enhancement. Because the most common malignant solid tumor (mucoepidermoid carcinoma[71]) may initially appear sonographically similar to a pleiomorphic adenoma, all solid lesions should be referred for definitive assessment and diagnosis.

SIALOLITHIASIS

A salivary duct stone or calculus will appear as a hyperechoic focus with prominent posterior acoustic shadowing. It will most typically be found within the salivary duct of the submandibular gland, and occasionally within the ductal hilum. Less commonly, a calculus may be encountered within the parotid duct or gland. The salivary duct in such cases will typically be quite dilated and will appear in long-axis as a prominent rectangular or tubular anechoic region leading up to the stone. The gland itself may appear enlarged with dilatation of the hilum of the gland giving the gland a somewhat "hydronephrotic" appearance (Figures 16-77 and 16-78).

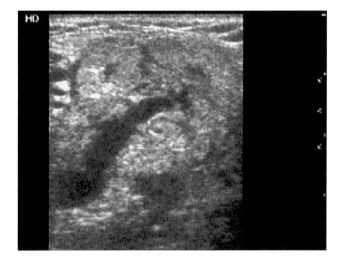

Figure 16-77. Submandibular gland in a patient with calculus sialadenitis. The gland is enlarged and there are hypoechoic regions within the gland and hilum caused by ductal dilatation from the distal outflow obstruction caused by the stone. The salivary duct exits from the gland and courses up and over the lateral border of the mylohyoid muscle.

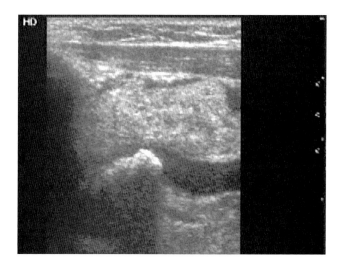

Figure 16-78. Long-axis sonogram of the distal submandibular duct. The dilated submandibular duct is seen in long-axis as an anechoic channel in the far field. A large echogenic salivary duct calculus is lodged in the distal duct; posterior acoustic shadowing is noted in the far field beneath the stone. The hypoechoic and striated mylohyoid muscle is seen just beneath the skin and subcutaneous tissue at the top of the image and its insertion onto the mandible is seen on the left side of the image. The inferior and posterior edge of the mandible appears as a curved echo with posterior acoustic shadowing on the far left of the image. For orientation purposes it is important to remember that the top of the head is at the bottom of the image.

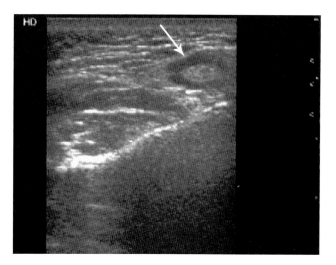

Figure 16-79. Longitudinal sonogram of an enlarged preauricular lymph node. A tender mass was clinically palpable in front of the ear; the sonogram demonstrates an enlarged intraparotid preauricular lymph node (elliptical in long-axis with a hypoechoic periphery and a hyperechoic central hilum). The node is surrounded by a thin rim of granular mid gray echogenicity that corresponds to normal parotid tissue.

LYMPH NODES

Finally, a preauricular mass or tenderness will sometimes be due to a reactive and enlarged lymph node. The lymph node has a characteristic elliptical shape with a hypoechoic periphery and an echogenic fatty central hilum (Figure 16-79).

▶ PITFALLS

The major pitfall with ultrasound imaging of the salivary glands is failure to consider a malignant etiology as a cause for a solid lesion. Since benign and malignant lesions may have similar sonographic appearances, all solid lesions should be referred for definitive workup. The role of the bedside ultrasound examination should be to identify if a lesion is present, to establish whether it is intraglandular or not, and to identify if calculus disease is the cause of the swelling or pain. Nearly all other pathologies should be considered for referral and further evaluation with the exception of diffuse polyglandular enlargement (as seen with mumps), diffuse uniglandular enlargement and tenderness (as seen in sialadenitis),

sialolithiasis, an obvious abscess cavity, and a reactive lymph node.

▶ MAXILLARY SINUSITIS

CLINICAL CONSIDERATIONS

Rhinosinusitis is one of the 10 most common diagnoses in ambulatory practice and the fifth most common diagnosis for which antibiotics are prescribed.[74] Bedside diagnosis of bacterial sinusitis, for which antibiotics are recommended, is difficult by history and physical examination alone, however. At most, only 50% of patients presenting to emergency or general care settings with sinus complaints will actually have bacterial sinusitis.[75] Signs and symptoms of bacterial sinusitis are nonspecific and may be indistinguishable from the clinically similar presentation that occurs with viral rhinosinusitis. Although radiography improves diagnostic accuracy somewhat, neither plain radiography nor CT is recommended for evaluating uncomplicated sinusitis in ambulatory patients because the additional time, cost, and radiation exposure produce little additional diagnostic accuracy.[76] A fluid-filled maxillary sinus can readily be identified by ultrasound, however. Ultrasound may, therefore, be employed as a rapid and safe diagnostic aid at the bedside when evaluating a patient suspected of having maxillary sinusitis. Sinusitis is also an important occult cause of fever and nosocomial pneumonia in patients undergoing prolonged mechanical ventilation.[77] In the ICU setting, bedside sinus ultrasound is a well-established screening test for detecting suspected maxillary sinusitis in intubated patients.

CLINICAL INDICATIONS

The primary indications for sinus ultrasound in emergency and ambulatory practice are as follows:

- Confirm or exclude clinically suspected maxillary sinusitis in patients with upper respiratory symptoms
- Detect maxillary sinus fluid in intubated ICU patients to screen for suspected nosocomial sinusitis.

Maxillary Sinusitis

Although CT and MRI are sensitive imaging modalities for diagnosing sinusitis, the presence of sinus fluid or mucosal thickening alone does not necessarily indicate bacterial infection (low specificity and low positive predictive value). The true "gold standard" for diagnosing bacterial sinusitis is a positive culture from fluid obtained on sinus puncture. Ultrasound, while less sensitive for mucosal changes and small amounts of fluid, is probably more specific for clinically important disease because a positive study requires the presence of a significant amount of fluid in the sinus. Studies evaluating the diagnostic characteristics of ultrasound for bacterial sinusitis vary substantially in terms of the population studied (general practice, subspecialty, or ICU), the criterion standard employed (sinus puncture, radiography, MRI), and methodologic quality. A summary of studies conducted in the 1980s and 1990s in which sinus ultrasound was compared to sinus puncture found a weighted mean sensitivity and specificity for ultrasound of 85% and 82%, respectively. This compares favorably to the 87% sensitivity and 89% specificity found for plain radiography.[78] A systematic review of these early studies concluded that operator skill and experience had a large effect on how well ultrasound performed.[79]

Three contemporary studies have been conducted in the ambulatory and emergency care setting comparing bedside ultrasound to radiography or MRI for diagnosing acute maxillary sinusitis. A study found that, using MRI as the gold standard, ultrasound was 64% sensitive and 95% specific compared to 73% sensitive and 100% specific for plain film radiography.[80] The authors concluded that a positive ultrasound examination confirmed the diagnosis of maxillary sinusitis. If the ultrasound examination was negative and clinical suspicion was high, however, they recommended that plain-film radiographs be obtained. A study found that ultrasound was 92% sensitive and 95% specific compared to plain film radiography. In the primary care setting in which their study was conducted, the addition of bedside sinus ultrasound to the history and physical examination would have reduced antibiotic prescriptions for sinusitis by one half.[81] Finally, Price and colleagues compared emergency physician–performed ultrasound to CT in 48 emergency department patients with suspected maxillary sinusitis. Sensitivity was 81% and specificity 89%.[82]

Maxillary Sinus Fluid in Intubated Patients

In the ICU setting, bedside ultrasound has emerged as a convenient screening test for nosocomial sinusitis, both because plain film radiographs are inaccurate assessing for sinus fluid in recumbent patients, and because obtaining CT imaging in intubated patients is particularly time and labor intensive. Ultrasound can be used at the bedside to assess for the presence of fluid in the maxillary sinus. If fluid is present, rhinoscopy or sinus puncture is subsequently performed to obtain fluid for culture. The reported prevalence of infected sinus fluid varies widely among different studies, ranging from 5% to 60% of cases.[77,83,84] Among the numerous studies investigating the use of maxillary sinus ultrasound in the ICU setting, the three best compared ultrasound to radiography or sinus puncture (presence of fluid), and found a sensitivity of 67–100% and specificity of 86–97%.[83,85,86] Specificity was 100% when all sinus walls were seen, which generally correlates with complete sinus opacification on radiography.

ANATOMIC CONSIDERATIONS

The maxillary sinuses are paired and somewhat pyramidal-shaped airspaces within the maxillary bone on either side of the nose. They are bordered by the orbital floor superiorly, the lateral nasal wall medially, the alveolar process and hard palate inferiorly, and the zygoma laterally. The maxillary sinus is typically 2–4 cm in anteroposterior depth, and fluid within the sinus renders the posterior wall of the sinus visible by ultrasound. The ethmoid sinuses lie superomedially, and the sphenoid sinus lies in the midline deeper within the skull. The frontal sinuses, which would seem to be sonographically accessible, are not well visualized by ultrasound, likely because the anterior surface of the frontal bone is quite thick.

▶ TECHNIQUE AND NORMAL ULTRASOUND FINDINGS

Maxillary sinus ultrasound may be performed with a wide array of transducers ranging from a phased array or microconvex 3.5 MHz transducer (e.g., a typical cardiac transducer) to a 3–10 MHz linear array transducer. A small skin contact footprint is preferred, however, for scanning on the curved, relatively solid surface over the anterior maxilla. Although one might think that lower frequencies would be required to adequately penetrate the anterior bony wall of the sinus, this does not appear to be the case in practice, and a fluid-filled sinus will be apparent with either transducer type. The patient should sit upright or lean slightly forward to ensure that sinus fluid, if present, layers out against the anterior wall. The sinus should be scanned in both sagittal and transverse planes, midway between the nose and the zygoma, just below the orbital rim. When using a linear array transducer, the sagittal image is easier to obtain by angling the transducer slightly superomedially, parallel to the nasolabial fold. Attention should be paid to proper depth settings (typically 5–7 cm) so that the image of the sinus fills about three fourths the screen. Comparison with the uninvolved sinus should be routine and can be useful in equivocal cases.

In the normal air-filled sinus, a prominent periodic resonance artifact will be apparent, consisting of an evenly spaced series of echogenic lines that parallel the shape of the anterior surface of the maxilla and diminish in intensity at increased depth. Beneath the distinct echo of the anterior wall of the sinus, an indistinct "snowstorm" appearance will be noted on the sonogram and the posterior wall of the sinus will *not* be apparent. Of note, it is important not to confuse one of the deeper periodic resonance artifacts as representing the posterior wall of the sinus (Figure 16-80).

► COMMON AND EMERGENT ABNORMALITIES

Acute viral rhinosinusitis produces abnormalities within the maxillary sinuses in up to 87% of cases, typically a thickening of the sinus mucosa along with some secretions. Occasionally, a significant amount of fluid will accumulate within the sinus and produce an air-fluid level on CT.[87] An ultrasound examination of the sinus at this point would appear positive for fluid, and would represent a false-positive result for the diagnosis of bacterial maxillary sinusitis. Bacterial sinusitis is said to supervene in 1–2% of cases of viral rhinosinusitis[75] and typically occurs after 5–7 days of symptoms. It may be accompanied by mucopurulent nasal discharge and signs of maxillary inflammation (such as focal, often unilateral sinus pain and tenderness). As the inflammatory process evolves, pus accumulates in the sinus, giving rise to air–fluid levels or complete opacification on radiography, decreased transillumination, and a positive sinus ultrasound examination.

In the patient with a completely fluid-filled sinus, the curved posterior wall of the sinus will be clearly apparent in the far field of the image and no periodic resonance artifact will be noted (Figure 16-81). If the sinus is only partially filled with fluid, a mixed picture

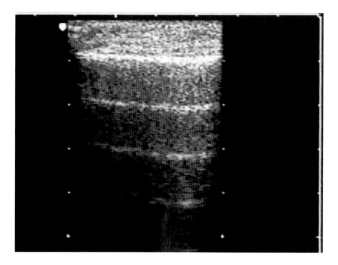

Figure 16-80. Sagittal sonogram of a normal sinus taken with a linear array transducer. Skin and subcutaneous tissue appear diffusely hyperechoic in the near field. A bright echo is seen at the level of the anterior surface of the maxillary sinus. The series of evenly spaced horizontal echoes that diminish in intensity at increasing depth represent a periodic resonance artifact emanating from the anterior wall of the sinus. A "snowstorm" pattern of echogenicity is normally seen within the nonopacified sinus.

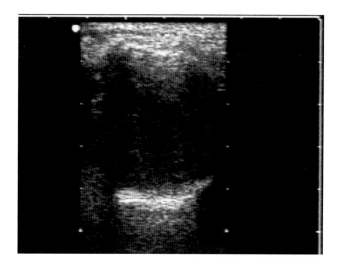

Figure 16-81. Sagittal sonogram of a patient with acute maxillary sinusitis. The brightly echogenic curve in the far field of the image represents the posterior wall of the sinus. The sinus cavity is hypoechoic and no periodic resonance artifacts are seen.

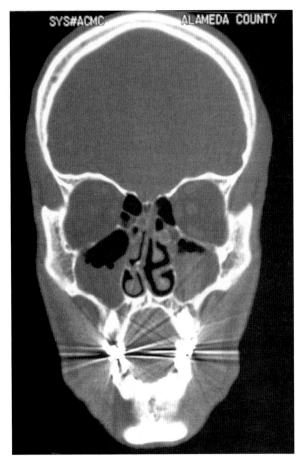

A

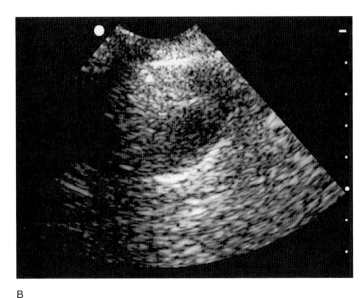

B

Figure 16-82. A *coronal* CT image of a patient with bilateral maxillary and ethmoid sinusitis (A). The left maxillary sinus is nearly completely fluid-filled; the one on the right is only partially opacified. Although this is the preferred orientation for CT imaging of the sinuses, it should be noted that the sonogram obtained when scanning the maxillary sinus will be orthogonal to this scan plane. Sagittal sonogram of the partially opacified right maxillary sinus (B). Image taken with a microconvex 3.5 MHz transducer. On the right side of the image (corresponding with the inferior fluid-filled portion of the sinus), the posterior wall of the sinus is apparent as a brightly echogenic line. On the left side of the image (corresponding with the air filled portion of the sinus) the image is indistinct and the posterior wall of the sinus is not apparent. A large amount of near field artifact is present because gain settings are too high.

will be seen. The posterior wall of the sinus will be apparent only in the lower fluid-filled portion of the sinus (right side of the image on a sagittal sonogram) and a periodic resonance artifact may be seen in the upper air-containing region of the sinus (left side of the image). An example of partial sinus opacification on CT and its corresponding sonographic representation are illustrated in Figure 16-82a,b. A continuous brightly echogenic line along the posterior wall of the sinus on sagittal imaging correlates well with complete sinus opacification on radiography. This has been referred to as a "sinusogram."[85] A discontinuous line, and some persistence of the periodic resonance artifact from the anterior wall, correlates with partial sinus opacification.[83,85]

▶ PITFALLS

The most important potential pitfall when evaluating suspected maxillary sinusitis with ultrasound is failure to consider the results of imaging in the context of the pretest likelihood of disease and other clinical indicators of severity. The sensitivity of ultrasound for maxillary sinusitis is not more than 85% and involvement of other sinuses cannot be assessed. Thus, in the patient with severe symptoms, in the elderly or diabetic patient, or when the clinical suspicion for sinusitis is high, a more sensitive imaging study such as CT should be obtained for definitive diagnosis. On the other hand, evidence of maxillary sinus fluid in what otherwise appears to be

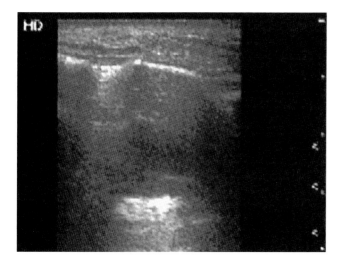

Figure 16-83. Sagittal sonogram of a patient with a polyp filling the lower half of the right maxillary sinus. The posterior wall of the sinus is visible in the inferior portion of the sinus (right side of the image) and posterior acoustic enhancement is evident. The upper portion of the sinus (left side of the image) has more of a "snowstorm" appearance with subtle reverberation and periodic resonance artifacts and no visualization of the posterior wall of the sinus.

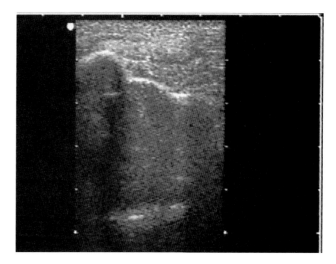

Figure 16-84. Sagittal sonogram of a patient with fractures of the anterior wall of the maxilla and a blood-filled maxillary sinus. Note the marked soft tissue swelling and the cortical irregularity of the anterior wall of the maxilla in the near field. The posterior wall of the sinus is clearly seen in the far field.

an acute viral rhinosinusitis should be treated conservatively with decongestants. It should also be noted that a number of conditions other than sinusitis will allow transmission of the insonating beam through the sinus and will result in a positive scan of the posterior wall of the sinus. Significant mucosal thickening, polyps, fluid-filled cysts, occasional solid masses, as well as blood from facial trauma and sinus fractures can all give rise to a positive "sinusogram" (Figures 16-83 and 16-84). Technical pitfalls include scanning with the patient in a supine position, failure to accurately set the image depth to a level that would include the posterior sinus, and misinterpreting a periodic resonance artifact as an image of the posterior wall of the sinus.

▶ SKIN AND SOFT TISSUE INFECTIONS

CLINICAL CONSIDERATIONS

Emergency and ambulatory care physicians evaluate patients with skin and soft tissue infections on a daily basis. These infections include cellulitis, subcutaneous abscess, and, on rare occasion, necrotizing fasciitis. The diagnosis of cellulitis by physical examination alone is usually straightforward when erythema, warmth, and tenderness are present. Similarly, determining that a subcutaneous abscess exists is simple when fluctuance or focal skin necrosis is present. Clinical findings can be misleading,

however, when a cutaneous abscess is small, deep to the skin surface, early in its formation, or where there is preexisting scar tissue from a prior abscess drainage procedure in that anatomic area. An occult abscess may coexist with what appears clinically to be a simple case of cellulitis. Ambiguous clinical findings may direct the clinician away from performing a drainage procedure when it is, in fact, indicated. Ultrasound has emerged as a valuable tool for assessing soft tissue infections at the bedside, and it is being used with increasing frequency in the emergency setting to correctly diagnose and localize occult abscesses, and to facilitate abscess drainage by providing the clinician with an anatomic road map for safely guiding the incision.

CLINICAL INDICATIONS

The clinical indications for the use of ultrasound in the management of soft tissue infections include

- detection of an occult subcutaneous abscess when ambiguous clinical findings are present and
- localization of an optimal site for incision and drainage or aspiration of an abscess

Detection of Occult Abscess

The ability of ultrasound to detect soft tissue abscesses and guide subsequent incision and drainage has been appreciated since the 1980s.[88–92] In reports focusing on injection drug users, particularly those with inflammatory lesions of the groin, ultrasound has been shown to successfully differentiate cellulitis from abscess, in addition to being useful for detecting adenitis, septic thrombophlebitis, and pseudoaneurysm.[88,91] Ultrasound has also been found to be of value in the diagnosis and treatment of odontogenic facial abscesses.[93]

Three studies conducted in the emergency department setting have examined the utility of bedside ultrasound for evaluation of skin and soft tissue infections.[94–96] All three studies examined the impact ultrasound assessment has on the accuracy of abscess diagnosis, with cases stratified by pretest likelihood of an abscess being present. Overall, ultrasound assessment led to a change in management in 17–56% of cases. A consistent finding was that among cases categorized as *unlikely* to have an abscess present, ultrasound frequently revealed an unsuspected pus pocket that was confirmed by a drainage procedure (this scenario occurred in 14–58% of "low" likelihood cases). It has been demonstrated that ultrasound has utility when an abscess is clinically judged likely to be present. In such cases, a negative ultrasound evaluation often correctly excludes abscess, thus preventing an unnecessary drainage procedure. With the addition of ultrasound to physical examination alone, the positive predictive value increased from 81 to 93% and the negative predictive value increased from 77 to 97%. However, because of methodologic limitations, the actual false-negative rate for detecting abscess cannot be determined with confidence from these studies.

ANATOMIC CONSIDERATIONS

A thorough understanding of the regional anatomy of the area being scanned is essential for the clinician evaluating for an abscess. Subcutaneous abscesses may be encountered nearly anywhere and are commonly seen on the hand, face, neck, forearm, groin, lower extremity, buttocks, and the perianal region. They may be found in close proximity to veins, arteries, nerves, tendons, and within muscles. Awareness of the proximity of adjacent structures, familiarity with their normal sonographic appearance, and an understanding of preferred lines for elective incision are mandatory.

▶ TECHNIQUE AND NORMAL ULTRASOUND FINDINGS

Sonographic evaluation of the skin and subcutaneous tissue for a suspected subcutaneous abscess is optimally performed with a 5–10 MHz linear array transducer, although an annular array or sector transducer may also be utilized. An acoustic stand-off pad may improve image resolution if a lower frequency transducer is being used or if the abscess is very superficial and no linear array transducer is available. Depth and focus settings are adjusted to place the area of interest within the transducer's optimal focal zone. Transducer pressure should be kept to a minimum to avoid collapse and nonvisualization of superficial veins. The soft tissue area being evaluated should be systematically scanned in two perpendicular planes.

General soft tissue normal ultrasound findings are reviewed as follows. Normal **skin** typically appears as a thin, homogeneous, and somewhat hyperechoic layer immediately beneath the transducer. **Subcutaneous** tissue, composed primarily of subcutaneous fat, lies immediately below and appears hypoechoic with a reticular pattern of thin echogenic connective tissue seen between the fat lobules. **Fascia** and connective tissue planes are usually seen as echogenic horizontal or gently curved lines that follow the contour of the underlying muscle. **Arteries and veins** appear as anechoic circular or rectangular structures, depending on the orientation of the transducer relative to the vessel; use of color flow or Doppler may aid in their identification. Veins typically compress easily with transducer pressure. **Muscle** appears relatively hypoechoic with a regular pattern of

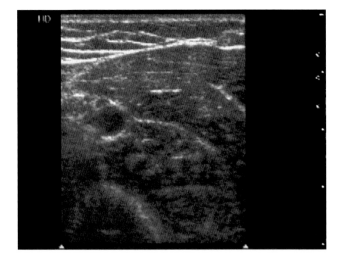

Figure 16-85. Short-axis sonogram of a normal arm. A thin layer of hyperechoic skin (epidermis) is seen adjacent to the transducer. Just below, a layer of hypoechoic subcutaneous tissue is seen with hyperechoic bands of connective tissue between the fat (dermis). A thin echogenic layer of muscle fascia is seen overlying hypoechoic muscle tissue below; the latter will appear striated or speckled depending on the angle of insonation relative to the direction of the muscle fibers. Some curved fascial planes are seen within the muscle belly and some hypoechoic vessels are seen in short-axis in the mid left portion of the image. The curved echogenic surface of a portion of the humerus is seen in the far field.

internal striations in long-axis and a speckled appearance in short-axis. The anterior cortex of **bone** is brightly echogenic with far-field acoustic shadowing. The normal sonographic appearance of the various layers of soft tissue within the forearm is seen in Figure 16-85.

► COMMON AND EMERGENT ABNORMALITIES

CELLULITIS

Although nonspecific, familiarity with the sonographic appearance of cellulitis is important for two reasons. First, a rim of cellulitic tissue nearly always surrounds an abscess cavity, and second, cellulitis is the usual diagnosis of exclusion when performing ultrasound on an undifferentiated skin and soft tissue infection. Cellulitis is a diffuse infection of the skin and subcutaneous tissue and the sonographic findings in cellulitis likely arise from the accumulation of edema fluid. Findings include thickened and abnormally hyperechoic skin, swelling and diffusely increased echogenicity of the subcutaneous tissue, and areas of hypoechoic edema that traverse the subcutaneous fat in a reticular pattern (Figure 16-86).[97–99] Comparison to the unaffected side may aid in the recognition of subtle findings. It should be emphasized that sonographic findings in cellulitis are simply indicative of edema and are therefore nonspecific; both necrotizing fasciitis and the inflamed tissue surrounding an abscess may take on the sonographic appearance of cellulitis. In a patient with chronic lymphedema, the subcutaneous

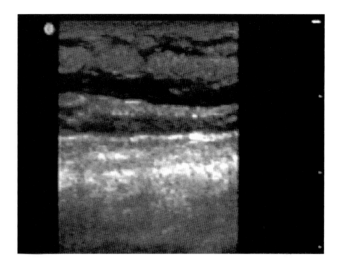

Figure 16-87. Sonogram of a leg with chronic lymphedema. The skin and subcutaneous tissue are thickened and somewhat more hyperechoic than normal but not as echogenic as seen with cellulitis. Prominent predominantly horizontal bands of edema fluid are seen below the subcutaneous tissue.

tissue appears hyperechoic relative to normal tissue but usually not as echogenic as that seen in cellulitis. With lymphedema, prominent horizontally layered bands of hypoechoic edema fluid will be seen traversing the subcutaneous tissue (Figure 16-87).

ABSCESS

A subcutaneous abscess may have a variety of sonographic appearances[91,97,99,100] but will almost universally be surrounded by a rim of edematous soft tissue or cellulitis that appears hyperechoic relative to normal subcutaneous tissue (Figures 16-88a,b). Abscess cavities are most often spherical or elliptical-shaped and the liquefied contents of the abscess cavity will typically demonstrate posterior acoustic enhancement (Figures 16-89, 16-90, and 16-91). Not uncommonly, however, abscesses may also appear irregular or lobulated, and the abscess cavity may interdigitate between tissue planes or take an irregular path within the hyperechoic surrounding cellulitic tissues (Figures 16-92 and 16-93). Although the contents of an abscess cavity may exhibit a wide range of sonographic patterns, they will most commonly appear hypoechoic or anechoic relative to the surrounding tissues. In some cases, however, the purulent abscess cavity contents may be isoechoic or hyperechoic, making the collection more difficult to identify. Abscesses may contain hyperechoic debris, septae, or gas; the latter will appear as brightly hyperechoic regions within the abscess cavity with an associated ring-down or reverberation artifact (Figures 16-94 and 16-95). Gentle transducer pressure over the abscess site may induce motion

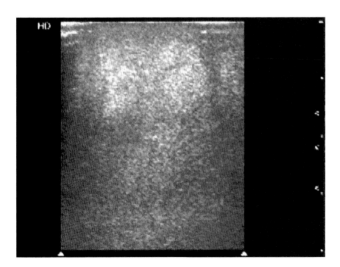

Figure 16-86. Sonogram of a region of cellulitis on a buttock. The skin and subcutaneous tissues appear diffusely hyperechoic and no soft tissue detail is appreciated. Some fine reticular areas of hypoechoic stranding are seen and are likely due to edema within the tissue.

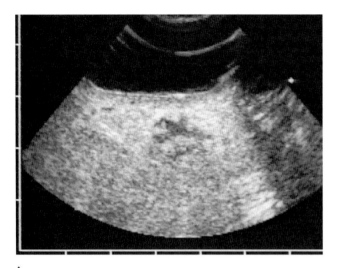

A

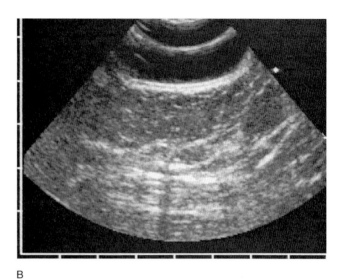

B

Figure 16-88. Sonogram of a patient with cellulitis of the lateral chest wall (A). The image was taken with an annular array transducer and an acoustic stand-off. The tissues are diffusely hyperechoic with little detail resolution. A small region of hypoechogenicity is seen in the center of the image and represents early abscess formation. Sonogram of the contralateral normal chest wall of the same patient (B). The skin layer is hyperechoic and the subcutaneous tissue relatively hypoechoic with much greater detail resolution than the abnormal side.

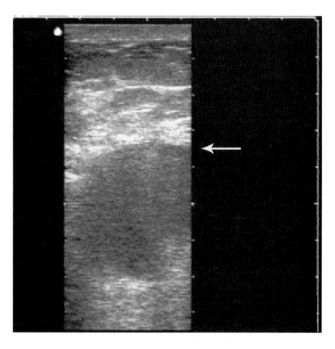

Figure 16-90. Long-axis sonogram of a deep midline buttock abscess in the region of the gluteal fold. The skin and immediate subcutaneous tissue appear to be of relatively normal echogenicity. The deeper tissues surrounding the rounded abscess cavity appear more hyperechoic and edematous. Note that the superior edge of this large abscess cavity is 3.5 cm from the skin surface (arrow). Knowledge of the depth of this abscess cavity is crucial to the individual performing the drainage procedure.

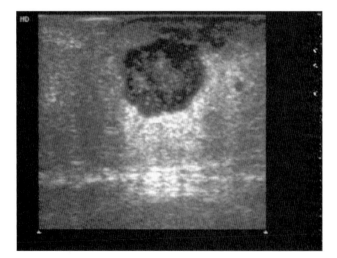

Figure 16-89. Typical appearance of a subcutaneous abscess on a thigh. The abscess cavity is rounded and hypoechoic with mixed internal echogenicity. There is posterior acoustic enhancement that reflects the liquid nature of the abscess contents. The surrounding skin is hyperechoic because of adjacent tissue edema and possibly cellulitis.

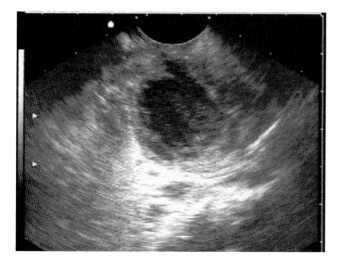

Figure 16-91. Sonogram of a peritonsillar abscess using a 7.5 MHz fingertip probe. The abscess cavity appears rounded with hypoechoic contents of mixed echogenicity. There is posterior acoustic enhancement and two vessels are seen in short-axis beneath the thick posterior wall of the abscess cavity. Peritonsillar abscesses are discussed in further detail in Chapter 20.

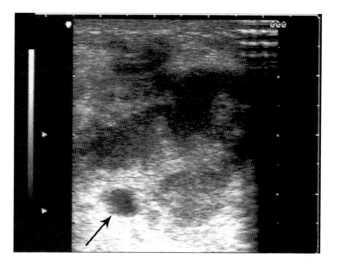

Figure 16-93. Short-axis sonogram of the antecubital fossa of an injection drug user with an abscess. The abscess cavity is large, irregular in shape, interdigitates between tissue planes and has both hypoechoic and isoechoic components. Swirling of abscess contents was apparent on real-time scanning. The deep brachial artery is seen in short-axis in the far field (arrow).

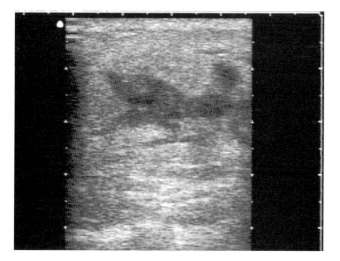

Figure 16-92. Sonogram of an irregularly shaped hypoechoic thigh abscess surrounded by hyperechoic skin and subcutaneous tissues.

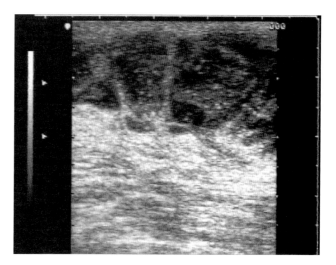

Figure 16-94. Sonogram of a postoperative abdominal wall wound infection. Multiple septae are seen in the hypoechoic collection immediately beneath the skin. Motion of the abscess contents was seen with gentle transducer pressure on real-time scanning. Posterior acoustic enhancement is also present.

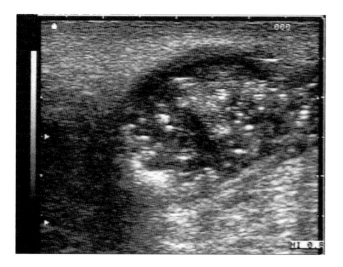

Figure 16-95. Hyperechoic foci with some associated ring-down artifact are seen within the mixed echogenicity contents of this abscess cavity. These hyperechoic regions on this sonogram correspond to small gas pockets within the abscess cavity.

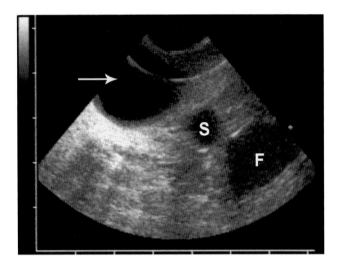

Figure 16-96. Short-axis sonogram of an abscess cavity in the left groin of an injection drug user. The thick walled hypoechoic abscess cavity (arrow) is seen on the left of the image; adjacent are the hypoechoic saphenous (S) and common femoral veins (F). Although I and D was simple, careful pre-procedure ultrasound mapping provided useful information to guide the incision.

of purulent material within the abscess cavity and helps confirm the liquid nature of the material being scanned, especially in cases where the abscess contents are relatively isoechoic with the surrounding tissue or muscle.[97] Color flow Doppler may demonstrate hyperemia adjacent to the abscess cavity and can help confirm absence of flow within it.[99] If a hypoechoic fluid collection is seen adjacent to a long bone, the diagnosis of osteomyelitis should be entertained. Finally, abscesses may be found situated adjacent to anatomic structures such as blood vessels, muscles, and tendons; recognition of the sonographic appearance of anatomically adjacent structures is essential prior to embarking on a drainage procedure (Figure 16-96).

▶ COMMON VARIANTS AND SELECTED ABNORMALITIES

NECROTIZING FASCIITIS

Necrotizing fasciitis is a rare soft tissue infection defined by tissue necrosis (particularly involving fascia) and a fulminant course. While rapid recognition and treatment can favorably affect outcome,[101] making the diagnosis of necrotizing fasciitis on clinical grounds alone is often difficult. The role of ultrasound as a diagnostic test for necrotizing fasciitis has never been studied systematically, and it should not be used to exclude the diagnosis.

However, sonographic findings thought to be characteristic of the disease have been described by two groups of investigators in Taiwan reporting on a total of 21 cases of necrotizing fasciitis in adults and children.[102,103] Invariably, the subcutaneous fascia, normally seen as a thin, brightly hyperechoic line, was greatly thickened and edematous-appearing, as was the overlying subcutaneous tissue. An anechoic fluid layer measuring greater than 4 mm adjacent to the deep fascia is considered diagnostic of necrotizing fasciitis.[102] In some cases, discreet masses were seen in and around the fascial plane from which pus was aspirated.[16] The presence of subcutaneous gas (which typically appears as "dirty" acoustic shadowing with a reverberation artifact) may also be rapidly confirmed with bedside ultrasound in such cases. It should be borne in mind, however, that this is a nonspecific finding and that gas pockets may also be seen within an abscess cavity.

▶ PITFALLS

1. **Abscesses are not always hypoechoic**. They can on occasion be sonographically subtle to detect. An isoechoic collection of pus, especially one that is in or around muscle tissue, or an abscess that is deep and obscured by overlying hyperechoic soft tissues may give rise to a false-negative ultrasound examination. Operator experience may also play a role. Optimization of the image with appropriate frequency, focus, and depth settings, and gentle transducer pressure to assess for any potential swirling or movement of the isoechoic region being evaluated may help avoid this pitfall. In the face of a strong clinical suspicion for an abscess and an apparently negative ultrasound result, an attempt at a needle aspiration for further assessment may be considered.

2. **Necrotizing soft tissue infections**. An uncommon, but potentially disastrous pitfall is failure to consider a necrotizing soft tissue infection once an abscess has been excluded by ultrasound. Studies examining the use of bedside ultrasound in the diagnosis of necrotizing fasciitis are limited. Ultrasound should not be used to exclude the presence of necrotizing fasciitis.

3. **Failure to recognize adjacent structures.** Abscesses may occur in close proximity to tendons, nerves, arteries, and veins. Although ultrasound is extremely helpful in diagnosing and mapping the location of an abscess, the decision to drain an abscess that is surrounded by these structures should be guided by the experience and comfort level of the sonographer.

REFERENCES

1. Nguyen K, Sauerbrei E, Nolan R, et al.: The abdominal wall, In: *Diagnostic Ultrasound*, Rumack C, Wilson S, Charboneau J et al., eds. 3rd ed., St. Louis, MO: Mosby, Inc., 2005, Chapter 13.

2. Hodgson T, Collins M: Anterior abdominal wall hernias: Diagnosis by ultrasound and tangential radiographs. *Clin Radiol* 44:185–188, 1991.

3. Engel J, Deitch E: Sonography of the anterior abdominal wall. *AJR* 137:73–77, 1981.

4. Alexiades G, Lambropoulou M, Deftereos S, et al.: Abdominal wall endometriosis-ultrasound research: A diagnostic problem. *Clin Exp Obst Gyn* 28:121–122, 2001.

5. Greher M, Eichenberger U, Gustorff B: Sonographic localization of an implanted infusion pump injection port: Another useful application of ultrasound in pain medicine. *Anesthesiology* 102:243, 2005.

6. Drescher M, Conrad F, Schamban N: Identification and description of esophageal intubation using ultrasound. *Acad Emerg Med* 7:722–725, 2000.

7. Ma G, Chan TC, Vilke GM, et al.: Confirming endotracheal intubation using ultrasound. *Ann Emerg Med* 36:S20–S21, 2000.

8. Raphael D, Conrad R: Ultrasound confirmation of endotracheal tube placement. *J Clin Ultrasound* 15:459–462, 1987.

9. Hsieh KS, Lee CL, Lin CC, et al.: Secondary confirmation of endotracheal tube position by ultrasound image. *Crit Care Med* 32:S374–S377, 2004.

10. Weaver R, Lyon M, Blaivas M: Confirmation of endotracheal tube placement after intubation using the ultrasound sliding lung sign. *Acad Emerg Med* 13:239–244, 2006.

11. Friedman E: Role of ultrasound in the assessment of vocal cord function in infants and children. *Ann Otol Rhinol Laryngol* 106:199–209, 1997.

12. Sidhu S, Stanton R, Shahidi S, et al.: Initial experience of vocal cord evaluation using grey-scale, real-time, B-mode ultrasound. *ANZ J Surg* 71:737–739, 2001.

13. Ooi LL, Chan HS, Soo KC: Color Doppler imaging for vocal cord palsy. *Head Neck* 17:20–23, 1995.

14. Werner S, Jones R, Emerman C: Sonographic assessment of the epiglottis. *Acad Emerg Med* 11:1358–1360, 2004.

15. Griffith JF, Rainer TH, Ching ASC, et al.: Sonography compared with radiography in revealing acute rib fracture. *AJR* 173:1603–1609, 1999.

16. Bitschnau R, Gehmacher O, Kopf A, et al.: Ultraschall-diagnostik von Rippen-und Sternumfrakturen. *Ultraschall Med* 18:158–161, 1997.

17. Wischhofer E, Fenkl R, Blum R: Sonographischer Nachweis von Rippenfrakturen zur Sicherung der Frakturdiagnostik. *Unfallchirurg* 98:296–300, 1995.

18. Fenkl R, Garrel T, Knaepler H: Notfalldiagnostik der Sternumfraktur mit Ultraschall. *Unfallchirurg* 95:375–379, 1992.

19. Dulchavsky S, Henry S, Moed B, et al.: Advanced ultrasonic diagnosis of extremity trauma: The FASTER examination. *J Trauma* 53:28–32, 2002.

20. Marshburn T, Legome E, Sargsyan A, et al.: Goal-directed ultrasound in the detection of long-bone fractures. *J Trauma* 57:329–332, 2004.

21. Brooks A, Price V, Simms M, et al.: Handheld ultrasound diagnosis of extremity fractures. *J R Army Med Corps* 150:78–80, 2004.

22. Thiede O, Kromer JH, Rudack C, et al.: Comparison of ultrasonography and conventional radiography in the diagnosis of nasal fractures. *Arch Otolaryngol Head Neck Surg* 131:434–439, 2005.

23. Danter J, Klinger M, Siegert R, et al.: Ultrasonographische Darstellung von Nasenbeinfrakturen mit einem 20-MHz-Ultraschallgerat. *HNO* 44:324–328, 1996.

24. Akizuki H, Yoshida H, Michi K: Ultrasonographic evaluation during reduction of zygomatic arch fractures. *J Cranio-Maxillo-Facial Surg* 18:263–266, 1990.

25. Hunter JD, Franklin K, Hughes PM: The ultrasound diagnosis of posterior shoulder dislocation associated with Erb's palsy. *Pediatr Radiol* 28:510–511, 1998.

26. Benson LS, Donaldson JS, Carrol NC: Use of ultrasound in management of posterior sternoclavicular dislocation. *J Ultrasound Med* 10:115–118, 1991.

27. Pollock RC, Bankes MJK, Emery RJH: Diagnosis of retrosternal dislocation of the clavicle with ultrasound. *Injury* 27:670–671, 1996.

28. Graif M, Stahl-Kent V, Ben-Ami T, et al.: Sonographic detection of occult bone fractures. *Pediatr Radiol* 18:383–385, 1988.

29. Chern TC, Jou IM, Lai KA, et al.: Sonography for monitoring closed reduction of displaced extra-articular distal radial fractures. *J Bone Joint Surg* 84-A:194–203, 2002.

30. Durston W, Swartzentruber R: Ultrasound guided reduction of pediatric forearm fractures in the ED. *Am J Emerg Med* 18:72–77, 2000.

31. Grechenig W, Clement HG, Fellinger M, Seggl W: Scope and limitations of ultrasonography in the documentation of fractures—An experimental study. *Arch Orthop Trauma Surg* 117:368–371, 1998.

32. Anderson MA, Newmeyer WL, Kilgore ES, Jr. Diagnosis and treatment of retained foreign bodies in the hand. *Am J Surg* 144(1):63–67, 1982.

33. Trautlein JJ, Lambert RL, Miller J: Malpractice in the emergency department—Review of 200 cases. *Ann Emerg Med* 13(9, Pt 1):709–711, 1984.

34. Rockett MS, Gentile SC, Gudas CJ, et al.: The use of ultrasonography for the detection of retained wooden foreign bodies in the foot. *J Foot Ankle Surg* 34:478–484, 1995.

35. Graham DD, Jr.: Ultrasound in the emergency department: Detection of wooden foreign bodies in the soft tissues. *J Emerg Med* 22(1):75–79, 2002.

36. Orlinsky M, Knittel P, Feit T, et al.: The comparative accuracy of radiolucent foreign body detection using ultrasonography. *Am J Emerg Med* 18:401–403, 2000.

37. Gilbert FJ, Campbell RSD, Bayliss AP: The role of ultrasound in the detection of non-radiopaque foreign bodies. *Clin Radiol* 41:109–112, 1990.

38. Turner J, Wilde CH, Hughes KC, et al.: Ultrasound-guided retrieval of small foreign objects in subcutaneous tissue. *Ann Emerg Med* 29:731–734, 1997.

39. Schlager D, Sanders AB, Wiggins D, Boren W: Ultrasound for the detection of foreign bodies. *Ann Emerg Med* 20(2):189–191, 1991.

40. Schlager D: The use of ultrasound in the emergency department. *Emerg Med Clin North Am* 15:895–912, 1997.

41. Manthey D, Storrow AB, Milbourn JM, et al.: Ultrasound versus radiography in the detection of soft-tissue foreign bodies. *Ann Emerg Med* 28:7–9, 1996.

42. Jacobson JA, Powell A, Craig JG, et al.: Wooden foreign bodies in soft tissue: Detection at US. *Radiology* 201:45–48, 1998.

43. Hill R, Conron R, Greissinger P, et al.: Ultrasound for the detection of foreign bodies in human tissue. *Ann Emerg Med* 29:353–356, 1997.

44. Ginsburg MJ, Ellis GL, Flom LL, et al.: Detection of soft-tissue foreign bodies by plain radiography, xerography, computed tomography, and ultrasonography. *Ann Emerg Med* 19(6):701–703, 1990.

45. Fornage BD, Schernberg FL: Sonographic diagnosis of foreign bodies of the distal extremities. *AJR* 147:567–569, 1986.

46. Crawford R, Matheson AB: Clinical value of ultrasonography in the detection and removal of radiolucent foreign bodies. *Injury* 20:341–343, 1989.

47. Bray PW, Mahoney JL, Campbell JP, et al.: Sensitivity and specificity of ultrasound in the diagnosis of foreign bodies in the hand. *J Hand Surg* 20:661–666, 1995.

48. Bonatz E, Robbin ML, Weingold MA: Ultrasound for the diagnosis of retained splinters in the soft tissue of the hand. *Am J Orthopedics* 27:445–459, 1998.

49. Banerjee B, Das RK: Sonographic detection of foreign bodies of the extremities. *Br J Radiol* 64:107–112, 1991.

50. Lyon M, Brannam L, Johnson D, Blaivas M, Duggal S: Detection of soft tissue foreign bodies in the presence of soft tissue gas. *J Ultrasound Med* 23(5):677–681, 2004

51. Friedman DI, Forti RJ, Wall SP, Crain EF: The utility of bedside ultrasound and patient perception in detecting soft tissue foreign bodies in children. *Pediatr Emerg Care.* 21(8):487–492, 2005.

52. Dean AJ, Gronczewski CA, Costantino TG: Technique for emergency medicine bedside ultrasound identification of a radiolucent foreign body. *J Emerg Med* 24(3):303–308, 2003.

53. Leech SJ, Gukhool J, Blaivas M: ED ultrasound evaluation of the Index Flexor Tendon: A comparison of Water-bath Evaluation Technique (WET) versus direct contact ultrasound. *Acad Emerg Med* 10(5):573, 2003.

54. Leech SJ, Blaivas M, Gukhool J: Water-bath vs direct contact ultrasound: A randomized, controlled, blinded image review. *Acad Emerg Med* 10(5):573–574, 2003.

55. Blaivas M, Lyon M, Brannam L, Duggal S, Sierzenski P: Water bath evaluation technique for emergency ultrasound of painful superficial structures. *Am J Emerg Med.* 22(7):589–593, 2004.

56. Grassi W, Filippucci E, Busilacchi P: Musculoskeletal ultrasound. *Best Pract Res Clin Rheumatol* 18:813–826, 2004.

57. Filippucci E, Unlu Z, Farina A, et al.: Sonographic training in rheumatology: a self teaching approach. *Ann Rheum Dis* 62:565–567, 2003.

58. Hoglund M, Tordai P, Engkvist O: Ultrasonography for the diagnosis of soft tissue conditions in the hand. *Scand J Plast Reconstr Hand Surg* 25:225–231, 1991.

59. Taboury J: Etude echographique des tendons des muscles rotateurs de l'epaule. *Annales de Radiologie* 38:275–279, 1995.

60. Vick CW, Bell SA: Rotator cuff tears. Diagnosis with sonography. *AJR* 154:121–123, 1990.

61. Farin P, Jaroma H: Sonographic detection of tears of the anterior portion of the rotator cuff (subscapularis tendon tears). *J Ultrasound Med* 16:221–225, 1996.

62. Fornage BD: Musculoskeletal evaluation, In: Mittelstaedt CA ed. *General Ultrasound.* New York: Churchill Livingstone, 1992:157.

63. Adler R, Sofka C: Percutaneous ultrasound-guided injections in the musculoskeletal system. *Ultrasound Q* 19:3–12, 2003.

64. Chen M, Lew H, Hsu T, et al.: Ultrasound-guided shoulder injections in the treatment of subacromial bursitis. *Am J Phys Med Rehabil* 85:31–35, 2006.

65. Bianchi S, Martinoli C, Abdelwahab I: Ultrasound of tendon tears. Part 1; general considerations and upper extremity. *Skeletal Radiol* 34:500–512, 2005.

66. Kalebo P, Sward L, Karlsson J, et al.: Ultrasonography in the detection of partial patellar ligament ruptures (jumper's knee). *Skeletal Radiol* 20:285–289, 1991.

67. Hashimoto BE, Kramer DJ, Wiitala L: Applications of musculoskeletal sonography. *J Clin Ultrasound* 27:293–318, 1999.

68. Martinoli C, Bianchi S, Zamorani M, et al.: Ultrasound of the elbow. *Eur J Ultrasound* 14:21–27, 2001.

69. Mahlfeld K, Kayser R, Mahlfeld A, et al.: Wert der Sonographie in der Diagnostik von Bursopathien im Bereich der Achillessehne. *Ultraschall Med* 22:87–90, 2001.

70. Finlay K, Ferri M, Friedman L: Ultrasound of the elbow. *Skeletal Radiol* 33:63–79, 2004.

71. Howlett D: High resolution ultrasound assessment of the parotid gland. *Br J Radiol* 76:271–277, 2003.

72. Alyas F, Lewis K, Williams M, et al.: Diseased of the submandibular gland as demonstrated using high resolution ultrasound. *Br J Radiol* 78:362–369, 2005.

73. Lamont J, McCarty T, Fisher T, et al.: Prospective evaluation of office-based parotid ultrasound. *Ann Surg Oncol* 8:720–722, 2001.

74. McCaig LF, Hughes JM: Trends in antimicrobial drug prescribing among office-based physicians in the United States. *JAMA.* 273(3):214–219, 1995.

75. Piccirillo JF, Mager DE, Frisse ME, Brophy RH, Goggin A: Impact of first-line vs. second-line antibiotics for the treatment of acute uncomplicated sinusitis. *JAMA* 286(15):1849–1856, 2001.

76. Hickner JM, Bartlett JG, Besser RE, Gonzales R, Hoffman JR, Sande MA: Principles of appropriate antibiotic use for acute rhinosinusitis in adults: background. *Ann Emerg Med* 37(6):703–710, 2001.

77. Geiss HK: Nosocomial sinusitis. *Intens Care Med* 25(10):1037–1039, 1999.

78. Engels EA, Terrin N, Barza M, Lau J: Meta-analysis of diagnostic tests for acute sinusitis. *J Clin Epidemiol* 53(8):852–862, 2000.

79. Varonen H, Makela M, Savolainen S, Laara E, Hilden J: Comparison of ultrasound, radiography, and clinical examination in the diagnosis of acute maxillary sinusitis: a systematic review. *J Clin Epidemiol* 53(9):940–948, 2000.

80. Puhakka T, Heikkinen T, Makela MJ, et al.: Validity of ultrasonography in diagnosis of acute maxillary sinusitis.

Arch Otolaryngol Head Neck Surg 126(12):1482–1486, 2000.

81. Varonen H, Savolainen S, Kunnamo I, Heikkinen R, Revonta M: Acute rhinosinusitis in primary care: a comparison of symptoms, signs, ultrasound, and radiography. *Rhinology* 41(1):37–43, 2003.

82. Price D, Park R, Frazee B, et al.: Emergency department ultrasound for the diagnosis of maxillary sinus fluid. *Acad Emerg Med* 13(3):363–b–364, 2006.

83. Hilbert G, Vargas F, Valentino R, et al.: Comparison of B-mode ultrasound and computed tomography in the diagnosis of maxillary sinusitis in mechanically ventilated patients. *Crit Care Med* 29(7):1337–1342, 2001.

84. Kaups KL, Cohn SM, Nageris B, Lavelle WG: Maxillary sinusitis in the surgical intensive care unit: a study using bedside sinus ultrasound. *Am J Otolaryngol* 16(1):24–28, 1995.

85. Lichtenstein D, Biderman P, Meziere G, Gepner A: The "sinusogram," a real-time ultrasound sign of maxillary sinusitis. *Intensive Care Med* 24(10):1057–1061, 1998.

86. Vargas F, Bui HN, Boyer A, et al.: Transnasal puncture based on echographic sinusitis evidence in mechanically ventilated patients with suspicion of nosocomial maxillary sinusitis. *Intens Care Med* 32(6):858–866, 2006.

87. Gwaltney JM, Jr., Phillips CD, Miller RD, Riker DK: Computed tomographic study of the common cold. *N Engl J Med* 330(1):25–30, 1994.

88. Yiengpruksawan A, Ganepola GA, Freeman HP: Acute soft tissue infection in intravenous drug abusers: its differential diagnosis by ultrasonography. *J Natl Med Assoc* 78(12):1193–1196, 1986.

89. Yeh HC, Rabinowitz JG: Ultrasonography of the extremities and pelvic girdle and correlation with computed tomography. *Radiology* 143(2):519–525, 1982.

90. vanSonnenberg E, Wittich GR, Casola G, Cabrera OA, Gosink BB, Resnick DL: Sonography of thigh abscess: detection, diagnosis, and drainage. *AJR Am J Roentgenol* 149(4):769–772, 1987.

91. Sandler MA, Alpern MB, Madrazo BL, Gitschlag KF: Inflammatory lesions of the groin: ultrasonic evaluation. *Radiology* 151(3):747–750, 1984.

92. Gitschlag KF, Sandler MA, Madrazo BL, Hricak H, Eyler WR: Disease in the femoral triangle: sonographic appearance. *AJR Am J Roentgenol* 139(3):515–519, 1982.

93. Peleg M, Heyman Z, Ardekian L, Taicher S: The use of ultrasonography as a diagnostic tool for superficial fascial space infections. *J Oral Maxillofac Surg* 56(10):1129–1131, 1998; discussion 1132.

94. Tayal VS, Hasan N, Norton HJ, Tomaszewski CA: The effect of soft-tissue ultrasound on the management of cellulitis in the emergency department. *Acad Emerg Med* 13(4):384–388, 2006.

95. Squire B, Fox CJ, Zlidenny A, Barajas G: ABSCESS: applied bedside sonography for convenient evaluation of superficial soft tissue infections. California Chapter, Amercian College of Emergency Physicians, Scientific Assembly, Squaw Valley; 2004.

96. Page-Wills C, Simon B, Christy D: Utility of ultrasound on emergency department management of suspected cutaneous abscess. *Acad Emerg Med* 7:493, 2000.

97. Loyer EM, DuBrow RA, David CL, Coan JD, Eftekhari F: Imaging of superficial soft-tissue infections: sonographic findings in cases of cellulitis and abscess. *AJR Am J Roentgenol* 166(1):149–152, 1996.

98. Craig JG: Infection: ultrasound-guided procedures. *Radiol Clin North Am* 37(4):669–678, 1999.

99. Bureau NJ, Chhem RK, Cardinal E: Musculoskeletal infections: US manifestations. *Radiographics* 19(6):1585–1592, 1999.

100. Loyer EM, Kaur H, David CL, DuBrow R, Eftekhari FM: Importance of dynamic assessment of the soft tissues in the sonographic diagnosis of echogenic superficial abscesses. *J Ultrasound Med* 14(9):669–671, 1995.

101. Lille ST, Sato TT, Engrav LH, Foy H, Jurkovich GJ: Necrotizing soft tissue infections: obstacles in diagnosis. *J Am Coll Surg* 182(1):7–11, 1996.

102. Yen ZS, Wang HP, Ma HM, Chen SC, Chen WJ: Ultrasonographic screening of clinically-suspected necrotizing fasciitis. *Acad Emerg Med* 9(12):1448–1451, 2002.

103. Chao HC, Kong MS, Lin TY: Diagnosis of necrotizing fasciitis in children. *J Ultrasound Med* 18(4):277–281, 1999.

CHAPTER 17

Ocular Ultrasound

Matthew Lyon and Michael Blaivas

In many acute ocular conditions, physical examination can be difficult and unreliable; persistent efforts to examine the eye may also be deleterious to the patient. Specialized equipment and ophthalmologic expertise are frequently unavailable, particularly during nontraditional business hours. In these circumstances, ultrasound can be an important tool for assessing a wide variety of ocular and orbital diseases, including penetrating injuries, retinal detachment, and evaluation for papilledema.[1-3]

The eye is an ideal structure for ultrasound interrogation since the anterior chamber and vitreous cavity are essentially fluid filled. With ultrasound, the globe, orbit, and retrobulbar structures can each be evaluated accurately and safely.[2] Because a cooperative patient can move the eye, all aspects of the globe can be evaluated when coupled with transducer angulation and movement. While ophthalmologists typically use highly specialized ultrasound transducers in their clinics, ocular ultrasound may be performed using transducers readily available to physicians using bedside ultrasound.[4-6] This technology accurately differentiates between pathology requiring immediate ophthalmologic consultation and that which can be followed up on an outpatient basis.

▶ CLINICAL CONSIDERATIONS

Physical examination incorporating ophthalmoscopic and slit lamp examination is the primary diagnostic approach to most ocular complaints. There are many situations in which the physical examination may be limited and imaging is required. Ophthalmologists have been using ultrasound to examine the structures of the eye for decades, while emergency physicians have reported only the utility of ocular ultrasound in the past 5 years.[2,7]

Ultrasound examination of the eye is potentially useful in many situations encountered in emergency or acute care practice. Since physical examination requires a clear visual axis to examine the structures of the eye, any obstruction that obscures this visual axis also limits physical examination. Ultrasound allows imaging beyond the obstruction. There is little attenuation of the ultrasound signal. Detailed, high-resolution images can be obtained of posterior structures even when direct visualization is difficult or impossible.

Situations in which direct visualization of intraocular structures may be difficult or impossible include lid abnormalities due to facial trauma, severe edema, subcutaneous air, or previous surgeries. In cases of facial trauma and swelling, it may be difficult to assess the eye without significant manipulation that can be painful and even harmful if there is globe perforation. Visual axis obstruction can also occur in the presence of corneal scars, cataracts, hyphema, or hypopyon, or with vitreous hemorrhage. Furthermore, normal conditions such as miosis make visualization of the retina difficult without pharmacologic agents.

Ultrasound may also be helpful in situations where physical examination alone is inadequate. An example is peripheral retinal detachment. Patients presenting with a history consistent with retinal detachment may have an unremarkable ophthalmologic examination. However, performing an examination of a dilated pupil is not always feasible. Ultrasound allows for visualization of the entire retina.

Computed tomography (CT) is frequently employed for evaluating the globe after trauma. CT is highly sensitive for orbital fractures, foreign bodies, and retrobulbar hematomas. Fine-cut CT scans with 2-mm sections are able to localize foreign bodies as small as 0.7 mm.[8] In contrast, ultrasound has been demonstrated to have a slightly lower sensitivity but a comparable positive predictive value for detecting similar size metal foreign bodies in a porcine model.[9] Thus, if an ultrasound examination is positive, the findings are likely true; otherwise, further orbital imaging with CT is warranted.

► CLINICAL INDICATIONS

The clinical indications for ocular ultrasound are as follows:

- eye trauma and facial trauma potentially involving the eye,
- acute change in vision, and
- head injury or altered mental status.

► EYE TRAUMA

Trauma is one of the leading causes of unilateral loss of vision in the United States and accounts for an estimated $200 million in cost per year.[10] Vision-threatening injuries include retrobulbar hematoma, retinal detachment, lens dislocation, traumatic optic neuropathy, and open as well as closed globe injuries.[11] The most common presentation for vision-threatening injuries is blindness after the injury. However, vision loss may occur gradually because of unrecognized trauma, or the patient may not be able to report vision loss due to lid swelling or alteration in mental status. As a consequence, ocular injuries are often missed by nonophthalmologists during the initial evaluation of trauma patients. A retrospective review of injured patients with potential ocular injury demon-

strated that nonophthalmologists frequently missed or underestimated potential eye trauma, diagnosing only 72% of eye injuries and referring only 27% for ophthalmologic evaluation.[12]

Significant swelling of the periorbital tissues can be encountered with midface or craniofacial fractures, injuries that increase the risk of concomitant ocular injury. One study found that out of 283 patients presenting with facial fractures, 71 had ocular injury, with 32 (12%) suffering a serious ocular injury.[13] While it is ideal for all facial trauma patients with suspected eye injury to have an examination performed immediately by an ophthalmologist, this is not feasible in most situations. There may be more serious, life-threatening injuries that require diagnosis and treatment first.

Ocular ultrasound can be performed at the bedside. It is noninvasive; hence, there is little risk for exacerbating an injury when performed correctly. The examination can also yield results even when medication, drugs, or hypoxia alters pupilary function. This is important in the initial clinical assessment of the eye where pupil size, reaction to light, and the presence or absence of a relative afferent papillary defect are assessed.[11] Retrobulbar hemorrhage can be diagnosed clinically when a significant hematoma is present.[14] However, this vision-threatening emergency often goes unrecognized, especially in trauma victims with a decreased level of consciousness. Delayed diagnosis may result in irreversible damage to the optic nerve. CT typically reveals stretching of the optic nerve and a tented posterior sclera. Retrobulbar hematoma may cause damage to the optic nerve either through direct compression leading to ischemia or through traction by propelling the globe forward and stretching the nerve. The hematoma occurs as a result of bleeding within or around the cone formed by the extraocular muscles. This cone of muscles combined with the bony orbit forms a compartment in which the ongoing hemorrhage leads to elevated intraorbital pressure. As the pressure rises, compression of the ophthalmic and retinal vessels can occur, resulting in ischemia and ultimately blindness.[11] Any potential injury must be treated rapidly as irreversible damage has been estimated to occur after only 60 minutes of ischemia.[15]

An open globe injury is defined as a full thickness wound involving the corneo-scleral wall of the eye. This type of injury is typically caused either by blunt force, particularly to the anterio-lateral part of the orbit, or due to laceration by a foreign body.[11,16] While some open globe injuries are obvious with vitreous extrusion, a significant proportion is not readily apparent. Clues to an open globe injury include blood-stained tears, lid lacerations, presence of a subconjunctival hemorrhage, or hyphema. However, none of these are pathognomonic for globe rupture. Furthermore, in cases involving small high-velocity projectiles, there may be no external signs of perforation.[11] CT evaluation for open globe injury has been shown to have a sensitivity and specificity of 75% and 93%, respectively.[17] Ultrasound has a similar sensitivity, but subtle findings consistent with open globe injury such as scleral discontinuity are more readily identified using 2-mm axial high-resolution CT with reconstruction.

CT is the test of choice for intraocular foreign body localization.[8] In contrast to CT, ultrasound has limitations when used for the detection of intraocular foreign bodies. In animal models, the sensitivity and specificity for the detection of the foreign body was 87.5% and 95.8%, respectively.[9] One study compared CT with ultrasound in a prospective study of traumatized eyes with opaque ocular media. The findings indicated that ultrasound had complete concurrence with surgical or clinical follow-up in 90% of their 61 cases. The study concluded that ultrasound was useful even though CT was more accurate in detecting the intraocular foreign bodies because ultrasound was superior to CT in demonstrating intraocular damage associated with an intraocular foreign body.

▶ ACUTE CHANGE IN VISION

Acute change in vision is a fairly common complaint in emergency and acute care settings. Symptoms may include floaters, flashing lights, double vision, and even complete blindness.

Although these symptoms may be indicative of nonocular problems, they require rapid attention to exclude such processes as lens dislocation, vitreous hemorrhage, retinal detachment, and vitreous detachment.

Lens dislocation is a condition frequently caused by blunt trauma. In a series of 71 consecutive patients presenting with ocular trauma, 12 were noted to have a lens dislocation.[18] However, lens dislocation can also occur without trauma and be idiopathic or hereditary (Marfan's syndrome). Ultrasound easily identifies the lens due to its anterior location. Using ultrasound, the clinician is able to evaluate the lens-supporting structures to determine whether the lens is subluxed or completely dislocated. Subtle lens subluxation can be a difficult diagnosis for even experienced sonographers.

The incidence of spontaneous vitreous hemorrhage is about 7 cases per 100,000 people.[19] Proliferative diabetic retinopathy, posterior vitreous detachment with or without retinal tear, and retinal detachment are the most common causes. Symptoms of a spontaneous vitreous hemorrhage typically include "floaters" or a clouding of vision. Other symptoms such as flashes of lights may be present, but these symptoms are usually due to the underlying cause of the hemorrhage, such as retinal detachment. As a vitreous hemorrhage ages, a membrane may form with attachments to the retina. When this membrane contracts, a retinal detachment may occur weeks after the initial hemorrhage. Ultrasound allows for visualization of the hemorrhage as well as the potential cause. In fact, there is no other imaging modality that can reliably ascertain the anatomic position of the retina.[19]

Retinal detachments and retinal tears, which may be a precursor to detachment, are common causes of vitreous hemorrhage. Both represent a separation between the retinal sensory and pigment layers. There are three types of retinal detachment: rhegmatogenous, tractional, and exudative. Most cases of rhegmatogenous retinal detachment are associated with a posterior vitreous separation; the detachment is caused by fluid seeping into a break in the sensory layer of the retina. Tractional retinal detachment occurs when fibrous membranes in the vitreous pull the retina from the underlying retinal pigment epithelium and is typically seen with proliferative diabetic retinopathy or as a common sequela of aging. However, this condition is also associated with retinopathy of prematurity, sickle cell retinopathy, and prior vitreous hemorrhage. Exudative retinal detachment occurs with conditions that disturb the blood–retinal barrier. This allows fluid to collect underneath the layers of the retina causing a separation.

In most cases of retinal detachment, patients will complain of seeing flashing lights, floaters, or a curtain-like veil-causing vision loss.[20] As the retinal tear progresses, retinal vessels may tear, producing a vitreous hemorrhage. This is a common occurrence and is why patients with retinal detachment frequently complain of floaters, typically prior to the onset of peripheral or total vision loss.

Posterior vitreous detachment is a separation of the vitreous humor from the retina. The separation is painless and usually abrupt; patients complain of new floaters in conjunction with the onset of flashing lights. The clinical history can be similar to retinal detachment as both patients complain of flashing lights at onset. In approximately 15–30% of cases of vitreous detachment, a retinal hole is formed that may lead to retinal detachment. Posterior vitreous detachment is also associated with vitreous hemorrhage.[21] Ultrasound is a choice modality for evaluating the retina and vitreous. When hemorrhage is present, ultrasound may be the only method for detecting posterior vitreous detachment.

▶ HEAD INJURY OR ALTERED MENTAL STATUS

Headache and alteration in mental status are common presenting complaints in the ED. These complaints may, in some cases, be associated with elevated intracranial pressure resulting from intracranial hemorrhage secondary to trauma or stroke. While many modalities are available to evaluate possible elevated intracranial pressure, each method may have significant limitations. In the acute trauma patient, evaluating for the presence of papilledema with an ophthalmoscope is difficult. Furthermore, papilledema can take hours to develop. Performing a lumbar puncture to measure cerebrospinal fluid pressure can be dangerous. CT is not always available. When unstable patients are taken directly to the operating suite for abdominal injuries, there may not be time for a head CT. In these cases, ocular ultrasound can provide a method for grossly assessing the intracranial pressure. In addition, multiple examinations can be readily performed on the same patient with an evolving clinical picture.

A direct communication between the subarachnoid space of the ventricles and the optic nerve sheath has been described in cadavers and an animal model. In an experimental model using rhesus monkeys, change in the optic nerve sheath diameter in response to changing intracranial pressure was demonstrated by varying the pressure in balloons placed in the subarachnoid space.[22] Multiple clinical studies have demonstrated this effect in actual patients. One study comparing CT to ultrasound measurement of the optic nerve sheath diameter in patients with suspected intracranial hemorrhage showed a sensitivity and specificity of 100% and 95%, respectively.[23] This procedure has also been described in pediatric patients where a different cutoff point for the maximal measurement of the optic nerve sheath diameter exists.[24]

▶ ANATOMIC CONSIDERATIONS

The globe is an oblong structure with a mean vertical diameter of 23.5 mm and mean anteroposterior diameter of 24 mm. The eye is embedded in the orbit and covered by the eyelids. On ultrasound evaluation the surrounding facial bones appear as bright reflectors with deep posterior shadowing. The lid is echogenic and divided into 2 by the hypoechoic tarsal plate.

The eye is divided into two segments. The anterior segment is in turn divided into the anterior and posterior chambers. The anterior chamber consists of the cornea and lens. The cornea appears as a thin, hyperechoic structure attached to the sclera at the periphery. The sclera is a dense membrane to which the extraocular muscles attach, but is indistinguishable from the lateral structures of the eye sonographically. Echolucent aqueous humor fills the anterior chamber; echoes are seen in pathologic states only. The iris separates the anterior chamber from the posterior chamber, which consists of the posterior surface of the iris, the anterior aspect of the lens, and its supporting ligaments. The lens appears as a hyperechoic reflector, which is concave, and may show reverberation artifact at the anterior surface (Figure 17-1).

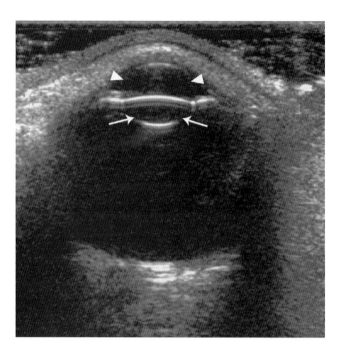

Figure 17-1. Normal ultrasound of the eye. The anterior chamber (arrow heads) is clearly seen as well as the lens (arrows). The vitreous appears black.

The posterior segment comprises the majority of the globe, about 80%. It contains the vitreous body, which consists of a colorless apparently structureless transparent gel, approximately 99% of which is water. The normal vitreous body is echolucent (dark on ultrasound); however, ultrasound artifacts may occasionally be seen.

The posterior layers of the eye consist of the retina and choroid, which are bounded by the sclera. The retina is the neural, sensory stratum of the globe. It is very thin, varying from 0.56 mm near the optic disk to 0.1 mm anteriorly. Its anterior surface is in contact with the vitreous body and the posterior surface is strongly adherent to the choroid. Near the center of the posterior aspect of the retina is the oval macula, where visual resolution is the greatest. At the macula, the retina is only a few cell layers thick. The choroid is a thin, highly vascular membrane lining the posterior globe. It is firmly adherent to the sclera and is thicker posteriorly where it is penetrated by the optic nerve. Its internal surface is firmly attached to the pigmented layer of the retina. On ultrasound interrogation of the normal eye, the three posterior layers (retina, choroid, and sclera) blend into one homogeneous structure. If separation occurs as with retinal detachment, the layers may be distinguished from one another.

The optic nerve and sheath may be seen posterior to the globe, traveling toward the optic chiasm. On ultrasound the nerve appears homogeneous with low internal reflectivity (Figure 17-2). This is in contrast to the more reflective sheath.[25] Measurement of the sheath is

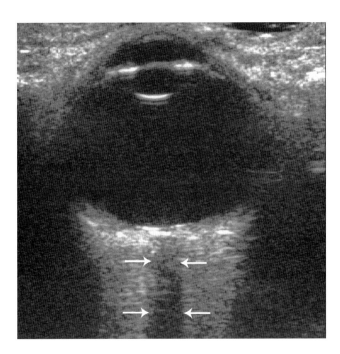

Figure 17-2. The optic nerve is seen posterior to the globe and is hypoechoic (arrows). Minimizing the gain is advisable to decrease echoes that can result in difficulty defining borders of the optic nerve sheath.

made 3 mm posterior to the globe (Figure 17-3). Normal measurements vary by age from 5 mm and less in adults, 4.5 mm in children (1–15 years), and 4 mm or less in children less than 1 year of age.[23–25] Since the optic nerve sheath is connected to the subarachnoid space and is

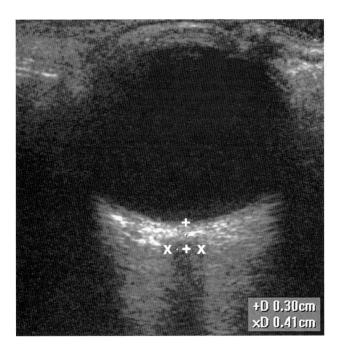

Figure 17-3. Normal measurement of the optic nerve sheath is shown. The measurement should take place 3 mm behind the globe.

+D 0.30cm
xD 0.41cm

easily distensible, conditions that elevate the intracranial pressure lead to dilation of the optic nerve sheath. Arterial and venous structures of the eye can be identified using color Doppler. The largest artery in the orbit is the ophthalmic artery, which runs parallel to the optic nerve.[26] The central retinal artery is located in the anterior part of the optic nerve shadow. The central retinal vein is found near the central retinal artery and is distinguishable from the central retinal artery with pulse wave Doppler examination.[27]

▶ GETTING STARTED

As with most examinations, the ultrasound machine is placed to the patient's right. Patient positioning will vary, with a trauma patient typically flat and supine while other patients may be sitting partially reclined or upright. Patients with potential penetrating injury may be reclined at 45 degrees. The patient should be made comfortable; this may require topical anesthetic in some cases and oral or parenteral medications in cases involving more significant trauma. If a ruptured globe is suspected, antiemetics may be considered to prevent retching and a resultant rise in intraocular pressure.

A linear array transducer in the 7.5–15 MHz frequency range (the same transducer utilized for line placement, soft tissue examinations, and musculoskeletal studies) will be used. Higher transducer frequencies may produce better images, but decreased penetration may limit visualization of retro-orbital structures. An endocavity transducer could be employed if a linear transducer is not available[1]; however, balancing an endocavity transducer can be difficult and imaging is somewhat limited. Color and spectral Doppler capacity allows for the evaluation of orbital vasculature and may be helpful in specific cases.

A small parts setting is available on most machines. Other presets such as thyroid, musculoskeletal, and superficial structure settings may also be useful. Sterile gel is typically not required but can be utilized. The gel supplied is small and utilized for pelvic and rectal examinations will work well as ultrasound gel and is also sterile and bacteriostatic.

A large amount of gel is used to fill the preorbital space, while the eye is kept closed during the examination (Figure 17-4). This allows an ultrasound examination to occur without ever touching the transducer to the eyelid. If the lid is not touched and no pressure is transmitted to the globe, the possibility of vitreous extrusion from a perforated globe is minimized. The spacing between the transducer and the eye can be seen during the ultrasound examination as an echo free space between the top of the screen and lid. It is advisable to have the patient keep both eyes closed so they will be less likely to inadvertently open the eye being scanned.

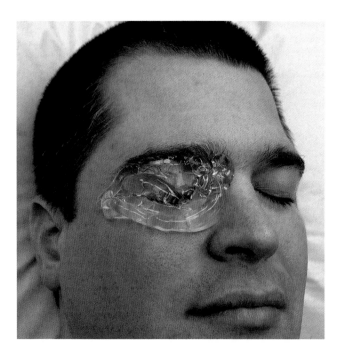

Figure 17-4. A generous amount of gel is placed on top of the closed lid. This much gel allows the sonologist to make no direct contact between the transducer and the eyelid itself.

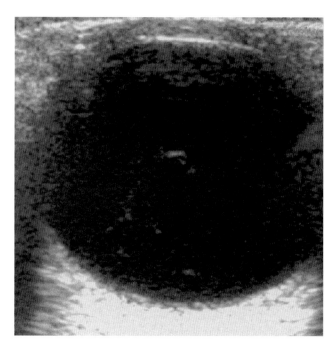

Figure 17-5. Artifacts are created by overgaining this image, and are seen in the near field as well as the periphery.

▶ TECHNIQUE AND NORMAL ULTRASOUND FINDINGS

The transducer should be gently placed into the gel with the normal conventions applying to probe orientation (probe indicator points to the top of the head for longitudinal views or to the patient's right for transverse views). After placing the probe into the gel, the sonologist must pay particular attention to the ultrasound image, leaving a stripe of echolucent gel anterior to the eyelid. This gel separation must be maintained if there is a possibility of globe rupture. Simply suspending the transducer over the patient's eye will inevitably lead to a shaky image and compression of the globe as the sonologist's arm grows tired. By resting a portion of the hand holding the transducer on a bony structure such as the ridge of the nose or the patient's eyebrow, the sonologist can stabilize the transducer and avoid resting the probe directly on the globe.

The gain on the ultrasound machine will need to be adjusted several times throughout the examination. If the gain is turned up too high initially, artifacts will be created making the examination difficult (Figure 17-5). However, a gain setting that is too low will cause a small vitreous hemorrhage or subtle detachment to be missed. Thus, if the examination is started with normal gain settings, at some point the gain should be turned up to evaluate for subtle pathology (Figure 17-6). The focal position should also be adjusted to the area of interest.

This will change throughout the examination as the sonologist changes his interest from near to far field.

Ultrasound imaging almost always involves visualizing structures in two orthogonal planes. Since each plane creates only a two-dimensional (2-D) image, by

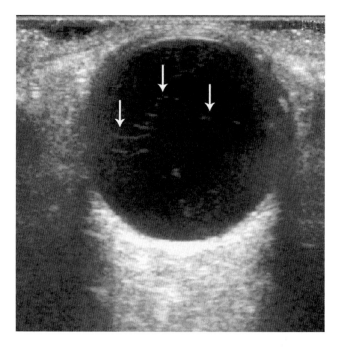

Figure 17-6. A subtle web-like abnormality is seen within the eye when the overall gain is increased (arrows).

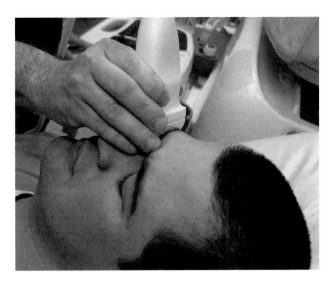 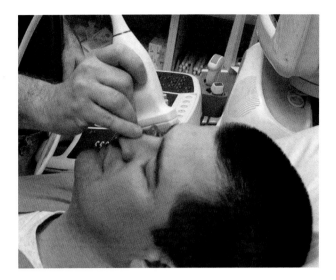

Figure 17-7. Longitudinal and short-axis view probe positions are shown.

combining these a mental 3-D image is built. The transverse probe position and the longitudinal probe position are both necessary for an adequate examination (Figure 17-7). It is important to sweep the transducer from side to side in both positions to demonstrate the full extent of the ocular structures, especially when the retinal periphery is being examined. If the patient is cooperative, he may be able to aid the sonologist by moving the eye, looking up and down, and then side to side. This allows the entire retina to be examined with less panning and probe movement. Sometimes movement of the eye will actually unmask subtle pathology (e.g., a small vitreous hemorrhage waving in the posterior aspect of the globe). Similarly, an imaging artifact will remain relatively unchanged with eye movements, whereas a retinal detachment will undulate with eye movements and appear to float in the vitreous.[16]

The optic nerve is seen traveling away from the globe posteriorly. The nerve itself is not seen with any great detail. Minor probe angulations are used to visualize the optic nerve sheath as crisply as possible. Measurement of the optic nerve sheath diameter is typically made 3 mm posterior to the optic disc. A measurement greater than 5 mm in adults is considered abnormal. Occasionally, the optic nerve sheath may appear dilated despite normal intracranial pressure. When measurements are in doubt, the 30 degree test can be used. Measurement of the optic nerve sheath is made in primary gaze and then after the patient shifts gaze 30 degrees from primary. In cases of elevated intracranial pressure, the nerve and sheath are stretched and the fluid is distributed in the extended nerve sheath resulting in a smaller diameter than in primary gaze. If nerve sheath enlargement is secondary to parenchymal infiltration or thickening of the optic nerve, there will be no change in the nerve sheath measurement when the gaze shifts.

Color and spectral Doppler measurements are helpful in the diagnosis of several conditions. With color or power Doppler, flow in the retina and the region just posterior to the eye is readily identified. With pulse wave Doppler, graphical representation of the blood flow is depicted. Typically, the optic nerve is located first. Then, the vessels are identified using color and spectral Doppler, as each vessel will have a typical waveform.[26] When interrogated with pulse wave Doppler, the ophthalmic artery tracing is similar in form to that of the internal carotid artery, containing a dicrotic notch. The central retinal artery waveform on pulse wave Doppler examination is more rounded and flat compared with that of the ophthalmic artery.

▶ COMMON AND EMERGENT ABNORMALITIES

RETROBULBAR HEMATOMA/HEMORRHAGE

A retrobulbar hematoma is seen as an echolucency just posterior to the globe. Since the orbit is a closed space, pressure may be exerted on the posterior globe by the hematoma. This pressure can be seen sonographically as a distortion in the posterior aspect of the eye. As the blood accumulates, retinal vasculature may become compressed and changes in the spectral Doppler pattern of the retinal vessels may also be seen.

IRIS EVALUATION

In some instances of facial trauma, assessing ocular and pupillary movements is difficult because of facial swelling. Using ultrasound, the iris is easily evaluated if the patient is able to cooperate with the examination. The patient is asked to look superiorly and the probe is placed on the inferior portion of the globe. The iris can be measured and function assessed by shining a light in the uninjured eye. By visualizing eye movement in the orbit, extraocular muscle function can also be assessed. If a muscle is entrapped by a fracture, movement will be limited.

VITREOUS HEMORRHAGE

Vitreous hemorrhage frequently accompanies trauma to the face but can be spontaneous, occur with retinal detachment or as a complication of diabetes mellitus, and with central vein occlusion. The echographic pattern of a vitreous hemorrhage depends upon the age and severity of the hemorrhage. In fresh mild hemorrhages, small areas of low reflective mobile vitreous opacities are seen (Figure 17-8). As the hemorrhage ages, particularly with severe hemorrhages, the blood organizes and forms membranes. Sonographically, this appears as a vitreous filled with multiple large opacities of high re-

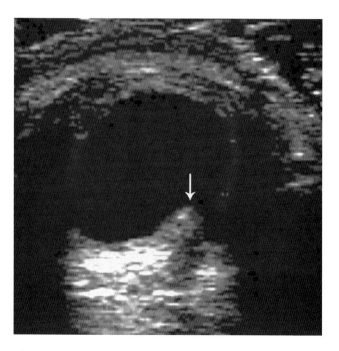

Figure 17-9. A collapsed globe from a penetrating injury showing a posterior fold (arrow).

flectivity. These opacities may layer because of gravity. Occasionally, with a penetrating foreign body, a membrane will form over the tract. If present, the tract may assist in localizing the foreign body.

▶ GLOBE PERFORATION

Globe perforation is typically associated with some type of trauma. Sonographically, the globe may be decreased in size, indicating loss of pressure or vitreous. Buckling of the sclera may be seen posteriorly and vitreous hemorrhage is frequently present (Figure 17-9). Subtle perforations may be missed if little vitreous has been lost. A careful look at the anterior chamber is warranted as it may be collapsed from a small perforation while little else is seen on ultrasound.

▶ FOREIGN BODIES

Ocular foreign bodies are easily identified with ultrasound in most cases. Even if previously detected with another imaging modality, foreign bodies can be more precisely localized with ultrasound.[28] Intraocular foreign bodies typically appear as highly reflective objects that may be located in the vitreous (accompanied by a vitreous hemorrhage) or embedded in the retina or in the posterior orbital fat (Figure 17-10). If embedded in the posterior orbital fat, the foreign body may be missed

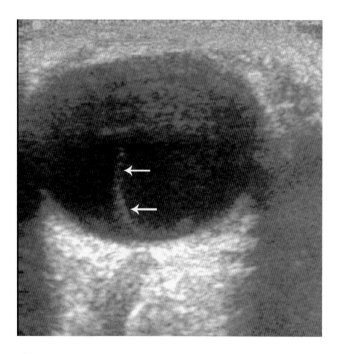

Figure 17-8. This vitreous hemorrhage could not be seen at normal gain settings. Turning the gain up significantly helped identify this strand of hemorrhage (arrows), which moved to and fro with eye movements.

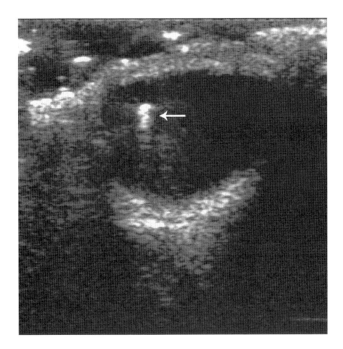

Figure 17-10. A metallic foreign body (arrow) is seen in an eye that is starting to lose some of its shape due to vitreous extrusion.

because of similar highly reflectivity.[16] If color Doppler is available a strongly reflective foreign body may produce a "twinkling" artifact (Figure 17-11), which appears as a rapidly changing mixture of red and blue.[29] Twinkling occurs with any strong reflector including calcifications.

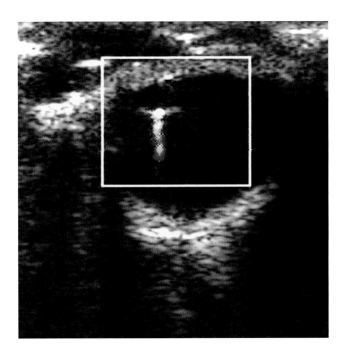

Figure 17-11. The same foreign body is outlined with color Doppler, making detection much easier due to the comet-like artifact.

▶ DISLOCATION OF THE LENS

Dislocation of the lens is easily visualized when it is significant. Dislocations may be partial (subluxation) or complete. With a subluxation, the lens may initially appear to be normal. However, with eye movement, the lens appears to move independently of the surrounding structures. A complete dislocation is more obvious as the lens will be out of its usual position.

▶ VITREOUS DETACHMENT

Vitreous detachment may occur after trauma, intraocular surgery, or spontaneously. A vitreous detachment generally has a V-shaped appearance sonographically, does not float with eye movements, and may be accompanied by hemorrhage (Figure 17-12).[16] A fibrinous vitreous membrane is sometimes seen when a vitreous hemorrhage leads to a retinal detachment.[16]

▶ CHOROIDAL DETACHMENT

Choroidal detachment is the separation of the choroid from the sclera due to blood accumulation from ruptured vessels. This condition is occasionally seen after trauma to the eye or face. It occurs most frequently after intraocular surgery. Choroidal detachment appears as a smooth, dome-shaped, thick structure (or structures, if multiple hemorrhages occur simultaneously) separated from the posterior aspect of the eye (Figure 17-13). If

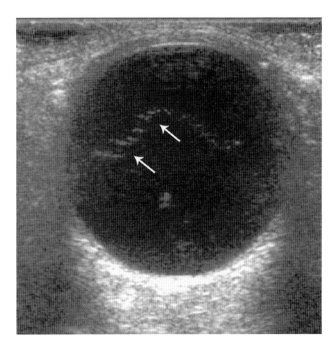

Figure 17-12. A web-like structure is seen (arrows), representing the detached vitreous membrane.

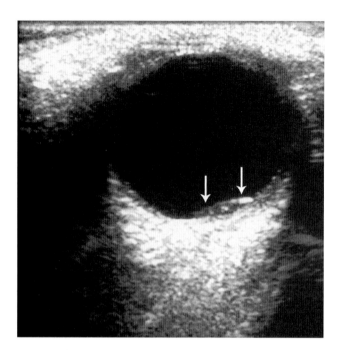

Figure 17-13. A small choroid detachment is seen posteriorly in the eye (arrows).

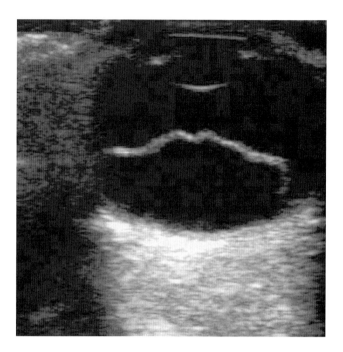

Figure 17-14. A prominent retinal detachment seen across the middle portion of the globe.

these domes become large enough to touch in the vitreous, this is referred to a "kiss."

▶ RETINAL DETACHMENT

Retinal detachments are important to recognize early as they may progress to full detachments and loss of vision if untreated. Retinal tears, the precursor to detachments, are difficult to see unless substantial. When visualized, retinal tears appear to be short, reflective, linear structures protruding into the vitreous.[16] Another clue to a retinal tear is the identification of subretinal fluid. Retinal detachments appear as a highly reflective membrane, which seems to "float" in the vitreous (Figure 17-14). In contrast to a choroidal detachment that does not change with eye movements, fresh or recent retinal detachments are very mobile with eye movements.[16] As the retinal detachment ages, this flexibility is lost and the membrane will become stiff and may appear more funnel shaped. When a retinal detachment becomes complete, a connection to the ora serrata is maintained anteriorly as well as posteriorly to the optic nerve head. The membrane will have a V shape in the vitreous cavity sonographically.

OPTIC NERVE

The optic nerve and its surrounding sheath are seen posterior to the globe (Figure 17-2). When evaluating for possible elevation in intracranial pressure, optic nerve

sheath diameter measurements are taken 3 mm posterior to the optic disc. Maximum measurements vary with age. The upper limit of normal in adults is less than 5 mm. Children over 1 year of age should be under 4.5 mm and 4 mm is the maximum in children less than 1 year of age.[2,25] Intracranial pressure elevation correlates well with increasing optic nerve sheath diameter (Figure 17-15). Measurements typically plateau at approximately

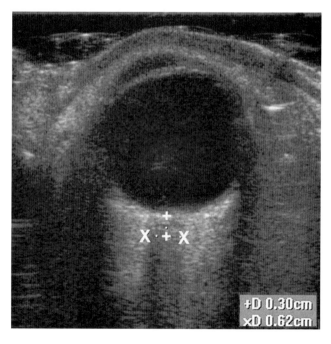

+D 0.30cm
xD 0.62cm

Figure 17-15. A wide optic nerve sheath is measured posterior to the globe (0.62 cm).

7.5 mm even in significantly increased intracranial pressures. In more severe cases, one can see an echolucent circle within the optic nerve sheath separating the sheath from the optic nerve. This is referred to as the "crescent sign."

► COMMON VARIANTS AND SELECTED ABNORMALITIES

MASSES

During the emergency ocular ultrasound examination, other nonemergent abnormalities may be encountered. One example is the incidental discovery of a mass. Symptoms of primary ocular cancer or metastatic disease involving the eye include blurry vision, distorted vision, blind spots, white pupils, red eye, eye pain, and vision loss. Many of these symptoms are neither specific nor sensitive for cancer. Furthermore, many ocular tumors produce no symptoms at all. The review and description of ocular tumors is beyond the scope of this chapter. The detection of a potential mass requires ophthalmologic follow-up.

RETINOSCHISIS

Retinoschisis is a separation in the layers of the retina and may occasionally be encountered in the emergency setting. Differentiating retinoschisis from a retinal detachment is difficult. By ultrasound, retinoschisis is more focal, smooth, and dome-shaped than a retinal detachment. In the emergency setting, differentiation between the two processes is not as critical as identifying the abnormality on ultrasound and obtaining ophthalmologic consultation.

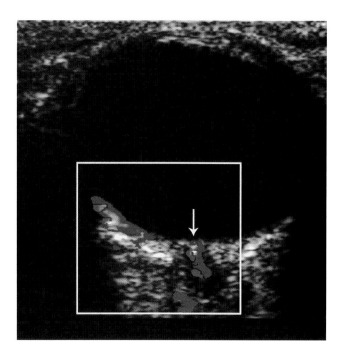

Figure 17-16. Normal arterial and venous flow is detected posterior to the globe (arrow).

CENTRAL RETINAL ARTERY AND VEIN

Central retinal vein or artery occlusion may present as painless visual loss that may or may not be complete. Utilizing color and pulsed wave Doppler just behind the globe will allow an evaluation of the blood supply to the eye (Figure 17-16). Color Doppler typically shows two directions of blood flow (opposite colors such as blue and red). Placing a pulsed wave Doppler gate over each flow direction will allow observation of venous and arterial flow patterns (Figure 17-17). The absence of either arterial or venous flow on the pulse wave Doppler strongly suggests a vascular cause in the patient with

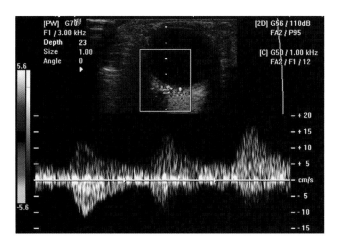 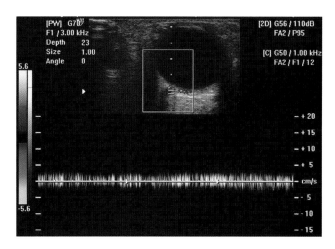

Figure 17-17. Pulse wave Doppler is utilized to confirm normal arterial and venous flow posterior to the globe.

sudden and painless loss of vision. Evaluation of these conditions requires an experienced ocular sonographer. However, since these processes are usually unilateral, comparison with the unaffected eye can be used to detect subtle differences.[26]

VITREOUS CHANGES

With age, the vitreous undergoes syneresis and low reflective vitreous opacities can be detected; the posterior vitreous may separate. Another benign condition occasionally detected by ultrasound is asterhyalosis. This appears as multiple pinpoint, highly reflective vitreous opacities due to reflective calcium salts that accumulate in the vitreous.

INTRAOCULAR PRESSURE ELEVATION

Elevated intraocular pressure may be noted with pulse wave Doppler. As the intraocular pressure rises, the central retinal artery is compressed. With progressive compression, the peak systolic velocity (PSV) and the end-diastolic velocity (EDV) of the central retinal artery decrease. However, the resistive index (RI) of the central retinal artery increases. The resistive index is the ratio of the difference in the PSV and the EDV divided by the PSV (RI = PSV − EDV/PSV).[27] One study that evaluated a healthy eye model showed that these measured differences in flow could accurately predict the presence of elevated intraocular pressure.[30]

▶ PITFALLS

1. **Safety issues.** From the standpoint of worsening an underlying injury, an ultrasound examination of the eye is safe if the techniques described in this chapter are followed. Like any ultrasound examination the amount of energy exposure of any tissue should be limited to what is necessary for the examination. This is especially true when using Doppler ultrasound. Pulse wave Doppler in particular is of higher intensity than normal B-mode ultrasound. Modern diagnostic ultrasound machines are manufactured with a maximum output power that is very unlikely to produce heating or damage to the tissues; however, there are no long-term data available with regard to the absolute safety of ocular ultrasound. Until further studies are available, when using this highly focused ultrasound examination, the time of the interrogation should be limited and the transmit power reduced to the minimum required.

2. **Inadequate amount of gel.** Ultrasound gel is essential for an adequate examination and should

be used liberally. The gel acts as a medium to couple the transducer to the skin surface, decreasing the impedance between these two interfaces. When an inadequate amount of gel is used, artifacts are more frequent and image quality deteriorates. Furthermore, the sonologist may be tempted to push harder on the globe to increase contact. With a perforated globe, this can be disastrous; in a conscious patient, this can be painful.

3. **Confusing pathology.** In clinical practice, there can be overlap in sonographic findings among various retinal abnormalities. A retinal detachment can be confused on ultrasound with a posterior vitreous detachment. Both have similar initial presentations. However, posterior vitreous detachments are often a benign process whereas a retinal detachment can be an ophthalmologic emergency. The development of a fixed visual field deficit along with a mobile membrane seen on ultrasound suggests retinal detachment.

4. **Retinal tears**. Ocular ultrasound is more sensitive than direct visualization for the detection of retinal detachments. This is also true for the detection of vitreous hemorrhage. However, retinal tears can be quite small and difficult to locate. Therefore, when the history is indicative of a retinal tear or detachment, but none is visualized using ultrasound, the emergency physician should consider ophthalmologic consultation or urgent referral.

▶ CASE STUDIES

CASE 1

Patient Presentation

A 32-year-old woman presented from the scene of a motor vehicle crash. She was an intoxicated, unrestrained driver who collided head on with another car. The patient was unconscious on arrival and had been hypotensive en route despite 2 litres of saline through large-bore catheters. Shortly after the primary survey, a trauma ultrasound examination was performed and showed a large amount of free intraperitoneal fluid in all four quadrants. As the patient's blood pressure continued to drift down, a transfusion was initiated. The patient had obvious facial trauma and a midface fracture prior to intubation. There was concern about the possibility of severe head injury, but the trauma surgeon wanted to take the patient to the operating room immediately.

Management Course

An ocular ultrasound examination is performed and reveals normal ocular structures. The optic nerve sheaths measure 6.4 mm on the right and 6.3 mm on the left. Given this information, the trauma surgeon elects to divert for head CT while the patient continues to receive blood. Head CT shows a large epidural hematoma and the neurosurgeon joins the operating team. The patient is found to have a large splenic laceration and her spleen is removed. Her epidural hematoma is evacuated. Despite repeated setbacks and two more trips to the operating room, the patient recovers and leaves the hospital 5 weeks later, and is able to care for herself and resume her office job.

Commentary

Case 1 represented an example of a very high risk and unstable patient. Risking a trip to the radiology suite for CT could have been disastrous if the patient had uncontrolled intraperitoneal hemorrhage. However, an expanding epidural hematoma would also have rapidly led to the patient's demise if not treated expeditiously. A rapid and noninvasive evaluation of intracranial pressure through optic nerve sheath measurement allowed the treating physicians to suspect a space occupying lesion that required immediate attention.

CASE 2

Patient Presentation

A 35-year-old man presented with complaints of left visual difficulties. He stated that for the last 12 hours his vision in the left eye had been considerably worse than before. He was not specific about any deficits. He denied trauma or prior visual problems. He did not wear glasses and denied any other medical problems.

Management Course

Visual acuity testing reveals 20/200 vision in the left eye and 20/20 in the right eye. Ophthalmoscopic examination shows a normal-appearing fundus and generally normal-appearing retina. No detachment is noted. A bedside ultrasound examination is performed on the affected eye. The anterior chamber and lens appear to be intact. The retina is detached on the nasal side of the eye with the central portion extending toward the macula. A consulting ophthalmologist is contacted regarding the patient. The ophthalmologist sees the patient in the emergency department and reviews the images, agreeing with the diagnosis. The patient is taken to the ophthalmology suite for laser treatment

Commentary

Case 2 demonstrated how ocular ultrasound can significantly improve upon the physical diagnosis that can be performed in the emergency department. The globe is an ideal organ to scan and ophthalmologists rely on it

heavily in many cases. A rapid and reliable diagnosis can be made.

CASE 3

Patient Presentation

A 59-year-old diabetic woman presented to the emergency department, complaining of waxing and waning vision in her right eye. It started approximately 12 hours before the presentation. The patient denied anything similar in the past. She had not had any facial or head trauma. The patient did not wear corrective lenses and normally had good vision. Physical examination revealed the patients to have 20/20 vision in the left eye with normal fields. In the right eye the patient is able to see light and some general shapes, but cannot read the Snelling chart. There is no tenderness on palpation of the globe, corneal staining does not reveal any abnormalities, and intraocular pressures are normal.

Management Course

An ocular ultrasound examination was performed and showed no structural abnormality in the right eye. The lens was in good position and there was no retinal or vitreous detachment. Color Doppler interrogation posterior to the globe revealed blood flow in the area of the central retinal vein and artery. However, only one color (blue) was noted and denoted flow away from the globe (Figure 17-18). Pulse wave Doppler was added

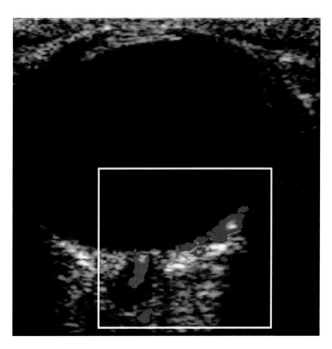

Figure 17-18. This patient had only venous flow visualized on color Doppler (blue, or leading away from the transducer). Pulse wave Doppler interrogation confirmed absence of arterial waveforms.

and showed an obvious venous tracing but no arterial flow could be located. The ophthalmologist was consulted and agreed with the diagnosis of central retinal artery occlusion. The patient was treated emergently by the ophthalmologist and regained partial vision.

Commentary

Case 3 demonstrated the expanded diagnostic capability of the ocular ultrasound. Structures posterior to the globe lent themselves readily to color and power Doppler interrogation as well as pulse wave Doppler, allowing for confirmation of appropriate blood flow to and from the eye.

REFERENCES

1. Blaivas M: Bedside emergency department ultrasonography in the evaluation of ocular pathology. *Acad Emerg Med* 7:947–950, 2000.

2. Blaivas M, Theodoro D, Sierzenski P: A study of bedside ocular ultrasonography in the emergency department. *Acad Emerg Med* 9:791–799, 2002.

3. Orawiec B, Gralek M, Stefanczyk L, Niwald A: Applicability of ultrasound in ocular tumors in children and adolescents. *Klin Oczna* 107:437–441, 2005.

4. Costantino TG, Parikh AK, Satz WA, Fojtik JP: Ultrasonography-guided peripheral intravenous access versus traditional approaches in patients with difficult intravenous access. *Ann Emerg Med* 46:456–461, 2005.

5. Brannam L, Blaivas M, Lyon M, Flake M: Emergency nurses' utilization of ultrasound guidance for placement of peripheral intravenous lines in difficult-access patients. *Acad Emerg Med* 11:1361–1363, 2004.

6. Theodoro D, Blaivas M, Duggal S, Snyder G, Lucas M: Real-time B-mode ultrasound in the ED saves time in the diagnosis of deep vein thrombosis (DVT). *Am J Emerg Med* 22:197–200, 2004.

7. Lizzy F, Coleman D: History of opthalmic ultrasound. *J Ultrasound Med* 23:1255–1266, 2004.

8. Papadopoulos A, Fotinos A, Maniatis V, Kavadias S, Michaelides A, Avouri M, Kalamara C, Stringaris K: Assessment of intraocular foreign bodies by helical CT multiplanar imaging. *Eur Radiol* 11:1502–1505, 2001.

9. Shiver SA, Lyon M, Blaivas M: Detection of metallic ocular foreign bodies with handheld sonography in a porcine model. *J Ultrasound Med* 24:1341–1346, 2005.

10. Larian B, Wong B, Crumley RL, Moeinolmolki B, Muranaka E, Keates RH: Facial trauma and ocular/orbital injury. *J Cranio-Maxillofacial Trauma* 5:15–24, 1999.

11. Perry M, Dancey A, Mireskandari K, Oakley P, Davies S, Cameron M: Emergency care in facial trauma—A maxillofacial and ophthalmic perspective. *Injury, Int J Care Injured* 36:875–896, 2005.

12. Pelletier CR, Jordan DR, Braga R, McDonald H: Assessment of ocular trauma associated with head and neck injuries. *J Trauma* 44:350–354, 1998.

13. Grossman MD, Roberts DM, Carr CC: Ophthalmologic aspects of orbital injury. *Clin Plast Surg* 19:71–85, 1992.

14. Rosdeutsher JD, Stadelmann WK: Diagnosis and treatment of retrobulbar hematoma resulting from blunt periorbital trauma. *Ann Plastic Surg* 41:618–622, 1998.

15. Bailey, Kuo, Evans. Diagnosis and treatment of retrobulbar haemorrhage. *J Oral Maxillofac Surg* 51:780–782, 1993.

16. Fielding J: Ultrasound imaging of the eye through the closed lid using a non-dedicated scanner. *Clin Radiol* 38:131–135, 1987.

17. Joseph DP, Pieramici DJ, Beauchamp NJ: Computed tomography in the diagnosis and prognosis of open-globe injuries. *Ophthalmology* 107:1899–1906, 2000.

18. Kwong JS, Munk PL, Lin DTC, Vellet AD, Levin M, Buckley AR: Real-time sonography in ocular trauma. *Am J Roentgenol* 158:179–182, 1992.

19. Rabinowitz R, Yagev R, Shoham A, Lifshitz T: Comparison between clinical and ultrasound findings in patients with vitreous hemorrhage. 18:253–256, 2004.

20. Gariano R, Kim C: Evaluation and management of suspected retinal detachment. *Am Fam Physician* 69:1691–1698, 2004.

21. Brod RD, Lightman DA, Packer AJ, et al.: Correlation between vitreous pigment granules and retinal breaks in eyes with acute posterior vitreous detachment. *Ophthalmology* 98:1366–1369, 1991.

22. Hayreh S: The sheath of the optic nerve. *Ophthalmologica* 189:54–63, 1984.

23. Blaivas M, Theodoro D, Sierzenski P: Elevated intracranial pressure detected by bedside emergency ultrasonography of the optic nerve sheath. *Acad Emerg Med* 10:376–381, 2003.

24. Tsung J, Blaivas M, Cooper A, Levick N: A rapid noninvasive method of detecting elevated intracranial pressure using bedside ocular ultrasound: Application to 3 cases of head trauma in the pediatric emergency department. *Pediatr Emerg Care* 21:94–98, 2005.

25. Newman W, Holliman A, Dutton G, Carachi R: Measurement of optic nerve sheath diameter by ultrasound: a means of detecting acute raised intracranial pressure in hydrocephalus. *Br J Ophthalmol* 86:1009–1113, 2002.

26. Williamson T, Harris A: Color Doppler ultrasound imaging of the eye and orbit. 40:255–267, 1996.

27. Martini E, Guiducci M, Campi L, Cavallini G: Ocular blood flow evaluation in injured and healthy fellow eyes. *Eur J Ophthalmol* 15:48–55, 2005.

28. McNicholas MM, Brophy DP, Power WJ, Griffin JF: Ocular trauma: evaluation with US. *Radiology* 423–427, 1995.

29. Ustymowicz Andrzej, Jaroslaw Krejza, and Zofia Mariak. Twinkling artifact in color doppler imaging of the orbit. *J Ultrasound Med* 21:559–563, 2002.

30. Chung H, Harris A, Evans D, Kagemann l, Garzozi H, Martin B: Vascualr aspects in the pathophysiology of glaucomatous optic neuropathy. *Survey Ophthalmol* 43:s43–s50, 1999.

CHAPTER 18

Pediatric Applications

Daniel D. Price and Michael A. Peterson

Ultrasound is an especially appealing imaging modality in children. Examinations can be performed at the bedside, at times with the child being held by a parent. This diagnostic test is noninvasive, involves no contrast or ionizing radiation, and is considered virtually risk-free.[1] Also, pediatric patients generally have less body fat and thinner abdominal walls, which enhances the ultrasound examination.

▶ PEDIATRIC TRAUMA

Trauma remains the most common cause of morbidity and mortality in children. Traumatic injuries result in hospital admission for approximately 600,000 children each year.[2] In the pediatric age group, blunt trauma is more prevalent than penetrating injuries. Twenty to 30% of pediatric trauma cases involve the abdomen.[2] Timely, accurate, and cost-effective evaluation of children suffering from blunt abdominal trauma remains a challenge for physicians.

The history and physical examination form the foundation of patient evaluation; however, they may be difficult or impossible to obtain in children who have altered mental status, central nervous system trauma, or distracting injuries. In one study of children with blunt abdominal trauma, an initial physical examination was considered reliable in only 41% of cases.[3] The physical examination has been reported to be misleading in up to 45% of injured children.[4,5] Although the physical examination is an important piece in the diagnostic puzzle, the clinician must resort to other modalities to adequately evaluate and treat the pediatric blunt abdominal trauma patient.

▶ CLINICAL CONSIDERATIONS

In the 1960s, diagnostic peritoneal lavage became a popular procedure for detecting blood or bowel contents in the peritoneal cavity. It can be performed at the bedside and is relatively rapid and safe, with a complication rate of approximately 1%.[6–8] Studies of diagnostic peritoneal lavage in children have demonstrated a high sensitivity in detecting injury (96%), but have noted the findings to be too nonspecific. Positive diagnostic peritoneal lavage studies do not provide information on which organ is injured or how severely, and have led to nontherapeutic laparotomy rates between 13% and 19%.[9,10] Since these studies were published, the trend toward nonoperative management of pediatric abdominal injuries has increased significantly.[11–24] In the 1980s, the direction shifted away from the use of diagnostic peritoneal lavage and toward the use of abdominal computed tomography (CT).

CT is now the most commonly used modality in evaluating pediatric abdominal injuries.[25–34] The primary advantage of CT is that it identifies and characterizes most abdominal injuries and provides important information to guide the management of the patient. CT is noninvasive and can evaluate intraperitoneal and retroperitoneal structures. The primary disadvantage of CT is that the test requires the transportation of the patient to the medical imaging department; consequently, its use is inadvisable in the hemodynamically unstable patient.[6] In addition, CT often requires sedation of pediatric patients. CT involves the administration of intravenous (IV) and oral contrast. This results in filling the stomach in a patient already at risk for vomiting, and possibly necessitates insertion of a nasogastric tube. CT also exposes patients to significant doses of ionizing radiation, and this has led to a more cautious approach recently. Children are 10 times more sensitive to the induction of cancer than adults, and one study estimated that an abdominal CT in a young girl results in a risk of fatal cancer later in life of about 1 in 1,000.[35] This becomes significant when the small individual risk is multiplied by the 2.7 million scans performed annually. CT interpretation may be more difficult in children because they lack the adipose tissue that helps differentiate anatomic planes. Furthermore, CT can be an expensive screening tool.[36] These considerations have led some trauma surgeons to advocate for the use of ultrasound in evaluating pediatric blunt abdominal trauma patients.[37,38]

The focused assessment with sonography for trauma (FAST) examination is a noninvasive and safe diagnostic tool for detecting hemoperitoneum, hemopericardium, and hemothorax.[1] The examination can be performed at the bedside in 3 minutes or less[39–42] and is easily repeatable. Use of the FAST examination has been well established in adults (see Chapter 5). Although the examination is less sensitive than CT for identifying solid organ injuries, the immediate identification of free fluid provides a useful operative triage tool.[43,44]

Over one third of pediatric solid organ injuries are not associated with free intraperitoneal fluid[45,46] and may not be identified by ultrasonography. When solid organ injuries are identified, they are more commonly managed nonoperatively. However, the diagnosis of solid organ injuries is important in determining the need for hospitalization, duration of bed rest, resumption of activity, and need for follow-up. In addition, one study demonstrated that results of CT scanning led to changes in management in 44% of patients.[47]

The sensitivity of the FAST examination in detecting intraperitoneal fluid and solid organ injury is difficult to determine (Table 18-1). Studies supporting the use of ultrasound have demonstrated sensitivities ranging from 71 to 100%.[32,37,41,46,48–54] Some of these studies evaluated only for free fluid, and they often lacked a gold standard by which to compare ultrasound results. Other

▶ TABLE 18-1. **STUDIES OF ULTRASOUND IN PEDIATRIC TRAUMA**

Year	Lead Investigator	Patients	Sonographer	Sensitivity
2005	Soundappan	85	Surgeon	81
2004	Soudak	313	Rad tech	93
2001	Holmes	224	Rad tech	82
2000	Corbett	47	EM res/faculty	75
2000	Benya	51	Rad tech/faculty	59
2000	Coley	107	Rad faculty	55
1999	Mutabagani	46	Rad faculty	44
1999	Patel	94	Rad res	45
1998	Partrick	230	Surg/EM res	71
1998	Thourani	192	Surg res/faculty	80
1997	Richardson	26	Rad faculty	86
1997	Akgur	217	Rad res/faculty	100
1997	Krupnick	32	Rad tech	80
1996	Katz	121	Rad	91
1993	Luks	81	Rad res/faculty	89
1993	Akgur	109	Rad res	95
1987	Filiatrault	170	Rad	80

studies have demonstrated sensitivities ranging from 31% to 65%,[3,55–58] but they often focused on detection of all injures and included injuries one would not expect to be detected by ultrasound, such as pneumoperitoneum.[55] When investigators focused on hypotensive patients, ultrasound was found to be very sensitive in identifying free intraperitoneal fluid.[51,55] Authors of studies showing low sensitivity for detecting injury have also endorsed a potential role for ultrasound in hemodynamically unstable pediatric blunt trauma patients.[57] A scoring system for predicting the need for laparotomy based upon ultrasound findings was evaluated in a group of 37 children with positive FAST examinations.[59] The ultrasound score was defined as the depth of the deepest pocket of fluid measured in centimeters plus the number of additional spaces where fluid was seen. Only 1 of the 22 patients with a score of 3 or less required therapeutic laparotomy compared to 8 of 15 patients with a score greater than 3. The sensitivity of the score for predicting the need for laparotomy was 89% with a specificity of 75%.

Ultrasound evaluation for pneumothorax has been shown to be more sensitive in adults (98%) than a supine chest radiograph (76%) when compared to CT as the gold standard.[60] A case report from the neonatal special care nursery had a similar finding.[61] The pneumothorax examination is simple and rapid, and has been studied as part of an extended FAST examination.[62]

▶ CLINICAL INDICATIONS

A focused bedside ultrasound examination is indicated in children with

- significant blunt abdominal or thoracic trauma and

- significant penetrating abdominal or thoracic trauma.

An algorithm developed in Denver is useful for delineating an appropriate role for the FAST examination in the emergency evaluation of pediatric blunt trauma patients (Figure 18-1).[46] Viewing the FAST examination as a triage tool is the key to understanding the role of ultrasound in the evaluation of children. The FAST examination helps determine which patients should go directly to the operating suite, which are less likely to decompensate during CT scanning, and which stable patients can be observed without CT scanning. Since the FAST examination lacks sensitivity for identifying specific solid organ injuries, the FAST examination cannot replace CT scanning for stable patients with clinical findings suggestive of intra-abdominal injury.

The FAST examination should be performed in all patients with significant blunt abdominal trauma as part of the secondary survey. If free intraperitoneal fluid is identified, and the patient remains hypotensive after a 20 mL/kg bolus of crystalloid, the decision to perform exploratory laparotomy should be made. If the patient's vital signs respond to the fluid bolus, abdominal CT scanning can be performed and is used to guide selective laparotomy. Patients who are hemodynamically stable and have a negative FAST examination should undergo abdominal CT scanning if they demonstrate peritoneal signs, abdominal distention, seat belt abrasion, hematuria, or persistent tachycardia. Patients who have sustained a significant mechanism of trauma but who have normal vital signs, a normal abdominal examination, and a negative FAST examination should be admitted for observation. These patients should receive serial abdominal examinations and FAST examinations.

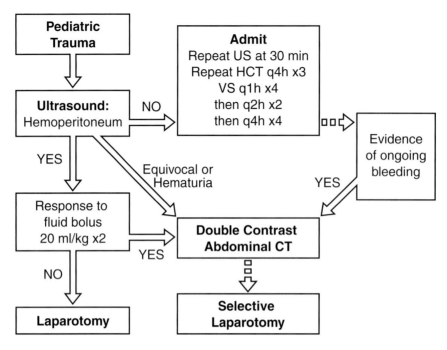

Figure 18-1. Diagram: Pediatric trauma management algorithm.

The FAST examination may also be applied in cases of penetrating trauma. In one study, six children who sustained penetrating trauma were evaluated with a FAST examination, and then followed by CT or laparotomy as part of a larger study.[52] Ultrasound identified one of two cases of intraperitoneal fluid and confirmed negative results in four cases. The missed injury involved a small hemoperitoneum noted on laparotomy in a 17-year-old gunshot wound victim who required a partial small bowel resection. Although virtually all patients who sustain a gunshot wound to the abdomen will be explored, blood in the abdomen, thorax or around the heart may be detected by ultrasound and help guide the surgeon. Ultrasound evaluation for pneumothorax can be performed as part of the routine trauma examination or reserved for cases of suspected pneumothorax.

▶ ANATOMIC CONSIDERATIONS

The FAST examination was designed to assess the three primary dependent areas of the peritoneal cavity in the supine trauma patient: right upper quadrant, left upper quadrant, and pelvis. The location of the fluid depends primarily upon the source of the bleeding but may be affected by the position of the patient. Some authors refer to seven dependent spaces in the abdomen.[63] For the purpose of understanding the anatomy as it relates to the FAST examination, the abdomen should be thought of being divided into quadrants by the mesentery of the transverse colon horizontally and by the spine vertically (Figure 18-2).

In the right upper quadrant, Morison's pouch is the potential space between the liver and the right kidney and represents the most dependent supramesocolic area. Blood from a liver laceration will accumulate in this area; blood from a splenic injury may also spill over the lumbar spine into Morison's pouch. Blood from an inframesocolic injury can spread over the sacral promontory into Morison's pouch as well via the right paracolic gutter. Since most major blunt abdominal injuries involve the liver and spleen, the right upper quadrant view of Morison's pouch is regarded as the most important of the four views in the FAST examination.[63] Alone, it has been found to be 51%–82% sensitive in detecting free fluid.[64–66]

Blood from a splenic injury will accumulate first in the subphrenic space. It may then spread to the potential space between the spleen and kidney (splenorenal recess), which is analogous to Morison's pouch. Blood from this area can flow into Morison's pouch, and it will preferentially reach the pelvis by spilling down the right paracolic gutter because the left upper quadrant is separated from the left paracolic gutter by the phrenicocolic ligament.[67]

Blood from inframesocolic injuries will accumulate first in the rectovesicular pouch in boys and the retrouterine pouch of Douglas in girls. These areas are the most dependent portions of the peritoneal cavity.[67] One study found an isolated pelvic view to be 68% sensitive in detecting free intraperitoneal fluid.[64]

Ultrasound examination for pneumothorax is based on observation of sliding of the visceral pleura of the lung on the parietal pleura of the chest wall. In a supine

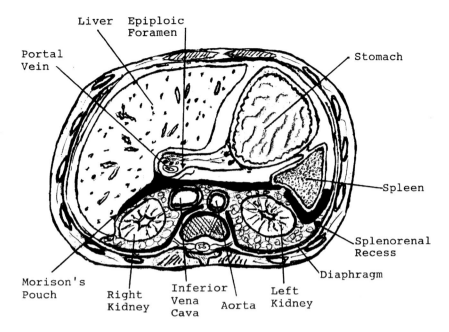

Figure 18-2. Transverse illustration of the upper abdomen that demonstrates the dependent compartments where free intraperitoneal fluid may collect. (Courtesy of Mark E. Hoffmann, MD)

trauma patient, thoracic air tends to accumulate between the anterior chest wall and the lung, separating the parietal and visceral pleurae.

► TECHNIQUE AND NORMAL ULTRASOUND FINDINGS

The classic FAST examination consists of right and left upper quadrant, suprapubic, and subxiphoid views (Figure 18-3). Time permitting, views of the hemidiaphragms and caudal thorax can be examined for blood. A 3.5 MHz transducer can be used in both children and adults. Some authors recommend using a 5.0 MHz (or even 7.5 MHz) transducer for finer resolution.[37,57] Because children tend to have less body fat and a thinner abdominal wall, the focus may be appropriate for a 5.0 MHz transducer, which will provide a higher quality image. The FAST examination should be performed with the patient supine, which is how the patient is transported on a backboard after blunt trauma. By convention, the index marker on the transducer should be directed cephalad or to the patient's right. The transducer may be moved up or down one or more rib spaces to optimize the view. Though not imperative, a partially darkened room will aid the sonologist's ability to discern more subtle findings.

Hemoperitoneum results from splenic or hepatic injuries 74% of the time in pediatric blunt trauma.[68] The right upper quadrant view can be performed first in pediatric blunt trauma patients because it will be the most sensitive in detecting free fluid. With the index marker

cephalad, the transducer should be placed in a coronal plane in the mid to anterior axillary line at the 10th intercostal space or below (Figure 18-3). The kidney lies retroperitoneal, so the transducer should be directed dorsally to maximize the view of the liver–right kidney

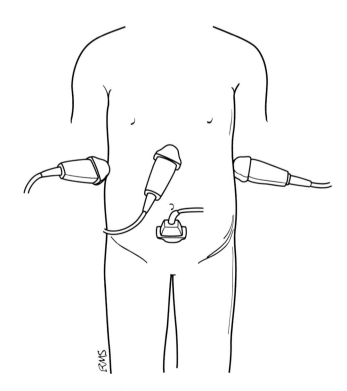

Figure 18-3. FAST examination transducer placement.

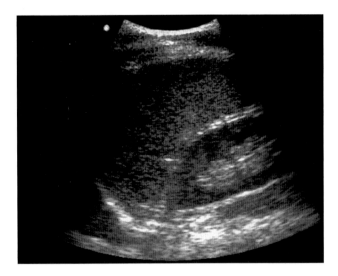

Figure 18-4. Ultrasound: Normal RUQ view.

interface (Figure 18-4). The transducer can be rotated 45 degrees counterclockwise to fit between the ribs and minimize shadowing. Sliding the transducer cephalad should bring the lower thorax into view where blood may appear on the monitor as a dark area cephalad to the bright, hyperechoic hemidiaphragm.

The left upper quadrant view is generally more difficult to obtain. The goal is to examine the potential space between the spleen and the diaphragm and the splenorenal recess where blood may accumulate (Figure 18-5). With the index marker cephalad, the transducer should be placed in the posterior axillary line in the coronal plane at the 9th intercostal space or below (Figure 18-3). The transducer may be rotated 45 degrees clockwise to minimize rib shadows. The diaphragm and lower thorax can be inspected for intrathoracic blood, as described above.

The solid organs—liver, spleen, and kidneys—should be quickly examined by rotating the transducer in a fanning motion to image through the entire organ. Although the goal of the FAST examination is to detect free intraperitoneal fluid, evidence of organ injury is helpful when identified.

An attempt should be made to obtain the suprapubic view prior to insertion of a Foley catheter. Urine in the bladder provides an important acoustic window through which to view the pelvic anatomy more accurately. The transducer should be placed just superior to the symphysis pubis in the midline sagittal plane with the index marker cephalad, and in the transverse plane with the index marker to the patient's right (Figure 18-3). Urine appears dark and is well circumscribed by the bladder wall (Figure 18-6). The uterus in girls and prostate in boys can be seen dorsal to the bladder. The transition in tissue densities between urine in the bladder and the surrounding soft tissue can produce bright echoes, so reducing the far gain will enhance subtle soft tissue details and help avoid missing free fluid in this area.

The subxiphoid view of the heart completes the classic 4-view FAST examination. Some sonologists recommend obtaining this view first. It certainly should be the initial view obtained in penetrating trauma patients in whom cardiac tamponade is suspected. The transducer should be placed in the coronal plane adjacent and depressed below the xiphoid process with the index marker to the patient's right. It should be directed toward the left shoulder with as flat an angle as possible (relative to the abdominal skin) using the liver as an acoustic window. This provides a four-chamber view of the heart surrounded by a hyperechoic pericardium (Figure 18-7). Pericardial fluid will appear as a dark stripe

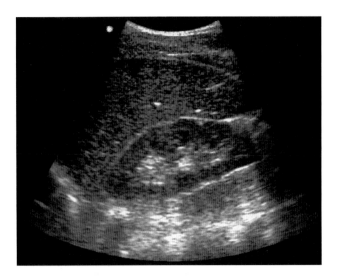

Figure 18-5. Ultrasound: Normal LUQ view.

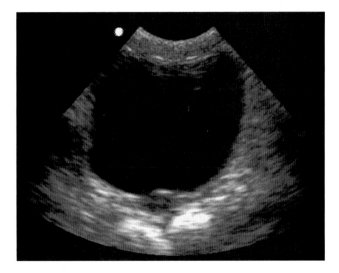

Figure 18-6. Ultrasound: Normal transverse suprapubic view.

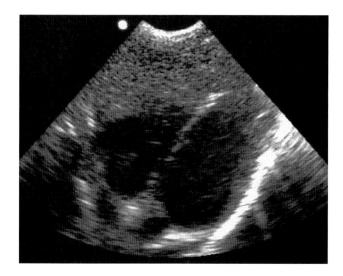

Figure 18-7. Ultrasound: Normal subxiphoid view. The right ventricle is closest to the probe and left ventricle is below with a bright posterior pericardial reflection. Only a portion of the posterior atria are seen in this example.

between the bright pericardium and the contracting, gray myocardium.

Some sonologists include views of the left and right paracolic gutters in their FAST examinations. These views can be obtained by placing the transducer, with index marker pointing cephalad, in the coronal plane below the 11th rib in the mid to posterior axillary line. Transverse views can also be obtained.

The amount of fluid that can be reliably detected in children has not been studied. In adults, 400 mL is a fair estimate.[69,70] One study suggests that placing the patient in Trendelenburg or decubitus positions allows sonolo-

gists to detect intraperitoneal fluid with only two thirds of the amount of fluid required in the supine position.[71] The reverse Trendelenburg position may help with identification of pleural or pelvic free fluid.

The ultrasound examination for pneumothorax can be performed with a linear transducer or with the curved probe used for the FAST examination with a higher frequency selected. The transducer should be placed in a longitudinal orientation with the hyperechoic, shadow-producing ribs as landmarks on either side of the image. Depth should be decreased to optimize the view of the pleural interface. With the transducer in the mid-clavicular line, the anterior chest is scanned from the clavicle to below nipple level on both sides. The interface of the visceral and parietal pleurae is a thin line just deep to the ribs and appears bright and echogenic. The normal findings indicating the absence of a pneumothorax are pleural sliding and comet-tail artifacts. Pleural sliding is seen in real time as scintillating, to-and-fro movement at the pleural line synchronized with respiration. Comet-tail artifacts are hyperechoic reverberation artifacts arising from the pleura and extending into the far field. If pleural sliding is not obvious, the patient should be observed for at least 3 respiratory cycles. Color Doppler and M mode (Figure 18-8) are potential adjuncts to help evaluate pleural movement.

▶ COMMON AND EMERGENT ABNORMALITIES

HEMOPERITONEUM

An anechoic stripe of blood separates the liver from the right kidney in Morison's pouch (Figure 18-9). This may

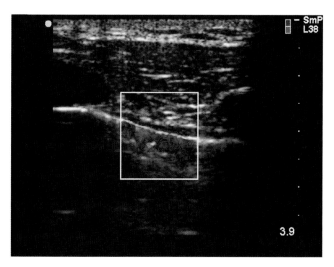

A

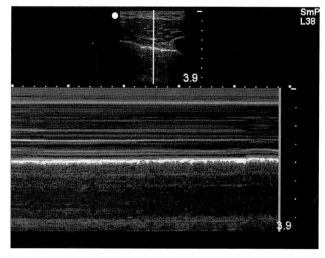

B

Figure 18-8. Ultrasound: Normal lung movement on Doppler (A) and M mode (B) demonstrating the absence of pneumothorax (the "seashore sign").

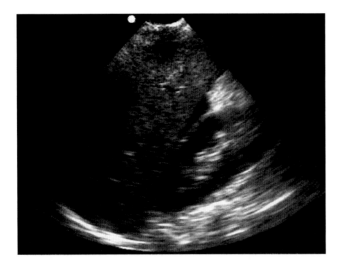

Figure 18-9. Ultrasound: RUQ hemoperitoneum. A thin echolucent stripe of fluid is seen in Morison's pouch.

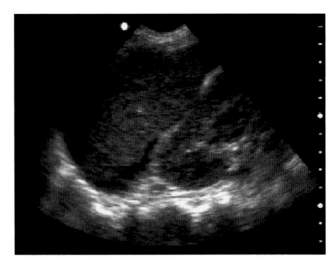

Figure 18-11. Ultrasound: Hemoperitoneum in a left upper quadrant view. Free fluid outlines the superior and inferior borders of the spleen.

extend to separate the liver from the overlying abdominal wall if large amounts of blood are present (Figure 18-10). Similarly, an anechoic stripe of blood may separate the spleen from the left kidney; however, blood more often accumulates between the spleen and the left diaphragm (Figure 18-11). Blood in the pelvic region may be seen floating above and outlining the loops of bowel (Figure 18-12) or it may assume a dependent position in the pelvis. On paracolic gutter views, free fluid appears as an anechoic pocket of fluid below the lower pole of the kidney and lateral to the psoas muscle. Also,

free fluid in the pararenal retroperitoneum can be identified as an echolucent stripe between the psoas muscle and medial renal border in this view.

HEMOPERICARDIUM

Unclotted blood in the pericardial space will appear as an anechoic stripe lying between the two brightly, echogenic layers of the pericardium (Figure 18-13). Clotted blood is more complex and gray, but can generally be distinguished from the contracting myocardium and the thin, white layers of the pericardium.

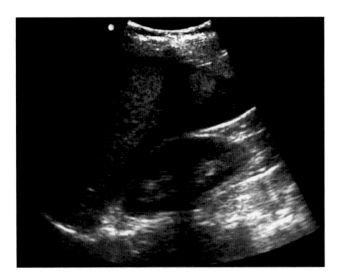

Figure 18-10. Ultrasound: RUQ hemoperitoneum. A large fluid collection is noted inferior to the liver edge and a small stripe extends between the liver and abdominal wall. A rib shadow is projecting down the center of the image.

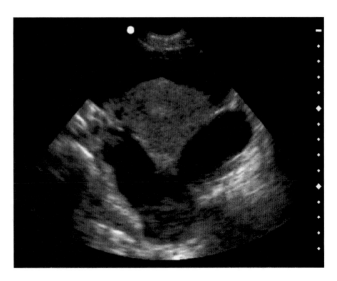

Figure 18-12. Ultrasound: Hemoperitoneum in a transverse suprapubic view. The uterus is outlined above and below with large pockets of fluid.

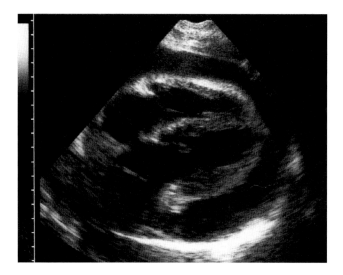

Figure 18-13. Ultrasound: Subxiphoid view demonstrates a large fluid collection within the pericardium. (Courtesy of James Mateer, MD)

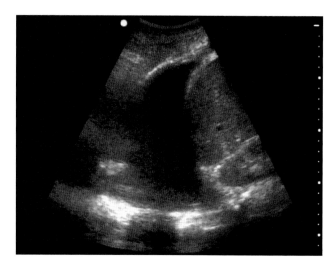

Figure 18-14. Ultrasound: Hemothorax RUQ view. A large pleural fluid collection is noted superior to the diaphragm with lung artifact on the left side of the image.

HEMOTHORAX

Blood in the chest appears as an anechoic area cephalad to the bright echogenic hemidiaphragm (Figure 18-14).

PNEUMOTHORAX

Absence of both normal lung sliding and comet-tail artifacts are the diagnostic criteria for pneumothorax. Absence of color on Doppler scanning, and linear, laminar lines deep to the pleura in M mode (Figure 18-15), re-

sembling those of the overlying stationary anterior chest wall, support the diagnosis of pneumothorax.

▶ COMMON VARIANTS AND SELECTED ABNORMALITIES

Certain aspects of normal anatomy can be easily mistaken for positive findings. In the upper quadrant views, dark rib shadows must not be interpreted as anechoic blood. Since all fluid appears black (anechoic) on ultrasound, bile in the gallbladder and blood in the inferior

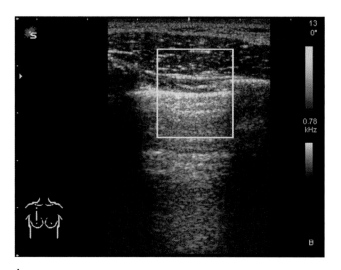

A

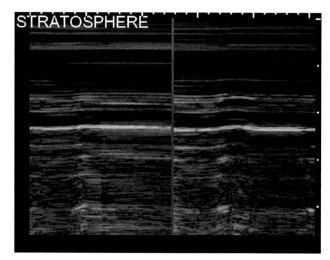

B

Figure 18-15. Ultrasound: Pneumothorax. Absence of lung movement on power Doppler (A) and M mode with linear, laminar lines deep to the pleura (B) support the diagnosis of pneumothorax. (Courtesy of James Mateer MD, (A), and Andrew W. Kirkpatrick MD, (B))

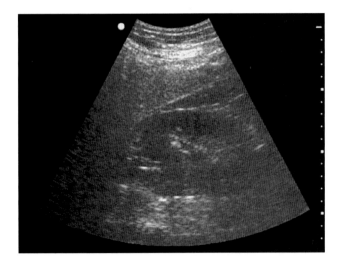

Figure 18-16. Ultrasound: Right upper quadrant view. A hypoechoic wedge of perinephric fat is seen anterior to the kidney.

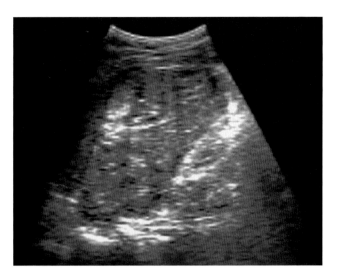

Figure 18-17. Ultrasound: LUQ subcapsular hematoma. A wide hyperechoic hematoma is located along the lateral border of the spleen (area closest to the probe).

vena cava can be erroneously interpreted as intraperitoneal free fluid. In each of the abdominal views, and especially in the suprapubic view, fluid-filled loops of bowel can be mistaken for free intraperitoneal fluid.[58] If viewed carefully, peristaltic movements often help identify the bowel. Perinephric adipose tissue may be hypoechoic relative to surrounding structures and can be mistaken for free fluid or clotted blood (Figure 18-16). Comparison with the area around the other kidney may help distinguish this; also, perinephric fat does not move separately from the kidney with respirations and is more homogenous than clotted blood.

A subcapsular hematoma may be visible between the bright reflection of the splenic capsule and the homogenous parenchyma, which may be disrupted by injury. Blood is often clotted, appearing more echogenic, but may be distinguished from the splenic parenchyma (Figure 18-17). Intraparenchymal blood is often isoechoic with the splenic parenchyma on initial evaluation.[72] Over time, a hematoma will become primarily hypoechoic.

▶ PITFALLS

1. **Contraindications.** The only absolute contraindication to performing the FAST examination is when immediate surgical management is clearly indicated. Subcutaneous emphysema, gas-filled bowel, or morbid obesity may render the examination indeterminate.
2. **Overreliance on the FAST examination.** The FAST examination is one data point in a continuum of clinical decision making. The initial FAST examination (and often repeat examina-

tions) may not detect intraperitoneal bleeding or significant injury. CT is generally required to characterize abdominal injuries, since most of them will be managed nonoperatively in children. The algorithm (Figure 18-1) provides a guideline for the appropriate utilization of trauma ultrasound in the pediatric population.

3. **Limitations.** Air and adipose tissue scatter sound waves and make the ultrasound image more difficult to interpret. Ascites is rarely a problem in children, and free fluid identified in the chest or abdomen in an injured child should be regarded as blood until proven otherwise. Ultrasound has not been found to be as accurate as CT for identifying solid organ injuries or hollow viscus injuries.[38,73] When the FAST examination is used solely to evaluate for intraperitoneal fluid, it suffers from limitations similar to diagnostic peritoneal lavage and has been regarded simply as a noninvasive diagnostic peritoneal lavage.[74]
4. **Technical difficulties with the FAST examination.** The view of Morison's pouch is generally the easiest for sonologists to locate and interpret. In children, however, this view is often more caudad than in an adult. For the left upper quadrant view, sonologists often fail to place the transducer far enough posteriorly (dorsally). The splenorenal recess is also more cephalad than Morison's pouch. Missed subcapsular hematomas and blood between the spleen and diaphragm are often the causes of false-negative scans. It is recommended that at least 50% of the left hemidiaphragm be visualized to avoid missing blood in this area. The suprapubic view may

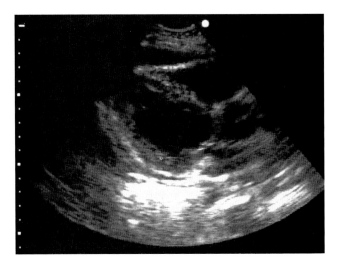

Figure 18-18. Ultrasound: Pericardial fluid in a parasternal long-axis view.

yield the most errors.[52,58,75] A bladder containing little urine provides no acoustic window. Sterile normal saline in quantities appropriate for the patient's age can be introduced into the bladder through the Foley catheter, if necessary. Finally, it can also be difficult to adequately visualize the heart in the subxiphoid view, especially when the child is obese or their abdomen is tender. Flattening the angle of the probe and having the patient breathe deeply can bring the heart into view. If adequate visualization is still not possible, parasternal long- or short-axis views of the heart are recommended (Figure 18-18).

5. **Too few interspaces viewed in pneumothorax examination.** Small pneumothoraces may be evident in only one interspace. Even small pneumothoraces are clinically significant in an intubated patient because positive pressure ventilation will expand a pneumothorax and may lead to cardiopulmonary compromise. For this reason, it is recommended that intercostal spaces from the clavicles to below the nipple line be scanned.

► CASE STUDIES

CASE 1

Patient Presentation

A 2-year-old boy was unbelted in a child seat when his car was struck on the side, throwing him against the driver's seat. He lost consciousness briefly and had a Glasgow Coma Scale (GCS) of 12 on arrival to the emergency department. His initial blood pressure was 90/60 mmHg, with a heart rate of 140 beats per minute, respi-

ratory rate of 20 per minute, and an oxygen saturation of 94% on room air.

On physical examination, the patient's skin was red as he cried for his mother. He opened his eyes and localized to painful stimuli. Pupils were equal and reactive, and an abrasion was noted on his forehead. His neck, lung, and heart examinations were normal except for tachycardia. His abdomen was firm as he cried, and it was difficult to discern tenderness because of his agitation.

Management Course

A 20 mL/kg bolus of normal saline was administered for his tachycardia, and CT scans of his head and abdomen were ordered. However, his GCS dropped to 7, and his next systolic blood pressure read 70 mmHg. He underwent rapid sequence intubation, and the FAST examination revealed free intraperitoneal fluid in the left upper quadrant with suspected disruption of the splenic parenchyma. After the FAST examination, he was taken directly to the operating room where a portion of his lacerated spleen was removed and a 1 cm tear in the small bowel was repaired. His hospital course was uncomplicated and he recovered completely.

Commentary

Case 1 demonstrated the difficulty in adequately examining young children during the initial trauma resuscitation. The abdominal examination was unreliable in the face of a severe injury. His acute decline in mental status was due to hypovolemia, not a head injury. His postoperative head CT scan was normal. This patient was unstable and could not be transported to the medical imaging department for abdominal CT scanning. Bedside emergency ultrasound rapidly revealed the cause of his hypotension and directed his care toward appropriate surgical intervention.

CASE 2

Patient Presentation

An 8-year-old boy showed a classmate his father's handgun stored in the night stand drawer. The gun discharged, and his classmate was shot in the abdomen. The patient's systolic blood pressure was 80 mmHg in the ambulance and he complained of abdominal pain. He received a bolus of normal saline en route, and on arrival to the emergency department his systolic blood pressure was 90 mmHg, heart rate was 120 beats per minute, respiratory rate was 22 per minute, and oxygen saturation 96% on room air. The patient was agitated, but his lung sounds were clear and equal. His heart was tachycardic with a regular, distinct S_1 and S_2. An entrance wound was noted in his epigastrium and this area was tender. The rest of his examination was normal.

Management Course

During the secondary survey, while the operating room was preparing for an exploratory laparotomy, a FAST examination quickly identified hemopericardium but no free intraperitoneal fluid. Shortly thereafter, the patient lost pulses and consciousness. A thoracotomy was performed in the emergency department while the patient was intubated. The pericardium was incised and the tamponade relieved. Closure of a large hole in the right atrium was quickly attempted with pledgeted, horizontal mattress sutures. The patient was rushed to the operating room, but died during surgery.

Commentary

Although the bullet entered the abdomen, it traveled cephalad, penetrating the diaphragm and injuring the heart. The FAST examination identified the true cause of the patient's cardiac arrest, which was pericardial tamponade, and directed the trauma team away from its focus on the abdomen as the source of possible exsanguinating injury.

► APPENDICITIS

Acute appendicitis is the most common indication for emergency surgery in children, representing approximately 80% of emergent cases. The diagnosis is made in 60,000–80,000 children each year in the United States.[76-78] Appendicitis is thought to result from luminal obstruction by hard concretions, fecal impaction, or appendiceal calculi. The lumen becomes distended, leading to ischemia and bacterial infection. Left untreated, this leads to necrosis, perforation, and abscess formation in 36–48 hours.[79]

Delays in diagnosis have been associated with higher rates of perforation and an increase in the rate of overall morbidity from 6 to 36%.[80] Studies of pre–school-aged children report a perforation rate of 30–60% at laparotomy.[81,82] If the diagnosis is delayed, the perforation rate increases to 65% or higher, and mortality increases as well.[83] The long-term sequelae are not well characterized, but a history of ruptured appendix has been shown to convey a three- to fivefold increased risk of infertility.[84] Failure to diagnose appendicitis is one of the most frequently successful malpractice claims against emergency physicians.[85] Timely diagnosis is the only proven means of decreasing morbidity and mortality.[86] In the pediatric patient, the diagnosis is often elusive for even the most astute clinician.

► CLINICAL CONSIDERATIONS

The classic presentation of appendicitis includes right lower quadrant abdominal pain associated with peritoneal signs, fever, vomiting, and anorexia. Together, these signs and symptoms have been found to be highly sensitive for appendicitis.[87] Younger children are often unable to adequately express themselves, and the physical examination may be nondiagnostic. Although frequently requested, the white blood cell (WBC) count[88] and plain abdominal radiograph[89,90] are neither sensitive nor specific for appendicitis. In light of the risks of misdiagnosis and subsequent perforation, pediatric surgeons have been quick to proceed to surgery. Negative laparotomy rates as high as 20% have been reported, with rates of 10–15% widely accepted.[91-93] Negative laparotomies come at significant costs, both financially and in terms of morbidity. Morbidity includes adhesions, hospitalization, and time away from school. Children with equivocal findings represent 25 to 30% of all cases of acute appendicitis.[94,95] This diagnostic challenge forces clinicians to rely on ancillary studies in equivocal cases.

Multiple ancillary studies have been used to help diagnose acute appendicitis, but each has its limitations. Barium enema has been used in the past, but is limited in an unprepared bowel. Barium enema's limitations include nonvisualization of the appendix, patient discomfort, time consumption, and radiation exposure. The barium enema is neither sensitive nor specific, except for the occasional appendicolith.[90] Leukocyte scintigraphy is also time consuming and difficult to perform.[96] Recently, the advent of laparoscopy has made minimally invasive surgery another tool for both the diagnosis and treatment of appendicitis in children.[97,98] However, laparoscopy requires general anesthesia and is an invasive study. Currently, ultrasound and CT are most commonly used to help diagnose appendicitis in patients with equivocal presentation.

Deutsch and Leopold reported the first demonstration of an inflamed appendix by ultrasound in 1981.[99] Development of the graded compression examination by Puylaert in 1986 established a technique and criteria for the diagnosis of appendicitis.[92] Ultrasound has several advantages, including lower cost, widespread availability, and no patient exposure to ionizing radiation. Ultrasound is noninvasive and there is no need for sedation or contrast material.

Studies of ultrasound use in children for detecting appendicitis have sensitivities ranging from 44 to 90% and specificities from 88 to 100% (Table 18-2).[78,92,100-110] The wide range in sensitivity likely reflects the operator-dependent nature of ultrasound, particularly for this examination. The right lower quadrant examination for signs of appendicitis is one of the more technically difficult ultrasound examinations. It may be difficult for a physician or part-time sonographer to gain the skills and

▶ TABLE 18-2. STUDIES OF ULTRASOUND IN PEDIATRIC APPENDICITIS

Year	Investigator	Patients	Ultrasound Sensitivity (%)	Ultrasound Specificity (%)	CT Sensitivity (%)	CT Specificity(%)
2002	Kaiser	600	80	94	97	93
2001	Lowe	76	100	88	97	100
2000	Karakas	360	74	94	84	99
2000	Sivit	386	78	93	95	93
2000	Horton	106	76	90	97	100
1999	Garcia pena	139	44	93	97	94
1999	Rice	103	87	88		
1999	Lessin	99	88	96		
1998	Roosevelt	231	88	95		
1998	Nahn	3859	90	97		
1994	Zaki	56	67			
1993	Crady	98	85	94		
1991	Siegel	178	82			
1988	Jeffrey	245	90	96		
1986	Puylaert	60	89	100		

experience necessary to reliably locate the appendix and recognize findings consistent with appendicitis.[111] Regardless of specialty, clinicians who are trained in right lower quadrant ultrasound examinations should not allow findings of a normal appendix, or inability to identify the appendix, to influence their clinical decision making.

Emergency physicians in Taiwan compared their evaluation of patients for appendicitis using ultrasound to the surgeons' clinical impressions without sonographic examinations and found sensitivities of 94.6% and 86.2%, respectively.[112] Swiss surgeons who performed ultrasound examinations in the emergency evaluation of patients with abdominal pain achieved a sensitivity of 91% for detecting appendicitis.[113] Surgical residents in Germany reached a sensitivity of 83%.[114] Another investigation used "specially trained pediatricians" and achieved 90% sensitivity.[101]

Studies of the use of helical CT for the diagnosis of appendicitis in children have produced sensitivities of 84–97% and specificities of 89–98%.[78,102,107,109,110,115] Although these ranges of sensitivity and specificity overlap with those of ultrasonography, the reliability of sonography is less consistent. When CT and ultrasonography are compared directly, CT has been superior in each study,[78,95,102,107,109,110] except for one study in which patients undergoing noncontrast CT were compared to a historic cohort who underwent graded compression sonography.[110] In a prospective, randomized trial comparing ultrasound with and without CT, ultrasound had a sensitivity of 80% and CT 97%.[109] Another study found that in 20 of 84 (24%) patients who had discordant CT and ultrasound readings, the CT diagnosis was correct 85% of the time.[107] When radiologists were asked to rate their confidence in reading ultrasound and CT images evaluating for appendicitis in children, sonography was interpreted with very low, low, or medium confidence in 59 of 139 (42.4%) patients. This is in comparison to 9 of 108 (8.3%) patients with CT.[116] In comparing ultrasound to CT for the diagnosis of appendicitis, Horton and coinvestigators asserted that a key to managing patients is the negative predictive value of each study. This was 56% for an ultrasound examination compared to 92% for CT scan.[95] Patients with negative CT scans were sent home from the emergency department, whereas those with negative ultrasound examinations required further testing and observation.

▶ CLINICAL INDICATIONS

An ultrasound examination is indicated when a clinician suspects that a child might have appendicitis, the physical examination is equivocal, and the patient is not sent directly to the operating room. Signs and symptoms typically last less than 48 hours and may include

1. Abdominal pain—especially pain that migrates from the periumbilical area to the right lower quadrant with accompanying peritoneal signs
2. Fever,
3. Vomiting, and
4. Anorexia.

Garcia Pena and colleagues evaluated a protocol for managing children with suspected appendicitis.[116] In their study, this protocol led to a beneficial change in management (i.e., a child with appendicitis who would have been discharged from the hospital or admitted for inpatient observation but was instead taken directly to the operating room) in 86 of 139 (62%) of their patients with equivocal clinical presentations. Roughly one third of patients who clinically appeared to have appendicitis were taken directly to the operating room for appendectomy. Another one third of patients for whom appendicitis was doubtful were discharged if no other diagnosis was identified other than nonspecific abdominal pain. The remaining one third, who had equivocal clinical presentations, underwent graded compression ultrasonography. When findings consistent with appendicitis were identified, patients were taken to the operating room. If the ultrasound results were negative or equivocal, context limited CT with rectal contrast was performed. Patients with positive findings on CT underwent appendectomy, and patients with normal findings were discharged from the emergency department. This resulted in a mean cost savings of $565 per patient. When the investigators studied the effect of implementing this protocol on clinical outcomes, they found a marked decrease in the perforation rate from 35 to 16%, and a significant decrease in the rate of negative appendectomies from 15 to 4%.[117]

▶ ANATOMIC CONSIDERATIONS

The vermiform appendix is a hollow lymphoid organ whose function is not well understood. The blind-ended appendix typically arises from the cecum, 1 to 2 cm distal to the ileum in the right lower quadrant (Figure 18-19). It is rarely congenitally absent.[118] Clinically, maximum pain from an inflamed appendix may localize to McBurney's point, which is the mid-point of an imaginary line between the umbilicus and the anterior–superior iliac crest. This should not be used as a rigid anatomic landmark because the appendix and the umbilicus are too variable in position. The appendix lies anterior to the psoas muscle.[118] A 1933 study reported

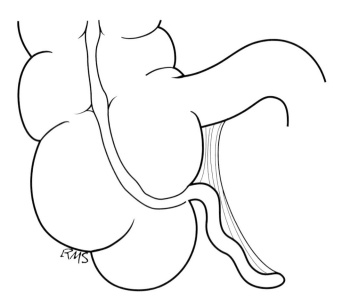

Figure 18-19. Line drawing: Normal appendix.

a classic pelvic orientation of the appendix in only 31% of 10,000 autopsies.[119] The appendix was retrocecal in 65% of cases; in this position, the ultrasound view is frequently obscured by overlying bowel gas.

The appendix averages 6 to 9 cm in length, but it can be twice as long. The normal diameter is less than 6 mm.[79] The appendiceal wall is composed of the serosa, muscularis, submucosa, and mucosa. These layers are typical of the intestinal wall, except that, in the appendix, the submucosa is heavily infiltrated with lymphoid tissue. The appendix is partially covered by a peritoneal fold known as the mesoappendix, which contains the appendicular artery, a branch of the ileocolic artery. The fold is often short, so the appendix may be folded or kinked.[118]

▶ TECHNIQUE AND NORMAL ULTRASOUND FINDINGS

A 5.0 MHz or 7.5 MHz linear-array transducer should be used, depending on the child's body habitus and need for penetration. The index marker should point cephalad or to the patient's right by convention. The graded compression technique is now the standard technique for the evaluation of appendicitis. It improves the quality of the examination and minimizes patient discomfort.[92]

With the patient supine, the transducer should be placed at the lateral edge of the right lower quadrant in a sagittal plane. It should be moved gently toward the midline to find the area of maximum tenderness. Gradual, gentle compression should be applied in the area of maximum tenderness, slowly advancing during expiration. Graded compression helps displace gas out of the cecum and ascending colon and moves the transducer closer to the appendix. Adequate compression has been achieved when the iliac vessels and psoas muscle are visualized, as the appendix will always be anterior to those structures.[79] Once the appendix is identified, the diameter should be measured in both transverse and longitudinal planes with electronic calipers.[101] A normal appendix will collapse with compression and should be observed for peristaltic activity.

▶ COMMON AND EMERGENT ABNORMALITIES

Appendicitis is diagnosed when the following findings are present (Figure 18-20):

- **Target shape:** Inflammation gives the appendix a classic targetoid or "bull's eye" appearance when viewed transversely. This results from anechoic fluid in the lumen, surrounded by an echogenic

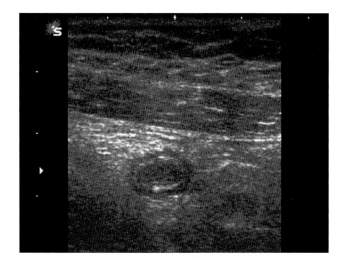

Figure 18-20. Ultrasound RLQ: short-axis view shows appendicitis with targetoid appearance. (Courtesy of James Mateer, MD)

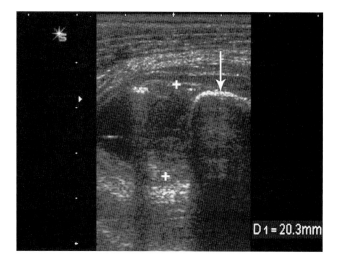

Figure 18-21. Ultrasound RLQ: A large appendicolith (>1 cm) is visible within the appendix (arrow). The appendix measures 20.3 mm and contains a small gas bubble with shadowing (just to left of top cursor). (Courtesy of James Mateer, MD)

ring of mucosa and submucosa, and an outer ring of hypoechoic muscularis externa.[96]
- **Diameter > 6 mm:** The diameter will be greater than 6 mm due to inflammation.
- **Noncompressible:** Inflammation and appendicoliths impede change in the shape of the appendix during graded compression.
- **No peristaltic activity:** The inflamed appendix is no longer able to contract sequentially.

► COMMON VARIANTS AND SELECTED ABNORMALITIES

The most important variant is that a normal appendix is rarely seen on ultrasound examination, which would render that study indeterminate. In his original work, Puylaert never identified a normal appendix.[92] One study reported that only 2% of normal appendices were seen on ultrasound.[78] One study was able to identify a normal appendix in 67% of healthy controls; however, 98% of histologically proven cases of appendicitis were not visualized on ultrasound. Consequently, they cautioned against concluding that a nonvisualized appendix is not inflamed.[101]

An appendicolith, when seen, helps make the diagnosis of appendicitis (Figure 18-21). An appendicolith resemble gallstones. They are dense and brightly echogenic, and produce acoustic shadowing.

The appendix loses its targetoid appearance when it perforates and is more difficult to identify. It may be surrounded by anechoic fluid or a developing abscess. A pericecal abscess usually demonstrates anechoic fluid with bright, hyperechoic debris (Figure 18-22). The ap-

pearance often varies, and the abscess may be loculated and more complex.

► PITFALLS

1. **Contraindications.** Children with a high clinical suspicion for appendicitis should be evaluated immediately by a pediatric surgeon in

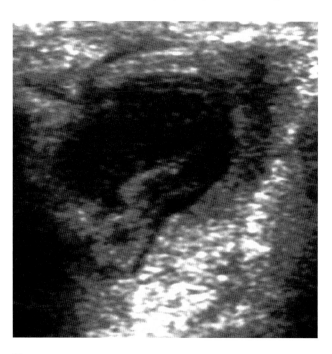

Figure 18-22. Ultrasound RLQ: Pericecal abscess. (Courtesy of Paul A Nancarrow, MD Children's Hospital Oakland, CA)

anticipation of expeditious appendectomy. They should not incur a delay in the emergency department or elsewhere for any unnecessary tests.

2. **Overreliance.** An ultrasound examination for this diagnosis has a limited sensitivity. A positive examination is an indication for operative management. A negative examination is not adequate to exclude appendicitis. Further evaluation with CT should be obtained.

3. **Perforation.** Sonography has a much lower sensitivity for recognizing appendicitis once perforation has occurred.[120–122] Peritonitis associated with perforation may inhibit adequate compression, and necrosis of the appendix may render it difficult to visualize.[120]

4. **Technical difficulties.** Air and adipose tissue scatter sound waves and make the ultrasound image difficult or impossible to distinguish. In an obese child, a 5.0 MHz transducer should be used to improve tissue penetration. An ultrasound examination may be complicated by an overlying gas-filled cecum and ascending colon or a location that is difficult to visualize, such as the retrocecum. While one study asserts that if the psoas muscle is visualized on graded compression, even a retrocecal appendix should be seen,[79] this has not been conclusively demonstrated.

► CASE STUDIES

CASE 1

Patient Presentation

An 18-month-old boy was brought into the emergency department by his mother complaining of 4 episodes of emesis and increased irritability since lunch. She stated he did not eat dinner, and she was concerned he might have a fever. In triage, his blood pressure was 87/50 mmHg, heart rate 130 beats per minute, respiratory rate 24 per minute, oxygen saturation 97% on room air, and temperature 38.5°C. His mucous membranes were mildly dry, and his heart and lungs sounds were normal. His abdomen was firm while crying.

Management Course

The child was administered a 20 mL/kg bolus of normal saline. A complete blood count (CBC) and basic metabolic panel were sent to the laboratory. The patient was reexamined after IV hydration and, without crying, exhibited guarding on abdominal examination. The pediatric surgeon was called in from home. While she drove in, the emergency physician performed a graded compression ultrasound examination of the right lower

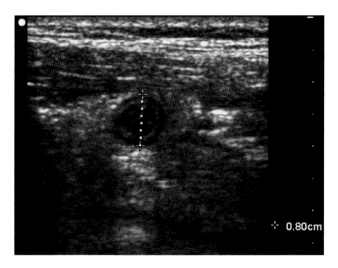

Figure 18-23. Case 1. Ultrasound: Appendicitis with a diameter of 8 mm in short-axis view.

quadrant. The emergency physician identified a classic targetoid appendix that measured 8 mm in diameter (Figure 18-23). The appendix was noncompressible, although the patient was not able to cooperate optimally with the examination. She relayed these results to the pediatric surgeon on arrival, and the patient was taken to the operating room where an inflamed appendix was resected.

Commentary

In Case 1, there was ample clinical evidence of appendicitis, and the patient could have been taken directly to the operating room. In this case, it was reasonable to perform an ultrasound examination while waiting for the pediatric surgeon. This did not delay definitive care. The positive results might have helped reassure the pediatric surgeon of the diagnosis. Graded compression can be difficult in children, especially younger children who understand only the pain.

CASE 2

Patient Presentation

An 8-year-old girl was brought to the emergency department by her father with a "tummy ache" after eating dinner. She had not been febrile or nauseated. Her last bowel movement occurred in the morning and was normal. Her blood pressure was 95/55 mmHg, heart rate 100 beats per minute, respiratory rate 22 per minute, oxygen saturation 98% on room air, and temperature 38.0°C. She did not appear ill. Her mucous membranes were moist, and her heart and lung examinations were normal. Her abdomen was soft but diffusely tender to palpation. No peritoneal signs were appreciated.

Management Course

The emergency physician sent blood to the laboratory for CBC, metabolic panel, liver function tests, and lipase. Urine was dip negative for infection or blood, but was sent for urinalysis and culture. The emergency physician performed a bedside ultrasound examination but was unable to confidently identify the appendix. Still concerned with the patient's abdominal pain, he administered broad-spectrum antibiotics and ordered an abdominal CT with IV contrast. The CT showed possible stranding in the periappendiceal fat. The child was thin, and the radiologist recommended clinical correlation. The pediatric surgeon decided to admit the patient for observation. Her pain worsened overnight, and she was taken to the operating room where a focally inflamed appendix was resected.

Commentary

In Case 2, the emergency physician recognized the limits of the ultrasound examination in detecting appendicitis and his limited experience in using this imaging modality. Because of his concern and these limitations, it was important that he followed up with a more definitive test. A formal ultrasound evaluation of the right lower quadrant could have been ordered, but CT is arguably a better study because it is more sensitive and specific. In this case, the CT showed possible signs of early inflammation but was not conclusive. The emergency physician ordered IV contrast for the CT, which is standard in many institutions. Other protocols involving oral, IV, and rectal contrast, alone or in combination, are also used. One study found CT without any contrast enhancement to have a sensitivity of 97%,[110] although this has not been definitively confirmed, and conflicting evidence exists.[123]

▶ PYLORIC STENOSIS

Idiopathic hypertrophic pyloric stenosis (IHPS) is an infrequent but serious problem encountered in any emergency department or pediatric clinic. Although there is usually no doubt about the need to hospitalize infants with symptoms suggestive of IHPS, the need to diagnose this entity rapidly stems from the desire to involve surgical consultants as early as possible.

IHPS is the pathologic hypertrophy of the muscle of the gastric pylorus that occurs for unknown reasons. The disorder has been associated with elevated gastrin levels as well as dysfunction of the pyloric ganglion cells.[124,125] Exposure to erythromycin has been associated with development of IHPS as well.[126] It does not appear to be a congenital disease.[127] The hypertrophied muscle obstructs outflow from the stomach, leading to persistent vomiting, classically projectile in nature. The disease occurs in 1:200–300 births,[128–130] with the typical age range of presentation between 4 and 6 weeks. IHPS has been reported as early as 10 days of age and as late as 20 weeks of age. The mean age of presentation is around 5 weeks, with males affected 3 to 6 times more than females.

IHPS is the most common surgical condition in infants.[131] Treatment consists of a pylorotomy, in which an incision is made into the hypertrophied pyloric muscle. Pylorotomy can be done as an open or laparoscopic procedure. Endoscopic pylorotomy done as an outpatient procedure under conscious sedation has recently been described.[132] Pylorotomy is curative and long-term sequelae are rare.[127] Atropine has been successfully used in Japan to reverse pyloric stenosis nonoperatively, but this treatment requires a prolonged hospital stay and a course of oral medication as an outpatient.[133] Atropine treatment has not been widely used in the United States.[134] Left untreated IHPS is typically fatal, as infants continue to vomit and become severely dehydrated with a hypochloremic, hypokalemic metabolic alkalosis.[125,131]

▶ CLINICAL CONSIDERATIONS

Most experts agree that the diagnosis of IHPS can be made in the appropriate age group (10 days to 20 weeks) on clinical grounds alone by palpation of the classic olive-shaped mass in the right upper quadrant in combination with the typical history of vomiting.[127,128,130] The positive predictive value of this combination of findings is nearly 100%. Though the number of patients presenting with these classic findings has declined somewhat over the last few decades, possibly because of patients presenting earlier in the course of the disease, it is still estimated that from 70 to 90% of cases meet the criteria for clinical diagnosis.[130] These patients can be referred directly for surgery without any imaging studies. Despite these recommendations, the majority of patients with suspected IHPS receive some type of imaging study prior to surgery.

The choice of imaging studies for IHPS is generally between a fluoroscopic upper gastrointestinal (GI) series and an ultrasound examination. Neither study seems to be clearly superior from a sensitivity or specificity standpoint. Sensitivities for ultrasound range from 85 to 100% and for upper GI series range from 90 to 100%.[135] One approach is to start with an ultrasound examination, and follow it with an upper GI series if the ultrasound examination is nondiagnostic or the ultrasound is negative but the patient's signs and symptoms persist. Sensitivity with this approach is 100%.[128] Another approach is to perform an ultrasound examination, and repeat the ultrasound if the initial study is nondiagnostic or symptoms persist. This approach has a sensitivity of 97%.[136]

The pros and cons of an upper GI series versus an ultrasound examination should be considered when deciding which imaging study to request initially for evaluation of the infant with projectile emesis. An upper GI series involves administration of contrast and exposure to small amounts of radiation but is a safe procedure. Despite concerns over potential complications, such complications were found to be nonexistent in a study looking at more than 600 patients undergoing an upper GI series.[128] An advantage of the upper GI series is that it more frequently defines other etiologies of vomiting; the most common being gastroesophageal reflux. In one study, when an upper GI series was the initial imaging study, only 6% of patients needed a second study (ultrasound) as part of their evaluation, as opposed to 17% when sonography was the first imaging study.[128] Despite the apparent advantage of using an upper GI series as the initial diagnostic study, ultrasound predominates as the study of choice for suspected IHPS.[129,137]

Ultrasound is a rapid and noninvasive means of assessing for a hypertrophic pyloric segment using measurements of the pyloric width and length. Unlike an upper GI series, which only implies a hypertrophied muscle by visualization of a thinned channel of barium through the pylorus, the ultrasound examination actually views the hypertrophied muscle itself. Infants are excellent candidates for ultrasound imaging because of their small size and limited body fat, which allows for the use of a higher frequency transducer producing higher resolution examinations. The examination is well tolerated by the ill infant and can be done at the bedside with the parent holding the infant, if necessary. No sedation is usually required and there is no exposure to contrast media or radiation.

► CLINICAL INDICATIONS

The ultrasound examination for IHPS is indicated in any patient aged 10 days to 20 weeks who presents with persistent painless, nonbilious vomiting where the clinical diagnosis is uncertain. Patients may or may not have a palpable olive-sized mass in the right upper quadrant or peristaltic stomach waves.

One third of infants presenting with symptoms suggesting IHPS will be found to have the disease. Anywhere from 50 to 90% of patients with IHPS have the classic olive-sized right upper quadrant mass, which is pathognomonic for the disease in the correct clinical setting. The hypertrophic pylorus may be found during palpation by locating the inferior border of the liver in the right upper quadrant, following it to the midepigastrium, then moving the hand caudally while pressing against the vertebral column. The olive-sized mass should roll under the finger tips.[125] An abdominal mass may not be palpated in some patients with IHPS, possibly because

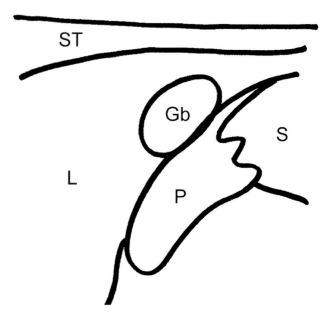

Figure 18-24. Line drawing with oblique cross section as depicted in Figure 18-25: location of pylorus in abdomen. ST = soft tissue, L = liver, Gb = gallbladder, P = pylorus, S = stomach.

of a stomach distended with air or tense abdominal wall musculature due to crying. When the diagnosis is not clear clinically, imaging should be employed.

► ANATOMICAL CONSIDERATIONS

The pylorus is contiguous with the stomach and usually lies just to the right of the midline and just caudal to the gallbladder (Figure 18-24). The stomach lies just to the left of the pylorus. Because of the inability of the stomach to pass fluid through the pylorus, the stomach may be distended with fluid, which makes its identification even easier. The hypertrophic pylorus itself is usually a linear structure lying along a line passing roughly from the right shoulder to the left hip (Figure 18-25).

► GETTING STARTED

This particular examination should be attempted only by more experienced examiners. It is not considered one of the "primary" applications in focused ultrasonography.

► TECHNIQUE AND NORMAL ULTRASOUND FINDINGS

The ultrasound examination for IHPS consists of identifying the hypertrophied pyloric wall muscle and

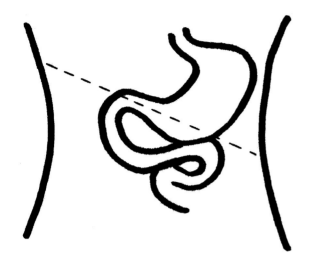

Figure 18-25. Line drawing: Orientation line for pylorus. The plane for imaging the pylorus along its length (represented by dotted line) is intermediate between the transverse and sagittal planes.

measuring the muscle wall thickness (MWT) as well as observing the dynamic function of the pylorus over 5–10 minutes.[124] The normal pyloric sphincter is a thin ring of muscle separating the pyloric antrum from the duodenum, with a MWT of <3 mm and a length of no more than a few millimeters. As the pyloric muscle pathologically hypertrophies, it both lengthens and thickens.

The examination should be performed with a 5.0–10 MHz linear or sector probe from an anterior approach on the supine patient. A warmed standoff pad (a latex glove with water or intravenous fluid bag will work) may be used to place the area of interest in the focal zone of the transducer. The pylorus is a cylindrical structure with an echogenic center surrounded by a sonolucent wall and is found between the gastric antrum and the duodenal bulb. The pylorus can be found in the transverse plane in the subxiphoid area by identifying the esophagus just anterior to the aorta, then sweeping the beam caudally to identify the stomach and then the pylorus.[131] The stomach is often filled with fluid from the obstruction, facilitating localization of the pylorus. If the stomach is empty, it may be filled orally with up to 100 mL of clear fluid. If the stomach is overly distended with fluid preventing visualization of the pylorus, rolling the patient in to the supine or left posterior oblique position may aid the examination.[131] Alternatively, a nasogastric tube may be placed to remove excess gastric fluid.

When making measurements, care should be taken to only measure the hypoechoic muscle layer and not the more echogenic mucosa, and measurements should be taken only on a perpendicular cross section of the pylorus or in the midline on a longitudinal section. The pylorus should be observed for at least 5 minutes to ensure that the MWT does not change. A changing MWT

that falls below 3 mm or obvious passage of gastric contents into the duodenum indicates pylorospasm and not IHPS.

► COMMON AND EMERGENT ABNORMALITIES

A pyloric MWT greater than 3 mm that does not vary over time is considered diagnostic for IHPS (Figure 18-26). Although several more complicated measurements that take into account patient weight, pyloric length, or

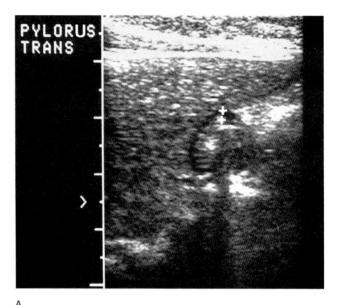

A

B

Figure 18-26. Ultrasound: Normal pylorus in cross section (A). The MWT was measured as 1.5 mm. Transverse view of pylorus in IHPS (B). The MWT was measured at 4.7 mm.

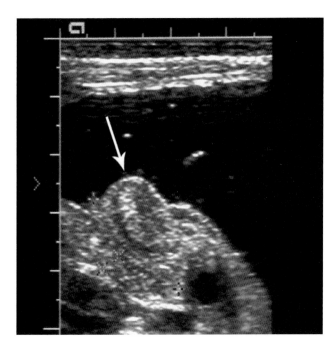

Figure 18-27. Ultrasound: Antral nipple sign. The nipple-shaped mass (arrow) protruding into the fluid-filled gastric antrum is formed by thickened gastric mucosa adjacent to the pylorus.

pyloric volume have been used to diagnose IHPS, the fact remains that the pyloric MWT remains the most widely accepted diagnostic standard and has a very high accuracy rate.[137,138] In addition, a functional assessment may support or refute the diagnosis of IHPS. In IHPS, no gastric contents should be seen transiting the pylorus to the duodenum during the ultrasound examination. Strong gastric peristaltic contractions may also be observed. The "antral nipple sign" has also been described with IHPS. The nipple-shaped mass found protruding into the gastric antrum is formed by thickened gastric mucosa adjacent to the pylorus (Figure 18-27).

▶ COMMON VARIANTS AND OTHER ABNORMALITIES

When performing the IHPS ultrasound examination, it is essential to recognize common normal variants that may mimic positive findings. The most important normal variant to exclude is pylorospasm. The MWT in pylorospasm may exceed 3 mm initially, but if observed over time the MWT varies, often dropping below 3 mm. Pylorospasm resolves without any surgical intervention.[139] Fluid in the colon or small bowel may appear to represent the stomach, leading to the presumption that a portion of the bowel is the pylorus. Also, a normal pylorus viewed tangentially instead of in true cross section may give falsely elevated muscle thickness measurements simulating IHPS.

If the cause of vomiting is not IHPS, clues to an alternate diagnosis may be seen. In malrotation with midgut volvulus, obstruction occurs past the pylorus so that a fluid-filled dilated proximal duodenum is present. Other rare causes of vomiting such as duodenal duplication, duodenal stenosis, or hiatal hernia may be visualized as well. The most common alternative diagnosis in patients suspected of IHPS is gastroesophageal reflux disease.

▶ PITFALLS

1. **Measurement error.** The difference between normal and abnormal may be 1 mm in size or less, so accurate measurement is key. In one study, 7 of 8 false-negative examinations were due to inaccurate measurements from poor technique.[136] Only the hypoechoic muscle layer should be measured, not the mucosa. Measurements should be taken only on a perpendicular cross section of the pylorus, or in the midline on a longitudinal section (Figure 18-28). A tangential cut on cross section will exaggerate the muscle thickness, as will a longitudinal view taken off the midline.

2. **Bilious vomiting.** Bilious vomiting suggests obstruction more distally than the pylorus, and malrotation with midgut volvulus should be considered in such cases. An upper GI series, not an ultrasound, would be the initial study of choice.

3. **Pylorospasm.** A pylorus with an elevated MWT should be observed for 5–10 minutes to ensure that the MWT does not vary into the normal range, indicating pylorospasm and not IHPS.

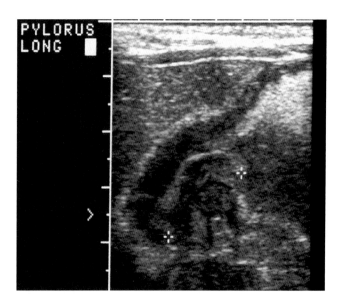

Figure 18-28. Ultrasound: Longitudinal view of the pylorus in IHPS. Measurement cursors are locating the borders of the pylorus (not MWT).

4. **Dehydration.** Significant dehydration may affect the muscle thickness of the pylorus, and it is recommended that the child be fluid resuscitated first in order to obtain a more accurate measurement. A falsely small measurement can be seen with significantly dehydrated patients.

► CASE STUDIES

CASE 1

Patient Presentation

A 1-month-old male infant was brought to the emergency department by his mother after the infant vomited everything he had eaten four times over the last 12 hours, and had been crying more than usual. The mother reported the child was otherwise acting normally, had an unremarkable birth history, and was on no medications. She had been bottle-feeding the infant milk-based formula.

On physical examination, vital signs were normal, although the infant did appear mildly dehydrated. He was alert and active. His head, neck, pulmonary, and cardiovascular examinations were unremarkable. The abdomen was soft, slightly distended and tympanitic, and nontender, and had good bowel sounds. No right upper quadrant mass was palpated.

Management Course

An intravenous line was established and 10 mL/kg of crystalloid was infused. A CBC and an electrolyte panel were sent, and an ultrasound examination was performed to evaluate the patient for IHPS. A 3.5-mm pyloric MWT was detected. The pylorus was observed for 5 minutes and did not demonstrate passage of gastric contents or change in MWT. The diagnosis of IHPS was confirmed and the patient was admitted to the hospital for intravenous hydration and surgical consultation for pylorotomy.

Commentary

The ultrasound examination was necessary only because the classic right upper quadrant mass was lacking on physical examination. Had this mass been present, it would have been reasonable to proceed directly to surgical consultation.

CASE 2

Patient Presentation

A 20-day-old female infant presented to the emergency department with 2 days of profuse vomiting, described as projectile. The grandmother (the patient's caretaker) reported that the infant had been well prior to the start of the vomiting, and other than being a 36-week premature infant, the birth history was unremarkable. The infant was fed on breast milk from a bottle since her mother worked full-time.

On physical examination, the child's vital signs included a blood pressure of 75/50 mmHg, heart rate 160 beats per minute, respiratory rate 36 per minute, and temperature 37.0°C rectally. The infant was alert and active although she appeared mildly dehydrated. Her head, neck, and pulmonary examinations were unremarkable. Cardiovascular examination showed capillary refill time of 3 seconds but was otherwise normal. Abdominal examination was normal and no mass could be palpated.

Management Course

An intravenous line was established and 20 mL/kg of crystalloid was administered. An ultrasound examination of the abdomen was performed and was negative for IHPS. Serum chemistries and CBC were unremarkable, as was the urinalysis. After fluid hydration, the patient vomited a challenge of oral electrolyte solution and was admitted to the hospital for continued hydration and observation.

The patient was observed for 6 hours. When the vomiting persisted, the patient's primary physician ordered a repeat ultrasound examination. The repeat ultrasound examination showed a MWT of 4 mm, which did not change with time. The diagnosis of IHPS was made and surgical consultation was then obtained for pylorotomy.

Commentary

Case 2 was an example of the imperfect negative predictive value of a single ultrasound examination. Repeat imaging was indicated (either an ultrasound or upper GI series) when symptoms consistent with IHPS did not resolve over time. Most infants with a significant history of vomiting and dehydration deserve a period of observation in the hospital regardless of the cause.

► INTUSSUSCEPTION

Intussusception is an uncommon but serious diagnosis in children, occurring in about 50 per 100,000 children per year.[140] Intussusception occurs when one piece of bowel invaginates and telescopes into a more distal segment, causing intermittent pain whenever the bowel peristalses on itself. The inciting event is believed to be an anatomical mass attached to the bowel ("lead point"), such as a Meckel's diverticulum or a lymphoma, that is pushed in to the distal segment of bowel by peristalsis. A lead point can be identified in only about 20% of intussusceptions in children, however. It is hypothesized that because a common site of intussusception in children is the ileocecal junction, that lymphoid hyperplasia in Peyer's patches may serve as the lead points.[141] Recently there has been an association of intussusception with an exposure to a particular rotavirus vaccine, which has since been removed form the market.[142,143]

Ages at the time of presentation typically range from 6 weeks to 1 year, but intussusception has been reported up to age 7 years.[144] The incidence peaks at 10–14 months, with 65% of patients younger than 1 year.[145] Patients present with a history of severe, intermittent abdominal pain. In the younger age group, a depressed level of alertness may be present. Up to 20% of younger children may present with vomiting as the only symptom. Although up to 75% of patients have some blood in the stool, the classic triad of intermittent abdominal pain, vomiting, and "currant jelly" stools occurs in less than 20% of cases.[145–147] Half of these patients have a palpable abdominal mass, usually in the right upper quadrant. Ninety-four percent of all pediatric patients with intermittent abdominal pain suspicious for intussusception that had a right upper quadrant mass on physical examination proved to have intussusception.[146]

Delays in diagnosis may lead to increasing bowel wall edema, ischemia, and bowel perforation, and makes the need for surgical intervention more likely.[148] In the 19th century, intussusception was usually a fatal disorder, but with current diagnostic and treatment tools mortality has been reduced to less than 1%. If diagnosed early, intussusception can be easily treated with hydrostatic or pneumatic enema reduction under fluoroscopic or ultrasound guidance.[149] Short-term recurrence rates of intussusception are between 5% and 10%, although this can be lowered by concomitant administration of dexamethasone.[150] Surgical intervention is indicated in cases of suspected bowel ischemia, perforation, or clinical instability.[151]

▶ CLINICAL CONSIDERATIONS

The imaging modalities commonly used in the evaluation of intussusception include plain abdominal radiographs, contrast enemas, and ultrasound. Plain films are appropriate in clinical situations suggestive of obstruction or perforation and demonstrate some abnormalities consistent with intussusception in 45–73% of cases. Typical plain radiograph findings include a "target" or "crescent" lucency soft tissue mass in the right side of the abdomen caused by intussuscepted mesenteric fat, lack of cecal gas, or a small bowel obstructive pattern.[147,152,153] Plain radiograph findings are nonspecific and further imaging studies are needed when intussusception is suspected. Plain films are helpful if free air is detected since liquid contrast studies are contraindicated in the

case of bowel perforation and surgical exploration is mandatory. Unfortunately, free air was not usually seen on the plain radiographs of children with intussusception and proven perforation.[141] Some authors advocate skipping plain radiography in children with a high index of suspicion for intussusception who do not have peritonitis.

The gold standard for the diagnosis of intussusception has been the contrast enema using barium or air. Not only are these studies diagnostic for the condition but they can be therapeutic as well. Despite being mildly invasive, enema studies are relatively safe. Radiation exposure is low, on the order of 4–7 rads. Although perforation of the bowel can occur, unless the bowel is completely obstructed or the patient is unstable, the risk of perforation is less than 1%.[146] Currently, the use of air enemas seems to be favored over barium or other liquid enemas. Air enemas are less messy and require less radiation. Although they have a slightly higher perforation rate than barium enemas (1.4% vs 0.2%), perforation associated with air enemas are smaller and leakage of air into the peritoneal space causes fewer problems than barium leakage.[152] The disadvantages of enema studies are their invasive nature, radiation exposure, and the requirement to move patients to the medical imaging suite. The major advantage to enema studies is that should intussusception be diagnosed, it can usually be reduced during the same procedure. Reduction of the intussusception involves infusing fluid or air rectally under fluoroscopic or ultrasound guidance, and pushing the telescoped segment out of the bowel into which it is invaginated.

Ultrasound has recently gained favor over enema studies as the initial diagnostic study for suspected intussusception. It has the distinct advantage of being entirely noninvasive, requiring no radiation exposure, and can be performed at the bedside if needed. The sensitivity of an ultrasound examination for intussusception ranges from 98 to 100%.[127,144,146,147,152] In addition, an ultrasound examination can locate pathologic lead points responsible for the intussusception; contrast enemas usually cannot. Ultrasound can also assess blood flow to the involved segment, although the clinical utility of this information has not yet been determined. The major disadvantage of an ultrasound examination is that if intussusception is diagnosed, the patient still requires a contrast enema for reduction.

There exists some controversy as to whether an ultrasound examination or contrast enema study should be done as the initial imaging choice. In one study, 20% of patients with suspected intussusception did not have the disease.[147] If an ultrasound examination is employed as the initial imaging modality, 20% of these patients will have been spared the radiation and invasiveness of a contrast enema. On the other hand, the 80% of patients diagnosed with intussusception would be subjected to both an ultrasound examination and a contrast enema study.

► CLINICAL INDICATIONS

An ultrasound examination is indicated in any patient suspected of intussusception. These patients usually present with severe, intermittent abdominal pain, often associated with vomiting, a right upper quadrant mass, or guaiac-positive stool.

► ANATOMICAL CONSIDERATIONS

Most cases of pediatric intussusception involve the terminal ileum invaginating into the cecum. The cecum is located in the right lower quadrant and is the gas-filled structure sandwiched between the anterior abdominal musculature and the large posterior psoas muscle. Continued pulling of the terminal ileum into the cecum pulls the cecum up into the right upper quadrant, giving rise to the classically described mass. In 45% of children aged 5 years or younger, the sigmoid colon loops into the right lower quadrant, and must not be confused with the cecum.[141]

► GETTING STARTED

Like the IHPS examination, this particular examination should be attempted only by more experienced examiners. It is not considered one of the primary applications in focused emergency ultrasonography.

► TECHNIQUE AND NORMAL ULTRASOUND FINDINGS

The highest frequency ultrasound probe, preferably linear, that still has the depth of penetration to focus on the area of interest should be used. In older children, this may be as low as 3.5 MHz; in smaller children, up to a 7.5 MHz probe may be used. The child should be examined supine. As with all children, a warmed conducting gel should be applied. If an abdominal mass can be palpated, this should be imaged in multiple planes. If no mass is palpated, then the path of colon should be followed from the cecum and terminal ileum to as far distally as possible, looking for a mass just deep to the abdominal wall. On an ultrasound examination, normal bowel appears as a hypoechoic ring (bowel wall) around a hyperechoic center (bowel contents, often with small gas bubbles causing a bright reflection and shadowing). Normal bowel should show peristalsis if observed for a short period of time. Imaging of the bowel may be more difficult in patients who have copious bowel gas due to bowel obstruction.

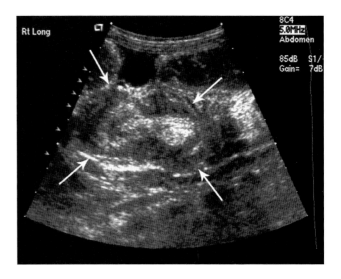

Figure 18-29. Longitudinal image of intussuception (arrows) demonstrating the "pseudokidney sign". Hypodense areas of intussuception are edematous bowel wall. Hyperechoic central area is caused by bowel contents (and possibly intussucepted mesenteric fat).

► COMMON AND EMERGENT ABNORMALITIES

When imaged along its longitudinal plane, the segment of intussuscepted bowel may appear to have multiple thick hypoechoic layers that are distinctly different from normal proximal and distal bowel, or may have the general appearance of a kidney ("pseudokidney sign") (Figure 18-29). Another well-described finding is of a sonodense center (bowel contents) surrounded by a sonolucent ring (bowel wall), which is known as the "target sign." This is seen on transverse cuts of the bowel (Figure 18-30). The typical intussusception is 3–5 cm in diameter.[141] Thickened bowel from a variety of causes, including inflammatory bowel disease, may give a similar appearance; however, if the bowel wall shows multiple echolucent layers, then intussusception must be suspected.

► COMMON VARIANTS AND OTHER ABNORMALITIES

In up to 20% of cases of suspected intussusception, another diagnosis is made. In a quarter of these cases, the ultrasound examination will find alternate abnormalities, including nonspecific bowel wall thickening (Crohn's disease, Henoch–Schönlein purpura, or enterocolitis), dilated loops of bowel filled with fluid, free intra-abdominal fluid, enlarged mesenteric lymph nodes, ovarian cysts, or volvulus. Free fluid does not necessarily imply perforation as long as no debris is seen in the free fluid.

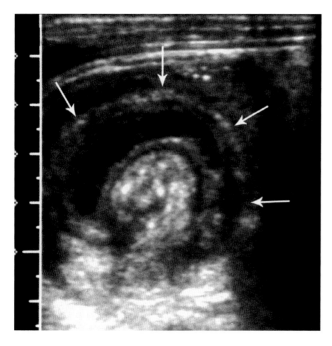

Figure 18-30. A transverse scan through ascending colon demonstrates the "donut" appearance of intussuception. The outer ring (arrows) is the intussuscipiens, while the central echoes are the intussusceptum. (From: Cohen HJ, Sivit CJ. *Fetal and pediatric ultrasound.* New York: McGraw-Hill, 2001; 287.)

In 10–20% of pediatric intussusception cases, a lead point exists and may be seen on an ultrasound examination. Meckel's diverticula, duplication cysts, polyps, or lymphoma may serve as lead points. An ultrasound examination may pick up other masses, such as a polycystic kidney, IHPS, or Wilm's tumor, or identify complications such as pneumoperitoneum.

▶ **PITFALLS**

False-positive ultrasound examinations are usually due to a sonologist's inexperience. In one study, the most common imitator of intussusception was fecal matter in the colon.[144] Other reported false-positive findings include hematoma of the bowel wall associated with Henoch–Schönlein purpura and nonspecific bowel wall edema or inflammation (such as with inflammatory bowel disease).

▶ **CASE STUDIES**

CASE 1

Patient Presentation

A previously healthy 2-year-old boy was brought to the emergency department by his parents after a 2-hour his-

tory of severe intermittent abdominal pain during which the patient squats to partially relieve the pain. The parents reported that the episodes lasted for 10 minutes and then subsided. He had vomited four times.

On physical examination, his vital signs were normal. He was alert and appeared in no distress. His head, neck, pulmonary, and cardiovascular examinations were unremarkable. The abdominal examination was soft and without tenderness, but with a palpable right upper quadrant mass. Rectal examination was guaiac negative. Just after the examination, the patient exhibited another episode of severe distress secondary to abdominal pain that lasted 5 minutes and then resolved.

Management Course

A complete blood count, chemistry panel, and urinalysis were ordered, and an intravenous line was established. The patient was administered a 10 mL/kg bolus of normal saline. An ultrasound examination demonstrated the mass to have the typical multilayered hypodense rings consistent with intussusception (Example: Figure 18-30). A subsequent fluoroscopic hydrostatic reduction was successful. The patient was admitted to the hospital overnight for observation.

Commentary

Case 1 was an example of a patient presenting to the emergency department with a history suggestive of intussusception and an abdominal mass on physical examination. The differential diagnosis of abdominal pain with an abdominal mass in children is lengthy and includes various tumors, adrenal pathology, pancreatitis, enteric duplication, various cysts, pyloric stenosis, polycystic kidneys, and hydronephrosis. Ultrasound is helpful in differentiating these general categories in a rapid and noninvasive manner. Prior to enema reduction of intussusception, adequate hydration is essential.[151]

▶ **URINE COLLECTION**

CLINICAL INDICATIONS

Both urethral catheterization and suprapubic aspiration for collection of urine may be considered in situations where uncontaminated urine collection for urinalysis and culture is paramount to patient evaluation. Both techniques have been shown to be safe and accurate, and both may be performed rapidly.[154] Urethral catheterization seems to be the favored method for uncontaminated urine collection, possibly due to its somewhat less invasive nature, as well as the fact that urethral catheterization is typically performed by nursing personnel. Without the use of ultrasound to assist with these procedures, reported success rates for suprapubic aspiration and urethral catheterization range widely from 46 to 90%[154–156] and from 31 to 100%, respectively.[154,156–158] Studies, however, have consistently shown improvement in success rates using ultrasound. For suprapubic aspiration, ultrasound improved the success rates from 64 to 90%,[159] 60 to 96%,[160] and 52 to 79%.[161] For urethral catheterization, ultrasound improved success rates from 72 to 96%[157] and 68 to 94%.[158]

Complication rates with either procedure are very low, on the order of 0.2%.[162] The most common complication of suprapubic aspiration is microhematuria, which occurs in up to 4% of cases and clears spontaneously within 24 hours.[159] Bowel perforation or gross hematuria during suprapubic aspiration are rare occurrences and tend to resolve without further sequelae.[155,163] Complications of urethral catheterization are rare and consist primarily of microhematuria, which usually resolves spontaneously, and cystitis.

ANATOMICAL CONSIDERATIONS

The bladder is located in the midline of the lower abdomen and is mostly hidden behind the symphysis pubis when empty, although it grows spherically and becomes exposed above the symphysis when filled with urine (Figure 18-31). In younger infants the bladder enlarges more posteriorly as it fills (as opposed to cephalad), which may make suprapubic aspiration more diffi-

cult. The bladder is anterior to the peritoneal space and, when full or partially full, is the first abdominal structure encountered when passing from anterior to posterior at a level just above the symphysis. This relationship makes it possible to insert a needle into the bladder from the anterior abdomen without placing any of the other abdominal organs at risk for puncture.

GETTING STARTED

If urine is present, the bladder can be located just above the symphysis pubis in the midline. If there is uncertainty as to whether or not the bladder is being visualized, the bladder is most likely empty or nearly empty. Free fluid in the pelvis may occasionally be mistaken for urine in the bladder. Fluid in the bladder can be identified by its rounded edges (typical for any fluid contained within a hollow cavity or structure). Collections of free abdominal fluid tend to have sharp edges and corners, as the fluid inserts itself around abdominal structures. Intraintestinal fluid is recognized by its echogenic gas bubbles or movement from bowel peristalsis.

▶ TECHNIQUE AND NORMAL ULTRASOUND FINDINGS

BLADDER IMAGING

The technique takes very little training and can be learned in less than 10 minutes. The bladder is imaged using a 5.0–7.5 MHz sector probe (a stand-off pad may be used if necessary) in a sagittal orientation in the midline of the lower abdomen. The probe should be placed just above the symphysis pubis (Figure 18-32). The probe is correctly placed if caudal movement of

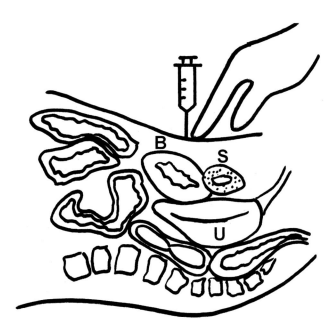

Figure 18-31. For suprapubic aspiration the needle is initially directed perpendicularly to the skin one finger breadth above the symphysis pubis. Bladder (B), Symphysis (S), Uterus (U), all bordered by bowel and rectum.

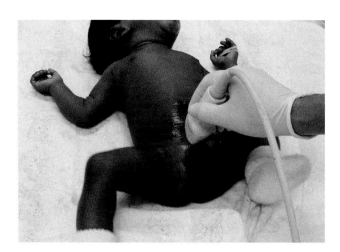

Figure 18-32. Probe position for bladder imaging in the infant.

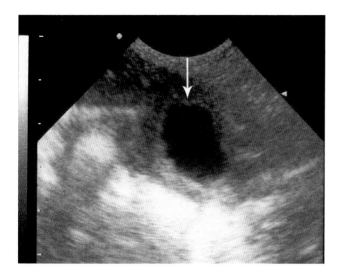

Figure 18-33. Sagittal midline image of the bladder (arrow) in an infant. Note that the bladder is about 1 cm in diameter (compare to centimeter scale to left of image), probably holding less than 1 cc of urine. SPA in this situation is less likely to be successful.

the probe causes the symphysis to shadow most of the screen. The bladder can be identified as a triangular-shaped (if mostly empty) or more spherically shaped (if mostly full) midline cystic structure (Figure 18-33).

URETHRAL CATHETERIZATION

Ultrasound can be used to assist with the collection of urine by urethral catheterization by viewing the bladder just prior to the procedure, ensuring that sufficient urine exists in the bladder to guarantee a successful catheterization. Ultrasound is especially helpful in cases where there is suspicion of an empty bladder (such as evidence of recent voiding or significant dehydration).

Several methods have been described for estimating adequacy of bladder volume (defined as a minimum of 2.0- to 2.5-mL urine). One-dimensional, two-dimensional, and three-dimensional measurement techniques result in approximately the same success rates, ranging from 94 to 100%.[157,158,164] Sample sizes in these studies are too low to show any real differences between the techniques. The simplest technique is to measure the transverse bladder diameter and postpone catheterization until the diameter is greater than or equal to 2 cm.[158]

SUPRAPUBIC ASPIRATION

Urethral catheterization may be contraindicated (urethral pathology) or unsuccessful (unable to locate meatus or pass catheter) in certain instances. Ultrasound-assisted or guided suprapubic aspiration of urine may be the procedure of choice in such cases. *Ultrasound-assisted* means that ultrasound is used primarily to determine whether sufficient urine exists in the bladder to perform a successful suprapubic aspiration, and secondarily to confirm the best location to insert the needle; ultrasound is not used during the needle insertion. *Ultrasound-guided* implies continuous ultrasound visualization of the needle during placement. For the initial attempt at the procedure, there appears to be no significant advantage of choosing ultrasound-guided over an ultrasound-assisted suprapubic aspiration in terms of success rate.[160]

Although blind suprapubic aspiration has success rates quoted as low as 46%, hydration for 15 minutes prior to the procedure along with observation for any spontaneous urination and percussion of the suprapubic are for dullness (indicating a full bladder) can increase the success rate to about 80%.[165] In one study, limiting the procedure to patients with a percussible bladder and no evidence of voiding for 1 hour prior to the procedure increased the success rate in blind suprapubic aspiration to over 90%.[155] To date, there have not been any studies to determine whether ultrasound improves success rates over these techniques.

EQUIPMENT

- Povidone-iodine solution
- 22- or 23-gauge needle, 1-inch length
- 3- to 10-mL syringe

PROCEDURE

It must first be determined with ultrasound that the bladder has sufficient volume for a successful suprapubic aspiration. In one study, when suprapubic aspiration was performed in infants who had a minimum bladder diameter of 2 cm in both the anteroposterior and transverse planes, success rate was 79%.[161] In another study, success of suprapubic aspiration correlated best with the transverse diameter of the bladder alone. Suprapubic aspiration was always successful if the transverse diameter exceeded 3.5 cm, and was never successful with diameters less than 3.0 cm.[166] If urine volume is insufficient, at least 30 minutes should elapse before attempting to rescan the bladder. The bladder should always be scanned in the transverse plane to confirm midline position prior to inserting the needle.

Under sterile conditions, the needle is inserted directly over the bladder and perpendicularly to the skin, one finger breadth above the symphysis pubis (Figure 18-31). While the needle is slowly advanced, constant negative pressure should be maintained on the syringe. If no urine is aspirated, then the needle should continue to be slowly advanced all the way to the hub. If unsuccessful, the needle should be backed out until the tip is just under the skin, and readvanced 30 degrees more caudad, again with negative pressure maintained as the needle is inserted slowly to the hub. If unsuccessful again, another attempt should be made with 30 degrees of cephalad angulation. If no urine is returned after the third attempt, the patient should receive further hydration and the procedure should be performed with ultrasound guidance.

▶ PITFALLS

1. **Complications.** Although a procedure with a very low complication rate, suprapubic aspiration does present the potential for serious misadventure if careful attention is not paid to the insertion site and direction of needle advancement.
2. **Other fluid.** Although unlikely, it is possible that another fluid-filled structure may be misidentified as the bladder. Fluid collections that are off the midline or more posterior in the abdomen should be regarded with suspicion. Free intra-abdominal fluid collections tend to have acute angles with "sharp edges" created by the fluid tracking around organs, as opposed to the more rounded edges of fluid inside a walled structure such as the bladder. Bowel will show intermittent peristalsis if observed for a short time, and usually will display a more heterogeneous content, often with shadow-forming gas bubbles.

REFERENCES

1. *Bioeffects and safety of diagnostic ultrasound.* Baltimore, MD: American Institute of Ultrasound in Medicine; 1997.
2. Childhood injuries in the United States. Division of Injury Control, Center for Environmental Health and Injury Control, Centers for Disease Control. *Am J Dis Child* 144(6):627–646, 1990.
3. Patel JC, Tepas JJ, III: The efficacy of focused abdominal sonography for trauma (FAST) as a screening tool in the assessment of injured children. *J Pediatr Surg* 34(1):44–47; discussion 52–44, 1999.
4. Jaffe D, Wesson D: Emergency management of blunt trauma in children. *N Engl J Med* 324(21):1477–1482, 1991.
5. Rodriguez A, DuPriest RW, Jr. Shatney CH: Recognition of intra-abdominal injury in blunt trauma victims. A prospective study comparing physical examination with peritoneal lavage. *Am Surg* Sep 48(9):457–459, 1982.
6. Davis JW, Hoyt DB, Mackersie RC, McArdle MS: Complications in evaluating abdominal trauma: diagnostic
7. peritoneal lavage versus computerized axial tomography. *J Trauma* 30(12):1506–1509, 1990.
7. Fischer RP, Beverlin BC, Engrav LH, Benjamin CI, Perry JF, Jr. Diagnostic peritoneal lavage: fourteen years and 2,586 patients later. *Am J Surg* Dec 136(6):701–704, 1978.
8. Soderstrom CA, DuPriest RW, Jr. Cowley RA: Pitfalls of peritoneal lavage in blunt abdominal trauma. *Surg Gynecol Obstet* Oct 151(4):513–518, 1980.
9. Rothenberg S, Moore EE, Marx JA, Moore FA, McCroskey BL: Selective management of blunt abdominal trauma in children—The triage role of peritoneal lavage. *J Trauma* 27(10):1101–1106, 1987.
10. DuPriest RW, Jr. Rodriguez A, Shatney CH: Peritoneal lavage in children and adolescents with blunt abdominal trauma. *Am Surg* Sep 48(9):460–462, 1982.
11. Trunkey D, Federle MP: Computed tomography in perspective. *J Trauma* 26(7):660–661, 1986.
12. Oldham KT, Guice KS, Ryckman F, Kaufman RA, Martin LW, Noseworthy J: Blunt liver injury in childhood: evolution of therapy and current perspective. *Surgery* 100(3):542–549, 1986.
13. Wisner DH, Blaisdell FW: When to save the ruptured spleen. *Surgery* 111(2):121–122, 1992.
14. Taylor GA, Guion CJ, Potter BM, Eichelberger MR: CT of blunt abdominal trauma in children. *AJR Am J Roentgenol* 153(3):555–559, 1989.
15. Knudson MM: Definitive care phase: pediatric trauma. In: LJ G, M M, Oldham KT ea, eds. *Surgery: Scientific Principles and Practice.* 2nd ed. Philadelphia, PA: JB Lippincott, 1997:377–386.
16. Karp MP, Cooney DR, Pros GA, Newman BM, Jewett TC, Jr.: The nonoperative management of pediatric hepatic trauma. *J Pediatr Surg* Aug 18(4):512–518, 1983.
17. Kohn JS, Clark DE, Isler RJ, Pope CF: Is computed tomographic grading of splenic injury useful in the nonsurgical management of blunt trauma? *J Trauma* 36(3):385–389; discussion 390, 1994.
18. Brick SH, Taylor GA, Potter BM, Eichelberger MR: Hepatic and splenic injury in children: role of CT in the decision for laparotomy. *Radiology* 165(3):643–646, 1987.
19. Bensard DD, Beaver BL, Besner GE, Cooney DR: Small bowel injury in children after blunt abdominal trauma: is diagnostic delay important? *J Trauma* 41(3):476–483, 1996.
20. Haller JA, Jr. Papa P, Drugas G, Colombani P: Nonoperative management of solid organ injuries in children. Is it safe? *Ann Surg* Jun 219(6):625–628; discussion 628–631, 1994.
21. Le Neel JC, Guiberteau B, Khosrovani C, et al.: [Traumatic hemoperitoneum of splenopancreatic origin. Apropos of 155 cases. Can a non-surgical treatment be proposed?]. *Chirurgie* 117(5–6):437–444, 1991.
22. Rossi D, de Ville de Goyet J, Clement de Cléty S, et al.: Management of intra-abdominal organ injury following blunt abdominal trauma in children. *Intensive Care Med* 19(7):415–419, 1993.
23. Giacomantonio M, Filler RM, Rich RH: Blunt hepatic trauma in children: experience with operative and nonoperative management. *J Pediatr Surg* 19(5):519–522, 1984.
24. Luna GK, Dellinger EP: Nonoperative observation therapy

for splenic injuries: a safe therapeutic option? *Am J Surg* 153(5):462–468, 1987.

25. Taylor GA, Fallat ME, Potter BM, Eichelberger MR: The role of computed tomography in blunt abdominal trauma in children. *J Trauma* 28(12):1660–1664, 1988.

26. Taylor GA, Kaufman RA: Commentary: emergency department sonography in the initial evaluation of blunt abdominal injury in children. *Pediatr Radiol* 23(3):161–163, 1993.

27. Meyer DM, Thal ER, Coln D, Weigelt JA: Computed tomography in the evaluation of children with blunt abdominal trauma. *Ann Surg* 217(3):272–276, 1993.

28. Turnock RR, Sprigg A, Lloyd DA: Computed tomography in the management of blunt abdominal trauma in children. *Br J Surg* 80(8):982–984, 1993.

29. Feliciano DV: Diagnostic modalities in abdominal trauma. Peritoneal lavage, ultrasonography, computed tomography scanning, and arteriography. *Surg Clin North Am* 71(2):241–256, 1991.

30. Goldstein AS, Sclafani SJ, Kupferstein NH, et al.: The diagnostic superiority of computerized tomography. *J Trauma* 25(10):938–946, 1985.

31. Mohamed G, Reyes HM, Fantus R, Ramilo J, Radhakrishnan J: Computed tomography in the assessment of pediatric abdominal trauma. *Arch Surg* 121(6):703–707, 1986.

32. Richardson MC, Hollman AS, Davis CF: Comparison of computed tomography and ultrasonographic imaging in the assessment of blunt abdominal trauma in children. *Br J Surg* 84(8):1144–1146, 1997.

33. Sivit CJ, Kaufman RA: Commentary: sonography in the evaluation of children following blunt trauma: is it to be or not to be? *Pediatr Radiol* 25(5):326–328, 1995.

34. Stylianos S: Commentary: the role of sonography in the initial evaluation of children after blunt abdominal trauma. *Pediatr Radiol* 23(3):164, 1993.

35. Hall EJ: Lessons we have learned from our children: cancer risks from diagnostic radiology. *Pediatr Radiol* 32(10):700–706, 2002.

36. Taylor GA, Eich MR: Abdominal CT in children with neurologic impairment following blunt trauma. Abdominal CT in comatose children. *Ann Surg* 210(2):229–233, 1989.

37. Akgur FM, Aktug T, Olguner M, Kovanlikaya A, Hakguder G: Prospective study investigating routine usage of ultrasonography as the initial diagnostic modality for the evaluation of children sustaining blunt abdominal trauma. *J Trauma* 42(4):626–628, 1997.

38. Akgur FM, Tanyel FC, Akhan O, Buyukpamukcu N, Hicsonmez A: The place of ultrasonographic examination in the initial evaluation of children sustaining blunt abdominal trauma. *J Pediatr Surg* 28(1):78–81, 1993.

39. Rozycki GS, Ochsner MG, Jaffin JH, Champion HR: Prospective evaluation of surgeons' use of ultrasound in the evaluation of trauma patients. *J Trauma* 34(4):516–526; discussion 526–517, 1993.

40. Price DD, Wilson SR, Murphy TG: Trauma ultrasound feasibility during helicopter transport. *Air Med J* 19(4):144–146, 2000.

41. Soundappan SV, Holland AJ, Cass DT, Lam A: Diagnostic accuracy of surgeon-performed focused abdominal sonography (FAST) in blunt paediatric trauma. *Injury* 36(8):970–975, 2005.

42. Boulanger BR, McLellan BA, Brenneman FD, et al.: Emer-gent abdominal sonography as a screening test in a new diagnostic algorithm for blunt trauma. *J Trauma* 40(6):867–874, 1996.

43. Liu M, Lee CH, P'Eng FK: Prospective comparison of diagnostic peritoneal lavage, computed tomographic scanning, and ultrasonography for the diagnosis of blunt abdominal trauma. *J Trauma* 35(2):267–270, 1993.

44. Tso P, Rodriguez A, Cooper C, et al.: Sonography in blunt abdominal trauma: a preliminary progress report. *J Trauma* 33(1):39–43; discussion 43–34, 1992.

45. Taylor GA, Sivit CJ: Posttraumatic peritoneal fluid: is it a reliable indicator of intraabdominal injury in children? *J Pediatr Surg* 30(12):1644–1648, 1995.

46. Partrick DA, Bensard DD, Moore EE, Terry SJ, Karrer FM: Ultrasound is an effective triage tool to evaluate blunt abdominal trauma in the pediatric population. *J Trauma* 45(1):57–63, 1998.

47. Neish AS, Taylor GA, Lund DP, Atkinson CC: Effect of CT information on the diagnosis and management of acute abdominal injury in children. *Radiology* 206(2):327–331, 1998.

48. Akgur FM, Aktug T, Kovanhkaya A, et al.: Initial evaluation of children sustaining blunt abdominal trauma: ultrasonography vs. diagnostic peritoneal lavage. *Eur J Pediatr Surg* 3(5):278–280, 1993.

49. Katz S, Lazar L, Rathaus V, Erez I: Can ultrasonography replace computed tomography in the initial assessment of children with blunt abdominal trauma? *J Pediatr Surg* 31(5):649–651, 1996.

50. Luks FI, Lemire A, St-Vil D, Di Lorenzo M, Filiatrault D, Ouimet A: Blunt abdominal trauma in children: the practical value of ultrasonography. *J Trauma* 34(5):607–610; discussion 610–601, 1993.

51. Holmes JF, Brant WE, Bond WF, Sokolove PE, Kuppermann N: Emergency department ultrasonography in the evaluation of hypotensive and normotensive children with blunt abdominal trauma. *J Pediatr Surg* 36(7):968–973, 2001.

52. Corbett SW, Andrews HG, Baker EM, Jones WG: ED evaluation of the pediatric trauma patient by ultrasonography. *Am J Emerg Med* 18(3):244–249, 2000.

53. Thourani VH, Pettitt BJ, Schmidt JA, Cooper WA, Rozycki GS: Validation of surgeon-performed emergency abdominal ultrasonography in pediatric trauma patients. *J Pediatr Surg* 33(2):322–328, 1998.

54. Soudack M, Epelman M, Maor R, et al.: Experience with focused abdominal sonography for trauma (FAST) in 313 pediatric patients. *J Clin Ultrasound* 32(2):53–61, 2004.

55. Mutabagani KH, Coley BD, Zumberge N, et al.: Preliminary experience with focused abdominal sonography for trauma (FAST) in children: is it useful? *J Pediatr Surg* 34(1):48–52; discussion 52–44, 1999.

56. Benya EC, Lim-Dunham JE, Landrum O, Statter M: Abdominal sonography in examination of children with blunt abdominal trauma. *AJR Am J Roentgenol* 174(6):1613–1616, 2000.

57. Krupnick AS, Teitelbaum DH, Geiger JD, et al.: Use of abdominal ultrasonography to assess pediatric splenic trauma. Potential pitfalls in the diagnosis. *Ann Surg* 225(4):408–414, 1997.

58. Coley BD, Mutabagani KH, Martin LC, et al.: Focused

abdominal sonography for trauma (FAST) in children with blunt abdominal trauma. *J Trauma* 48(5):902–906, 2000.

59. Ong AW, McKenney MG, McKenney KA, et al.: Predicting the need for laparotomy in pediatric trauma patients on the basis of the ultrasound score. *J Trauma* 54(3):503–508, 2003.

60. Blaivas M, Lyon M, Duggal S: A prospective comparison of supine chest radiography and bedside ultrasound for the diagnosis of traumatic pneumothorax. *Acad Emerg Med* 12(9):844–849, 2005.

61. Liu DM, Forkheim K, Rowan K, Mawson JB, Kirkpatrick A, Nicolaou S: Utilization of ultrasound for the detection of pneumothorax in the neonatal special-care nursery. *Pediatr Radiol* 33(12):880–883, 2003.

62. Kirkpatrick AW, Sirois M, Laupland KB, et al.: Hand-held thoracic sonography for detecting post-traumatic pneumothoraces: the Extended Focused Assessment with Sonography for Trauma (EFAST). *J Trauma* 57(2):288–295, 2004.

63. Hilty W, Snoey ER: Trauma ultrasonography. In: Simon BC, Snoey ER, eds. *Ultrasound in Emergency and Ambulatory Medicine* St Louis, MO: Mosby, 1997:151–189.

64. Ma OJ, Kefer MP, Mateer JR, Thoma B: Evaluation of hemoperitoneum using a single- vs multiple-view ultrasonographic examination. *Acad Emerg Med* 2(7):581–586, 1995.

65. Jehle D, Guarino J, Karamanoukian H: Emergency department ultrasound in the evaluation of blunt abdominal trauma. *Am J Emerg Med* 11(4):342–346, 1993.

66. Hilty W, Wolfe RE, Moore EE, et al.: Sensitivity and specificity of ultrasound in the detection of intraperitoneal fluid (abstract). *Ann Emerg Med* 22(5):921, 1993.

67. Meyers MA: The spread and localization of acute intraperitoneal effusions. *Radiology* 95(3):547–554, 1970.

68. Taylor GA, Sivit CJ: Computed tomography imaging of abdominal trauma in children. *Semin Pediatr Surg* 1(4):253–259, 1992.

69. Branney SW, Wolfe RE, Moore EE, et al.: Quantitative sensitivity of ultrasound in detecting free intraperitoneal fluid. *J Trauma* 39(2):375–380, 1995.

70. Frezza EE, Solis RL, Silich RJ, Spence RK, Martin M: Competency-based instruction to improve the surgical resident technique and accuracy of the trauma ultrasound. *Am Surg* 65(9):884–888, 1999.

71. Abrams BJ, Sukumvanich P, Seibel R, Moscati R, Jehle D: Ultrasound for the detection of intraperitoneal fluid: the role of Trendelenburg positioning. *Am J Emerg Med* 17(2):117–120, 1999.

72. Lupien C, Sauerbrei EE: Healing in the traumatized spleen: sonographic investigation. *Radiology* 151(1):181–185, 1984.

73. Filiatrault D, Longpre D, Patriquin H, et al.: Investigation of childhood blunt abdominal trauma: a practical approach using ultrasound as the initial diagnostic modality. *Pediatr Radiol* 17(5):373–379, 1987.

74. Givre S, Kessler S: The evaluation of blunt abdominal trauma: the evolving role of ultrasound. *Mt Sinai J Med* 64(4–5):311–315, 1997.

75. Ingeman JE, Plewa MC, Okasinski RE, King RW, Knotts FB: Emergency physician use of ultrasonography in blunt abdominal trauma. *Acad Emerg Med* 3(10):931–937, 1996.

76. Lund DP, Folkman J: Appendicitis. In: Walker WA, Durie PR, Hamilton JR, et al, eds. *Pediatric gastrointestinal disease: pathophysiology, diagnosis and management* 2nd ed. St Louis: Mosby; 1996:907–915.

77. Lund DP, Murphy EU: Management of perforated appendicitis in children: a decade of aggressive treatment. *J Pediatr Surg* 29(8):1130–1133; discussion 1133–1134, 1994.

78. Garcia Pena BM, Mandl KD, Kraus SJ, et al.: Ultrasonography and limited computed tomography in the diagnosis and management of appendicitis in children. *JAMA* 282(11):1041–1046, 1999.

79. Sivit CJ: Acute appendicitis. In: Cohen HL, Sivit CJ, eds. *Fetal and pediatric ultrasound: a casebook approach* New York: McGraw-Hill; 2001:444–449.

80. Savrin RA, Clatworthy HW, Jr. Appendiceal rupture: a continuing diagnostic problem. *Pediatrics* 63(1):36–43, 1979.

81. Graham JM, Pokorny WJ, Harberg FJ: Acute appendicitis in preschool age children. *Am J Surg* 139(2):247–250, 1980.

82. Jess P, Bjerregaard B, Brynitz S, Holst-Christensen J, Kalaja E, Lund-Kristensen J: Acute appendicitis. Prospective trial concerning diagnostic accuracy and complications. *Am J Surg* 141(2):232–234, 1981.

83. Hartman GE: Acute appendicitis. In: Behrman RE, Kliegman RM, Alvin AM, eds. *Nelson Textbook of Pediatrics* 16th ed. Philadelphia, PA: WB Saunders, 1996:1109–1111.

84. Mueller BA, Daling JR, Moore DE, et al.: Appendectomy and the risk of tubal infertility. *N Engl J Med* 315(24):1506–1508, 1986.

85. Trautlein JJ, Lambert RL, Miller J: Malpractice in the emergency department—Review of 200 cases. *Ann Emerg Med* 13(9, Pt 1):709–711, 1984.

86. Ravitch MM: Appendicitis. *Pediatrics* 70(3):414–419, 1982.

87. Reynolds SL, Jaffe DM: Diagnosing abdominal pain in a pediatric emergency department. *Pediatr Emerg Care* 8(3):126–128, 1992.

88. Bolton JP, Craven ER, Croft RJ, Menzies-Gow N: An assessment of the value of the white cell count in the management of suspected acute appendicitis. *Br J Surg* 62(11):906–908, 1975.

89. Fee HJ, Jr. Jones PC, Kadell B, O'Connell TX:Radiologic diagnosis of appendicitis. *Arch Surg* Jun 112(6):742–744, 1977.

90. Lewis FR, Holcroft JW, Boey J, Dunphy E: Appendicitis. A critical review of diagnosis and treatment in 1,000 cases. *Arch Surg* 110(5):677–684, 1975.

91. White JJ, Santillana M, Haller JA, Jr.: Intensive in-hospital observation: a safe way to decrease unnecessary appendectomy. *Am Surg* Dec 41(12):793–798, 1975.

92. Puylaert JB: Acute appendicitis: US evaluation using graded compression. *Radiology* 158(2):355–360, 1986.

93. Bell MJ, Bower RJ, Ternberg JL: Appendectomy in childhood. Analysis of 105 negative explorations. *Am J Surg* 144(3):335–337, 1982.

94. Rothrock SG, Skeoch G, Rush JJ, Johnson NE: Clinical features of misdiagnosed appendicitis in children. *Ann Emerg Med* 20(1):45–50, 1991.

95. Horton MD, Counter SF, Florence MG, Hart MJ: A prospective trial of computed tomography and ultrasonography

for diagnosing appendicitis in the atypical patient. *Am J Surg* 179(5):379–381, 2000.

96. Abu-Yousef MM, Bleicher JJ, Maher JW, Urdaneta LF, Franken EA, Jr., Metcalf AM:High-resolution sonography of acute appendicitis. *AJR Am J Roentgenol* Jul 149(1):53–58, 1987.

97. Blewett CJ, Krummel TM: Perforated appendicitis: past and future controversies. *Semin Pediatr Surg* 4(4):234–238, 1995.

98. Lobe TE: Acute abdomen. The role of laparoscopy. *Semin Pediatr Surg* 6(2):81–87, 1997.

99. Deutsch A, Leopold GR: Ultrasonic demonstration of the inflamed appendix: case report. *Radiology* 140(1):163–164, 1981.

100. Crady SK, Jones JS, Wyn T, Luttenton CR: Clinical validity of ultrasound in children with suspected appendicitis. *Ann Emerg Med* 22(7):1125–1129, 1993.

101. Hahn HB, Hoepner FU, Kalle T, et al.: Sonography of acute appendicitis in children: 7 years experience. *Pediatr Radiol* 28(3):147–151, 1998.

102. Karakas SP, Guelfguat M, Leonidas JC, Springer S, Singh SP: Acute appendicitis in children: comparison of clinical diagnosis with ultrasound and CT imaging. *Pediatr Radiol* 30(2):94–98, 2000.

103. Lessin MS, Chan M, Catallozzi M, et al.: Selective use of ultrasonography for acute appendicitis in children. *Am J Surg* 177(3):193–196, 1999.

104. Rice HE, Arbesman M, Martin DJ, et al.: Does early ultrasonography affect management of pediatric appendicitis? A prospective analysis. *J Pediatr Surg* 34(5):754–758; discussion 758–759, 1999.

105. Roosevelt GE, Reynolds SL: Does the use of ultrasonography improve the outcome of children with appendicitis? *Acad Emerg Med* 5(11):1071–1075, 1998.

106. Siegel MJ, Carel C, Surratt S: Ultrasonography of acute abdominal pain in children. *JAMA* 266(14):1987–1989, 1991.

107. Sivit CJ, Applegate KE, Stallion A, et al.: Imaging evaluation of suspected appendicitis in a pediatric population: effectiveness of sonography versus CT. *AJR Am J Roentgenol* 175(4):977–980, 2000.

108. Zaki AM, MacMahon RA, Gray AR: Acute appendicitis in children: when does ultrasound help? *Aust N Z J Surg* 64(10):695–698, 1994.

109. Kaiser S, Frenckner B, Jorulf HK: Suspected appendicitis in children: US and CT—A prospective randomized study. *Radiology* 223(3):633–638, 2002.

110. Lowe LH, Penney MW, Stein SM, et al.: Unenhanced limited CT of the abdomen in the diagnosis of appendicitis in children: comparison with sonography. *AJR Am J Roentgenol* 176(1):31–35, 2001.

111. Promes SB: Miscellaneous applications. In: Simon BC, Snoey ER, eds. *Ultrasound in Emergency and Ambulatory Medicine* St Louis, MO: Mosby, 1997:151–189.

112. Chen SC, Wang HP, Hsu HY, Huang PM, Lin FY: Accuracy of ED sonography in the diagnosis of acute appendicitis. *Am J Emerg Med* 18(4):449–452, 2000.

113. Allemann F, Cassina P, Rothlin M, Largiader F: Ultrasound scans done by surgeons for patients with acute abdominal pain: a prospective study. *Eur J Surg* 165(10):966–970, 1999.

114. Zielke A, Hasse C, Sitter H, Kisker O, Rothmund M: "Sur-

gical" ultrasound in suspected acute appendicitis. *Surg Endosc* 11(4):362–365, 1997.

115. Sivit CJ, Applegate KE, Berlin SC, et al.: Evaluation of suspected appendicitis in children and young adults: helical CT. *Radiology* 216(2):430–433, 2000.

116. Pena BM, Taylor GA: Radiologists' confidence in interpretation of sonography and CT in suspected pediatric appendicitis. *AJR Am J Roentgenol* 175(1):71–74, 2000.

117. Pena BM, Taylor GA, Fishman SJ, Mandl KD: Effect of an imaging protocol on clinical outcomes among pediatric patients with appendicitis. *Pediatrics* 110(6):1088–1093, 2002.

118. O'Rahilly R, Muller F: *Anatomy: A Regional Study of Human Structure.* 5th ed. Philadelphia, PA: WB Saunders, 1986.

119. Wakely CPG: The position of the vermiform appendix as ascertained by an analysis of 10,000 cases. *J Anat* 67:277, 1933.

120. Borushok KF, Jeffrey RB, Jr. Laing FC, Townsend RR: Sonographic diagnosis of perforation in patients with acute appendicitis. *AJR Am J Roentgenol.* Feb 154(2):275–278, 1990.

121. Fa EM, Cronan JJ: Compression ultrasonography as an aid in the differential diagnosis of appendicitis. *Surg Gynecol Obstet* 169(4):290–298, 1989.

122. Puylaert JB, Rutgers PH, Lalisang RI, et al.: A prospective study of ultrasonography in the diagnosis of appendicitis. *N Engl J Med* 317(11):666–669, 1987.

123. Kaiser S, Finnbogason T, Jorulf HK, Soderman E, Frenckner B: Suspected appendicitis in children: diagnosis with contrast-enhanced versus nonenhanced Helical CT. *Radiology* 231(2):427–433, 2004.

124. Blumer SL, Zucconi WB, Cohen HL, Scriven RJ, Lee TK: The vomiting neonate: a review of the ACR appropriateness criteria and ultrasound's role in the workup of such patients. *Ultrasound Q* 20(3):79–89, 2004.

125. Letton RW, Jr.: Pyloric stenosis. *Pediatr Ann.* Dec 30(12):745–750, 2001.

126. Cooper WO, Griffin MR, Arbogast P, Hickson GB, Gautam S, Ray WA: Very early exposure to erythromycin and infantile hypertrophic pyloric stenosis. *Arch Pediatr Adolesc Med* 156(7):647–650, 2002.

127. Morrison SC: Controversies in abdominal imaging. *Pediatr Clin North Am* 44(3):555–574, 1997.

128. Hulka F, Campbell JR, Harrison MW, Campbell TJ: Cost-effectiveness in diagnosing infantile hypertrophic pyloric stenosis. *J Pediatr Surg* 32(11):1604–1608, 1997.

129. Mendelson KL: Emergency abdominal ultrasound in children: current concepts. *Med Health R I* 82(6):198–201, 1999.

130. Olson AD, Hernandez R, Hirschl RB: The role of ultrasonography in the diagnosis of pyloric stenosis: a decision analysis. *J Pediatr Surg* 33(5):676–681, 1998.

131. Hernanz-Schulman M: Infantile hypertrophic pyloric stenosis. *Radiology* 227(2):319–331, 2003.

132. Ibarguen-Secchia E: Endoscopic pyloromyotomy for congenital pyloric stenosis. *Gastrointest Endosc* 61(4):598–600, 2005.

133. Corner B: Intravenous atropine treatment in infantile hypertrophic pyloric stenosis. *Arch Dis Child* Jan 2003;88(1):87; author reply 87.

134. Nagita A, Yamaguchi J, Amemoto K, Yoden A, Yamazaki T, Mino M: Management and ultrasonographic appearance of infantile hypertrophic pyloric stenosis with intravenous atropine sulfate. *J Pediatr Gastroenterol Nutr* 23(2):172–177, 1996.

135. Leonidas JC: The role of ultrasonography in the diagnosis of pyloric stenosis: a decision analysis. *J Pediatr Surg* 34(10):1583–1584, 1999.

136. Godbole P, Sprigg A, Dickson JA, Lin PC: Ultrasound compared with clinical examination in infantile hypertrophic pyloric stenosis. *Arch Dis Child* 75(4):335–337, 1996.

137. Rohrschneider WK, Mittnacht H, Darge K, Troger J: Pyloric muscle in asymptomatic infants: sonographic evaluation and discrimination from idiopathic hypertrophic pyloric stenosis. *Pediatr Radiol* 28(6):429–434, 1998.

138. Lowe LH, Banks WJ, Shyr Y: Pyloric ratio: efficacy in the diagnosis of hypertrophic pyloric stenosis. *J Ultrasound Med* 18(11):773–777, 1999.

139. Cohen HL, Zinn HL, Haller JO, Homel PJ, Stoane JM: Ultrasonography of pylorospasm: findings may simulate hypertrophic pyloric stenosis. *J Ultrasound Med* 17(11):705–711, 1998.

140. Applegate KE: Clinically suspected intussusception in children: evidence-based review and self-assessment module. *AJR Am J Roentgenol* 185(3, suppl):S175–s183, 2005.

141. Daneman A, Navarro O: Intussusception. Part 1: a review of diagnostic approaches. *Pediatr Radiol* 33(2):79–85, 2003.

142. Bines JE: Rotavirus vaccines and intussusception risk. *Curr Opin Gastroenterol* 21(1):20–25, 2005.

143. Murphy TV, Gargiullo PM, Massoudi MS, et al.: Intussusception among infants given an oral rotavirus vaccine. *N Engl J Med* 344(8):564–572, 2001.

144. Verschelden P, Filiatrault D, Garel L, et al.: Intussusception in children: reliability of US in diagnosis—A prospective study. *Radiology* 184(3):741–744, 1992.

145. Brown L, Jones J: Acute abdominal pain in children: "Classic" presentations vs. reality. *Emerg Med Pract* 2(12):1–24, 2000.

146. Harrington L, Connolly B, Hu X, Wesson DE, Babyn P, Schuh S: Ultrasonographic and clinical predictors of intussusception. *J Pediatr* 132(5):836–839, 1998.

147. Shanbhogue RL, Hussain SM, Meradji M, Robben SG, Vernooij JE, Molenaar JC: Ultrasonography is accurate enough for the diagnosis of intussusception. *J Pediatr Surg* 29(2):324–327; discussion 327–328, 1994.

148. Meier DE, Coln CD, Rescorla FJ, OlaOlorun A, Tarpley JL: Intussusception in children: international perspective. *World J Surg* 20(8):1035–1039; discussion 1040, 1996.

149. Gu L, Zhu H, Wang S, Han Y, Wu X, Miao H: Sonographic guidance of air enema for intussusception reduction in children. *Pediatr Radiol* 30(5):339–342, 2000.

150. Lin SL, Kong MS, Houng DS: Decreasing early recurrence rate of acute intussusception by the use of dexamethasone. *Eur J Pediatr* 159(7):551–552, 2000.

151. Daneman A, Navarro O: Intussusception. Part 2: An update on the evolution of management. *Pediatr Radiol* 34(2):97–108; quiz 187, 2004.

152. Littlewood Teele R, Vogel SA: Intussusception: the paediatric radiologist's perspective. *Pediatr Surg Int* 14(3):158–162, 1998.

153. Stanley A, Logan H, Bate TW, Nicholson AJ: Ultrasound in the diagnosis and exclusion of intussusception. *Ir Med J* 90(2):64–65, 1997.

154. Pollack CV, Jr. Pollack ES, Andrew ME: Suprapubic bladder aspiration versus urethral catheterization in ill infants: success, efficiency and complication rates. *Ann Emerg Med.* Feb 23(2):225–230, 1994.

155. Saccharow L, Pryles CV: Further experience with the use of percutaneous suprapubic aspiration of the urinary bladder. Bacteriologic studies in 654 infants and children. *Pediatrics* 43(6):1018–1024, 1969.

156. Tobiansky R, Evans N: A randomized controlled trial of two methods for collection of sterile urine in neonates. *J Paediatr Child Health* 34(5):460–462, 1998.

157. Chen L, Hsiao AL, Moore CL, Dziura JD, Santucci KA: Utility of bedside bladder ultrasound before urethral catheterization in young children. *Pediatrics* 115(1):108–111, 2005.

158. Witt M, Baumann BM, McCans K: Bladder ultrasound increases catheterization success in pediatric patients. *Acad Emerg Med* 12(4):371–374, 2005.

159. Ozkan B, Kaya O, Akdag R, Unal O, Kaya D: Suprapubic bladder aspiration with or without ultrasound guidance. *Clin Pediatr (Phila)* 39(10):625–626, 2000.

160. Kiernan SC, Pinckert TL, Keszler M: Ultrasound guidance of suprapubic bladder aspiration in neonates. *J Pediatr* 123(5):789–791, 1993.

161. Gochman RF, Karasic RB, Heller MB: Use of portable ultrasound to assist urine collection by suprapubic aspiration. *Ann Emerg Med* 20(6):631–635, 1991.

162. Kimmelstiel FM, Holgersen LO, Dudell GG: Massive hemoperitoneum following suprapubic bladder aspiration. *J Pediatr Surg* 21(10):911–912, 1986.

163. Simon G: Suprapubic bladder puncture in a private pediatric practice. *Postgrad Med* 72(1):63–64, 66, 1982.

164. Milling TJ, Jr. Van Amerongen R, Melville L, et al.: Use of ultrasonography to identify infants for whom urinary catheterization will be unsuccessful because of insufficient urine volume: validation of the urinary bladder index. *Ann Emerg Med.* May 45(5):510–513, 2005.

165. Chu RW, Wong YC, Luk SH, Wong SN: Comparing suprapubic urine aspiration under real-time ultrasound guidance with conventional blind aspiration. *Acta Paediatr* 91(5):512–516, 2002.

166. Garcia-Nieto V, Navarro JF, Sanchez-Almeida E, Garcia-Garcia M: Standards for ultrasound guidance of suprapubic bladder aspiration. *Pediatr Nephrol* 11(5):607–609, 1997.

CHAPTER 19

Vascular Access

John S. Rose, Aaron E. Bair, and Aman K. Parikh

Establishing reliable vascular access in an emergency situation is of critical importance. Many factors, including body habitus, volume depletion, shock, history of intravenous drug abuse, congenital deformity, and cardiac arrest can make obtaining vascular access in the critically ill or injured patient extremely difficult. The introduction of real-time bedside ultrasound into emergency and acute care settings has been an important advance for facilitating rapid and successful vascular access.

▶ CLINICAL CONSIDERATIONS

For central access, the use of an anatomic landmark-guided approach has been the traditional practice. Internal jugular vein location traditionally relies on the sternocleidomastoid muscle and clavicular landmarks; the femoral vein relies on the inguinal ligament and femoral artery pulsation landmarks; and the subclavian vein relies on clavicular landmarks. In many patients, however, these landmarks may be distorted, obscured, or nonexistent. In addition, normal variations in the anatomic relationship of the internal jugular vein may make cannulation difficult.[1] In the emergent situation, attempting central vascular access with poor external landmarks is frequently approached using a "best guess" estimate of the vessel location. This may lead to multiple needle passes to locate the vessel. Excessive bleeding, inadvertent arterial puncture, vessel laceration, pneumothorax, and hemothorax are some of the potential complications of central vascular access. The incidence of complications increases when multiple attempts are required for cannulation.[2–5] In patients with an underlying coagu-

lopathy (pathologic or therapeutic), multiple attempts can carry significant morbidity due to hemorrhage.[6,7]

The introduction of portable bedside ultrasound has been very effective in assisting with the placement of central venous access catheters. For internal jugular vein cannulation, ultrasound use has been described by numerous disciplines, including emergency medicine, critical care medicine, anesthesiology, obstetrics/gynecology, nephrology, surgery, and radiology.[2,3,8–10] When compared to the external landmark approach, ultrasound-guided internal jugular vein cannulation results in fewer complications and is more effective in time-to-cannulation and first-attempt success.[2,6,11–14] For femoral vein cannulation, the ultrasound-guided approach was found to be more successful than the landmark approach in patients presenting in cardiac arrest.[15]

Peripheral venous access is less invasive and is used more commonly in the emergency department than central access. The inability to find an adequate peripheral vein generally requires that the clinician consider central venous access. Traditionally, successful peripheral venous cannulation requires that a vein first be visualized or palpated. Some peripheral veins that are not readily apparent on the skin surface can be clearly visualized with the use of ultrasound, which may obviate the need for central access.[15,16] The basilic and cephalic veins of the arm are superficial veins that are not generally visible but are readily cannulated using ultrasound guidance. Basilic vein cannulation has been shown to be very successful in the emergency department setting in patients in whom it was difficult to obtain other peripheral vascular access.[17] Basilic vein cannulation is readily learned by novice users.[18] In addition, basilic veins have been cannulated using ultrasound in patients requiring prolonged outpatient intravenous access.[19]

Evidence supporting the use of ultrasound for vascular access has become overwhelming. In 2001, a report published by the Agency for Healthcare Research and Quality (AHRQ) on patient safety in health care included a chapter strongly advocating the use of ultrasound in central venous catheterization.[20] The resulting scientific and policy positions favor the use of ultrasound for central venous access stronger than any other emergency ultrasound application. The National Institute for Clinical Excellence (NICE) has also recommended that central venous catheters be inserted under ultrasound guidance.[21]

► CLINICAL INDICATIONS

Indications for ultrasound guidance for vascular access are:

- **To confirm vessel location prior to landmark-based approach.** This is termed the *static* approach with ultrasound for intravenous access. The patient is positioned and the ultrasound transducer is placed on the patient to confirm the predicted landmark-based anatomy. The transducer is then removed, and the patient is prepped for vascular access via the standard landmark-based technique. This can be performed by a single operator and does not require additional adjunctive equipment such as a sterile transducer sleeve. This approach is particularly useful when the patient is unable to assume the standard position for cannulation and the operator wishes to confirm vessel location. One randomized trial demonstrated that the static technique is superior to traditional landmark technique for central venous cannulation.[13]

- **To assist in real-time cannulation under direct ultrasound visualization.** This is termed the *dynamic* approach. The ultrasound transducer is inserted into a sterile sleeve and placed on the patient after the sterile prep. The operator can then watch the needle enter the vessel under real-time ultrasound guidance. This technique can involve one or two operators.[22] With two operators, real-time vessel visualization can be maintained throughout the entire procedure. With a single operator, the transducer must be put down prior to guidewire insertion to free up the nondominant hand. This technique takes full advantage of the benefits of ultrasound-assisted vascular access. The dynamic technique is the approach advocated in the AHRQ report. Although this method may require more preparation time, it can save precious minutes when routine land-

marks are not evident in the critically ill or injured patient.

- **To minimize the number of vascular access attempts.** In certain clinical situations, definitive access is needed in patients at risk for significant complications from multiple vascular attempts. Patients with therapeutic anticoagulation, disseminated intravascular coagulation, thrombocytopenia, hemophilia, or any condition that adds significant risk to vascular access attempts can benefit from the higher first-attempt success rate afforded by ultrasound.

- **To assist in alternative peripheral access.** Alternative peripheral vascular access is important in many patients. Either static or dynamic ultrasound techniques can be used to locate and facilitate cannulation of peripheral vessels. Saphenous, basilic, and cephalic veins are all easily located with ultrasound but difficult to locate with surface visualization. Some clinical situations require vascular access but choosing a central approach may add unwarranted risk. Ultrasound-guided approach to peripheral veins allows for reliable access without the need for central venous access. This has been shown to be helpful in both adults and children.[15,23]

- **To facilitate arterial puncture or cannulation.** Ultrasound can be used to locate arteries for puncture or cannulation. Radial, brachial, and femoral arteries are easily located with ultrasound. Both dynamic and static techniques can be used to facilitate arterial puncture.

► ANATOMIC CONSIDERATIONS

At times it may not be easy to distinguish veins from arteries with B-mode ultrasound. Recognition of key sonographic characteristics can help distinguish veins from arteries. In comparison to arteries, veins have several distinct sonographic features: (1) they are more easily compressed, (2) have thinner walls, and (3) have no arterial pulsation. In addition, central veins possess characteristic triphasic venous pulsations that can be distinguished from arteries. The addition of color flow is a useful adjunct on ultrasound units used for vascular access.

CANNULATION OF THE INTERNAL JUGULAR VEIN

Ultrasound allows for easy localization of the internal jugular vein. In addition, the carotid artery can be distinguished from the adjacent internal jugular vein. The internal jugular vein lies deep to the sternocleidomastoid muscle and is lateral and superficial to the carotid

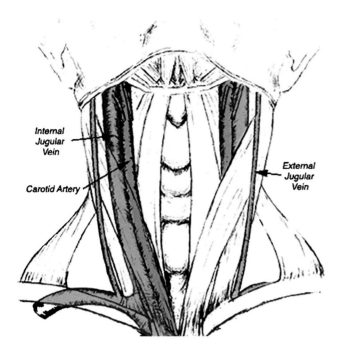

Figure 19-1. The anterior superficial structures of the neck.

CANNULATION OF THE SUBCLAVIAN VEIN USING A SUPRACLAVICULAR APPROACH

Placement of a central venous catheter into the subclavian vein at the take-off of the internal jugular vein is possible using ultrasound guidance (Figure 19-3). The use of ultrasound for the traditional infraclavicular approach to subclavian vein catheter placement is limited by the large acoustic shadow created by the clavicle. In contrast, the supraclavicular approach allows for adequate sonographic visualization of the proximal subclavian vein anatomy.

CANNULATION OF THE SUBCLAVIAN/AXILLARY VEIN USING AN INFRACLAVICULAR APPROACH

For this approach, the ultrasound transducer should be placed inferior and lateral to the clavicle. It is oriented in long axis over the proximal axillary vein. Although this is a more lateral approach than the traditional blind infraclavicular technique, it allows for excellent visualization of the axillary vein just before it technically changes name to the subclavian vein (Figure 19-4).

CANNULATION OF THE FEMORAL VEIN

The initial vascular survey is initiated by placing the transducer in a transverse position just below the midportion of the inguinal ligament. Identification of the key vascular structures begins just below the inguinal ligament and medial to the femoral arterial pulsation.

artery. Using the sternocleidomastoid muscle as the external landmark, the internal jugular vein sits below the bifurcation of the sternal and clavicular heads of the muscle (Figures 19-1 and 19-2). It is important to note that the relative relationship of the carotid artery to the internal jugular vein may change with head position. Specific technical details of internal jugular vein cannulation are provided below.

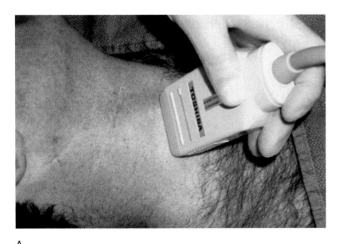
A

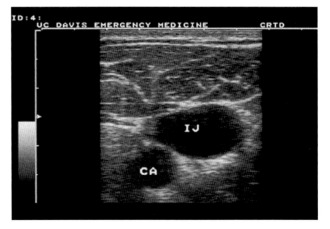
B

Figure 19-2. Ultrasound image of the large internal jugular vein and deeper carotid artery. Probe position (A) and corresponding ultrasound image (B). CA = Carotid artery, IJ = Internal Jugular vein.

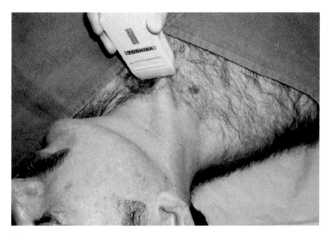

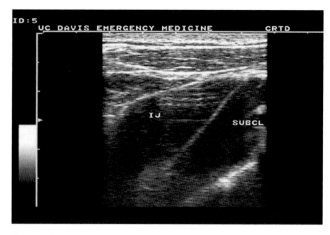

A

B

Figure 19-3. Placement of the transducer to facilitate visualization of the internal jugular/subclavian vein junction using a supraclavicular approach (A). In some patients, a more lateral probe position is required. Transverse view of the "venous lake" created by the combined subclavian vein and internal jugular vein (B).

The compression technique may be used to distinguish the readily compressible vein from the less compressible artery (Figure 19-5). In addition, appreciating the variable relationships of the vascular structures with respect to limb position is important. Either the static or dynamic technique can be utilized for femoral vein cannulation. Recent evidence has indicated that the routine use of the femoral vein for central venous access should be limited in adults because of higher complication rates.[20]

PERIPHERAL VENOUS CANNULATION

Ultrasound will permit localization of veins that often do not have consistent anatomic relationships or are too deep to be readily palpable. Of note, the super-

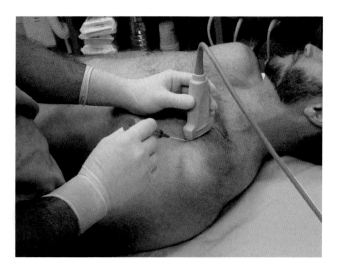

Figure 19-4. Probe placement for cannulation of the subclavian/axillary vein using the infraclavicular approach. (Courtesy of Michael Blaivas, MD)

ficial venous structures are easily collapsed with even slight pressure of the transducer on the skin. This feature of collapsibility is useful for distinguishing between veins and arteries. Superficial veins may not be identified, however, if they are collapsed by inadvertent excessive pressure on the transducer. Placing a tourniquet on the extremity to maximize vein dilation is also advisable. Once a suitable vein is identified, the process of intravenous catheter placement is largely unchanged from standard practice using routinely available venous catheters. With respect to ultrasound guidance in peripheral venous access, either the static or dynamic technique may be successfully utilized. Ultrasound use for peripheral IV access has been shown to decrease the number of needle sticks and time to successful cannulation, and can be readily used by novice users.[15,16]

CANNULATION OF THE EXTERNAL JUGULAR VEIN

Since the external jugular vein is superficial, it is often readily identified by visualization and palpation without ultrasound assistance (Figure 19-6). However, limited range of motion (i.e., cervical spine precautions) or adiposity may make this vessel difficult to cannulate without ultrasound guidance.

CANNULATION OF THE BRACHIAL AND CEPHALIC VEINS OF THE UPPER EXTREMITY

The antecubital veins of the arms are commonly used for venous access in the emergency setting, as are the

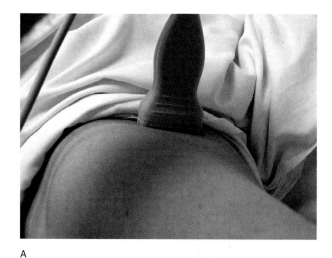

A

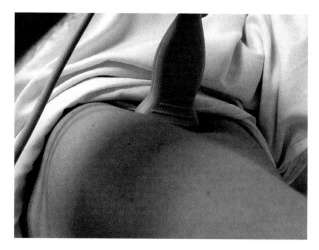

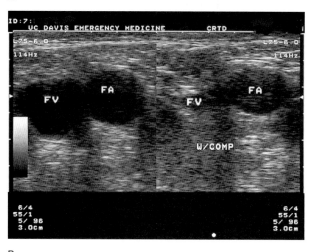

B

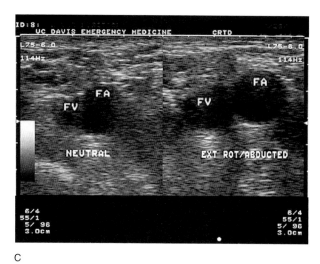

C

Figure 19-5. Femoral vein: Gentle pressure is applied to the transducer to identify venous structures by their easy compressibility (A). Femoral vein (FV) collapses with compression, and the femoral artery (FA) retains its shape even with compression (B). Femoral vein (FV) position is seen to vary with hip abduction and external rotation (C). In neutral position (left frame), the vein is closely opposed to the femoral artery (FA); however, when the hip is abducted and rotated, the vein is displaced from the artery (right frame). (Courtesy of Michael Blaivas, MD, (A))

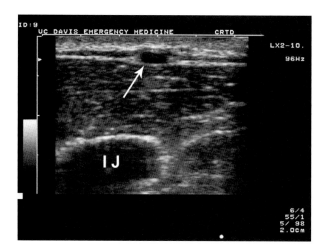

Figure 19-6. Transverse ultrasound of the external jugular vein (arrow) and internal jugular veins (IJ).

more proximal cephalic and brachial veins (Figure 19-7a). The cephalic and brachial veins lie deeper in the structures of the upper arm and are not readily palpable; consequently, these veins are not generally used for intravenous catheter placement in the absence of ultrasound guidance. Caution should be taken with the more proximal brachial vein since it lies immediately adjacent to the ulnar and median nerves. In most patients, the depth of these vessels and angle required for cannulation mandates that a longer catheter (2.5 inches) be used. An example of probe placement and vessel visualization for proximal vein cannulation is demonstrated in Figure 19-7.

ARTERIAL CANNULATION

In the absence of color flow Doppler, real-time arterial pulsation, thickness of arterial wall, and lack of arterial

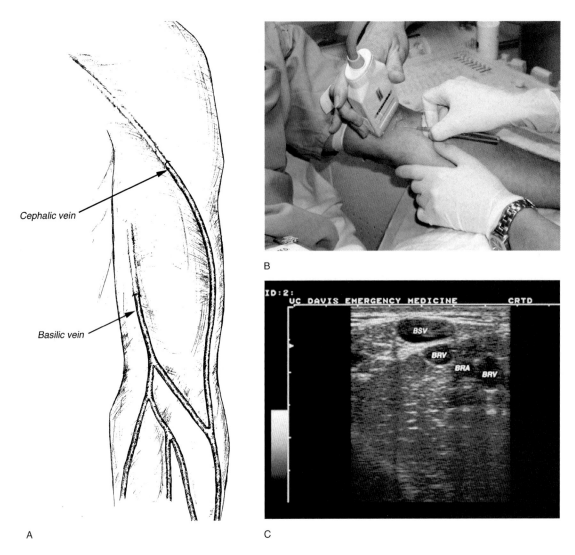

Cephalic vein

Basilic vein

A

B

C

Figure 19-7. The superficial veins of the proximal upper extremity (A). Demonstration of probe placement for cannulation of the basilic vein (B). An image demonstrating transverse ultrasound orientation (C) of the relatively superficial basilic vein (BSV) with deeper lying brachial artery and veins (BRV, BRA). Note the proximity of the brachial artery to its venous counterpart makes inadvertent arterial puncture a possibility.

compressibility are all sonographic features that help distinguish arterial from venous anatomy. The mechanics of placing an arterial catheter or simple arterial puncture can proceed along traditional technical guidelines once the pertinent anatomy has been recognized.

▶ TECHNIQUE AND NORMAL ULTRASOUND FINDINGS

Use of the dynamic technique can be summarized by the Four Ps: Pre-scan, Preparation, Poke, and Path. A 7.5 or 10 MHz, linear array transducer should be used.

The purpose of the **Pre-scan** is to survey the underlying vessels and confirm the target vessel appropriately (Figure 19-8). For internal jugular vein cannulation, three structures should be seen during the pre-scan: thyroid gland, internal jugular vein, and carotid artery. Generally, all three structures should be visualized before proceeding. The internal jugular vein can be easily compressed, especially in volume-depleted patients; confirming its presence in relationship to the other structures will ensure verification of the proper target vessel. When standing at the head of the bed, the position marker should be pointed toward the patient's left side. This will ensure the proper relationship of the underlying anatomy to the ultrasound image anatomy. For example, when cannulating the patient's right internal jugular vein,

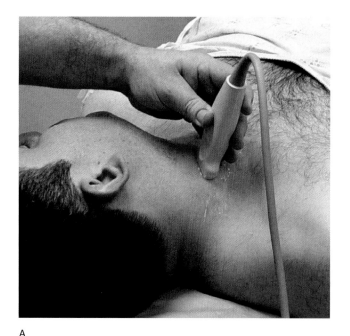

A

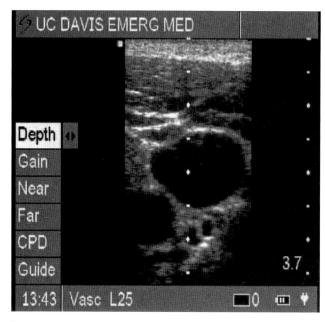

B

Figure 19-8. First P-Prescan of jugular vein (A). Transverse orientation of right internal jugular vein and right carotid artery (B). Note needle guide present.

the thyroid, carotid artery, and internal jugular vein will be from left to right anatomically as well as on the ultrasound monitor. Thus, when moving the needle more medially, or to the left, it will move left on the monitor. When moving the needle more lateral, or to the right, it will move to the right on the monitor.

The second P stands for **Preparation**. The patient's skin is prepared for a sterile procedure in the usual fashion. For dynamic cannulation, the transducer is prepared with a sterile sleeve and gel. Several types of sleeves are available for ultrasound transducers. Sleeves that cover the transducer and cable are preferred since they can be placed on the sterile field and easily located for single operator use (Figure 19-9). Careful application of coupling gel to the transducer prior to placement in a sterile sleeve is necessary to avoid entrapment of air bubbles. The sterile sleeve is placed and generally secured with elastic bands. Sterile coupling gel will then be applied to the outside of the transducer sleeve prior to further imaging. With the sterile barrier in place, the transducer is ready for use. The use of a sterile glove is an alternative to using a specialized sterile sleeve. The transducer cable will not be sterile and care is required to avoid contaminating the field.

The **poke** refers to the initial skin puncture (prior to actual venipuncture), which places the needle in the subcutaneous tissues where it is identified before further advancement. The initial insertion of the needle and its subsequent localization is an important step. Advancing the needle prior to localization can result in a misdirected

path. Figure 19-10 demonstrates proper needle position for the initial insertion. It should be noted how close the needle is to the transducer.

Following the **path** of the needle and adjusting the course are keys to successful placement. Tissue motion during real-time imaging of the procedure can help direct the advancing needle prior to visualization of the needle itself. The needle will subsequently be detectable

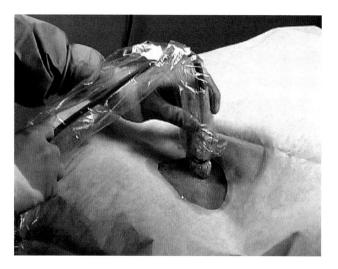

Figure 19-9. Second P-Preparation. Note the transducer with long sterile sleeve allowing easy use in a sterile field.

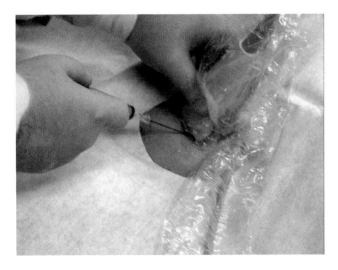

Figure 19-10. Third P-Poke. Note how close the needle is to the transducer in order to locate the needle tip immediately after the puncture.

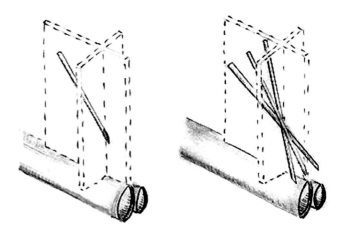

Figure 19-12. Drawing illustrating pitfall during the fourth P-Path. Note how in the transverse plane the three needles all converge in one point although their vectors are different. This illustrates why it is important to follow the tip of the needle into the vessel.

through ring-down artifact (Figure 19-11). The needle is directed toward the vessel while using the monitor display to locate the needle tip. Care must be taken to ensure that the needle *tip* has been located prior to advancement of the needle. A common error involves mistaking the needle shaft for the needle tip and thereby misjudging the actual tip location. Figure 19-12 illustrates scanning with three different needle vectors. Note the convergence of all three needle paths in the transverse plane. However, each needle tip is in a different loca-

tion in relation to the vessel. Prior to successful cannulation, the vein will be seen to deform with the pressure of the advancing needle (Figure 19-13). Confirmation of successful venipuncture proceeds as usual with a flash of venous blood into the syringe. With either static or dynamic technique, the mechanics of catheter placement (i.e., using the Seldinger technique) proceeds unchanged from routine technique.

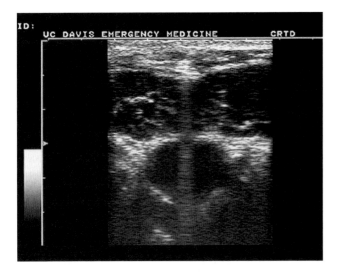

Figure 19-11. Ring-down artifact of needle after the initial puncture. This is used to localize the needle prior to advancing.

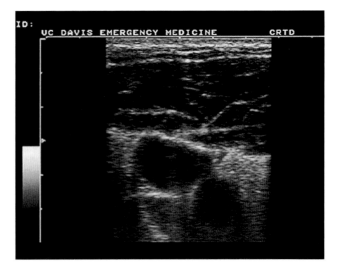

Figure 19-13. Tenting or deformity of the vessel will occur prior to needle penetration. In this example, the vessel is slightly collapsed. In real time, the vessel wall may briefly indent, then quickly rebound as the needle enters.

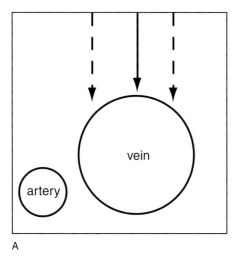

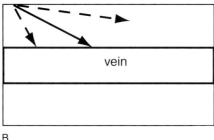

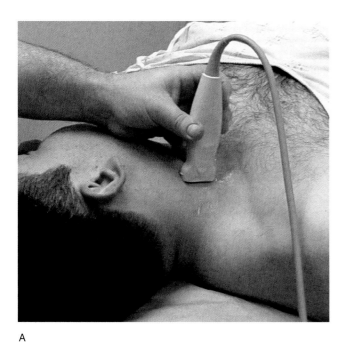

Figure 19-14. Diagram illustrating transverse and longitudinal orientation. Transverse gives better lateral/medial positioning (A). Longitudinal gives better slope and depth positioning (B).

TRANSDUCER ORIENTATION: LONGITUDINAL VERSUS TRANSVERSE

Variations of probe positioning will yield different information relative to vessel and needle placement. Transverse probe positioning gives information related to lateral orientation. The longitudinal probe position gives depth and slope information (Figure 19-14). The authors generally rely primarily on transverse short-axis imaging to assist with venous cannulation. The transverse short-axis orientation is most helpful with demonstrating relationships to other adjacent anatomy (Figure 19-8). Recent evidence supports the transverse short-axis approach for novice users.[24] The longitudinal orientation will help with needle orientation in the long axis of the vessel of interest (Figures 19-15). A potential danger with the short-axis approach is unseen penetration of the deep wall of the vein and any structure that lies deep to it. Long-axis orientation can be helpful when difficulty is encountered with the guidewire. The long-axis view may demonstrate the location of resistance and allow for subtle readjustments.

STATIC VERSUS DYNAMIC PLACEMENT TECHNIQUE

Techniques utilizing ultrasound-assisted venous cannulation may vary depending on the clinical scenario and

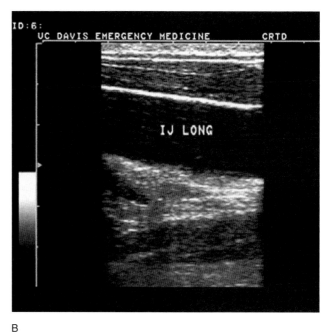

A   B

Figure 19-15. Transducer placement (A) and ultrasound image (B) of the longitudinal or long-axis plane of the internal jugular vein.

the availability of assistance as well as the necessity for strict sterile technique. The advantage of the dynamic technique is that it allows for real-time observation of the needle position and target vascular structures. The logistical simplicity of the static technique may be advantageous in the case where the landmark-based anatomy is straightforward. The static technique allows a brief inspection and confirmation of the vessel location without the reliance on a second operator. Both static and dynamic approaches have been found to be superior to the traditional landmark based approach.[13]

STERILE TECHNIQUE

There are several different options for maintaining sterile technique. The best option is to use prepackaged sterile probe sleeves that are manufactured solely for the purpose of handling the probe and transducer cord in a sterile fashion (figure 19-16). Alternatively, the use of a large sterile glove while positioning the probe and adequate amounts of conductive gel into the thumb of the glove can also be effective (Figures 19-17). If using the glove option, care must be taken to avoid compromising sterility by puncturing one of the "extra" fingers of the glove during the process of venipuncture. Sterile lubricant is sufficient as a conductive medium between the sleeve and the skin.

▶ COMMON VARIANTS AND OTHER ABNORMALITIES

VARIABILITY OF NORMAL VENOUS ANATOMY

The large central venous structures of the body have fairly constant anatomy whereas the peripheral veins are

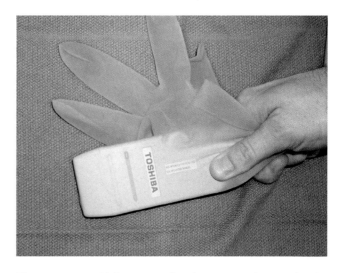

Figure 19-17. Using a sterile glove as an improvised transducer cover.

extremely variable in their position. It is helpful, however, to keep in mind the typical course of the veins and the important adjacent structures while using ultrasound to assist in vessel identification and cannulation.

EFFECT OF PATIENT POSITIONING

The usual considerations apply for patient preparation for central or peripheral venous cannulation. The Trendelenburg position is useful to provide slight venous distention in the veins of the head and neck. Furthermore, the use of ultrasound may help determine optimal patient position with respect to surrounding arterial anatomy.[25] It is apparent in individual patients that rotation or abduction of a limb will significantly alter the relationship of the vein and artery with respect to the skin. It merits emphasizing that in certain individuals leg position alone can cause the femoral artery to directly overlie the femoral vein. Hence, the use of a standard (non–ultrasound-assisted) technique, given certain patient positioning, may result in arterial injury or failed venous cannulation (Figure 19-5c).

▶ PITFALLS

There are no absolute contraindications to the use of ultrasound for vascular access; however, there are a few common pitfalls.

1. **Failure to identify the needle in tissue.** When using ultrasound for dynamic venous access, it is important to accurately view the needle ring-down artifact or venous tenting to confirm

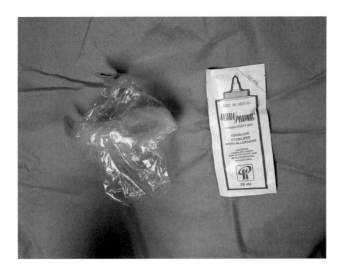

Figure 19-16. Sterile transducer cover and sterile coupling gel in prepack setup.

position. Whether using the transverse or longitudinal approach, it is important to identify the needle with ultrasound visualization before advancing into deeper structures. This is important to ensure successful cannulation while minimizing complications. Transverse orientation allows for better lateral positioning of the needle while longitudinal orientation provides better depth and needle-slope positioning.

2. **Failure to distinguish between vein and artery through compression testing or color-flow Doppler**. Since arterial pulsations at times may be subtle, veins and arteries may initially appear very similar (especially in the hypotensive patient). In the absence of color-flow Doppler capability, the vessel should be confirmed that it is a vein by using compression maneuvers. A vein will easily collapse with gentle external pressure. While color or power Doppler may be of some use, pulse wave Doppler will enable the sonologist to actually interrogate the vessel of choice and determine if venous or arterial flow is present.

3. **Locating the vessel with the static approach prior to the patient being in proper position.** The vessel should be located *after* the clinician has the patient properly positioned for the cannulation attempt. As emphasized earlier, many vessels will move slightly and change relationship depending on the patient's position.

4. **Failure to angle the transducer beam into the needle puncture area.** Since ultrasound provides a two-dimentional image, the beam should be angled toward the needle where it will enter the vessel. Occasionally, fanning the transducer beam may be required to identify the optimal location. Figure 19-12 demonstrates how in the short-axis the needle can appear over the vessel while the tip is not within the vessel. Note how three different needle vectors intersect over the vessel although the ultimate needle tip may be in a very different location.

► CASE STUDIES

CASE 1

Patient Presentation

A 50-year-old man who was morbidly obese presented complaining of chest pain. On examination, he was hypotensive and diaphoretic. A 12-lead EKG revealed him to be in complete heart block. Multiple attempts at peripheral access failed. The transcutaneous pacemaker

was intermittently capturing but had little effect on the patient's hemodynamic status. There were no good external anatomic landmarks due to his adiposity.

Management Course

The patient's right internal jugular vein was easily visualized under ultrasound guidance using a 7.5 MHz linear transducer. A dynamic real-time ultrasound-guided cannulation of the right internal jugular vein was successful on the first attempt. An intravenous pacemaker wire was then successfully placed (also under ultrasound visualization). Upon improved ventricular capture, the patient's blood pressure normalized.

CASE 2

Patient Presentation

An 18-year-old woman who was severely scarred and contracted from old burns to the neck, chest, arms, and legs, presented after ingesting a lethal quantity of a tricyclic antidepressant in a suicide attempt. On examination, the patient was hypotensive and lethargic. Numerous attempts at peripheral access failed. There were no appreciable anatomic landmarks for central access due to her old scars.

Management Course

Although a femoral arterial pulsation was difficult to palpate for the landmark-based approach, the femoral vein was easily visualized under ultrasound guidance. An ultrasound-guided femoral vein catheter was inserted on the first attempt. The patient was then administered induction agents for orotracheal intubation and successfully resuscitated.

CASE 3

Patient Presentation

A 40-year-old man with a long history of intravenous drug use presented for drainage of a deltoid abscess. It was determined that the abscess cauld be drained as an outpatient with the use of systemic sedation and analgesia. Numerous attempts at routine peripheral venous access failed. The patient was refusing a central venous line.

Management Course

The patient has a large right basilic vein easily visualized with ultrasound. A 2-inch 18-gauge catheter is inserted without difficulty. The patient's abscess is successfully drained after receiving adequate intravenous sedation and analgesia.

Commentary

Anatomic landmarks in patients may be distorted, obscured, or nonexistent. In the three cases, each patient presented with anatomic variations that made it difficult to obtain rapid peripheral venous access or landmark-based central venous access. Venous access was facilitated by the use of ultrasound in each case, thereby expediting patient resuscitation and care. Ultrasound use allowed the clinicians to obtain venous access on the first attempt and helped prevent complications associated with delays in obtaining venous access or multiple attempts to obtain central venous access.

REFERENCES

1. Denys BG, Uretsky BF: Anatomical variations of internal jugular vein location: Impact on central venous access. *Crit Care Med* 19:1516–1519, 1991.
2. Bagwell CE, Salzberg AM, Sonnino RE: Potentially lethal complications of central venous catheter placement. *J Pediatr Surg* 35:709–713, 2000.
3. Conz PA, Dissegna D, Rodighiero MP: Cannulation of the internal jugular vein: Comparison of the classic Seldinger technique and an ultrasound guided method. *J Nephrol* 10:311–313, 1997.
4. Lee W, Leduc L, Cotton DB: Ultrasonographic guidance for central venous access during pregnancy. *Am J Obstet Gynecol* 161:1012–1013, 1989.
5. Trottier SJ, Veremakis C, O'Brien J: Femoral deep vein thrombosis associated with central venous catheterization: Results from a prospective, randomized trial. *Crit Care Med* 23:52–59, 1995.
6. Farrell J, Gellens M: Ultrasound-guided cannulation versus the landmark-guided technique for acute haemodialysis access. *Nephrol Dial Transplant* 12:1234–1237, 1997.
7. Gallieni M, Cozzolino M: Uncomplicated central vein catheterization of high risk patients with real time ultrasound guidance. *Int J Artif Organs* 18:117–121, 1995.
8. Hudson PA, Rose JS: Real-time ultrasound guided internal jugular vein catheterization in the emergency department. *Am J Emerg Med* 15:79–82, 1997.
9. Meredith JW, Young JS, O'Neil EA: Femoral catheters and deep venous thrombosis: A prospective evaluation with venous duplex sonography. *J Trauma* 35:187–190, 1993.
10. Vucevic M, Tehan B, Gamlin F: The SMART needle. A new Doppler ultrasound-guided vascular access needle. *Anaesthesia* 49:889–891, 1994.
11. Caridi JG, Hawkins IF, Wiechmann BN: Sonographic guidance when using the right internal jugular vein for central vein access. *AJR Am J Roentgenol* 171:1259–1263, 1998.
12. Slama M, Novara A, Safavian A: Improvement of internal jugular vein cannulation using an ultrasound-guided technique. *Intensive Care Med* 23:916–919, 1997.
13. Milling TJ, Rose JS, Briggs WM, Birkhahn G, Melniker LM: Randomized, controlled clinical trial of point-of-care limited ultrasonography assistance of central venous cannulation: The Third Sonography Outcomes Assessment Program (SOAP-3) Trial. *Crit Care Med* 33:1764–1769, 2005.
14. Hilty WM, Hudson PA, Levitt MA: Real-time ultrasound-guided femoral vein catheterization during cardiopulmonary resuscitation. *Ann Emerg Med* 29:331–336, 1997.
15. Costantino TP, Parikh A: Ultrasonography-guided peripheral intravenous access versus traditional approaches in patients with difficult intravenous access. *Ann Emerg Med* 46:456–661, 2005.
16. Brannam l: Emergency nurses' utilization of ultrasound guidance for placement of peripheral intravenous lines in difficult-access patients. *Acad Emerg Med* 11:1361–1363, 2004.
17. Keyes LE, Frazee BW, Snoey ER: Ultrasound-guided brachial and basilic vein cannulation in emergency department patients with difficult intravenous access. *Ann Emerg Med* 34:711–714, 1999.
18. Rose JS, Norbutas CM: A randomized controlled trial comparing one-operator versus two-operator technique in ultrasound-guided basilic vein cannulation. *J Emerg Med* 2006 (in press).
19. Parkinson R, Gandhi M, Harper J: Establishing an ultrasound guided peripherally inserted central catheter (PICC) insertion service. *Clin Radiol* 53:33–36, 1998.
20. Rothschild JM: Ultrasound guidance of central vein catheterization: Making healthcare safer: A critical analysis of patient safety practices. Available at http://www.ahrq.gov/clinic/ptsafety/chap21.htm.
21. National Institute for Clinical Excellence: Guidance on the use of ultrasound locating devices for placing central venous catheters. *NHS* 49:1–24, 2002.
22. Milling TJ: Randomized controlled trial of single-operator vs. two-operator ultrasound guidance for internal jugular central venous cannulation. *Acad Emerg Med* 13:245–247, 2006.
23. Bair AE, Rose JS, Vance C, Kuppermann N: Ultrasound assisted peripheral intravenous access in pediatric emergency department patients: A randomized clinical trial. *Acad Emerg Med* 12:325–328, 2005.
24. Blaivas M: Short-axis versus long-axis approaches for teaching ultrasound-guided vascular access on a new inanimate model. *Acad Emerg Med* 10:1307–1311, 2003.
25. Armstrong PJ, Sutherland R, Scott DH: The effect of position and different maneuvers on internal jugular vein diameter size. *Acta Anaesthesiol Scand* 38:229–231, 1994.

CHAPTER 20

Additional Ultrasound-Guided Procedures

Andreas Dewitz, Robert Jones, and Jessica Goldstein

Invasive procedures are frequently performed in the emergency department. Traditionally, these invasive procedures have been performed by emergency physicians who relied on physical assessment for making the correct diagnosis and surface landmarks for determining the correct approach for an invasive procedure. In recent years, the use of bedside ultrasound has been incorporated into the practice of many emergency physicians to guide or assist in the performance of a variety of invasive procedures.

The use of ultrasound guidance (dynamic guidance) or ultrasound assistance (static guidance) to perform certain procedures can decrease complications when utilized correctly. Before performing any procedure under ultrasound guidance, it is imperative that clinicians have a thorough understanding of sonographic anatomy, the basic principles of ultrasound, and have practical training with phantoms or models to develop the hand–eye coordination required. Lack of familiarity with ultrasound and the orientation of the image on the screen can lead to complications even in the hands of a physician skilled at performing the procedure in a "blind" fashion.

▶ DYNAMIC GUIDANCE AND STATIC ASSISTANCE

Procedures can be performed using either ultrasound guidance (dynamic) or ultrasound assistance (static). In real-time ultrasound guidance, the procedure is performed while imaging the target during the procedure. In ultrasound assistance, the procedure is performed in the traditional fashion after the anatomy and any pathology has been mapped by ultrasound and the entry point marked.

The decision to perform a procedure under ultrasound guidance or ultrasound assistance is based on the procedure itself. Some procedures are simply inherently more dangerous when not performed under real-time guidance. In the case of others, there is only slightly more danger when real-time visualization is not utilized after an initial ultrasound assessment. For these procedures, it is often a matter physician experience and preference that may be the deciding factor. Procedures such as paracentesis, thoracentesis, and abscess drainage are frequently performed using ultrasound assistance since the fluid collections tend to be static, and once anatomy and pathology are marked out, it is typically safe to proceed blindly. Vascular access, paracentesis, and foreign body removal are examples of applications typically performed under ultrasound guidance.

▶ NUMBER OF OPERATORS

Ultrasound-guided procedures can be performed with the physician holding the transducer with one hand and using the free hand to perform the procedure. The free hand may be holding a needle, forceps, or be manipulating tissue itself. In the two-operator approach, one person holds the ultrasound transducer and another person performs the actual procedure. Physicians in many settings may not have the option of having a colleague assist them because of staffing levels or how busy a setting they work in. For others, it is a matter of personal preference. Having an additional person holding the transducer means coordinating actions with another person. Similar to ultrasound-guided vascular access, it may simply be easier for one person to do both in a dynamic setting such as when a needle or forceps are moving underneath the skin.

For those just learning to perform ultrasound-guided procedures, it is recommended that the one-operator technique be emphasized. The hand–eye coordination and neural feedback obtained by the single operator is much more accurate than the verbal communication that occurs between two operators. Changes in transducer placement or orientation by an assistant may go unnoticed by the operator with the needle until it is too late. This mishap may result in the need for another attempt or more significantly may result in the inadvertent puncture of an adjacent structure.

▶ PROCEDURE GUIDES

For some ultrasound-guided procedures involving placement of a needle into target locations for aspiration, mechanical needle guides that attach to the transducer are

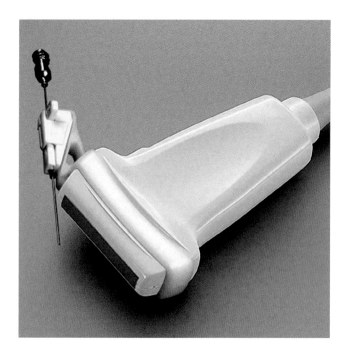

Figure 20-1. Mechanical needle guide.

commercially available (Figure 20-1). These guides are useful for keeping the needle in a predictable path so that intersection of the needle and ultrasound beam occurs at a known depth in case of a short-axis needle guide. For guides that place the needle in a long axis to the transducer, a needle will travel directly under the ultrasound beam for its full length, eliminating the requirement for some hand–eye coordination and adjustments. The main disadvantage of using mechanical guides is that the angle of entry is fixed on some guides (Figure 20-2). Furthermore, in the case of deep structures, the needle guide itself typically uses up a considerable length of the common needle, thus making it difficult to reach areas over 2–4 cm deep.

▶ NEEDLE TO TRANSDUCER ORIENTATION

Ultrasound-guided procedures can be performed using either a long-axis or short-axis approach. The orientation of the axis when performing an ultrasound-guided procedure refers to the relationship of the transducer to the needle. A long-axis approach indicates that the transducer is in line with the needle (Figure 20-3). A short-axis approach indicates that the transducer is 90 degree to the long-axis of the needle (Figure 20-4). The long-axis approach provides the advantage of allowing the needle to be visualized in its long axis, so the location of the needle tip in relationship to the target structure can be identified with certainty throughout the entire path taken by

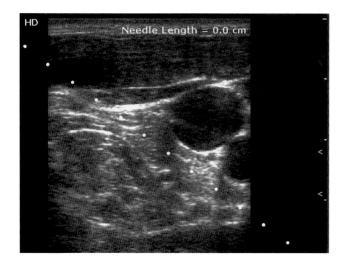

Figure 20-2. Note the fixed trajectory for needle entry when using a mechanical needle guide. The path of the needle is indicated by the dotted line. If the internal jugular vein was the desired target, then the transducer would need to be repositioned since the internal jugular vein is not currently in the path of the needle.

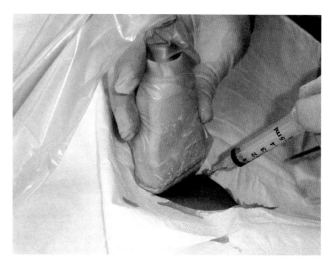

Figure 20-4. Short-axis approach. Note that the needle is perpendicular to the transducer beam.

the needle (Figure 20-5). The main disadvantage of this approach is that the needle must be kept in line with the ultrasound beam and this requires reasonable hand–eye coordination a steady hand and some practice. Failure to keep the beam in line with the needle (even slight movement of the probe) can result in complete loss of visualization of the needle (Figure 20-6A and 20-6B).

The short-axis approach relies on the centering of the vessel or target structure on the screen and using the center of the long face of the transducer as the entry point (Figure 20-7). Using this approach, the shaft of the

needle will be seen only in its short axis (Figure 20-8). The main disadvantage of this approach is that the tip of the needle may be hard to localize. When using this technique to perform ultrasound-guided vascular access, it is not uncommon to penetrate the anterior and posterior wall of the vessels and occasionally unintended underlying structures (Figure 20-9).

Regardless of the approach taken and the instrument used, the sonologist should always know where on the ultrasound screen the instrument should appear once under the skin. In the case of a long-axis approach, it is prudent to decide whether the needle will appear from the right or left side of the screen. This can be accomplished by setting the transducer in the desired orientation on whatever body surface the procedure will take

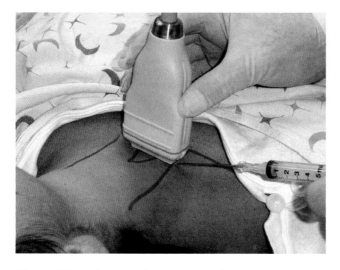

Figure 20-3. Long-axis approach. Note that the needle is in line with the transducer beam.

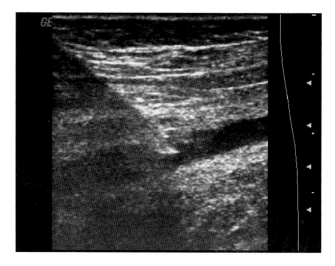

Figure 20-5. Long-axis approach with the needle tip visualized within the vessel lumen.

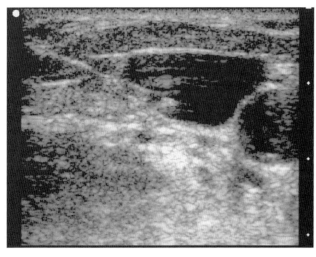

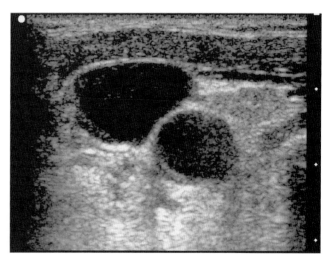

A   B

Figure 20-6. (A) Long-axis approach with the needle visualized. (B) Long-axis approach with complete loss of visualization of the needle due to slight movement of the transducer.

place. Using a finger, disturb the skin on the side of the transducer from which the instrument will penetrate the skin. The resulting disturbance on the ultrasound screen will indicate where on the screen the instrument will appear under the skin as long as the same orientation is maintained. For short-axis approach, the structure of interest should be aligned under the center of the transducer and the needle puncture done under the center of the transducer face. Some find it useful to place a permanent mark on the center of the linear array transducer to mark this location. Others use a technique of placing the needle flat between the transducer face and the skin to align the needle artifact with the intended structure

before tilting the needle up to the intended puncture angle.

▶ **TECHNICAL ASPECTS**

For ultrasound guidance or assistance to be successful, the desired structure must be easily and clearly visible with ultrasound. Difficulty in visualizing a structure that is normally readily imaged with ultrasound can be due to numerous technical factors such as difficult scanning plane, body habitus, inadequate gel use, and interference from adjacent structures. In these difficult patients,

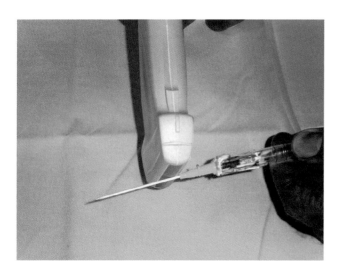

Figure 20-7. Short-axis approach. Note that the needle is perpendicular to the axis of the transducer beam.

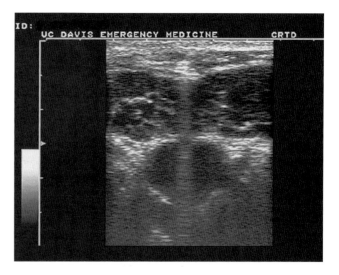

Figure 20-8. Image obtained using short-axis approach. Note needle artifact centered above vein. (Courtesy of John S. Rose, MD)

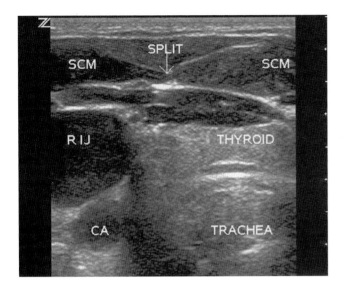

Figure 20-9. Structures surrounding the internal jugular vein. Transverse view of the neck with the carotid artery (CA) noted directly posterior to the right internal jugular vein (RIJ). SCM-sternocleidomastoid muscle.

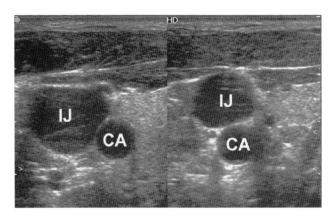

Figure 20-10. Split-screen image demonstrating the effect of head turning on the relationship of the internal jugular vein and the carotid artery. This emphasizes the importance of performing the procedure in the same position that the scan was performed. IJ = internal jugular vein, CA = carotid artery.

developing an alternative plan may be the best option if the target structure cannot be imaged despite addressing the pitfalls just listed. The chance of successfully targeting a structure with a needle or hemostat that cannot be reliably seen is lower and the chance of experiencing complications in these patients will be higher.

Once an initial scouting ultrasound examination confirms that the target is accessible, the next step involves procedure preparation and setup. These are essential aspects of an invasive procedure. The patient should be optimally positioned prior to beginning the procedure. Experiment with different patient positions prior to beginning in order to see which position will improve the chance of success. If ultrasound assistance is used to mark a location, it will be important for the patient to maintain the same body position between marking the invasive procedure. An obvious example of this is fluid marking for paracentesis. If the patient moves, fluid may shift away from the path of the needle and bowel penetration may occur. A more subtle example is the slight but important realignment of vascular structures that may occur with movement (Figure 20-10).

The location of the ultrasound machine in relationship to the operator and the patient must be carefully considered. The machine should be placed in a location where the operator can easily visualize the screen, ideally without turning his or her head and simply by glancing up or slightly to the side (Figure 20-11). Placing the machine in a location where the operator is forced to turn around or be in an awkward position will make the process less comfortable and increase the likelihood

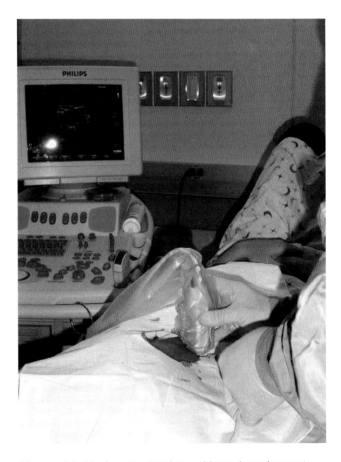

Figure 20-11. Appropriately positioned equipment. Note that the screen is in direct line with the operator's vision.

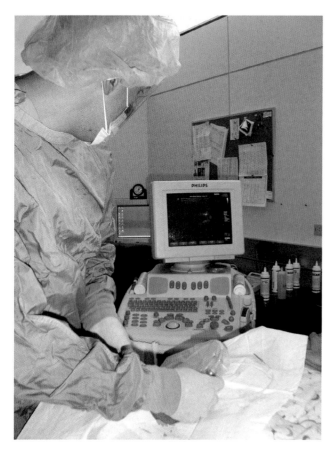

Figure 20-12. Inappropriately positioned equipment. Note that the operator has to turn his head to see the screen.

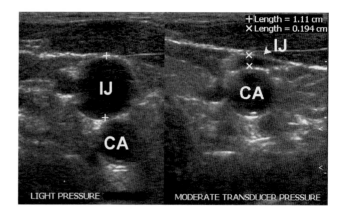

Figure 20-13. Split-screen image demonstrating the effect of compression of the internal jugular vein (arrowhead) by heavy transducer pressure. IJ = internal jugular vein, CA = carotid artery.

of failure (Figure 20-12). Correct ultrasound image adjustments should be done before the final preparations for the procedure so that both hands are free and can remain gloved and sterile.

► GETTING STARTED IN PROCEDURAL GUIDANCE

HOLDING THE TRANSDUCER

The development of good hand–eye coordination and control of the transducer are essential for success. Poor technique may not lead to failure in straightforward cases such as an abdomen filled with 10 liters of ascites. However, in the case of a small peritonsillar abscess, poor technique will lead to failure and possibly injury.

When scanning a patient, always have a comfortable grasp of the transducer and maintain light hand contact with the patient. Holding the transducer too close to the cable will limit fine-motor control and make it difficult to keep the transducer in one position on the patient's skin. This loss of fine motor control will cause the operator to apply more pressure on the skin with the transducer and may compress or distort the target struc-

ture (Figure 20-13). The ability to maintain alignment of the ultrasound beam and instrument requires that the transducer be held steadily, which is made possible by keeping a finger or edge of the hand in contact with the patient's skin.

CONTROLLING THE INSTRUMENT

The needle, hemostat, or other instrument should be moved in a slow, controlled fashion during an ultrasound-guided procedure. Fast movements may result in loss of instrument visualization or result in operator confusion. Using short, controlled movements is usually the best way to advance the instrument through the soft tissue. Occasionally a short jab may be called for to move the instrument through soft tissue. However, this must be performed with control to avoid over penetration and damage of vital tissues. One example is in the case of an interscalene nerve block where a spinal type needle is used to avoid cutting nerve tissue and must be gently thrust to penetrate the sheath surrounding the brachial plexus. Without sheath penetration, delivery of anesthetic will be compromised. At the same time uncontrolled jabbing with the needle may result in nerve injury, even with a noncutting needle.

FACTORS AFFECTING INSTRUMENT VISUALIZATION

Instrument visualization is critical in ultrasound-guided procedures, regardless of whether the instrument is a needle, hemostat, trocar, or some kind of probe. Despite what appears to be good alignment of the instrument and the ultrasound beam, visualization can occasionally be surprisingly difficult. Composition of the soft tissue, instrument type, needle gauge, bevel position,

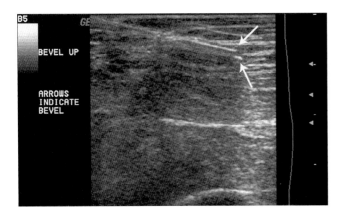

Figure 20-14. Good visualization of the needle tip (arrows) is noted with the needle bevel directed toward the transducer.

instrument movement, and the ultrasound beam angle all affect visualization.

Needle visualization will be improved by using a larger diameter needle and by keeping the needle as close to perpendicular to the axis of the ultrasound beam as possible. Unfortunately, a sonologist may not always be in a position to place the needle or other instrument perpendicular to the ultrasound beam in all situations. In these cases, keeping the ultrasound beam to instrument angle close to 60 degrees will improve visualization (see Figure 20-5).

A needle tip will be better visualized if the bevel of the needle faces either toward or away from the sound beam (Figure 20-14). When the bevel of the needle is rotated 90 degrees in either direction, the needle tip will not be clearly visualized. It has been suggested that scattering of the beam away from the transducer when the bevel is in the 90 degree position from the ultrasound beam results in the return of fewer echoes to the transducer. In difficult patients or in cases where the needle angle is suboptimal, the use of an echogenic needle may be beneficial (Figure 20-15). Traditional needles with a

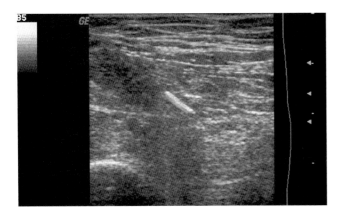

Figure 20-15. Echogenic needle with a roughened surface at the tip. Note the improved echogenicity at the tip.

smooth surface have a significantly smaller amount of echoes returning to the transducer due to the nonperpendicular angle.

LOCATING THE INSTRUMENT UNDER THE SKIN

When the instrument is difficult to visualize or cannot be visualized, the operator must first reassess the relationship of the instrument to the ultrasound beam. The most common reason for not visualizing a needle is lack of alignment of the needle and ultrasound beam. Continued advancement of the needle is inadvisable since needle advancement will not improve needle visualization if the needle and ultrasound beam are not aligned. The transducer should be gently repositioned, either panning or rocking from side to side, until the instrument is visualized. If the instrument cannot be clearly visualized at this point, the instrument can be gently wiggled to see if this improves visualization. Large motions should be avoided since this may allow a sharp instrument to lacerate deep structures. In long-axis procedures, once the instrument is visualized, move the transducer in the same plane toward the target. Redirect the instrument toward the target while keeping in mind which direction the transducer was moved. The decision to attempt the procedure from another entry location, changing the instrument angle after withdrawing it, or the use of a more echogenic instrument may be considered at this time.

▶ ARTHROCENTESIS

CLINICAL CONSIDERATIONS

Emergency and acute care physicians are commonly called upon to evaluate patients with a painful or swollen joint where definitive diagnosis will depend upon joint fluid being obtained for analysis or therapeutic reasons. While many physicians feel comfortable tapping a knee effusion, the comfort level for performing arthrocentesis in other joints is often much lower. On occasion, the provider's discomfort with the procedure may stem from the complete absence of recognizable landmarks due to the patient's morbid obesity. Whether because of lack of familiarity with the regional anatomy or unfamiliarity with the landmarks or techniques traditionally relied upon for the procedure, arthrocentesis of less commonly tapped joints such as the elbow, ankle, shoulder, hip, acromioclavicular, or metatarsophalangeal joints are often referred to rheumatologists, interventional radiologists, or orthopedists. The growing use of ultrasound for procedural applications is likely to change this historical pattern. Arthrocentesis of all these joints can easily be added to the armamentarium of procedures performed by the emergency physician if certain basic procedural principles are applied and a few basic anatomic and sonographic pointers for each area are noted.

CLINICAL INDICATIONS

- Diagnostic fluid sampling from a joint for laboratory testing
- Therapeutic fluid drainage from a joint

ANATOMIC CONSIDERATIONS

Joints in the human body, while built on similar principles, vary in their individual design and size. Sampling fluid from each requires knowledge of the particular anatomy of the specific joint. In the following section, each joint will have a brief discussion of anatomy specific to the individual application.

TECHNIQUE AND ULTRASOUND FINDINGS

Most ultrasound machines now purchased for use in acute, emergency, and critical care settings will be capable of supporting diagnostic presets and the transducers required for arthrocentesis. A 7.5–10 MHz linear array transducer will be used for most joints except the hip, where a curvilinear 5 MHz or lower frequency transducer may be utilized. Doppler evaluation should be performed to identify any vascular structures surrounding the effusion or along the planned aspiration approach in order that they may be avoided. Image depth should be adjusted appropriately for the joint in question (the 80/20 rule applies: 80% of the image should focus on the anatomic area of interest, with 20% left over in the far field so as to see adjacent anatomy) and image depth should be set to the level of the bony cortex of the relevant joints being imaged.

For precise localization, the joint fluid collection should be mapped in two orthogonal planes and the skin marked with indelible ink on either side of the transducer. Connecting the lines will create a target with the aspiration site in the center of the " + "; note should be taken of the optimal aspiration angle. The depth from the skin surface to the deepest portion of the effusion should be noted so that an appropriate length needle can be chosen for the procedure. Most effusions will be mapped and marked and then aspirated using a freehand technique. If real-time guidance is used, such marking will not be required, but the site should be prepared in a sterile manner and ultrasound transducer properly draped. Guiding the needle to a joint effusion in real time is little different from vascular access or abscess drainage techniques.

Graded compression and power Doppler can help distinguish synovial fluid from synovial proliferation. A color flow signal may be noted at the border between synovium and where joint fluid is moving because of compression caused by the transducer. Freely mobile loose bodies will occasionally be seen within a joint effusion and will typically reveal themselves by virtue of their hyperechoic acoustic profile and accompanying posterior acoustic shadowing. They are typically found in the suprapatellar bursa of the knee or in the elbow joint and can be seen to move with either gentle palpation of the effusion or pressure on the transducer.

Knee

The suprapatellar bursa is a large synovium lined pouch that is really an extension of the joint space of the knee. It is located at the anterior distal femur extending about a hand breadth above the adult knee joint, bounded superiorly by skin, subcutaneous tissue, and quadriceps tendon and inferiorly by prefemoral fat and the femur. When the knee joint is distended with fluid, the deepest collections will be found where the suprapatellar bursa bulges out on either side of the quadriceps tendon, particularly at the lateral suprapatellar recess. The suprapatellar bursa is the largest bursa in the body and can distend to accommodate a large volume of fluid. Numerous other bursae also surround the knee joint. Two that are of clinical relevance are the gastocnemiosemimembranosis bursa (found in the medial popliteal fossa), and the subcutaneous prepatellar bursa. The former often communicates with the knee joint, and when distended can cause pain and swelling in the popliteal fossa and is known as a Baker's cyst. The subcutaneous prepatellar bursa lies immediately below the skin over the lower patella, does not communicate with the knee joint, and may become swollen and infected due to local trauma.

The normal knee joint will have little or no fluid visible within the joint space. The highest yield sites for detection of an effusion will be in the lateral and medial recesses of the suprapatellar bursa. A simple effusion appears as a hypoechoic fluid collection separated from the brightly echogenic femoral cortex by a thin layer of hyperechoic prefemoral fat (Figure 20-16). With a more chronic process, inflammatory synovial changes (pannus) may be appreciated and will appear as a thickening of the synovium or lobulations within the joint space (Figure 20-17). An effusion due to intraarticular hemorrhage may initially appear echo-free but later exhibit a homogenous mid-level gray echotexture consistent with clotted or partially clotted blood (Figure 20-18). A knee joint effusion should not be confused with other fluid collections that can be found around this joint. A prepatellar bursitis appears as a hypoechoic fluid collection that is seen in the subcutaneous

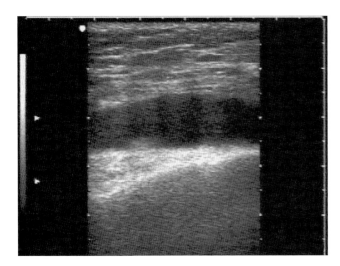

Figure 20-16. Transverse sonogram of a knee effusion at the lateral suprapatellar recess. Hyperechoic prefemoral fat is seen just below the hypoechoic effusion.

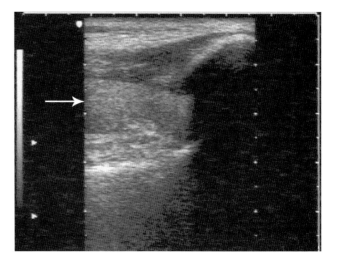

Figure 20-18. Midline sagittal sonogram of a knee hemarthrosis. The curved shadow of the patella is seen to the right of the image and the bright echo of the anterior femoral cortex below. Just above the prefemoral fat there is a homogenous mid-grey echotexture layer (arrow) consistent with hematoma.

tissue anterior to the patella and proximal patellar ligament and is often surrounded by hyperechoic edematous soft tissue typical of cellulitis (Figure 20-19). A Baker's cyst communicates with the knee joint and classically appears as a hypoechoic stomach-shaped fluid collection in the medial posterior fossa of the knee (Figure 20-20).

The knee is optimally scanned with the patient supine and the slightly flexed knee supported from behind with a sheet or towel for patient comfort. Scanning is most easily performed in a paramedian longitudinal plane just above the patella. Small volumes of fluid will first be seen in the lateral or medial recesses of the supra-

patellar bursa. Longitudinal and transverse scanning of the fluid collection is followed by marking of the skin with indelible ink to form a " + " designating the site for aspiration (Figure 20-21). Depth from the skin surface to the effusion and the optimal aspiration angle should be noted. From this point the procedure does not differ from blind aspiration unless real-time guidance is chosen by the sonologist. In this case, the transducer should be dressed in a sterile sheath, and sterile coupling gel

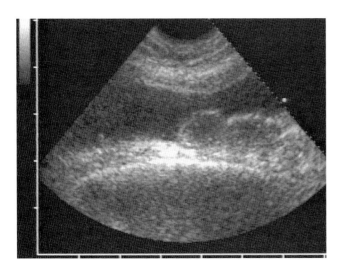

Figure 20-17. Transverse sonogram of a more chronic knee effusion with thickened, lobulated appearing synovium.

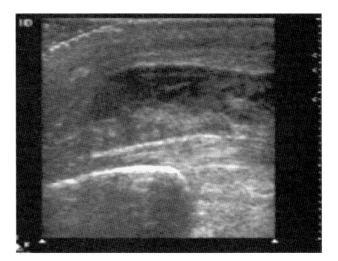

Figure 20-19. Sagittal midline sonogram of a prepatellar bursitis. Note the thickened hyperechoic skin, some debris within the fluid-filled prepatellar bursa, the shadow from the echogenic patella on the left inferior border of the image, and a portion of the fibrillar patellar ligament.

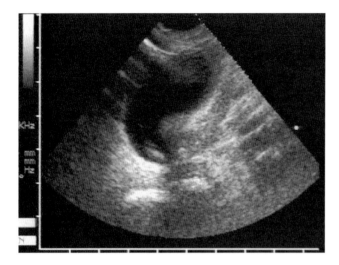

Figure 20-20. Transverse sonogram at the medial popliteal fossa demonstrating the characteristic stomach-shaped fluid collection of a Baker's cyst.

should be utilized. An approach allowing for long-axis visualization of the needle is best and is identical to other needle guidance techniques.

Hip

Sonographic evaluation of the hip joint can be successfully accomplished with a variety of transducers, ranging from a 3–5 MHz curved array or sector transducer to a 7.5–10.0 MHz linear array transducer. With the transducer aligned along the long axis of the femoral neck

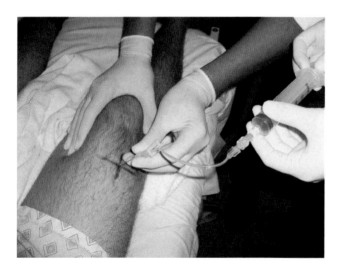

Figure 20-21. Knee aspiration technique at the lateral suprapatellar recess: two-person technique where pressure is applied to the contralateral recess for maximal joint cavity distension. Sterile drape omitted for purposes of illustration.

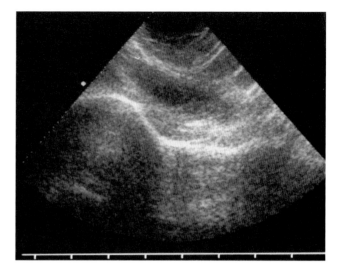

Figure 20-22. Ventral oblique sonogram of the normal hip. The prominent curve of the femoral head is seen on the left of the image and leads to a concave region along the femoral neck where an effusion will preferentially collect.

(orientation marker pointing toward the umbilicus), the normal hip will appear as a brightly curved line about 3–6 cm below the skin surface, convex along the surface of the femoral head on the left side of the image, then gently concave along the femoral neck to the right. The area just anterior to the femoral neck is termed the anterior synovial recess and represents the potential space between the femoral neck and the joint capsule where a hip effusion will preferentially collect (Figure 20-22). A thin line of hypoechogenicity may be noted adjacent to the cortex of the femoral head; this line corresponds to the articular cartilage. The acetabular labrum will often be seen as an echogenic area to the immediate left of and slightly superior to the femoral head. The joint capsule is of variable echogenicity, sometimes difficult to identify, other times clearly visible as an echogenic layer 3–8 mm in thickness extending from the acetabular labrum to the base of the femoral neck (Figure 20-23). The joint capsule is usually readily identified when an effusion is present. The commonly accepted sonographic criteria for defining a hip effusion in a native hip include (1) a convex bulging joint capsule with a fluid stripe greater than 5–6 mm; or (2) when compared to the asymptomatic joint, a greater than 2 mm increase in the distance from the cortical echo to the joint capsule. A perpendicular measurement of the effusion is taken at its widest anteroposterior dimension between the surface of the femoral neck and the inner surface of the joint capsule Comparison with the contralateral hip should be routine (Figure 20-24).

In the prosthetic hip the sonographic landmarks will obviously be different. Transducer alignment should still

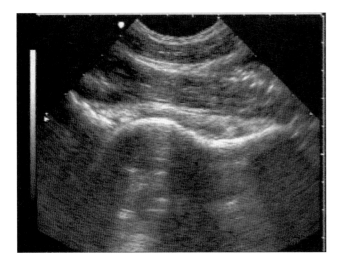

Figure 20-23. Ventral oblique sonogram of the hip. The joint capsule is seen as a hyperechoic, horizontally oriented layer extending from the acetabular labrum to the femoral neck. A small amount of joint fluid is noted below the joint capsule.

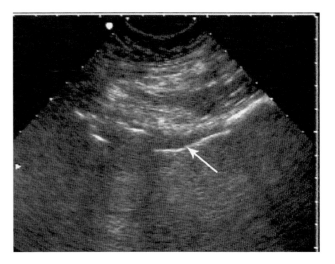

Figure 20-25. Ventral oblique sonogram of a normal prosthetic hip. Four echogenic lines are noted. From left to right: a short segment that corresponds to the acetabular component of the prosthesis; next, a wider more superficially located line that corresponds to the femoral head (a prominent metallic reverberation is noted below it); next, the long prosthetic femoral neck; and finally, a somewhat more anterior and more echogenic line that corresponds to the most proximal portion of the remaining native femur. A small amount of fluid is normally seen anterior to the prosthetic femoral neck (arrow).

be along the long axis of the now prosthetic femoral neck aiming toward the umbilicus. A series of four horizontally oriented hyperechoic lines will be noted. First, a short segment to the left of the image may be seen that corresponds to the acetabular component of the prosthesis. Adjacent to this line is a somewhat wider, more superficially located horizontal line that represents the head of the prosthesis. A prominent metallic reverberation or ring-down artifact will be seen behind the prosthesis during real-time scanning. Next, and to the immediate right, a longer and somewhat deeper echogenic horizontal line will be seen. This line corresponds to the neck of the hip prosthesis and a metallic ring-down artifact will be noted here as well. Finally, a bright and somewhat thicker echo will be noted to the right of the image. This echogenic line is located a few millimeters more superficially than the echo from the prosthetic femoral neck and represents the anterior surface of the most proximal portion of the remaining native femur where the prosthesis has been inserted. It is typical to see a small amount of hypoechoic fluid surrounding the neck of the prosthesis. As noted above, no joint capsule will be seen since it will have been removed during hip replacement surgery (Figure 20-25). A perpendicular measurement is taken of the width of the fluid collection located between the superior surface of the most proximal edge of the remaining native femoral cortex and the edge of the pseudocapsule above. A fluid collection with a width of greater than 3.2 mm at this location is considered to be abnormal (Figure 20-26).

In children, the sonogram of the hip appears somewhat different from that of the adult. The growth plate of the femoral capital epiphysis produces a curved notch in the convexity of the femoral head and, depending on

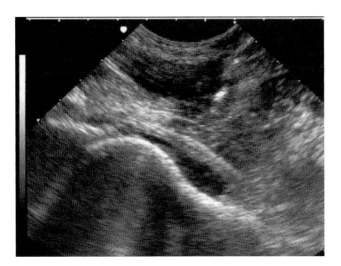

Figure 20-24. Ventral oblique sonogram of a hip effusion in a patient with reactive arthritis. The anterior synovial recess is distended with fluid and the capsule is seen to bulge anteriorly. The hyperechoic echo from the aspirating needle is seen in the upper right of the image.

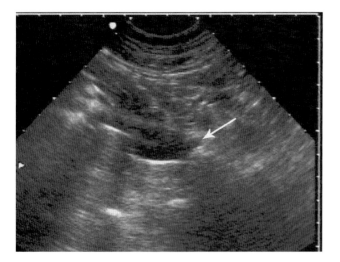

Figure 20-26. Ventral oblique sonogram of a septic prosthetic hip. A reverberation artifact is seen emanating from the prosthetic femoral head. A large fluid collection is seen anterior to the prosthetic femoral neck. A 5-mm fluid collection was measured between the most proximal native femur and the pseudocapsule above (arrow) (>3.2 mm is considered abnormal).

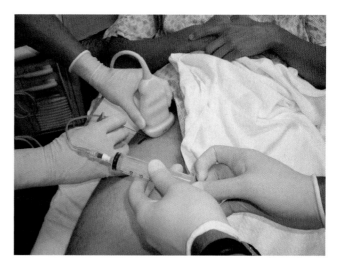

Figure 20-28. Ultrasound-guided hip aspiration technique. The needle is advanced in line within the long-axis scan plane of the transducer and its characteristic reverberation artifact is used to guide the needle tip into the effusion. For purposes of illustration, the sterile drape and probe cover are not shown.

the degree of ossification, a linear lucency in the anterior head of the femur. The hypoechoic region anterior to the notch represents the cartilaginous acetabulum and should not be mistaken for an effusion (Figure 20-27).

If a decision is made to aspirate the collection, either a mapping technique and a subsequent freehand aspiration or an aspiration under real-time guidance may

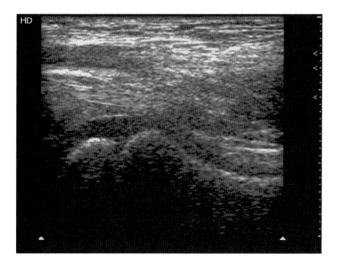

Figure 20-27. Ventral oblique sonogram of a pediatric hip. A notch is seen in the femoral head that corresponds to the growth plate of the femoral capital epiphysis. The hypoechoic area adjacent to this notch corresponds with the still cartilaginous acetabulum and should not be mistaken for an effusion.

be employed. With the ultrasound marking approach a line over the femur and best point of entry are marked and from there the procedure is a blind one like a typical hip aspiration. If a real-time aspiration technique is employed, a sterile sheath over the probe and sterile gel will be utilized. The transducer should be aligned along the long axis of the femoral neck as described previously and note should again be made of the location of the femoral vessels in order that they may be avoided by the aspirating needle. Once the effusion is identified and its most bulging portion centered in the monitor image the needle is inserted at one end of the probe and guided in long axis to the fluid collection just as in other aspiration and vascular access procedures (Figure 20-28).

Ankle

Scanning of the ankle is usually performed with a 5–10 MHz linear array transducer. In a sagittal scan plane over the distal tibia, a brightly echogenic horizontal line that corresponds to the anterior tibial cortex will be noted about 1 cm below the skin surface. As the transducer is moved further distally, a V-shaped recess will appear to the right of the image, formed by the distal tibia on the left and the dome of the talus on the right. This location is the region where the anterior synovial recess of the ankle joint is found and is normally filled by an anterior intracapsular fat pad (Figure 20-29). A small amount of echo-free fluid may be seen at the base of this recess and a collection of <3 mm in anteroposterior height is considered normal. In sagittal midline orientation, an

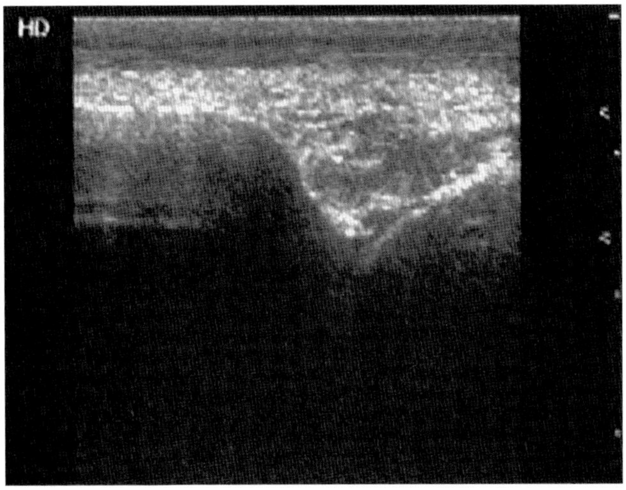

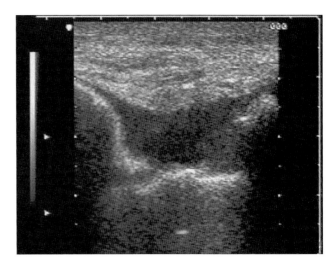

Figure 20-29. Sagittal midline sonogram of a normal ankle joint. The V-shaped recess is formed by the distal tibia on left and the talar dome on the right, and is filled by the anterior intracapsular fat pad. No fluid is seen in this example.

Figure 20-31. Sagittal medial paramedian sonogram of an ankle effusion. The ankle effusion in this location appears more rectangular in configuration.

ankle effusion will typically appear as a prominent triangular area of sonolucency that fills this V-shaped recess. The fibrous joint capsule is sometimes seen as a distinct and somewhat echogenic structure lying horizontally just anterior to the upper border of the effusion (Figure 20-30). More medially, the effusion will often take on a more rectangular configuration (Figure 20-31). On occasion, there may be significant associated soft tissue swelling of the overlying skin accompanying the inflammatory process within the joint. On a transverse image

through the joint line, the anterior tibial/dorsalis pedis artery will be located somewhat medial to the midline and appear as a hypoechoic circle just above the hypoechoic effusion (Figure 20-32).

Once a fluid collection has been identified in long-axis orientation, the transducer should be positioned so that the deepest portion of this V-shaped recess is located in the exact center of the image. A horizontal line can then be drawn on the skin with an indelible marker on either side of the transducer at the site that corresponds to the deepest portion of the effusion. Next, a transverse view should be obtained and the location of

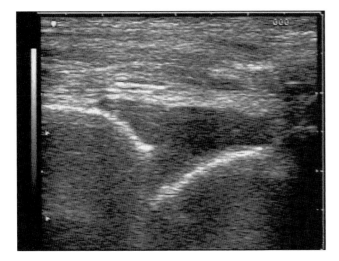

Figure 20-30. Sagittal midline sonogram of an ankle effusion. The joint capsule is seen as somewhat echogenic structure just above the hypoechoic effusion. The cortical echoes from the distal tibia and talar dome outline the posterior surface of the triangular effusion.

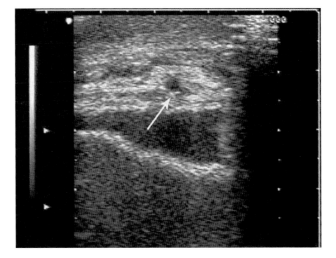

Figure 20-32. Transverse sonogram of an ankle effusion. The location of the hypoechoic anterior tibial/dorsalis pedis artery (arrow) should be marked on skin with a "Ø" so that it may by avoided during the aspiration. The deep peroneal nerve is located just medial to the artery.

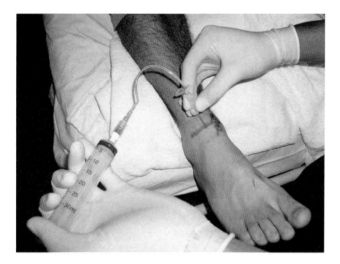

Figure 20-33. Freehand ankle aspiration technique. The location of both the deepest portion of the anterior recess and the anterior tibial/dorsalis pedis artery has been marked on the skin. Needle entry is laterally to the artery. When fluid is obtained, the needle can be held fixed in place with one hand while the syringe aspirates the effusion with the other. Sterile drape omitted for purposes of illustration.

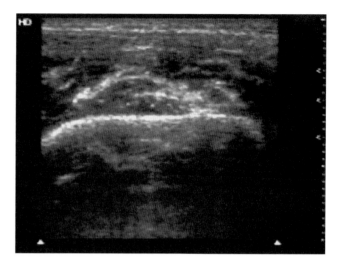

Figure 20-34. Transverse sonogram of posterior humerus at the level of the medial and lateral epicondyles. The brightly echogenic posterior humerus transitions from its rounded profile above to the flat profile seen here. As the transducer is moved a bit further distally, a U-shaped depression will be seen in the humerus that corresponds with the olecranon fossa.

the anterior tibial/dorsalis pedis artery should be marked on the skin with an "Ø" so that it may be avoided during the aspiration. Note should be taken of the angulation of the transducer, if any, as well as the degree of ankle plantar flexion and this information used to aim the needle in the appropriate direction during the aspiration. The patient is then sterilely prepped and draped, anesthetized, and the aspiration performed with a freehand technique (Figure 20-33). If a real-time technique is desired, the largest subjective image of the effusion is obtained in a transverse orientation with simultaneous visualization of the artery. The needle can be inserted under direct visualization somewhat lateral to the artery using a superior or inferior approach. This technique requires additional preparation and a sterile probe cover, however, and is usually not required.

Elbow

Ideally, the patient should be seated on a stretcher with the elbow held in 90 degrees of flexion and the forearm resting in neutral position a folded towel. In transverse orientation at the level of the medial and lateral epicondyles, the posterior echogenic surface of the humerus flattens (Figure 20-34) and then, somewhat more distally, forms a centrally located echogenic "U"-shaped depression that corresponds to the olecranon fossa (Figure 20-35). This space is normally filled with a posterior fat pad that exhibits a mid-level gray echotexture with some areas of increased internal echogenicity. In a longitudinal midline orientation over the distal el-

bow, the echogenic posterior surface of the humerus will be seen to the left of the image, the olecranon fossa and the posterior fat pad will appear in a "V"-shaped recess in the center, and the echogenic posterior surface of the olecranon will be located more superficially on the right side of the image. The triceps tendon may be apparent just below the skin as a horizontal, somewhat hyperechoic structure with a fibrillar echotexture. The

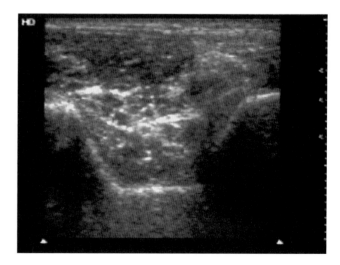

Figure 20-35. Transverse sonogram of the normal posterior elbow at the level of the olecranon fossa (also known as the posterior recess). The U-shaped depression in the humerus corresponds with the olecranon fossa and is filled by the posterior fat pad.

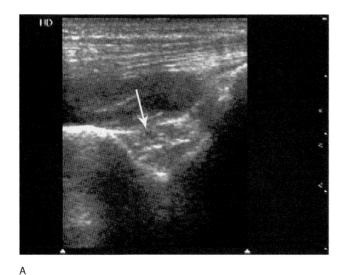
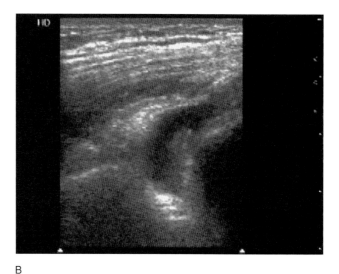

A   B

Figure 20-36. Sagittal sonogram of the normal posterior elbow (A). Humerus to the left, olecranon process to the right. The olecranon fossa is V-shaped in this orientation and the somewhat echogenic posterior fat pad is seen filling the recess (arrow). The fibrillar triceps tendon is seen just below the skin and it inserts on the echogenic olecranon on the right of the image. The hypoechoic region below the tendon is a portion of the triceps muscle. Sagittal sonogram of the posterior elbow in a patient with an anechoic effusion (B). The echogenic fat pad has been pushed superiorly and the joint capsule bulges posteriorly.

distal portion of the triceps muscle appears as a hypoechoic structure just beneath the tendon, superficial to the posterior fat pad (Figure 20-36A). In a longitudinal posterior midline orientation, an elbow effusion will appear as an anechoic fluid collection that pushes the posterior fat pad superiorly (to the left of the image) and distends the joint capsule posteriorly (Figure 20-36B). An effusion may appear hypoechoic or exhibit complex echogenicity depending on etiology (Figure 20-37).

If fluid is present, the horizontally aligned transducer should be positioned such that the largest subjective image of the fluid collection is centered on the monitor image. The skin should then be marked with indelible ink at both ends of the transducer and the ends connected with a horizontal line. Alternatively, the line may be constructed by scanning in a midline sagittal position (orientation marker facing up) and the deepest portion of the recess marked on either side of the transducer. This line will determine the optimum vertical location for the aspiration. Needle insertion should always be 1–2 cm lateral to the midline in order to remain remote from the medially located ulnar nerve and avoid the centrally located triceps tendon. The aspirating needle should be aimed toward the midline, however, in order to access the deepest portion of the always centrally located posterior recess. The skin is prepped, draped, and anesthetized as usual and the aspiration performed freehand (Figure 20-38). If a real-time technique is preferred, the needle tip should be inserted in an out-of-plane approach from above the transversely oriented transducer.

Shoulder

On the transverse sonogram of the anterior shoulder at the level of the coracoid process, an echogenic layer of skin and subcutaneous tissue will be seen overlying a thicker, hypoechoic, and horizontally striated layer that corresponds to the anterior portion of the deltoid muscle. Deep to the deltoid muscle lie two distinct, brightly

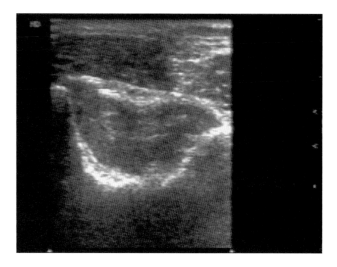

Figure 20-37. Transverse sonogram of the posterior elbow of a patient on warfarin with atraumatic elbow pain and an elevated INR. The olecranon fossa is filled with clotted blood. The bony outline of the fossa is brighter than usual because of posterior acoustic enhancement.

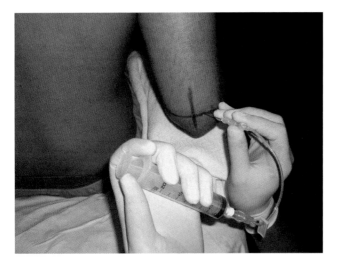

Figure 20-38. Elbow arthrocentesis technique—posterior approach. The effusion has been mapped and marked. Needle insertion is *lateral* to the midline to avoid the triceps tendon and to stay well remote from the ulnar nerve. The needle should be medially angulated so that it will reach the deepest portion of the centrally located recess.

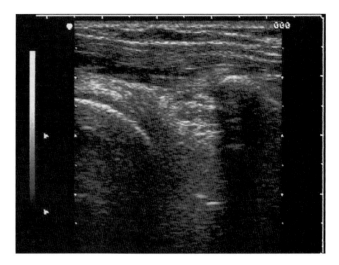

Figure 20-39. Transverse sonogram of the right anterior shoulder. The deltoid muscle is seen as a thin hypoechoic layer just below the skin. The curved medial humeral head appears on the left and the coracoid process with its pronounced posterior acoustic shadow on the right. The midline between these two structures represents the sagittal plane where the aspiration should occur (several centimeters below the level of the coracoid process, however).

echogenic lines that represent the medial humeral head (seen as a large, smoothly curved echo in the lateral portion of the image), and the anterior surface of the coracoid process (seen as a somewhat flatter, anterior echo medially). The hypoechoic rim surrounding the humeral head represents cartilage and should not be mistaken for a layer of fluid. The coracoid process is distinctive by virtue of the dense posterior acoustic shadow that it casts (Figure 20-39). If the profile of the medial humerus appears flat (Figure 20-40), the arm should be slightly externally rotated to obtain the more desirable rounded profile. The middle of the space between these two bony echoes will identify the vertical line where the effusion will be tapped, usually several centimeters inferior to the level of the coracoid. An effusion will appear as a hypoechoic collection that extends past the midline into the axillary recess of the joint capsule.

On the transverse sonogram of the posterior shoulder just below the posterior angle of the acromion, the echogenic layer of skin and subcutaneous tissue will be seen overlying a substantially thicker hypoechoic layer that represents the posterior portion of the deltoid muscle. Deep to the deltoid, the triangular or beak-shaped infraspinatus muscle (hypoechoic) and tendon (hyper- or hypoechoic, depending on the angle of insonation) will be seen pointing laterally over the curved echogenic line that corresponds to the humeral head (Figure 20-41). A thin hypoechoic rim that corresponds to articular cartilage may be noted adjacent to the hyperechoic head of the humerus. Medial to the humeral head, two additional lines will be noted: a slightly more superficial

echogenic line corresponding to the dorsal glenoid rim, and a somewhat deeper horizontal echogenic line corresponding to the posterior surface of the scapula (Figure 20-42). An effusion will appear as an anechoic region

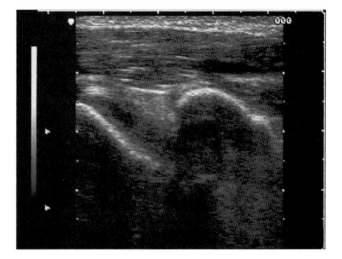

Figure 20-40. Transverse sonogram of the right anterior shoulder. The deltoid muscle appears more prominent in this example, and the coracoid process on the right is brightly echogenic. The profile of the medial humerus appears flat because the arm is too internally rotated. With slight external rotation, the more desirable curved profile of the humeral head will be obtained.

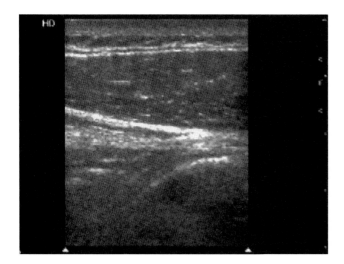

Figure 20-41. Transverse sonogram of the right posterior shoulder. The deltoid muscle is seen below the skin in the near field as a thick hypoechoic layer. The triangular or beak-shaped infraspinatus muscle (hypoechoic) and tendon (hyperechoic) are seen pointing to the right over the curved echogenic humeral head. The glenoid rim is seen as an indistinct echogenic line medial to the humeral head.

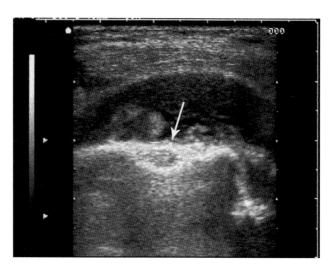

Figure 20-43. Transverse sonogram of the right anterior shoulder in a patient with a chronic subacromial (subdeltoid) bursitis. A large, complex hypoechoic collection is seen immediately beneath the deltoid muscle. The bursal fluid contains some echogenic debris within it and the synovium appears thickened and lobulated below. The echogenic anterior surface of the proximal humerus is seen beneath the effusion with the hypoechoic rounded biceps tendon resting within the bicipital groove (arrow). The bursal sac is seen to extend somewhat medial to the proximal humerus on the right side of the image.

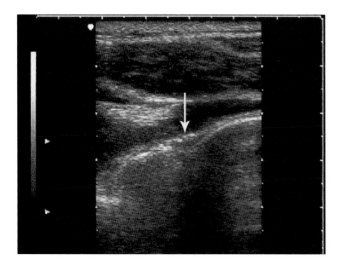

Figure 20-42. Transverse sonogram of the right posterior shoulder. In this example, the infraspinatus tendon is noted to be brightly echogenic on the left of the image but hypoechoic on the right; this is due to tendon anisotropy. With slight movement of the transducer, the entire tendon could be visualized. The glenoid rim is seen as a more distinct curved structure just medial to the larger curve of the head of the humerus. The site for the aspiration will be between the glenoid rim and the medial humeral head (arrow). The flatter echo to the left of the glenoid emanates from the surface of the scapula.

in the groove between the humeral head and the dorsal glenoid rim. Finally, a subacromial (or subdeltoid) effusion or bursitis will appear as a hypoechoic collection immediately beneath the deltoid muscle but superficial to the supraspinatus tendon (Figure 20-43). The effusion will best be seen from an anterior transverse approach at the level of the coracoid process (similar to the scan technique employed when assessing the biceps tendon for bursitis). The fluid collection seen with a subacromial (or subdeltoid) bursitis will not extend significantly inferior to the coracoid process; this characteristic can help distinguish it from an intra-articular effusion on an anterior view of the shoulder.

Shoulder arthrocentesis is typically performed from either an anterior or a posterior approach and can be ultrasound assisted or ultrasound guided. For the seated or supine patient, an anterior approach may be used (Figure 20-44). The arm is ideally extended in slight abduction with the palm facing up. A 7.5 MHz linear array transducer is placed in transverse orientation at the level of the coracoid process. The "V"-shaped recess seen between the medially located coracoid process and the laterally located medial head of the humerus is aligned in the center of the image. The skin on both sides of the transducer should be marked with an indelible marker at the precise location of the base of this recess and a

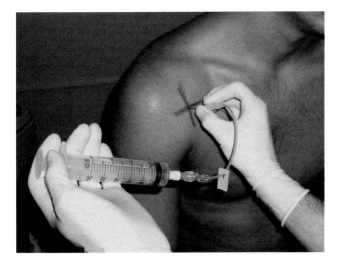

Figure 20-44. Shoulder arthrocentesis technique—anterior approach. The space midway between with coracoid process and the medial humeral head has been mapped and marked with a vertical line. The aspiration should occur perpendicular to the skin several centimeters below the level of the coracoid (at the horizontal line) and the needle should always remain lateral to the coracoid process.

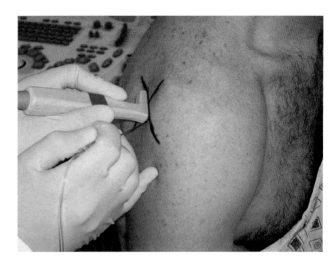

Figure 20-45. Shoulder arthrocentesis technique—ultrasound-guided posterior approach. The effusion is mapped and marked several centimeters inferior and medial to the bulge of the posterior angle of the acromion. The aspiration needle is guided to the space between the glenoid rim and the medial humeral head under ultrasound guidance. Sterile drape and probe cover are omitted for purposes of illustration.

vertical line drawn along this axis. The optimal site for aspiration will be on this line, but several centimeters inferior to the level of the coracoid process. If performed blindly, the needle should be advanced perpendicular to the skin surface.

For the posterior approach, the patient should be sitting with the elbow flexed and with the forearm resting at the side in neutral position (Figure 20-45). The transducer is placed in transverse orientation approximately 2–3 cm inferior and 1–2 cm medial to the bulge of the posterior acromion. The optimal image of the joint space can usually be obtained by tilting the lateral edge of the transducer slightly inferiorly from the horizontal plane. Beneath skin, subcutaneous tissue and deltoid muscle, the triangular or beak-shaped infraspinatus muscle and tendon will be seen overlying the echogenic curve of the medial humeral head. Slightly deeper and just medial to the humerus, a less distinct echo will be seen that corresponds to the dorsal glenoid labrum. An effusion will appear as an anechoic or hypoechoic collection adjacent to the curved head of the humerus, filling the groove between it and the medially located glenoid labrum.

The needle entry site should be from the lateral edge of the transducer in the plane of the ultrasound beam. The transducer is covered with a sterile sheath, and after a sterile prep, drape, and local anesthesia, the needle should be aimed toward the fluid collection in the groove between the medial humeral head and the glenoid rim. The aspiration path is fairly horizontal; this

will enhance visualization of the metallic needle and help guide precise placement of the needle tip. The joint capsule should be punctured along the medial border of the humeral head, slightly lateral to the glenohumeral joint so as to avoid contact with the circumflex scapular vessels and the suprascapular nerve that are located medial to the glenoid rim.

Other Joints and Bursae

Patients will occasionally present with joint pain that is ultimately discovered to be due to a pathologic process affecting the acromioclavicular, sternoclavicular, or first metatarsophalangeal joints. Ultrasound allows for precise mapping of these superficially located joints. The acromioclavicular and sternoclavicular joints are located on the lateral and medial end of the clavicle, respectively, and contain an articular disc that separates and cushions the clavicle from the abutting acromion or sternal articular surfaces. The fibrous capsule of the joint inserts on the bone immediately adjacent to the articular surfaces. The capsule of the first metatarsophalangeal joint surrounds the joint, extending from the nonarticular bony surfaces of the distal metatarsal bone to the proximal portion of the proximal phalanx.

The acromioclavicular and sternoclavicular joints are most easily scanned by first placing the transducer sagittally over the upper chest in order to identify the bright superficial echo from the clavicle (Figure 20-46).

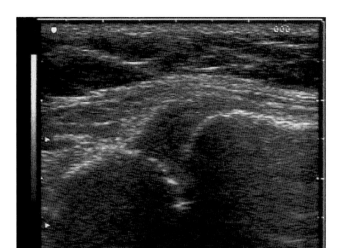

Figure 20-46. Longitudinal sonogram across the right acromioclavicular joint in a patient with gout. The hypoechoic V-shaped recess between the acromion on the left and the clavicle on the right represents the site where an aspiration or steroid injection would be directed.

The transducer is then slid either medially or laterally, and at the joint of interest, is rotated along the long axis of the clavicle spanning the relevant joint space. The hypoechoic V-shaped recess that corresponds to the joint space is marked on either side of the transducer, and then marked again with the transducer turned orthogonally. The two lines are connected and the center of the " + " marks the location for the aspiration. The first metatarsophalangeal joint is best scanned axially over the joint space and a similar mapping technique is utilized. Alternatively, the acoustic shadow of a paper clip can be used here to map the desired puncture site. After the usual sterile prep, drape, and local anesthesia, the mapped areas are vertically punctured at the mapped sites and aspirated.

▶ PITFALLS

1. Most problematic is the puncture of adjacent vascular or nerve structures. This can be avoided with real-time guidance, making it preferable in many situations to static imaging and marking.
2. Iatrogenic joint infection, although extremely are, is a possibility. There is some debated if real-time ultrasound guidance increases or decreases this risk.
3. Failure to aspirate fluid may occur if performing the procedure blindly and at this point real-time guidance may be helpful.
4. Vasovagal reactions may occur with needle penetration.

▶ LUMBAR PUNCTURE

CLINICAL CONSIDERATIONS

Lumbar puncture (LP) is a frequently performed procedure in any emergency department and in skilled hands is usually successful without the need for imaging assistance. There remains, however, a challenging subset of patients where even the skilled practitioner will be unable to successfully perform an LP. Procedural failure in these patients often occurs because of the clinician's inability to identify bony landmarks relied upon for performance of LP or because of degenerative changes in the interspinous structures. Ultrasound imaging can be used to assist with landmark localization, potentially obviating the need for such referral and facilitating successful performance of the procedure at the bedside.

Traditional landmark technique for performance of lumbar puncture relies upon the identification of midline lumbar spinous processes and the intercristal or Tuffier's line, an imaginary line drawn on the back between the highest points of the two iliac crests. Where the intersection of these two lines occurs is purported to represent the location of the L4 spinous process or the L4–L5 interspace. In one report on a series of 300 parturients receiving epidural anesthesia, prepuncture ultrasound of the lumbar spine created conditions that allowed for a more focused puncture process and for a significant reduction in the number of puncture attempts. Determination of an optimal skin puncture site, the ideal direction of needle advancement, and, most importantly, knowledge of the magnitude of the skin to epidural space distance were the factors that were felt to have contributed to this more focused and successful puncture technique.

Ultrasound has also found a role in the assessment of failed neonatal lumbar punctures. Because the relevant anatomic structures are more superficial and the posterior elements of the spine poorly ossified in this group of patients, high-resolution images of both intra- and extra-spinal anatomy can frequently be obtained. In a series of 32 patients aged 3–86 days referred for fluoroscopy after failed blind LP attempts, the authors emphasized the value of ultrasound for first assessing the thecal sac for a possible epidural or intrathecal hematoma. Because success rates in obtaining spinal fluid are low in patients with no definable cerebrospinal fluid (CSF) space, a fluoroscopic attempt would therefore be avoided or delayed.

ANATOMIC CONSIDERATIONS

Beginning from the skin in the midline of the lower lumbar region, the most posterior bony structure encountered will be the curved spinous processes of the lumbar vertebrae. They are located at varying depths below the skin surface depending on body habitus, are 3–8 mm in width with a triangular configuration in coronal section (widest portion caudal), 15–20 mm in height, have a quadrilateral shape (midline sagittal orientation) with a caudally slanting tilt of the superior and inferior borders, and are 3–4 cm in length. Of note, the fifth lumbar vertebra has a smaller spinous process than the other lumbar vertebrae (helpful for establishing a precise level for needle entry). In a cross-sectional view of the lumbar spine from behind, the spinous process is represented as the long handle of a "Y" that then flares out into the two broad laminal plates. The laminae form the bony posterior roof of the spinal canal, splay out 30–45 degrees laterally to each side of the spinous process on cross section, and have an anteroposterior tilt in vertical profile like shingles on a roof. The laminae are contiguous with the superior and inferior articular processes whose facets articulate with the articular processes of adjacent lumbar vertebrae. The two transverse processes are long and slender, project horizontally to each side, and arise from the junctions of the laminae and the pedicles in the upper lumbar vertebrae, and from the pedicles and vertebral body in the lower lumbar vertebrae. The two pedicles connect all the posterior elements of the lumbar vertebra to the body of the vertebra.

The range of distances from the skin surface to the epidural space in a series of 72 parturients was found to be quite broad, ranging from 20 to 90 mm, with an average distance from skin to ligamentum flavum of 51.2 mm. With caudal progression, the distance from skin to the epidural space was noted to increase.

CLINICAL INDICATIONS

- Lumbar puncture in a patient with no obvious anatomic landmarks visible or palpable.
- Lumbar puncture after failed attempts with limited anatomic detail on physical examination.

TECHNIQUE AND ULTRASOUND FINDINGS

The anatomic relationship of the spinous processes, laminae, ligamentum flavum and dura, and the recommended transducer positions for obtaining midline sagittal and paramedian images of the lumbar spine are clearly demonstrated in Figures 20-47A and B. Midline sagittal scans of the lumbar spine with a linear array transducer set at 4–5 cm field depth will demonstrate the hyperechoic, convex posterior surfaces of the lumbar spinous processes (Figure 20-48). The skin appears hyperechoic, the subcutaneous tissue hypoechoic and of variable thickness depending on body habitus (Figure 20-49), and the horizontally oriented thoracolum-

bar fascia and supraspinal ligament are seen as a somewhat hyperechoic layer that follows the course of the spinous processes. If the transducer is off midline, the longitudinally oriented paraspinal muscle fibers will be seen just below the echogenic layer of thoracolumbar fascia (Figure 20-50). When centered over the midline, the transducer may be moved superiorly and inferiorly to precisely locate the interspace between adjacent spinous processes. Portions of adjacent curved spinous processes will then be seen in the lateral portions of the image (Figure 20-51). As the linear array transducer moves down to the level of the L5 spinous process, the supraspinal ligament will be noted to transition from its horizontal course and will be seen curving downward on the right side of the image as it descends to its insertion on the sacrum (Figure 20-52).

For the deeper structures of interest—the ligamentum flavum, epidural space, and the posterior and anterior walls of the dural sac—a 6- to 8-cm field depth will be required. From the midline position the linear array transducer is lined up over the interspace between two adjacent spinous processes. A somewhat echogenic horizontal line representing the posterior midline dura will be found in the well between these interspaces, about 3–4 cm deep to the surface of the posterior spinous processes. In general, the imaging depth required and the narrow acoustic window afforded by this location make the images somewhat difficult to obtain (Figure 20-53). With the better penetration of the curved array transducer at this depth (also from the midline position) a succession of three horizontal lines may be noted at the base of this well representing first, the ligamentum flavum, next, the posterior and anterior walls of the dural sac, and occasionally an additional echo return will be seen from the posterior surface of the vertebral body itself.

The paramedian imaging location provides a larger acoustic window for visualizing the ligamentum flavum, epidural space, and dural sac. Image depth needs to be set at about 7–8 cm; the orientation marker is oriented cephalad as with midline imaging. On the left side of the linear array image a bright, slightly curved hyperechoic line will be seen with distinct posterior acoustic shadowing. This curved line represents the posterior cortical surface of a superior hemi-lamina that has been scanned in cross section. Just to the right of and several millimeters deep to the top of this curved echo two echogenic horizontal lines will be seen. These echogenic lines represent the posterior and anterior surfaces of the ligamentum flavum, respectively. The epidural space lies immediately below the ligamentum flavum, followed by another usually somewhat more echogenic horizontal line that represents the posterior wall of the dural sac. The echo from this structure is usually found about 8–10 mm deep to the posterior facing surface of the ligamentum flavum (Figure 20-54). A depth measurement taken

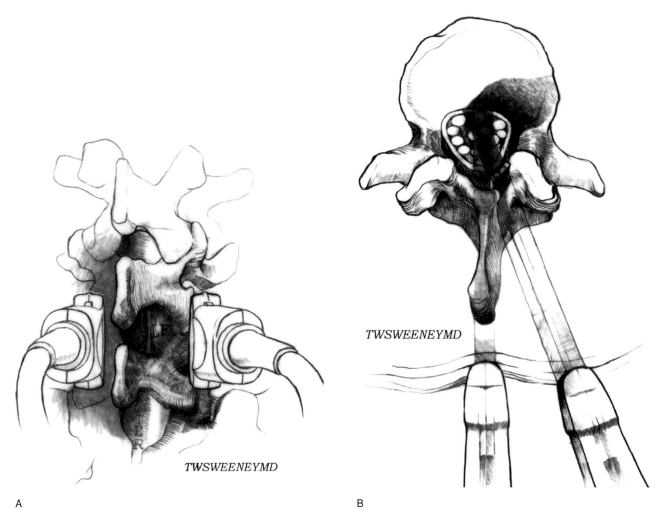

A   B

Figure 20-47. Sagittal (A) and transverse (B) drawings of the lumbar spine demonstrating the relationship of the spinous processes, laminae, ligamentum flavum, and dura mater as well as the recommended transducer positions for imaging the lumbar spine from both midline and paramedian locations. (Anatomic drawings kindly provided by artist and emergency physician Timothy W. Sweeney, MD)

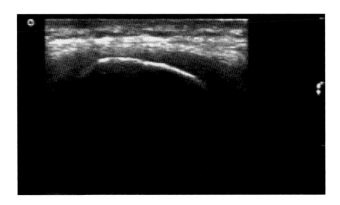

Figure 20-48. Midline sagittal linear array image of a lumbar spinous process in a patient with a normal habitus. The hyperechoic, convex posterior surface of a lumbar spinous process is seen in the near field of the image.

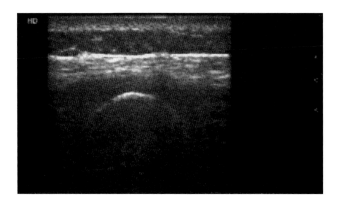

Figure 20-49. Midline sagittal linear array image of a lumbar spinous process in a patient in whom the spinous processes were not palpable. The skin appears hyperechoic, the subcutaneous tissue hypoechoic, and the thoracolumbar fascia and supraspinal ligament appear as a hyperechoic layer above the contour of the hyperechoic spinous process.

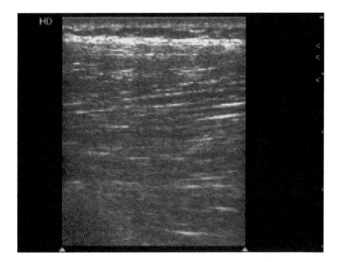

Figure 20-50. Longitudinally oriented paraspinal muscle fibers are seen just below the echogenic layer of thoracolumbar fascia on this sagittal sonogram that is no longer centered on the lumbar midline.

from the skin surface to this posterior dural sac echo will correlate highly with the depth needed to obtain CSF. With the broader field of view and the better penetration of the curved array transducer, both the superior and inferior laminae may be seen, along with the ligamentum flavum (sometimes), both walls of the dural sac, and occasionally the posterior surface of the corresponding body of the vertebra (Figure 20-55).

At the level of the intergluteal fold the midline sacrum will be seen as an echogenic linear structure, 3–5 cm below the skin surface, tilting either horizontally or down toward the left portion of the image (Figure 20-56A). A small V-shaped dip will often be noted near

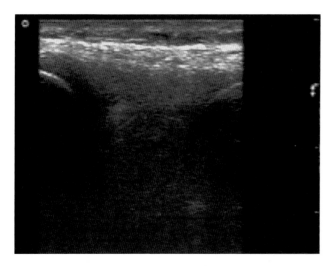

Figure 20-51. Midline sagittal linear array image of the interspinous space. The hyperechoic convexities of adjacent spinous processes are seen in the lateral portions of the image.

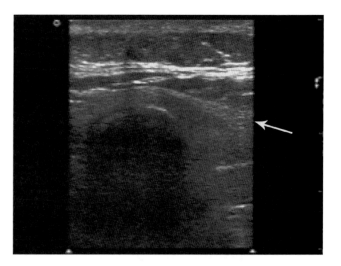

Figure 20-52. Midline sagittal linear array scan of the L5 spinous process. The supraspinal ligament is seen as mid-level grey structure just above the spinous process and is seen to descend on the right side of the image (arrow) as it proceeds to its insertion on the sacrum.

the top of the sacrum; this usually represents the recess just below the most superior ridge of the sacral crest. As one proceeds superiorly and just beyond this echogenic convexity, the next dip in the image corresponds to the L5–S1 interspace. The spinous processes can be counted upward from this reference point. As the transducer is moved cephalad, several spinous processes will be seen on a single curved array image (Figure 20-56B).

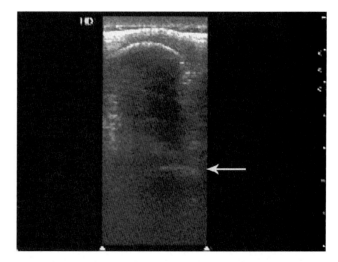

Figure 20-53. Midline sagittal linear array image of a lumbar spinous process. The somewhat echogenic horizontal line in the far field of the right side of the image represents the posterior facing surface of the midline dura (arrow). The narrow acoustic window afforded by this location makes the image somewhat difficult to obtain and interpret.

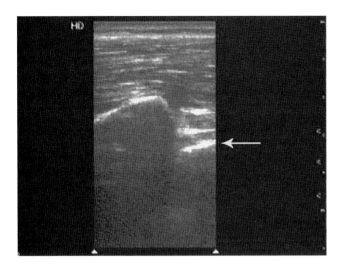

Figure 20-54. Paramedian sagittal linear array image. The echogenic posterior facing surface of the lamina is seen to the left of the image and a prominent posterior acoustic shadow is noted. The first two horizontal lines to the right of the lamina represent the two surfaces of the ligamentum flavum. Immediately below lies the epidural space, followed by another usually somewhat more echogenic horizontal line that represents the posterior wall of the dural sac (arrow). The distance from the posterior facing surface of the ligamentum flavum and the posterior facing wall of the dural sac is usually about 8–10 mm.

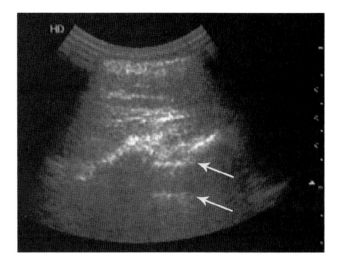

Figure 20-55. Paramedian sagittal curved array image. Laminae of adjacent vertebra are seen as brightly echogenic angulated lines with prominent posterior acoustic shadowing. The ligamentum flavum no longer appears as a distinct structure. Both walls of the dural sac (arrows) are apparent as horizontal echogenic lines in the space between and deep to adjacent laminae.

In transverse orientation with a curved array transducer, the hyperechoic posterior surface of a lumbar spinous process is often hard to visualize, but its location will be apparent by the midline posterior acoustic shadow that it casts. The paraspinal muscles will appear as two circular bundles on either side of the spinous

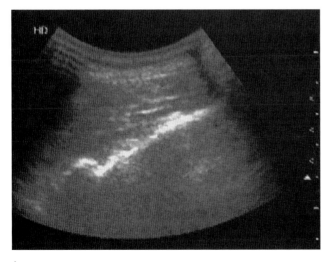

A

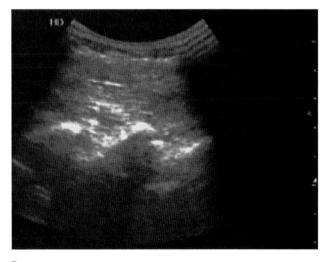

B

Figure 20-56. A midline sagittal curved array image at the level of the intergluteal fold will reveal the posterior surface of the sacrum as a hyperechoic line. The V-shaped dip to the left of the image represents the space below the superior sacral crest. The L5–S1 interspace is found just superior to this ridge, off to the left side of the image. Moving cephalad and paramedian (B), the L4 and L5 laminae are seen on a single sagittal curved array image as echogenic lines with prominent posterior acoustic shadowing. The echogenic posterior surface of the sacrum is seen to the right of the image.

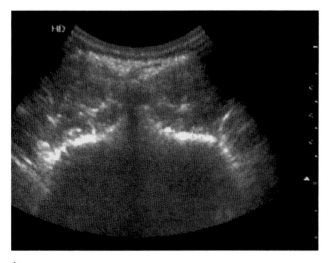

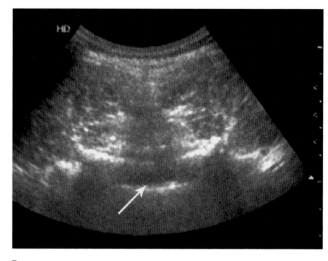

A

B

Figure 20-57. In this transverse curved array image (A), the lumbar spinous process is best found by following its midline posterior acoustic shadow up to the near field of the image. The paraspinal muscles appear as symmetric circular bundles on either side of the spinous process. The echogenic posterior-facing surfaces of the laminae appear as a cape-like structure with dense posterior acoustic shadowing below. In this somewhat more cephalad transverse curved array image (B), a series of echogenic lines is seen that correspond to the articular and transverse processes and the posterior facing surface of the vertebral body. The paired articular processes appear brightly echogenic and exhibit prominent posterior acoustic shadowing. To their immediate right and somewhat deeper are a pair of echogenic lines that correspond to the transverse processes. The bright echo from the posterior facing surface of the vertebral body lies somewhat deeper in the midline of the image. The spinal canal appears as the hypoechoic region just anterior to this vertebral body echo (arrow).

process. Over the lower portion of the vertebra, the laminae will appear as a cape-like structure, echogenic on the posterior facing surface, with a dense posterior acoustic shadow below (Figure 20-57A). When the transducer is moved somewhat cephalad, echogenic lines will be seen that correspond to the articular and transverse processes and the posterior facing surface of the vertebral body. The spinal canal will appear as a hypoechoic circle just anterior to this vertebral body echo (Figure 20-57B).

Depending on the patient's degree of illness, ability to cooperate, and the preference of the physician performing the procedure, the patient may be placed in either a seated position leaning forward over a tray table or in a lateral decubitus position with knees and back flexed. The most rapid approach is to locate the spinous processes in a midline sagittal orientation and mark this midline location above and below the transducer with indelible ink. When centered directly over a spinous process, its location and superior–inferior extent can be marked with a corresponding curve just lateral to the transducer (Figure 20-58). This should be done with the three lowest lumbar spinous processes encountered. A quick confirmation of the level of these mapped spinous processes can be achieved by placing the curved array transducer sagittally on the midline sacrum at the level of the intergluteal fold. The bright echo from the sacrum will be seen and as the transducer is moved cephalad,

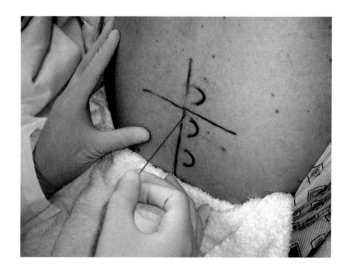

Figure 20-58. The precise location of the lumbar midline and the relative location of the curved spinous processes have been mapped and marked with an indelible marker. A horizontal line is used to indicate the L3–L4 interspace. Needle entry begins in the lower half of the interspace and the needle is angled cephalad both to avoid the spinous process above and to follow the cranial slanting path to the dural sac. For purposes of illustration, the sterile drape is not shown.

and the shorter spinous process of L5 noted. Counting of the spinous processes can proceed accordingly from this reference point and be correlated with what has already been mapped. A horizontal line should be placed at the level of the mid L3–L4 interspace to mark the optimal skin entry point. A paramedian view may simultaneously be made at this interspace and note made of the ideal trajectory and the magnitude of the distance to the dural sac in case a paramedian approach will be required. Once located and properly marked, the approach is the same as without ultrasound assistance. If the paramedian approach is employed, the puncture site may be several centimeters off the midline at the low to mid interspace level.

▶ PITFALLS

1. Morbidly obese patients may present so much soft tissue that most medical ultrasound gear available in an emergency setting will not penetrate deep enough to see bony structures.

▶ NERVE BLOCKS

CLINICAL CONSIDERATIONS

Regional nerve and plexus blocks have been integral to the practice of anesthesiology for over 50 years and are commonly used for hand, arm, knee, and foot surgery. Traditional training in regional anesthesia relies upon identification of anatomic landmarks and the use of a nerve stimulator to assist with accurate placement of the anesthetic delivery needle as close to the target nerve or nerve plexus as possible. The success of these regional anesthetic blocks is highly operator dependent, however, and even with the use of a nerve stimulator in skilled hands, a block failure rate of 10%–30% is not uncommon, depending on the site of the block.

In the past 10–15 years an emerging body of anesthesia literature has demonstrated the significant role ultrasound can play in enhancing both the performance and success rates of these various regional block techniques.[8–19] The development of more portable ultrasound equipment, higher resolution transducers, and improved picture-processing technology (such as compound imaging) have all helped accelerate this process, and the utilization of ultrasound for performance of regional anesthetic blocks is moving toward becoming standard of care. For all of the commonly performed nerve and plexus blocks, ultrasound imaging allows for real-time visualization of the target nerve in most patients. This, in turn, allows the operator to deposit the anesthetic agent in a precise location, simultaneously enhancing all the desirable operating characteristics of the procedure and minimizing complications.

In a series of 40 patients undergoing forearm or hand surgery, one study reported an ultrasound-guided brachial plexus block success rate of 95% at both the supraclavicular and axillary sites with no reported complications; this compares with an historical 70–80% block success rate at this site with a nerve stimulator. More importantly, the ultrasound-guided supraclavicular brachial plexus block provided the additional advantage of reliable anesthesia of the musculocutaneous nerve with a minimal risk of associated complications such as pneumothorax.

In a series of 40 patients with hip fracture receiving a femoral nerve block for analgesia prior to surgery, the onset of femoral nerve sensory blockade was noted to be significantly faster in the ultrasound group (16 minutes) compared with the nerve stimulator group (27 minutes), and overall block success improved from 85% in the nerve stimulator group to 95% with ultrasound guidance. In a subsequent study, 60 patients with hip fracture were randomized to receive a femoral nerve block for pre-op analgesia. The ultrasound group had higher procedural success rates (95% with ultrasound compared to 80% with nerve stimulator technique), an improved onset time of sensory loss, and a smaller overall volume of anesthetic required for the block (20 mL 0.5% bupivacaine in the ultrasound-guided group compared with 30 mL 0.5% bupivacaine in the nerve stimulator group).

Ultrasound guidance clearly leads to improved nerve block success rates, more rapid onset of complete analgesia, a decreased volume of anesthetic agent required for block performance, and fewer procedural complications. Complications from regional nerve and plexus blocks vary with the site being punctured and include pain from needle insertion and direct nerve irritation, prolonged procedure times if localization is difficult or if block onset is delayed, possible block failure, iatrogenic nerve damage from presumed intraneural sheath injection, reported spinal cord injury with the interscalene block, phrenic or recurrent laryngeal nerve paralysis as well as inadvertent lung puncture and pneumothorax with the interscalene and supraclavicular brachial plexus blocks, inadvertent vascular puncture and bleeding, systemic reactions to local anesthetics, infection, and vasovagal reactions.

ANATOMIC CONSIDERATIONS

Physicians performing these blocks should first refamiliarize themselves with the detailed regional anatomy of the area being punctured. The successive anatomic layers encountered in the supraclavicular region are as follows: skin, platysma muscle fibers coursing inferolaterally from the chin to the clavicle, sternoclei-domastoid muscle forming the medial border, the clavicle forming the anterior border, and the trapezius muscle forming the posterior border of this triangular shaped region. The C4–T1 nerve roots that make up the brachial plexus exit from their respective vertebral foramina between the anterior and middle scalene muscles and course inferolaterally where they coalesce into the upper, middle, and lower trunks of the brachial plexus in the supraclavicular region. The trunks subsequently divide into anterior and posterior divisions, and then into the medial, lateral, and posterior cords before ending as the terminal branches of the brachial plexus (the radial, median, and ulnar nerves) in the upper axillary region. The three scalene muscles (anterior, middle, and posterior) arise from the transverse processes of the cervical spine and insert on the superior surface of the first rib. At the anterior border of the supraclavicular fossa and immediately posterior to the clavicle the superficially located brachial plexus roots and trunks are clustered in a fascial plane that lies immediately lateral to the subclavian artery. The anterior scalene muscle—inserting on the medial aspect of the first rib—lies just medial to the subclavian artery; the first rib lies below or in close proximity to the combined artery and plexus cluster, and the middle scalene muscle lies just lateral to the plexus. The subclavian vein courses adjacent to or over the flattened surface of the first rib just *medial* to the anterior scalene muscle insertion. Lung tissue lies just below the rib with the cupula of the lung rising above the level of the first rib as one moves more medially and posteriorly. The phrenic nerve runs longitudinally along the anteromedial surface of the anterior scalene muscle.

At the level of the axillary crease in the uppermost anterior axilla, the axillary artery, vein, and the branches of the brachial plexus course just below the skin surface within a neurovascular fascial sheath, resting on a fascial plane known as the medial brachial intermuscular septum. This fascial plane separates the arm extensors (biceps and coracobrachialis muscles) from the arm extensors (triceps muscle). The terminal branches of the brachial plexus (median, ulnar, and radial nerves) are found within this neurovascular fascial sheath in close proximity to the axillary vessels, typically surrounding the axillary artery.

The distribution of anesthesia provided by these nerve blocks is typically as follows. An axillary brachial plexus block will provide complete anesthesia of the arm, elbow, forearm, and hand provided that the musculocutaneous nerve is successfully blocked at the axillary level. If the musculocutaneous nerve is not blocked, no anesthetic effect will be achieved in the region innervated by the lateral cutaneous nerve of the forearm (specifically, the radial aspect of the forearm as well as the radial half of the volar surface of the forearm). The

supraclavicular brachial plexus block has the advantage of providing a rapid and more consistent blockade of this entire territory and should be used when this larger field of anesthesia is desired. Note that these two blocks do not provide adequate analgesia for procedures of the shoulder.

In the femoral region at the level of the inguinal crease (just inferior to the inguinal ligament), the anatomic layers of relevance for the femoral nerve block are as follows: skin, subcutaneous tissue, fascia lata (dense connective tissue that covering the muscles of the hip and thigh), and from medial to lateral, the femoral vein, artery, and nerve. The femoral artery and vein are encased in a thick connective tissue sheath. The femoral nerve is found immediately lateral and somewhat deep to the femoral artery. Proximal to the inguinal ligament, the femoral nerve lies deep to and then somewhat lateral to the psoas major muscle. As the femoral nerve comes from behind the psoas muscle and approaches the inguinal region, it then runs deep to the iliopectineal arch. Despite its immediate proximity to the femoral artery, the femoral nerve is located in a separate fascial plane, physically separated from the vessels in the femoral sheath by the iliopectineal fascia. The latter is a thick connective tissue fascial layer that arises from the psoas minor tendon, covers the medial distal portion of the iliacus muscle and the femoral nerve, and then extends medially under the adjacent femoral artery and vein to the anterior surface of the pectineus muscle found inferior and medial to the femoral vein. The pubic bone and the iliopubic eminence of the acetabulum lie just deep to the femoral vessels and nerve. The lateral femoral cutaneous nerve and the obturator nerve that are included in the "three-in-one" block of the femoral nerve originate more proximally and course along the anterior surface of the iliacus muscle.

Peripheral nerves are not rigidly fixed and they may exhibit some degrees of mobility within the anesthetic solution that is injected around them. The shape of a given nerve or nerve plexus in short-axis orientation may vary from round to triangular to oval depending on where in its long-axis location it is scanned, and its relationship to underlying bony structures or fascial planes. Some of the commonly blocked nerves will be found to be located at a very shallow depth below the skin surface. In a study of 15 volunteers, the mean skin-to-nerve distance of the most superficial portion of the brachial plexus in the supraclavicular area was noted 0.9 ± 0.3 cm. Similar results were reported in the axillary region.

CLINICAL INDICATIONS

- Regional nerve blockade in any location

TECHNIQUE AND ULTRASOUND FINDINGS

Nerve tissue appears hypoechoic relative to surrounding subcutaneous tissue and nerves as small as 2 mm in diameter (such as the digital nerves at the proximal digital crease) may be visualized with a 10 MHz linear array probe. From anatomic correlation studies it is reported that a 15 MHz transducer will reveal approximately one third of the fascicles that are seen on microscopy. Cervical roots exhibit a sonographic pattern that is hypoechoic and described as monofascicular; in short axis, they appear as rounded hypoechoic shapes within the more brightly echogenic fascial tissue that surrounds them. Nerves are usually somewhat more echogenic than blood vessels and, unlike blood vessels, are not compressible. This feature, along with color or power Doppler interrogation, can help distinguish a nerve from an adjacent vessel.

As nerve bundles become larger, they will usually exhibit greater internal echogenicity. A more prominent internal fascicular pattern may be noted, due to the greater amount of echogenic connective tissue (epineurium and perineurium) holding the nerve bundles together. Depending on the size of the nerve being imaged and the resolution of the transducer being employed, nerve bundles will also exhibit some degree of anisotropy, although less so than tendons.

The median nerve is an excellent target nerve to image for improving one's skills at nerve recognition by ultrasound. It is readily visualized in cross section at the distal flexor wrist crease with a 10 MHz or higher frequency transducer. In short axis it appears as a superficial, hypoechoic oval structure with an echogenic rim; its fascicular pattern of internal echogenicity is differentiated from the more echogenic fibrillar internal echotexture of the underlying tendons in the carpal tunnel (Figure 20-59).

In the supraclavicular region, the bright echo of the first rib will be seen in the most distal portions of the sonogram with the rounded, anechoic subclavian artery located either just above or adjacent to the echogenic superior rib margin. The cluster of nerves that make up the brachial plexus at this level will always be found immediately lateral to and often somewhat superior to the level of the subclavian artery. The visualized roots and trunks of the brachial plexus appear as a cluster of many oval or rounded hypoechoic nodules set off by the more hyperechoic fascial tissue that surrounds them. The fascial sheath containing the brachial plexus is situated between two hypoechoic muscle bundles, the medially located anterior scalene muscle and the laterally located middle scalene muscle (Figures 20-60A, 20-60B, and 20-60C).

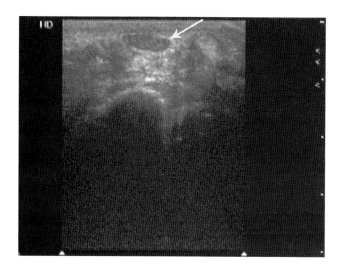

Figure 20-59. Median nerve in cross section. The median nerve at the level of the volar proximal wrist crease appears as a superficially located hypoechoic oval structure with a hyperechoic rim (arrow). The nerve is hypoechoic relative to the surrounding tendons.

In a short-axis view of the arm at the level of anterior axillary crease, the pulsatile axillary artery will appear as an anechoic circle in the near field, located about 1–1.5 cm below the skin surface (Figure 20-61). Since the axillary vessels are quite superficial at this level, even light probe pressure may collapse the axillary vein (or veins) and make it (or them) invisible. The axillary vein may therefore become apparent only if the patient performs a Valsalva maneuver (Figure 20-62). The axillary vessels and branches of the brachial plexus rest on an echogenic fascial plane known as the medial brachial intermuscular septum; this septum separates the arm extensors above (biceps and coracobrachialis) from the flexors below (triceps muscle). In short-axis orientation at the level of the axilla, the three terminal nerve branches of the brachial plexus (the median, ulnar, and radial nerves) will typically be seen as hypoechoic circles circumferentially surrounding the axillary artery; occasionally only two nerves will be noted.

In the femoral region, the femoral nerve may have a rounded, oval, or triangular shape in short-axis orientation and may exhibit somewhat greater echogenicity than the nerves seen in the brachial plexus. The femoral nerve can be found immediately lateral and somewhat deep to the anechoic common femoral artery, and is situated medial to the iliacus muscle (Figures 20-63A and 20-63B).

High-frequency linear array transducers in the 7.5–15 MHz range are recommended for supraclavicular and axillary brachial plexus blocks; 5–10 MHz linear array transducers have been used successfully for "three-in-one" femoral nerve blocks. The usual sterile prep, drape,

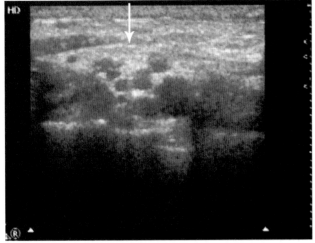

A

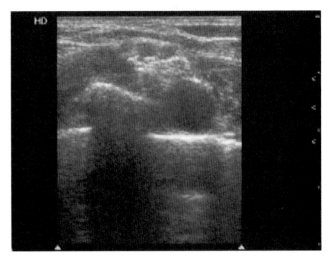

B

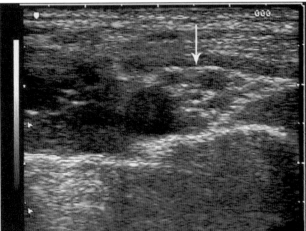

C

Figure 20-60. Supraclavicular brachial plexus. (A) Right supraclavicular brachial plexus with the nerve trunks and divisions appearing as a cluster of superficial hypoechoic circles within a more hyperechoic fascial sheath (arrow). The middle scalene muscle appears as a hypoechoic structure just lateral to the plexus (to the left, on this image), the subclavian artery is seen as the largest and most hypoechoic circle near the center of the image, and the anterior scalene muscle appears as a somewhat indistinct hypoechoic structure just medial to the subclavian artery (to the right, on this image). (B) Right supraclavicular brachial plexus with a prominent rib shadow from the first rib, and the brightly echogenic pleural line noted below the subclavian artery. The plexus is somewhat less distinct in this patient, and appears laterally adjacent and superior to the hypoechoic subclavian artery. (C) Left supraclavicular brachial plexus. The subclavian artery and brachial plexus (arrow) are seen overlying the brightly echogenic superior surface of the first rib.

and a sterile probe cover are assumed for all nerve blocks as well as appropriate anesthetic agents and needles. Typical cutting needles such as the average 18-gauge needle found in most settings are suboptimal for nerve blocks and a noncutting needle such as a spinal needle should be used.

For most nerve blocks the needle used for anesthetic deposition should be advanced in the plane of the ultrasound beam so that precise real-time needle tip localization can be performed. This is best accomplished with needle insertion on the outer end of the transducer so that the nerve or nerve bundle is seen in short axis and the needle in long axis. Thus, the tip of the needle can be visualized throughout its course and precise delivery of anesthetic can be assured. If paresthesias are elicited, the needle should be moved slightly so that an intraneural injection will be avoided.

Supraclavicular Brachial Plexus Block

The patient should be supine, with arms at the side in neutral position and the head turned 45 degrees away from the side of the block. The skin in the supraclavicular fossa is prepped and draped. The transducer is covered with a sterile probe cover and a sterile conductive medium is applied to the skin. The transducer is placed just posterior to the clavicle and lateral to the sternocleidomastoid in an oblique coronal plane with the transducer orientation marker facing left. The medial portion of probe will be angled more anteriorly than coronally, following the angle of the clavicle (Figure 20-64). Anesthetize the skin entry site with lidocaine under direct ultrasound visualization. Then use a 22–24-gauge 5–7-cm spinal type needle that has been attached to a short piece of extension tubing and connected to a

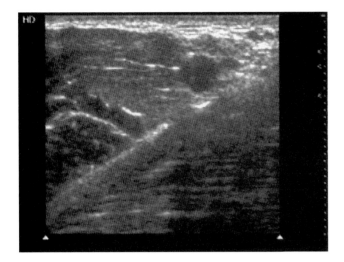

Figure 20-61. Right axillary brachial plexus. Typically, only the axillary artery will be apparent since even light probe pressure will collapse the superficially located axillary vein. The echogenic fascial plane on which the vessels and plexus rest (the medial brachial intermuscular septum) separate the arm extensors above from flexors below. This septum may be obliquely or horizontally situated in the image.

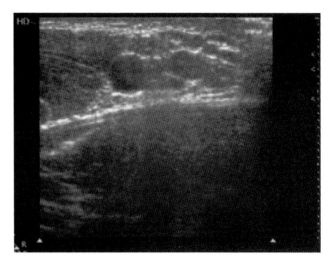

Figure 20-62. Right axillary brachial plexus. A valsalva maneuver has been performed and the distended axillary vein can be seen to the right of the axillary artery. Surrounding the artery are the hypoechoic branches of the brachial plexus that are found at this level (specifically, the radial, median and ulnar nerves).

20-mL syringe filled with the desired agent for anesthetic delivery. Introduce the needle from the posterolateral edge of the transducer and move the needle anteromedially toward the brachial plexus nerve cluster under real-time guidance. When the needle tip is in close contact to the cluster, the needle can be held fixed in place while an assistant delivers a test dose of 1–2 mL of anesthetic agent after first aspirating to ensure that no intravascular injection will occur. If the agent spreads around the target nerves, continue to slowly deliver the rest of the

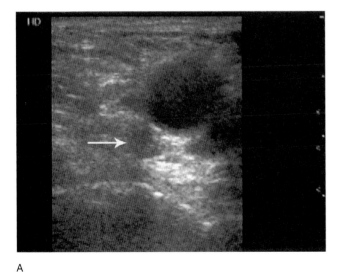

A

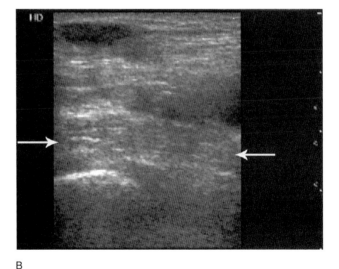

B

Figure 20-63. The right femoral nerve is seen in this short-axis image (A) as an ovoid hypoechoic circle (arrow) that lies just deep and slightly lateral to the common femoral artery. The somewhat deeper echogenic curve below the nerve represents the iliopubic eminence of the acetabulum. In a long-axis view of this same femoral nerve (B) the subtle fibrillar echotexture of the nerve is apparent as it courses approximately 5 mm above the echogenic iliopubic eminence (arrows).

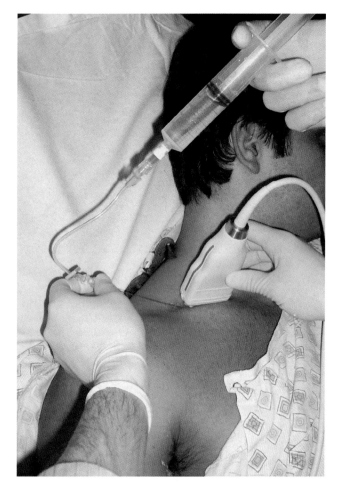

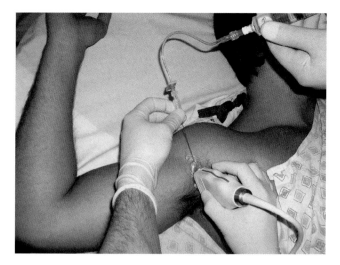

Figure 20-65. Axillary brachial plexus technique. The patient is in "high-5" position with transducer placed high in the anterior axilla at the level of the anterior axillary crease (at the border between the biceps and the deltoid muscle). The transducer is oriented vertically, perpendicular to the long axis of the humerus. The anesthetic delivery needle is inserted from the superior aspect of the transducer and positioned under direct ultrasound guidance. When the needle tip reaches the desired location, the operator can hold it in a fixed position while an assistant delivers a test dose (1–2 cc) of the anesthetic solution to confirm adequate needle tip placement. For purposes of illustration, the sterile drape and probe cover are not shown.

Figure 20-64. Supraclavicular brachial plexus technique. The patient's head is turned to the opposite side and the transducer is held in an oblique coronal plane just behind the clavicle. The anesthetic delivery needle is inserted on the lateral aspect of the transducer and positioned under direct ultrasound guidance. When the needle tip reaches the desired location, the operator can hold it in fixed position while an assistant delivers a test dose (1–2 cc) of the anesthetic solution to confirm adequate needle tip placement. For purposes of illustration, the sterile drape and probe cover are not shown.

anesthetic agent; if not, reposition the needle, deliver another test dose and proceed accordingly.

Axillary Perivascular Brachial Plexus Block

The patient should be supine with the head midline, arm abducted to 90 degrees, elbow flexed at 90–100 degrees, and the back of the hand resting on the bed facing upward ("High-5" position). The skin at the level of the anterior axillary crease is prepped and draped. The transducer is covered with a sterile probe cover and a sterile conductive medium is applied to the skin.

The transducer is placed high in the anterior axilla at the level of the anterior axillary crease (at the border between the deltoid and the biceps muscle). The transducer should be placed perpendicular to the long axis of the humerus with the orientation marker facing up so that a short-axis view of the vessels and nerves will be obtained (Figure 20-65). Anesthetize the skin entry site with lidocaine under direct ultrasound visualization. Then use a 22–24-gauge 5–7-cm noncutting needle that has been attached to a short piece of extension tubing and connected to a 20-mL syringe filled with the desired agent for anesthetic delivery. Introduce the needle from the lateral edge of the transducer and move the needle toward the axillary artery under real-time guidance, just like in long-axis vascular access. When the needle tip is either in close proximity to the axillary artery or ideally, between the artery and the vein, the needle can be held fixed in place while an assistant delivers a test dose of 1–2 mL of anesthetic agent after first aspirating to ensure that no intravascular injection will occur. If the agent spreads around the target nerves, continue to slowly deliver the rest of the anesthetic agent; if not, reposition the needle, deliver another test dose, and proceed accordingly.

Femoral Nerve Block

The patient is supine with both legs extended; the side on which the block is to be performed may be slightly externally rotated. The skin at the area of the femoral crease and femoral vessels is prepped and draped, and the transducer is covered with a sterile probe cover. Sterile conductive medium is applied to skin. The transducer is placed in an oblique transverse orientation at the level of and in line with the inguinal crease. The femoral nerve will be seen immediately lateral and somewhat deep to the common femoral artery; the nerve should be positioned in the center of the image (Figure 20-66). Anesthetize the skin entry site with lidocaine under direct visualization. Use a 22–24-gauge 5–7-cm noncutting needle attached to a short piece of extension tubing and connected to a 20-mL syringe filled with the desired anesthetic agent. Introduce the needle lateral to the edge of the transducer (long-axis approach) and advance the needle under real-time guidance. When the needle tip has punctured the iliopectineal fascia and is in close proximity to the femoral nerve, the needle can be held fixed in place while an assistant delivers a test dose of 1–2 mL of anesthetic agent after first aspirating

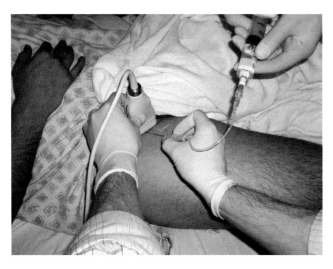

Figure 20-66. Femoral nerve block technique. The transducer is placed in an oblique transverse orientation at the level of and in line with the inguinal crease, orientation marker facing left. The femoral nerve is positioned in the center of the image and the anesthetic delivery needle is inserted below the center of the transducer in an out-of-plane approach. Under ultrasound guidance, the needle tip is positioned below the iliopectineal fascia as close to the femoral nerve as possible. When the needle tip reaches the desired location, the operator can hold it in a fixed position while an assistant delivers a test dose (1–2 cc) of the anesthetic solution to confirm adequate needle tip placement. For purposes of illustration, the sterile drape and probe cover are not shown.

to ensure that no intravascular injection will occur. If the anesthetic agent is seen to spread around the femoral nerve, continue to slowly deliver the rest of the anesthetic agent; if not, reposition the needle, deliver another test dose, and proceed accordingly. Pressure on the skin below the block during injection is said to augment cephalad deposition of the anesthetic agent. It should be noted that an inguinal paravascular injection technique will usually fail to block the femoral nerve both because the femoral sheath will impede the spread of anesthetic agent and because the nerve is physically separated from this sheath by the iliopectineal fascia.

▶ PITFALLS

1. Use of a cutting needle will make nerve injury much more likely. Use a noncutting needle like a spinal needle whenever possible.
2. Misidentification of vascular structures for nerves will lead to potential intravascular injection of large amount of anesthetic and failed blocks.
3. Failure to penetrate a nerve sheath and injection just outside of the nerve will lead to block failure.

▶ PARACENTESIS

CLINICAL CONSIDERATIONS

Confirming the presence and location of peritoneal fluid prior to paracentesis is simply an extension of the typical Focused Assessment with Sonography for Trauma (FAST) examination. Indications for performing abdominal paracentesis in the emergency department include the evaluation of the patient with new onset ascites, obtaining fluid for diagnostic purposes in the patient with suspected cancerous or spontaneous bacterial peritonitis, and as a therapeutic intervention to relieve discomfort or respiratory embarrassment in symptomatic patients with massive ascites. Occasionally, paracentesis may also play a role in clarifying the nature of the intraabdominal fluid found in a patient with a positive FAST examination but no clear history of trauma.

Ultrasound is considered a gold standard test for detecting ascites, reliably identifying as little as 100 mL of free fluid and occasionally able to detect volumes in the range of 5–10 mL around the bladder. Larger volumes are required for successful paracentesis, however, with reported success rates of only 44% when the volume of ascites is 300 mL, increasing to 78% at 500 mL. While the left lower quadrant has long been considered a standard location for blind paracentesis, patients with smaller volumes of ascites may have no sonographically demonstrable fluid present in this area. Routine bedside ultrasonography prior to every paracentesis that is performed in the emergency department is highly recommended. One reported series of 100 emergency department patients undergoing abdominal paracentesis demonstrated a significantly higher procedural success rate for ultrasound-assisted paracentesis compared to the traditional non–image-guided technique (95% vs 65%).

Diagnostic paracentesis typically involves the collection of small volumes of fluid for routine analysis (often <60 mL). Small volume therapeutic paracentesis is defined as removal of less than 2 liters of ascitic fluid; large volume paracentesis is commonly defined as more than 4 liters removed. Complications of paracentesis are infrequent but can include abdominal wall hematoma, inferior epigastric artery pseudoaneurysm, mesenteric hematoma, intraperitoneal hemorrhage, bladder and bowel perforation, abdominal wall abscess, persistent ascitic fluid leak, and peritonitis.

ANATOMIC CONSIDERATIONS

Although visualization of an accessible fluid pocket is paramount, guidelines for paracentesis also include a number of common-sense caveats. Avoid the upper quadrants, (hepatosplenomegaly), avoid surgical scars (possible adhesions and adherent bowel loops), stay remote and lateral to the rectus muscles (the superior and inferior epigastric vessels may inadvertently be punctured), avoid large collateral venous channels visible on the abdominal wall, avoid the right lower quadrant (gaseous distension at the cecum due to the use of lactulose is frequent, and there may be an appendectomy scar at this site), and finally, use a relatively small-gauge needle. A fluid collection of at least 3 cm in depth is considered adequate for the procedure. With the goal of finding a location for paracentesis that would simultaneously offer both the deepest pocket of fluid and the thinnest portion of the abdominal wall, one study obtained ultrasound images on 62 cirrhotic patients at two standard locations: the left lower quadrant (defined as 2 finger breadths medial and 2 finger breadths cephalad to the left anterior superior iliac spine) and the midline infraumbilical area (defined as 2 finger breadths inferior to the umbilicus). The abdominal wall exhibited a wide range of thickness in both locations (0.6–9.1 cm in the left lower quadrant and 0.9–9.5 cm in the infraumbilical midline), but was noted to be consistently thinner in the left lower quadrant (a mean of 1.8 cm compared to 2.4 cm in the midline). When the patient was positioned in the left lateral oblique position, the pool of ascites was noted to increase from an average of 2.86 to 4.57 cm.

CLINICAL INDICATIONS

- Diagnostic sampling of intraperitoneal fluid
- Therapeutic drainage of intraperitoneal fluid

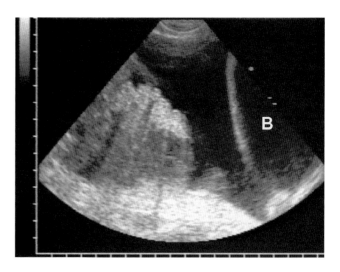

Figure 20-67. Midline sagittal view of a patient with a large amount of simple ascites. The echogenic bladder dome appears to the right of the image. Both urine and simple ascites appear similarly hypoechoic. Echogenic loops of bowel with "dirty" shadowing from intraluminal bowel gas are seen to the left of the image. B = bladder.

TECHNIQUE AND ULTRASOUND FINDINGS

Simple transudative ascites will appear as an anechoic extraluminal fluid collection within the peritoneal cavity. In a midline longitudinal orientation in the lower abdomen, the echogenic bladder dome may be seen to the right of the image with anechoic fluid and bowel loops noted adjacent to the bladder (Figure 20-67). Echogenic fibrinous strands may occasionally be noted within the fluid. Loops of peristaltic small bowel will usually be seen floating within the ascitic fluid and varying degrees of "dirty" shadowing may be present depending on the amount of intraluminal bowel gas present (Figure 20-68). A mesenteric stalk attached to the bowel loops may also be noted. It is important to remember that the presence of fluid on ultrasound examination does not always signify ascites. Acute hemoperitoneum (Figure 20-69) may also manifest as an entirely echo-free fluid collection. If any doubt exists as to the fluid identity, a diagnostic paracentesis or further imaging may be performed (Figure 20-70).

Ascitic fluid may occasionally appear particulate, exhibiting complex fluid characteristics with varying degrees of internal echogenicity that reflect the presence of either leukocytes, erythrocytes, protein particles, or fibrin within the fluid (Figure 20-71).

The ultrasound examination for ascites is typically performed with a 3.5 MHz curved linear array transducer. Gain settings should be adjusted to make the fluid appear black (assuming that the patient has simple ascites). If possible, the head of the bed should be

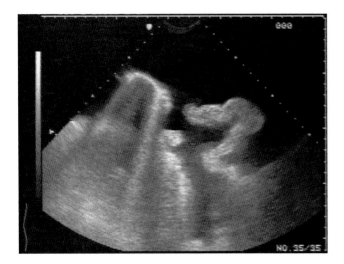

Figure 20-68. Large-volume simple ascites with hyperechoic loops of small bowel. Some "dirty" shadowing and hyperechoic reverberation artifacts from intraluminal bowel gas are noted. Gain settings have been adjusted to make the simple fluid appear uniformly black.

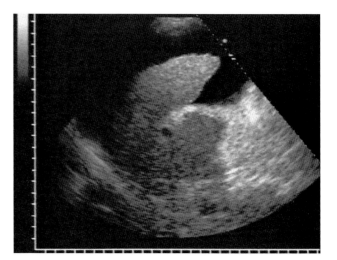

Figure 20-70. FAST orientation in the right upper quadrant. A large volume of anechoic intraperitoneal fluid is noted; given the hyperechoic, shrunken, and nodular appearance of the liver, one can reasonably assume that this fluid is ascites.

raised and, if needed, the patient turned slightly to the left lateral oblique position to maximize the depth of the fluid collection. Optimally, imaging should be performed just prior to the procedure with the patient remaining in the exact same position. The bladder dome should be noted so that it may be avoided during paracentesis if the planned site of paracentesis is in the midline infraumbilical region. The fluid pocket should be mapped in two orthogonal planes, and the skin entry site marked with indelible ink. The thickness of the abdominal wall, the

depth of the fluid pocket until bowel or bladder is encountered, and the anticipated puncture angle should all be noted. The volume of ascitic fluid being removed will dictate the type of equipment needed for the aspiration. For a diagnostic small volume aspiration, all that may be required is an 18-gauge needle or angiocatheter, a short piece of extension tubing and a 30–60-cc syringe (Figure 20-72). For a small volume therapeutic paracentesis, commercially available centesis kits with an 8 French catheter with multiple side holes, and a gravity feed collection bag (or vacuum bottles) may be used for the fluid

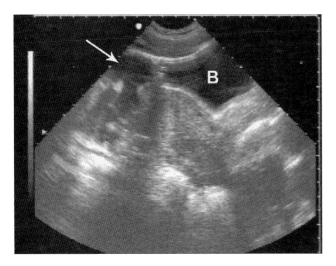

Figure 20-69. Midline sagittal view of a female with hemoperitoneum. The bladder and uterus are noted to the right of the image; the hypoechoic pocket of fluid (arrow) above the bladder dome represents unclotted blood and is sonographically indistinguishable from ascites. B = bladder.

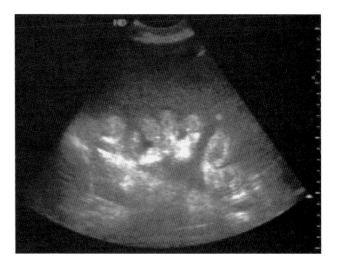

Figure 20-71. Hemorrhagic ascites; the ascitic fluid in this patient with known cirrhosis and ascites exhibits a complex pattern with increased echogenicity throughout. The patient presented with a 10-point drop in HCT from a recent prior visit; the search for a bleeding hepatoma proved positive.

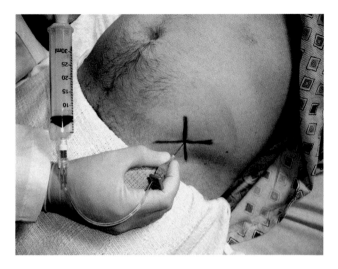

Figure 20-72. Paracentesis: small-volume aspiration technique. The fluid pocket has been mapped and marked in two orthogonal planes and the skin has been prepped in and anesthetized down to the peritoneum. The patient remains in the exact same position for the aspiration as when mapped and is asked to protrude the abdomen during the procedure to facilitate needle insertion and prevent inadvertent puncture of deeper structures. The extension tubing allows for manipulation of the syringe while the needle is held fixed in place. For purposes of illustration, the sterile drape is not shown.

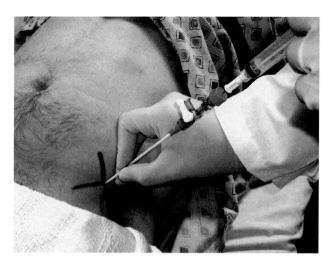

Figure 20-73. Paracentesis: Large-volume aspiration technique. Procedural details are similar to the small volume aspiration technique but with several additions. A skin stab wound is made to the beveled edge of the scalpel blade included in the centesis kit; this will facilitate passage of the 8 French catheter. Once ascitic fluid is aspirated, the catheter needle is held fixed while the catheter is advanced several centimeters. The large-gauge needle is then withdrawn from the catheter assembly and connector tubing may then be attached to the side port of the stopcock. Drainage may be passive, into a collection bag included in the kit, or vacuum assisted into evacuated glass containers. For purposes of illustration, the sterile drape is not shown.

collection (Figure 20-73). In the vast majority of paracentesis, the procedure can be successfully performed with prepuncture mapping only. Real-time guidance may be useful in patients where only a small volume of ascites has been found; in such cases, a sterile probe cover and sterile conductive medium will be needed.

▶ PITFALLS

1. Allowing the patient to move after fluid mapping may lead to a shift in fluid and result in a dry tap or bowel penetration
2. Mistaking large fluid-filled structures such as a large bladder, cyst, or fluid filled loop of bowel for part of an intraperitoneal fluid collection. It is important to verify the identity of all small fluid collections.

▶ PERICARDIOCENTESIS

CLINICAL CONSIDERATIONS

Cardiac tamponade is a life-threatening condition caused by the accumulation of fluid in the pericardial space,

resulting in reduced ventricular filling and subsequent hemodynamic compromise. Beck's classic triad of physical findings for diagnosing cardiac tamponade (hypotension, jugular venous distention, and muffled heart sounds) usually applies only to patients in whom the increase in intrapericardial pressure is rapid. Echocardiography is preferentially used to guide needle placement into the pericardial space for fluid removal. A study examining 1,127 consecutive ultrasound-guided pericardiocenteses demonstrated a 97% procedural success rate and an overall total complication rate of only 4.7%.

CLINICAL INDICATIONS

The clinical indication for pericardiocentesis is drainage of an ultrasound diagnosed pericardial effusion in cases of

- cardiac arrest with pericardial effusion and
- hypotension with rapid decompensation in the setting of a large pericardial effusion.

ANATOMIC CONSIDERATIONS

The two most common entry locations for pericardiocentesis are the subxiphoid and parasternal/apical approaches. The subxiphoid approach is most often used for pericardiocentesis that is performed without imaging ("blind"), while the parasternal/apical approach is a good choice for ultrasound guided pericardiocentesis. In the parasternal/apical approach, visualization of the fluid ensures that the lung and other vital organs are not in the pathway of the needle. Vascular structures to be avoided include internal mammary artery (3–5 cm lateral to parasternal border) and intercostal arteries (located along inferior rib margin).

TECHNIQUE AND ULTRASOUND FINDINGS

The sonographic findings of cardiac tamponade are the direct result of the progressive limitation of ventricular diastolic filling, and the reduction of stroke volume and cardiac output that occurs because of the increased intrapericardial pressure. Right ventricular diastolic collapse (Figures 20-74), right atrial collapse during systole, and dilated inferior vena cava with lack of inspiratory collapse (Figure 20-75) may be seen with cardiac tamponade. The presence of isolated left atrial collapse or left ventricular diastolic collapse may occur with localized left-sided compression or in severe pulmonary hypertension.

The patient should first be scanned using the standard cardiac windows with a phased array or microconvex transducer of appropriate frequency. One study

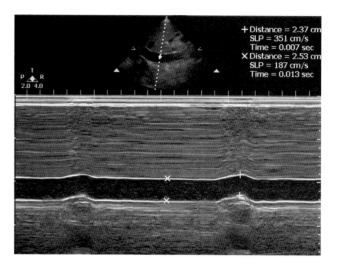

Figure 20-75. Subcostal, sagittal window with dilated inferior vena cava and and M-mode showing lack of respiratory phasicity.

found that the anterior thoracic approach was selected 79% of the time and was preferred over the subxiphoid approach based on the superficial location of the fluid collection, the maximal size of the fluid collection, and the lack of key structures within the path of the needle. Once an entry site is selected, the clinician must make appropriate preparations such as sterilizing the field prior to needle penetration and placing an appropriate sterile sheath on the transducer.

For the parasternal/apical approach the patient is positioned in the left lateral decubitus position if possible. The largest pocket of fluid is identified and will often be located somewhere between the traditional transducer position for a parasternal view and an apical view (Figure 20-76A and B). A long-axis orientation to the heart is recommended as well as longitudinal needle guidance. Vascular structures should be avoided (locations described above). Local anesthesia should be infiltrated first at the entry site and deeper infiltration should be done along the predetermined trajectory if clinical circumstances allow. The needle should be introduced adjacent to the transducer in the long-axis plane and opposite the probe orientation indicator. The needle to be inserted for aspiration should be a 14- to 18-gauge, 5.1- to 8.3-cm Teflon-sheathed angiocatheter. The larger catheter will allow for easier fluid removal especially if it happens to be viscous due to some degree of hemorrhage. A thicker needle will be visualized more easily during real-time guidance. Once the needle is visualized after initial penetration through the skin the same guidance principles apply as for needle placement in vascular access and abscess drainage applications. The needle's path can be tracked in long axis the entire way and be seen entering the pericardial effusion. Upon obtaining

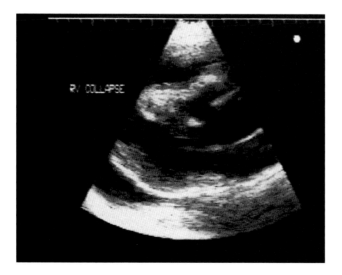

Figure 20-74. Parasternal long-axis view with RV collapse noted in a patient with cardiac tamponade. (Courtesy of James Mateer, MD)

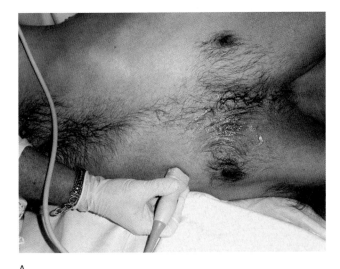

A

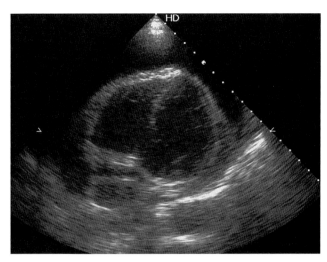

B

Figure 20-76. Transducer placement for the apical four chamber view (A). For direct needle guidance, the transducer should be rotated 90 degrees counterclockwise to the apical long-axis view. (B) Apical window with moderate to large pericardial effusion. The image is between an apical four-chamber and parasternal short-axis view. The maximum fluid pocket will often be located in this area for patients who are in a left lateral decubitus position. Note: absence of lung artifact at intended area of puncture.

fluid, the needle should be advanced several millimeters. The Teflon-sheath should then be advanced while the needle is removed. This may be especially useful in very large effusions that can take considerable time to drain.

As an alternative, the probe position, angle, and fluid depth can be noted and the procedure completed without direct needle guidance (static method). Be careful to avoid patient movement between sonographic mapping and needle insertion.

The subxiphoid window (Figure 20-77A) is obtained by placing the transducer in the subcostal space with the ultrasound beam directed into the patient's left chest and the transducer indicator directed to the patient's right (assuming an abdominal orientation preset is used). This window will provide a four-chamber view of the heart (Figure 20-77B). Because the liver may be prominent in the near field and the heart is located in the far field, it should be apparent that the needle will have to traverse other structures prior to reaching the

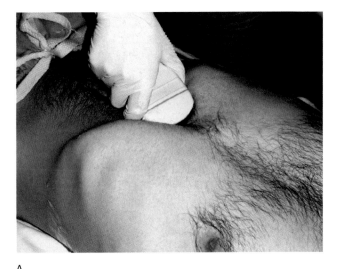

A

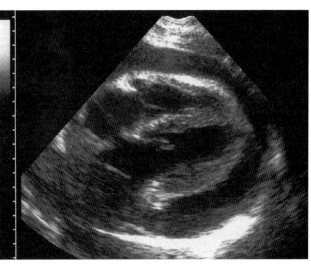

B

Figure 20-77. (a) Transducer placement for the subcostal window. (b) Four-chamber subcostal window. A moderate pericardial effusion is present. (Courtesy of James Mateer, MD (B))

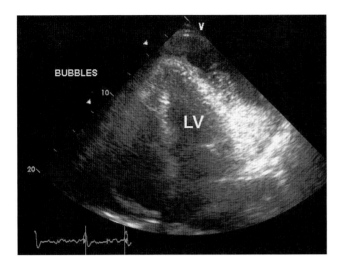

Figure 20-78. Apical four-chamber view with bubbles from aggitated saline injection into the pericardial fluid. LV = left ventricle.

pericardial fluid collection. For this approach, pericardiocentesis is most commonly performed using the static method.

If bloody fluid or no fluid is obtained, then 5 mL of agitated saline can be injected through the sheath. The agitated saline is prepared by connecting two 5-mL syringes to a three-way stopcock. One 5-mL syringe contains 5 mL of sterile saline while the other is empty. The saline should be aerated by rapid injection back and forth between the two syringes. The agitated saline is then rapidly injected through the sheath and the contrast effect is observed on ultrasound. If the echogenic appearing contrast is in the pericardial sac, then it should be safe to continue the procedure (Figure 20-78). If the echogenic-appearing contrast is deep to the myocardium, then the sheath should be withdrawn. If the catheter is not inserted far enough, simply putting the needle back in the sheath and advancing it further may be dangerous since there is a significant risk of shearing off the tip of the sheath. It may be best to repeat the procedure.

▶ PITFALLS

1. Failure to consider the location of the internal mammary artery and the neurovascular bundles located on the underside of the ribs when choosing an entry point.
2. Failure to confirm location of the needle when bloody fluid is obtained if the needle tip is not adequately visualized on ultrasound.
3. Failure to consider alternative approaches if there is significant obstruction from lung tissue in the parasternal approach.

▶ PERITONSILLAR ABSCESS DRAINAGE

CLINICAL CONSIDERATIONS

Peritonsillar abscesses are the most common deep space infection of the head and neck. In some cases, clinical examination cannot be used to reliably distinguish between peritonsillar cellulitis and peritonsillar abscess. The consequence of this is that some patients are inappropriately managed with antibiotics alone while others are inappropriately subjected to drainage attempts. Therefore, diagnostic needle aspirations are performed to determine the presence or absence of a fluid collection. This procedure is not without complications when performed in the "blind" fashion and has been associated with a false-negative rate of up to 12% or even higher.

Studies have shown that intra-oral ultrasound is useful in the diagnosis and management of peritonsillar abscess. Intra-oral ultrasound has a sensitivity of 89% and a specificity of 100% for the diagnosis of peritonsillar abscess while computed tomography has a sensitivity of 100% and a specificity of 75%. Ultrasound has emerged as an extremely valuable tool in the diagnosis and management of peritonsillar infections and is being used with increasing frequency in the emergency department.

CLINICAL INDICATIONS

The clinical indications for the use of ultrasonography in the management of peritonsillar infections include

- discriminating between peritonsillar cellulitis and peritonsillar abscess and
- real-time ultrasound needle guidance into the peritonsillar abscess for drainage.

ANATOMIC CONSIDERATIONS

The anatomy of the posterior pharynx and peritonsillar region is highly complex with numerous structures being visible on intra-oral ultrasound. Structures that may be visualized by intra-oral ultrasound include the palatine tonsil, the margin of the bony hard palate and styloid process of the temporal bone, the medial pterygoid muscle, various fascial planes, the internal jugular vein, and the internal carotid artery. In the sonographic evaluation for peritonsillar abscess, only the internal carotid artery and the palatine tonsil need be identified in every case. The internal carotid artery courses anterior to the internal jugular vein within the carotid sheath and is normally located posterolateral to the tonsil and within 5–25 mm of a peritonsillar abscess.

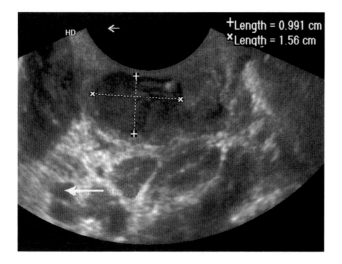

Figure 20-79. Right peritonsillar abscess. Note the presence of the hypoechoic, purulent fluid collection within the abscess cavity (cursors), and the proximity of the carotid artery (arrow).

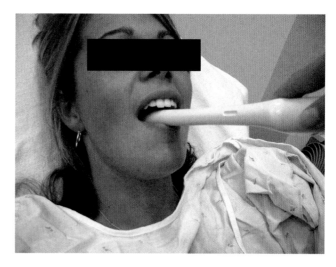

Figure 20-80. Intraoral transducer insertion for peritonsillar evaluation.

TECHNIQUE AND ULTRASOUND FINDINGS

Peritonsillar abscesses can have a variable echogenic appearance. Some will have an echogenic rim with a central area of hypoechogenicity (Figure 20-79). Depending on the composition of the purulent material, the fluid within the cavity may have an isoechoic or hyperechoic appearance. It is therefore important to recognize the relationship of the mass to the tonsil. An echogenic mass with mass effect adjacent to the tonsil should be considered sonographic evidence for the presence of an abscess. Gentle pressure can be utilized to assess for fluid movement within the cavity, but may not be well tolerated by most patients.

For this application an intracavitary transducer should be used. The procedure should be explained completely to the patient before performing it. An important aspect of intra-oral ultrasound is that it requires a cooperative patient. Topical anesthetic spray should be applied to the back of the throat prior to the examination. The transducer should be covered with a transducer sheath with gel appropriately applied similar to an endovaginal scan. The transducer should be gently inserted into the mouth until it contacts the posterior pharynx (Figure 20-80). The examination should typically be performed in a horizontal orientation, allowing visualization of much of the posterior pharynx. The relationship of the tonsil and peritonsillar abscess cavity to the internal carotid artery is best defined in the transverse plane (Figure 20-81). Scanning in a vertical orientation may be helpful in many situations to better define adjacent anatomy. In select cases, it can be helpful to scan the normal side for comparison.

If an abscess is visualized, a needle should be guided in real time to the cavity for drainage. This should typically be performed freehand, but use of a biopsy guide for the intracavitary transducer may be helpful. Inserting a long spinal needle into the oral cavity of a patient with trismus along side the transducer and maintaining alignment of the needle and ultrasound beam is technically challenging. The transducer should be held horizontally and an 18-gauge needle attached to a 5- to 10-mL syringe is placed lateral to the transducer tip. Ideally the needle should be placed in the middle of the transducer tip, exactly in the same plane as the ultrasound beam. Much like in vascular access, deciding from which side the needle will appear can be exceedingly

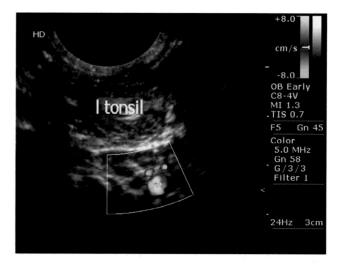

Figure 20-81. Transverse image of the posterior pharynx and left peritonsillar region with color Doppler identification of adjacent vascular structures.

helpful. The needle should be advanced slowly; no further advancement should be made if it slips out of the ultrasound plane at any point. A safety measure sometimes practiced for novice sonologists is cutting off the tip of the needle cap to control the depth of needle penetration. With ultrasound, the precise length of needle required to enter the abscess can be determined and thus carotid penetration made even more unlikely.

▶ PITFALLS

1. *Failure to recognize an isoechoic or a hyperechoic abscess cavity.* The purulent fluid within a peritonsillar abscess cavity is typically hypoechoic in appearance. The presence of an isoechoic or a hyperechoic abscess may result in the sonologist overlooking it.
2. *Failure to visualize the internal carotid artery.* The relationship of the internal carotid artery to the abscess cavity must be noted before commencing with the surgical drainage. The internal carotid artery courses posterolateral to the tonsil and is typically located within 5–25 mm of the abscess cavity.
3. *An uncooperative patient.* An intraoral ultrasound examination requires that the patient be cooperative.
4. *Losing track of the needle during insertion.* If the needle is lost on the ultrasound screen, the sonologists no longer knows where it is traveling and how deep it might be. At this point the needle should not be driven any deeper and the ultrasound transducer should be panned up and down to locate the needle. Once located, the physician can then assess how far out of plane the needle is and redirect it toward the abscess. All of these movements are small and incremental.

▶ SUPRAPUBIC BLADDER ASPIRATION

CLINICAL CONSIDERATIONS

Percutaneous bladder aspiration and catheterization are emergency procedures aided by ultrasound guidance. Suprapubic bladder aspiration traditionally was considered the gold standard method for obtaining a sterile urine culture in patients younger than 2 years although this practice is now less common. In cases of urethral trauma or inability to pass a urethral catheter, suprapubic catheter placement may be unavoidable.

CLINICAL INDICATIONS

- Urethral stricture or known false passage
- Inability to catheterize the urethra
- Suspected urethral trauma

Ultrasound can facilitate higher success rates of suprapubic aspiration by determining whether or not the bladder has sufficient urine to aspirate, guiding the needle or catheter to the greatest depth of the bladder, and identifying abnormalities or anatomic variations that may help reduce the risk of complications. Physical examination is insensitive for determining bladder fullness. Blind suprapubic aspiration has variable rates of success with estimates ranging from 36% to 80%. Complications of suprapubic aspiration or catheterization include bowel perforation and hematuria. Ultrasound saves time, prevents multiple attempts at aspirating an empty bladder, and decreases the complication rate, much as it does with vascular access and abscess drainage.

ANATOMIC CONSIDERATIONS

The bladder is fixed inferiorly. In the neonate, the bladder is an abdominal organ and distends anteroposteriorly. As the body grows, the pelvis rises above the bladder and in adults, the bladder is an intrapelvic organ. The bladder is a midline structure but may be shifted off of midline by pelvic or abdominal masses. Variability exists in the shape of the bladder and contributes to inaccuracy when estimating bladder volume with standard formulas. An obviously distended bladder can be readily cannulated under direct ultrasound guidance.

TECHNIQUE AND ULTRASOUND FINDINGS

The bladder is typically a midline elliptical structure with posterior enhancement (Figure 20-82). Any structures that are fluid filled but off midline may be distended loops of bowel or ovarian cysts (Figure 20-83). Limitations in bladder visualization are evident in morbidly obese patients or those with scar tissue.

A 3–5 MHz convex probe is used for a screening ultrasound examination to confirm an adequate volume of urine. A linear transducer may be used in small children. The cut-off value for an adequate volume to attempt aspiration varies in the literature from 1 cm × 1 cm in the transverse plane to 3.5 cm in the transverse plane to greater than 10 mL estimated volume when using a dedicated bladder scanner. A safe estimate is to use a minimum of 2 cm measured in at least 2 planes. If the bladder is empty on first view, the scan should be repeated every 15 minutes until an adequate volume is present.

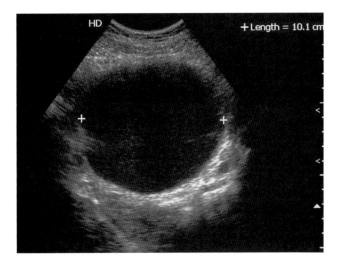

Figure 20-82. Transverse view of a round bladder—10 cm diameter, 9 cm height. If the length of this bladder is 10 cm, the volume can be estimated at 675 mL. (Using the simple formula: length × width × height × 0.75)

In neonates, minimal pressure should be applied to the skin to avoid irritating the bladder and having the patient urinate prior to the procedure.

The skin should be prepped in a sterile manner, and a sterile sheath should be placed over the transducer. Much like needle placement into an abscess cavity, the long-axis approach to the needle, which allows visualization throughout its length, is ideal. Line up the greatest depth of the bladder with the center of the probe in long or short axis and proceed under direct visualization. When bladder volumes are very small (neonates), the short-axis approach may be preferred (Figure 20-84). Proper local anesthetic is required for patient comfort. Aspirating urine and visualizing the needle within the

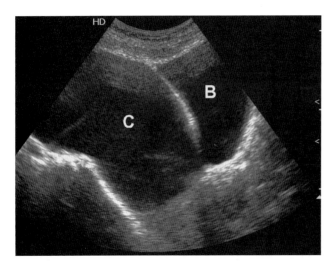

Figure 20-83. Bladder displacement due to a large ovarian cyst. B = bladder, C = cyst.

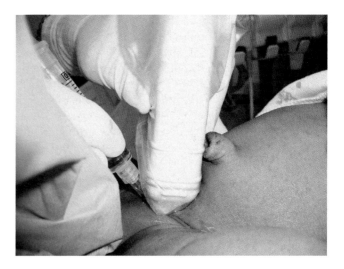

Figure 20-84. Hand and needle position for ultrasound-guided bladder aspiration (short-axis approach).

bladder should unequivocally confirm that the bladder has been successfully cannulated. At this point, catheterization should proceed (Seldinger technique), unless a simple bladder aspiration was only required.

▶ PITFALLS

1. Attempting to aspirate an empty bladder. Wait for an adequately filled bladder before attempting to aspirate, especially in a neonate.
2. Do not confuse the bladder with a distended loop of bowel or an enlarged ovarian cyst. Examining for peristalsis and tracing the extent of all fluid-filled structures should help differentiate bowel from bladder. A large ovarian cyst that crosses midline and compresses the bladder can be quite difficult to differentiate. Noting the presence of ureteral jets should reassure the sonologist. More extensive scanning may be required if the fluid-filled structure seems to extend to the adnexa.

▶ THORACENTESIS

CLINICAL CONSIDERATIONS

Bedside chest ultrasonography allows for rapid identification, characterization, and precise localization of pleural effusions. While percussion, tactile fremitus, and landmark identification play a role in the armamentarium of physical diagnosis skills, pre-procedure ultrasound assessment and marking landmarks prior to thoracentesis improves the performance characteristics of a procedure that can be associated with a complication rate as high as 20–50%. Chest sonography was shown to be significantly superior to the decubitus chest radiograph for detecting pleural fluid and assisting in collection of an adequate fluid sample for analysis in a series of 85 patients with small pleural effusions. In a group of 52 patients undergoing thoracentesis of large free-flowing pleural effusions, ultrasound guidance was associated with significantly fewer overall complications. While the pneumothorax rate was 19% overall, none occurred in the ultrasound-guided group. In a report on 26 patients where blind thoracentesis attempts had failed, subsequent ultrasound-guided aspiration was successful in 88% of the cases.

Patients who are mechanically ventilated may present a significant challenge as the inflation and deflation of the lung and their typically supine position make blind thoracentesis more hazardous. Ultrasound guidance may be especially helpful in such patients. In a clinical report on thoracentesis in 40 mechanically ventilated patients, the procedure was safely, easily, and rapidly performed. Usually very rapid to perform, the authors reported a 97% success rate for obtaining more than 5 mL of fluid. No pneumothorax or hemoptysis was observed in this series. The authors recommended that the following guidelines be followed: the width of the fluid collection (as measured by the parietal to visceral interpleural distance) should be at least 15 mm, and the fluid should be visible over at least 3 intercostal spaces. Of incidental note, pleural fluid was considered to be "absent" on the chest radiograph in 17 patients, in whom fluid was subsequently identified and obtained by ultrasound.

ANATOMIC CONSIDERATIONS

When performing thoracentesis, the anatomic area of interest will typically be the mid to lateral back below the level of the scapulae, or on occasion, the lateral chest wall in the mid axillary region. The broad latissimus dorsi muscles cover most of the posterior and lateral chest wall deep to the skin and subcutaneous tissue of the back below the scapulae. Deep to this muscular layer lie the lower ribs, curving inferolaterally, with the intercostal muscles spanning adjacent ribs. Coursing along the inner surface of each intercostal space just below the parietal pleura that lines the chest cavity are the intercostal vein (closest to the inferior edge of the rib above), the intercostal artery, and the intercostal nerve. This neurovascular bundle follows the curve of the interspace and can be avoided by the aspirating needle only by paying meticulous attention to performing the puncture *immediately* above the superior edge of the marked rib. From a lateral approach, the chest wall layers of the lower mid axillary region consist of skin and subcutaneous tissue, the external oblique muscle, and ribs, intercostals, neurovascular

bundle, and parietal pleura. Higher in the lateral mid axillary region, the muscular layer is made up of the slips of the serratus anterior muscle instead of the external oblique. The top of the diaphragm normally rests at the level of the 10th thoracic vertebra.

Pleural fluid will initially collect along the most dependent surfaces between the inferior surface of the lower lobes and the diaphragm in a potential space called the costodiaphragmatic recess. The recess can track as low at the 12th rib posteriorly and to the level of the 8th rib laterally. The exact location of the lung will depend on the size of the pleural effusion, the degree of atelectasis, and the timing of the respiratory cycle. Even though the liver, spleen, and kidneys lie inferior to the diaphragm, inadvertent puncture of these organs can occur when a blind thoracentesis technique is employed.

CLINICAL INDICATIONS

1. Sampling of thoracic fluid for diagnostic reason
2. Therapeutic drainage for pleural fluid

TECHNIQUE AND ULTRASOUND FINDINGS

A pleural effusion is sometimes first detected when performing abdominal scanning. On a transverse view of the abdomen, a pleural effusion will appear as an echo free collection in the most dependent portion of the image, in the costodiaphragmatic recess (Figure 20-85). The fluid collections are typically asymmetric in location and will be located on a somewhat lower scan plane on the left, and a somewhat higher one on the right. The echogenic inferior border of the lung may be seen within

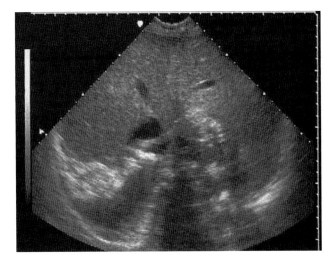

Figure 20-85. A right-sided pleural effusion is seen in the right costodiaphragmatic recess on this transverse sonogram of the upper abdomen.

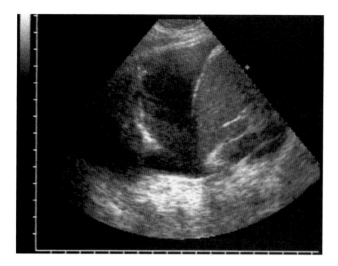

Figure 20-86. A large pleural effusion with somewhat increased fluid echogenicity; the echogenic inferior lung border is seen in the effusion on the left of the image.

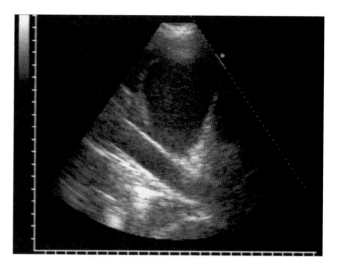

Figure 20-88. A more medially oriented longitudinal view of a left pleural effusion from the posterior chest; the tubular descending aorta is seen in the far field, and the inferior lung border to the left

the effusion, located somewhat above the diaphragm in a location that will vary depending on the respiratory cycle (Figure 20-86). When scanning the patient in long-axis orientation from the back (with the patient sitting upright), a simple pleural effusion will appear as an echo-free collection closest to the transducer just deep to the chest wall. In the left hemithorax, the heart will be seen in short-axis orientation in the far field of the image, the lower border of the lung to the left, and the diaphragm and spleen to the right (Figure 20-87). If the transducer is moved medially, the tubular appearance of the descending aorta will be noted in the far field of the

image with the inferior lung border to the left of the image and the effusion immediately below (Figure 20-88).

When marking the location for the thoracentesis from behind, the echogenic surface of the rib and its dense posterior acoustic shadow will be noted just deep to the subcutaneous tissue and the latissimus dorsi muscle. Deep to the rib, the brightly echogenic pleural line will be visually apparent and its depth within the image will precisely represent the amount of chest wall that must be traversed to enter the pleural cavity (Figure 20-89).

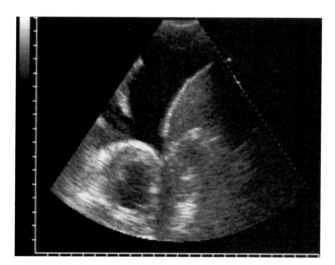

Figure 20-87. A longitudinal view of a left pleural effusion from the posterior chest. The heart is seen in short axis in the far field, the spleen to the right, the inferior lung border to the left, with the posterior chest wall closest to the transducer

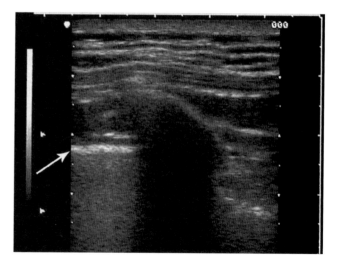

Figure 20-89. A linear array image of posterior chest wall showing skin, subcutaneous tissue, the thin muscular layer of the latissimus dorsi muscle, a rib with a prominent posterior acoustic shadow, and the brightly echogenic pleural line (arrow). No pleural effusion is seen in this image.

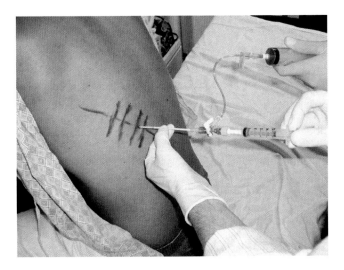

Figure 20-90. Thoracentesis procedural technique—dorsal approach. The rib interspace for the aspiration has been marked and mapped. Needle insertion is over the center of the rib; the aspirating needle is then moved to a point immediately above the superior border of the rib into the interspace. A commercially available self-sealing thoracentesis needle is employed, and an assistant is available to aspirate the pleural fluid sample or connect the side port to a drainage bag.

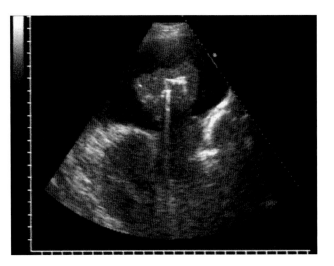

Figure 20-91. A transverse view of a pleural effusion from the posterior chest. An echogenic portion of atelectatic lung is noted within the effusion. Prominent reverberation artifacts are seen where air-filled.

A 2.5–4.0 MHz cardiac phased array transducer is commonly used for mapping the effusion, but a microconvex transducer of similar frequency range will suffice. Most emergency department patients requiring thoracentesis will have large effusions, are likely to be aspirated for both diagnostic *and* therapeutic purposes, and will have their aspiration performed from a dorsal approach (Figure 20-90). Mobile and cooperative patients should ideally be positioned on the edge of a bed leaning against a tray table, sitting as vertically as possible with their arms folded and head resting on a pillow. The relevant hemithorax should be scanned from the upper lumbar region to the inferior border of the scapula and from the paravertebral region to the posterior axillary line. When an adequately deep fluid collection is sonographically visualized at the anticipated puncture site throughout the respiratory cycle, its location and size should be systematically mapped to determine an optimal site for aspiration. The superior and inferior extents of the fluid collection should be noted and the fluid collection should routinely be assessed in two orthogonal scan planes. Since transverse scanning will be performed along the rib interspaces, the ultrasound beam will be positioned somewhat obliquely to a true transverse scan plane. The location of the diaphragm, underlying liver or spleen, and any interposed lung should clearly be noted. Particular attention should be paid to any changes in the position of the lung that occur with respiration (Figure 20-91).

It may be helpful to mark ribs surrounding the chosen interspace with indelible ink. The optimum depth for needle or catheter insertion can be predetermined by directly measuring the distance from the skin surface to the fluid collection or by estimation using the depth scale markers located on the ultrasound screen. In the debilitated or intubated patient, thoracentesis is commonly performed from a lateral approach with the puncture site in the lateral chest in the mid axillary line. Less frequently, a dorsal approach can be utilized with the patient in a lateral decubitus position. For the lateral approach, the patient is supine with the head of the bed elevated at about 45 degrees and the ipsilateral arm positioned as one would for a chest tube (arm abducted, elbow flexed with the hand behind the head). For the dorsal approach, the patient is placed in lateral decubitus position lying on the side of the effusion with the back next to the edge of the bed. Needle insertion for this position is just above the rib at the posterior axillary line. With both these positions, it is advantageous to have intubated patients deeply sedated during the procedure. The transducer should be angled slightly in all four directions from the anticipated puncture site checking specifically for the absence of interposed lung, heart, liver, or spleen during the respiratory cycle. Again, the distance from skin to parietal pleura, and the depth of the fluid collection itself, should be noted and the needle length, puncture depth, and aspiration angle adjusted accordingly.

For all of the above approaches, the thoracentesis should be performed immediately after the effusion is mapped with the patient remaining in the exact same position as when scanned. From this point the technique is the same as for blind aspiration including proper local anesthetic at the skin, rib, and pleura. Alternatively, real-time ultrasound guidance may be utilized to actually guide the needle to the fluid collection after entering the skin. This is not typically necessary with moderate to large fluid collections. If used, the needle should be inserted to one side of the phase array probe, which must be sterile for the procedure. The needle is seen in its long axis and the same basic principles apply that are utilized for vascular access and abscess drainage.

▶ PITFALLS

1. Cellulitis involving site of desired needle entry may lead to infection of an otherwise sterile collection of fluid. Needle puncture should not be undertaken through a site of skin infection.
2. Penetrating too deeply into the chest cavity with the aspirating needle is more likely to lead to lung or great vessel injury.
3. Morbidly obese patients provide such limited ultrasound visualization that safely determining effusion location may not be possible

▶ TRANSVENOUS PACEMAKER PLACEMENT

CLINICAL CONSIDERATIONS

Transvenous pacing is indicated in the emergency department for prolonged pacing or when transcutaneous pacing is ineffective or not tolerated by the awake patient. Traditional guidance of the transvenous pacemaker follows electrocardiographic monitoring of the pacer wire attached to one of the cardiac monitor leads. This may be too time consuming and inaccurate in an emergent situation. In hypotensive patients, a low-flow state may make it more difficult for the pacemaker wire to naturally flow into the right ventricle. Ultrasound is ideal for visualizing pacemaker wire advancement into the right atrium and right ventricle.

CLINICAL INDICATIONS

- To assist in correct placement of transvenous pacemaker insertion.
- To confirm pacemaker wire location in an inserted transvenous pacemaker that is no longer capturing.
- To confirm myocardial contraction from pacemaker firing.

ANATOMIC CONSIDERATIONS

The subxiphoid, parasternal, or apical windows can all be used to evaluate myocardial contraction in response to pacing. For pacemaker placement, the subxiphoid and four-chamber apical windows are the most useful for adequate visualization of pacer wire entry into the right atrium with progression into the right ventricle. A good four-chamber apical view is optimal for detecting and directing wire progress. The sonologist should be familiar with more than one approach to ensure adequate visualization.

TECHNIQUE AND ULTRASOUND FINDINGS

The transvenous pacemaker lead can be seen in both the subxiphoid four-chamber and apical four-chamber views as it enters the right atrium. The pacer wire can appear out of plane initially; some sonographic fanning through the atrium may be required to visualize the wire upon entry. In the subxiphoid view, the right ventricle is at the top left of the screen (Figure 20-92). In the apical four-chamber view the wire will appear in the bottom left as it enters the right atrium. A phased array cardiac probe is ideal for this application although a low-frequency convex probe can also be used. If the pacer wire is not visualized after an appropriate length of the pacemaker has been inserted, checking the inferior vena cava may reveal the pacer wire to be below the diaphragm. Scanning down through the liver, an adjustment should be made to locate the hepatic veins draining into the inferior vena cava. Panning through the inferior vena cava should help locate the misplaced pacer wire.

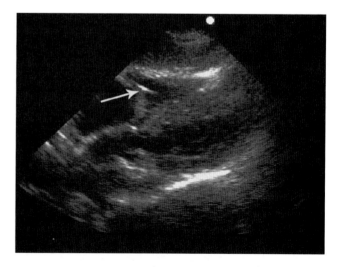

Figure 20-92. Subcostal cardiac view with pacemaker wire in right ventricle (arrow), just below the tricuspid valve. (Courtesy of Michael Blaivas, MD)

When the pacer wire first appears in the right atrium, ultrasound guidance is not yet complete because wire coiling in the right atrium is common. Slight retraction of the pacer wire may be required, followed by further incremental insertion. Careful coordination between the sonologist and the physician inserting the pacemaker is required in some low-flow situations. The pacer wire (with balloon up) can be brought up next to the tricuspid valve; when the valve opens, the pacer wire will flow into the right ventricle. The pacer wire can then be visualized as it enters the apex of the right ventricle.

▶ PITFALLS

1. The subxiphoid window is sometimes challenging to obtain because of bowel gas or a protuberant abdomen.
2. The apical four-chamber view may be difficult in very obese patients or those with emphysema.

BIBLIOGRAPHY

1. Aguilera PA, Durham BA, Riley DA: Emergency transvenous cardiac pacing placement using ultrasound guidance. *Ann Emerg Med* 36(3):224–227, 2000.
2. Bochman RF, Karasic RB, Bergin D, et al.: Echogenic polymer coating: Does it improve needle visualization in sonographically guided biopsy? *AJR Am J Roentgenol* 178(5): 1188–1190, 2002.
3. Bondestam S: The needle tip echo. *J Ultrasound Med* 11(6): 253–256, 1992.
4. Coley BD, Shiels WE, Hogan MJ: Diagnostic and interventional ultrasonography in neonatal and infant lumbar puncture. *Pediatr Radiol* 31:399–402, 2001.
5. Cork RC, Kryc JJ, Vaughan RW: Ultrasonic localization of the lumbar epidural space. *Anesthesiology* 52:513–516, 1980.
6. Fessell D, Jacobsen J, Craig J, et al.: Using sonography to reveal and aspirate joint effusions. *AJR* 174:1353–1362, 2000.
7. Grau T: Ultrasonography in the current practice of regional anesthesia. *Best Pract Clin Anesthesiol* 19:175–200, 2005.
8. Gray A: Ultrasound-guided regional anesthesia: Current state of the art. *Anesthesiology* 104:368–373, 2006.
9. Haeggstrom A, et al.: Intraoral ultrasonography in the diagnosis of peritonsillar abscess. *Otolaryngol Head Neck Surg* 108(3):243–247, 1993.
10. Heller M: Use of portable ultrasound to assist urine collection by suprapubic aspiration. *Ann Emerg Med* 20(6):631–635, 1991.
11. Hopkins RE, Bradley M: In-vitro visualization of biopsy needles with ultrasound: A comparative study of standard and echogenic needles using an ultrasound phantom. *Clin Radiol* 56(6):499–502, 2001.
12. Kapral S, Krafft P, Klemens E, et al.: Ultrasound-guided supraclavicular approach for regional anesthesia of the brachial plexus. *Anesth Analg* 78:507–513, 1994.
13. Rorie D, Byer D, Neslon D, et al.: Assessment of block of the sciatic nerve in the popliteal fossa. *Anesth Analg* 59:371–376, 1980.
14. Schafhalter-Zoppoth I, McCulloch CE, Gray AT: Ultrasound visibility of needles used for regional nerve block: An in vitro study. *Reg Anesth Pain Med* 29(5):480–488, 2004.
15. Sites B, Beach M, Gallagher J, et al.: A single injection ultrasound-assisted femoral nerve block provides effect-sparing analgesia when compared with intrathecal morphine in patients undergoing total knee arthroplasty. *Anesth Analg* 99:1539–1543, 2004.
16. Snoeck M, Vree T, Gielen M, et al.: Steady state bupivicaine plasma concentrations and safety of a femoral "3-in-1" nerve block with bupivicaine in patients over 80 years of age. *Int J Clin Pharmacol Therapeutics* 41:107–113, 2003.
17. Tsang TS, et al.: Consecutive 1127 therapeutic echocardiographically guided pericardiocenteses: Clinical profile, practice patterns, and outcomes spanning 21 years. *Mayo Clin Proc* 77(5):429–436, 2002.

INDEX